HANDBOOK OF ATTACHMENT-BASED INTERVENTIONS

Also Available

Clinical Applications of the Adult Attachment Interview
Edited by Howard Steele and Miriam Steele

Handbook of
Attachment-Based
Interventions

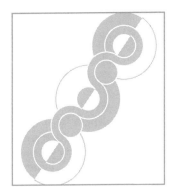

Edited by
Howard Steele
Miriam Steele

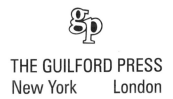

THE GUILFORD PRESS
New York   London

Library of Congress Cataloging-in-Publication Data
Names: Steele, Howard, 1959– editor. | Steele, Miriam, editor.
Title: Handbook of attachment-based interventions / edited by Howard Steele,
    Miriam Steele.
Description: New York: Guilford Press, 2018. | Inludes bibliographical
    references and index.
Identifiers: LCCN 2017028509 | ISBN 9781462532612 (hardcover : alk. paper)
Subjects: LCSH: Attachment disorder. | Attachment behavior.
Classification: LCC RC455.4.A84 H355 2018 | DDC 616.85/88—dc23
LC record available at *https://lccn.loc.gov/2017028509*

For our children, Gabi, Joe, and Miki

About the Editors

Howard Steele, PhD, is Professor and Chair of the Clinical Psychology faculty and Co-Director of the Center for Attachment Research in the Department of Psychology at The New School for Social Research. Dr. Steele is senior and founding editor of the journal *Attachment and Human Development* and founding and past president of the Society for Emotion and Attachment Studies. He has published more than 100 journal articles and book chapters, many in collaboration with Miriam Steele, in the areas of attachment theory and research, intergenerational patterns of attachment, mourning in response to trauma and loss, and attachment-based interventions to prevent child maltreatment and promote secure, organized attachments. With Miriam Steele and Anne Murphy, Dr. Steele has pioneered the development of Group Attachment-Based Intervention (GABI©), aimed at preventing child maltreatment and promoting attachment security. He is a recipient of the 2017 Bowlby–Ainsworth Award from the Center for Mental Health Promotion, which cited his contributions as a scientist, editor, and clinical innovator.

Miriam Steele, PhD, is Professor of Psychology and Co-Director of the Center for Attachment Research at The New School for Social Research. Dr. Steele trained as a psychoanalyst at the Anna Freud Centre. Her work aims to bridge the world of psychoanalytic thinking and clinical practice with contemporary research in child development. She initiated the London Parent–Child Project, a major longitudinal study of intergenerational patterns of attachment that gave rise to the concept of "reflective functioning." She has published more than 100 journal articles and book chapters, many in collaboration with Howard Steele. With Howard Steele and Anne Murphy, Dr. Steele has pioneered the development of GABI©. She is a recipient of the 2017 Bowlby–Ainsworth Award from the Center for Mental Health Promotion, which cited her innovative longitudinal studies and translational research on attachment and mental representation.

Contributors

Jessica Gorkin Albertson, MA, Doctoral Program in Clinical Psychology, City University of New York, New York, New York

Alessandro Albizzati, MD, ASST Santi Paolo and Carlo Hospital, Milan, Italy

Rebecca Atkins, MA, School of Psychology, London Metropolitan University, London, United Kingdom

Marian J. Bakermans-Kranenburg, PhD, Centre for Child and Family Studies, Leiden University, Leiden, The Netherlands

Tessa Baradon, MSc, Under 5s Development, Anna Freud Centre, London, United Kingdom

Kristin Bernard, PhD, Department of Psychology, Stony Brook University, Stony Brook, New York

Annie Bernier, PhD, Department of Psychology, University of Montréal, Montréal, Québec, Canada

David Kyle Bond, MA, Department of Psychology, Claremont Graduate University, Claremont, California

Karen Bonuck, PhD, Department of Family and Social Medicine, Albert Einstein College of Medicine, Bronx, New York

Jessica L. Borelli, PhD, Department of Psychology, Pomona College, Claremont, California

Karl Heinz Brisch, MD, Department of Pediatric Psychosomatic Medicine and Psychotherapy, Dr. von Hauner Children's Hospital of Ludwig Maximilian University of Munich, Munich, Germany

Sara Burstin, BA, Department of Psychology, Hebrew University, Jerusalem, Israel

Chloe Campbell, PhD, Research Department of Clinical, Educational and Health Psychology, University College London, London, United Kingdom

Jude Cassidy, PhD, Department of Psychology, University of Maryland, College Park, Maryland

Miriam Chriki, MA, Department of Psychology, Hebrew University, Jerusalem, Israel

Nancy Close, PhD, Yale Child Study Center, Yale School of Medicine, New Haven, Connecticut

Glen Cooper, MA, Circle of Security International, Spokane, Washington

Carolyn Pape Cowan, PhD, Department of Psychology, University of California, Berkeley, Berkeley, California

Philip A. Cowan, PhD, Department of Psychology, University of California, Berkeley, Berkeley, California

Chantal Cyr, PhD, Department of Psychology, University of Québec at Montréal, Montréal, Québec, Canada

Guy S. Diamond, PhD, PhD Program in Couple and Family Therapy and Center for Family Intervention Science, Drexel University, Philadelphia, Pennsylvania

Nancy Donelan-McCall, PhD, Department of Pediatrics, University of Colorado Denver School of Medicine, Aurora, Colorado

George Downing, PhD, Pitié-Salpêtrière Hospital, Paris, France

Mary Dozier, PhD, Department of Psychological and Brain Sciences, University of Delaware, Newark, Delaware

Karine Dubois-Comtois, PhD, Department of Psychology, University of Québec at Trois-Rivières, Trois-Rivières, Québec, Canada

Karen Dudley, BA, private practice, Los Angeles, California

Byron Egeland, PhD, Institute of Child Development, University of Minnesota, Minneapolis, Minnesota

Martha Farrell Erickson, PhD, Children, Youth, and Family Consortium, University of Minnesota, St. Paul, Minnesota

E. Stephanie Krauthamer Ewing, PhD, Department of Couple and Family Therapy, Drexel University, Philadelphia, Pennsylvania

Abel Fagin, MA, ADv Dip, Anna Freud National Centre for Children and Families, London, United Kingdom

Peter Fonagy, PhD, Research Department of Clinical, Educational and Health Psychology, University College London, London, United Kingdom

Tim Greacen, PhD, Research Laboratory, EPS Maison Blanche, Paris, France

Jonathan Green, MD, Division of Neuroscience and Experimental Psychology, University of Manchester, Manchester, United Kingdom

Antoine Guédeney, MD, Child and Adolescent Psychiatry, Paris 7 Diderot University, Paris, France

Nicole Guédeney, MD, Mutualist Institute, Montsouris, Paris Descartes University, Sorbonne Paris Cité, Paris, France

Danielle Guild, MA, Department of Clinical and Social Sciences in Psychology, Mt. Hope Family Center, University of Rochester, Rochester, New York

Hans-Peter Hartmann, MD, Department of Clinical Psychology, University of Giessen, Giessen, Germany

Kent Hoffman, RelD, Department of Psychology, Gonzaga University, Spokane, Washington

Jeannette Hollerbach, MA, Department of Pediatric Psychosomatic Medicine and Psychotherapy, University of Munich, Munich, Germany

Elena Ierardi, PhD, Department of Psychology, University of Milano-Bicocca, ASST Santi Paolo and Carlo Hospital, Milan, Italy

Femmie Juffer, PhD, Centre for Child and Family Studies, Leiden University, Leiden, The Netherlands

Marsha Kaitz, PhD, Department of Psychology, Hebrew University, Jerusalem, Israel

Judith Levy, BA, Department of Psychology, Hebrew University, Jerusalem, Israel

Suzanne A. Levy, PhD, Center for Family Intervention Science, College of Nursing and Health Professions, Drexel University, Philadelphia, Pennsylvania

Alicia F. Lieberman, PhD, Department of Psychiatry, University of California, San Francisco, San Francisco, California

Paul Meissner, MSPH, Montefiore Medical Center, Bronx, New York

Louisa C. Michl-Petzing, MA, Department of Clinical and Social Sciences in Psychology, Mt. Hope Family Center, University of Rochester, Rochester, New York

Catherine Mogil, PsyD, Semel Institute for Neuroscience and Human Behavior, University of California, Los Angeles, Los Angeles, California

Marlene M. Moretti, PhD, Psychology Department, Simon Fraser University, Burnaby, British Columbia, Canada

Ellen Moss, PhD, Center for Study of Attachment and the Family, Department of Psychology, University of Québec at Montréal, Québec, Canada

Anne Murphy, PhD, Rose F. Kennedy Children's Evaluation and Rehabilitation Center, Montefiore Medical Center, Bronx, New York

Katherine A. O'Donnell, MS, Department of Psychology, Simon Fraser University, Burnaby, British Columbia, Canada

David Olds, PhD, Prevention Research Center for Family and Child Health, Department of Pediatrics, University of Colorado Denver School of Medicine, Aurora, Colorado

Dave S. Pasalich, PhD, Research School of Psychology, College of Medicine, Biology and Environment, The Australian National University, Canberra, Australia

Victoria Ponce, BA, Department of Child and Adolescent Psychiatry, University of California, Los Angeles, Los Angeles, California

Bert Powell, MA, Circle of Security International, Spokane, Washington

Marsha Kline Pruett, PhD, School for Social Work, Smith College, Northampton, Massachusetts

Kyle Pruett, MD, Yale Child Study Center, Yale School of Medicine, New Haven, Connecticut

Cristina Riva Crugnola, PhD, Department of Developmental Psychology, University of Milano-Bicocca, Milan, Italy

Caroline K. P. Roben, PhD, Psychological and Brain Sciences, University of Delaware, Newark, Delaware

Trudie Rossouw, MD, Priory Group, North London Priory, London, United Kingdom

Frank C. Sacco, PhD, Community Services Institute, Boston and Springfield, Massachusetts, and Doctoral Field Placement, Springfield College, Springfield, Massachusetts

Lois Sadler, PhD, Yale Child Study Center, Yale School of Nursing, New Haven, Connecticut

Hermann Scheuerer-Englisch, PhD, Child Guidance Clinic, Katholische Jugendfürsorge Regensburg e.V., Regensburg, Germany

Syreeta A. Scott, PhD, ABFT Training Program, Drexel University, Philadelphia, Pennsylvania

Tanika Eaves Simpson, LCSW, IMH-E, Yale Child Study Center, Yale School of Medicine, New Haven, Connecticut

Arietta Slade, PhD, Yale Child Study Center, Yale School of Medicine, New Haven, Connecticut

Michelle Sleed, PhD, Department of Psychology, University College London, London, United Kingdom

Diane St-Laurent, PhD, Department of Psychology, University of Québec at Trois-Rivières, Trois-Rivières, Québec, Canada

Howard Steele, PhD, Department of Psychology, The New School for Social Research, New York, New York

Miriam Steele, PhD, Department of Psychology, The New School for Social Research, New York, New York

Gerhard J. Suess, PhD, Department of Social Work, Hamburg University of Applied Science, Hamburg, Germany

George M. Tarabulsy, PhD, School of Psychology, Laval University, Québec City, Québec, Canada

Susana Tereno, PhD, Institute of Psychology and Laboratory of Psychopathology and Health Process, Paris Descartes University, Sorbonne Paris Cité, Paris, France

Naomi Tessler, BSW, Department of Psychology, Hebrew University, Jerusalem, Israel

Sheree L. Toth, PhD, Mt. Hope Family Center, University of Rochester, Rochester, New York

Stuart W. Twemlow, MD, Research Department of Clinical, Educational and Health Psychology, University College, London, United Kingdom

Marinus H. van IJzendoorn, PhD, Centre for Child and Family Studies, Leiden University, Leiden, The Netherlands

Rachel van Schaick, DClinPsy, Hackney Children's Social Care, London, United Kingdom

Denise Webb, MSN, Yale Child Study Center, Yale School of Medicine, New Haven, Connecticut

Susan S. Woodhouse, PhD, Department of Education and Human Services, Lehigh University, Bethlehem, Pennsylvania

Preface

There is no shortage of attachment-based interventions, so there was inevitably a process of selection in determining which interventions are represented in the 21 chapters in this *Handbook of Attachment-Based Interventions*. The process was influenced by three considerations:

1. Does the theory informing the intervention rely in some significant way upon attachment theory?
2. Does the evidence base for the effectiveness of the intervention include reliable and previously validated attachment measures?
3. Is there a robust scientific inquiry (e.g., a randomized controlled trial) completed, under way, or planned?

Applying these three criteria yielded 12 chapters that report on interventions aimed at parents and their children ages 0–3 years; three chapters that report on interventions appropriate for preschool-age children (and their parents); one school-based intervention; four interventions aimed at adolescents, including one that focuses on adolescent parents and also addresses the young couple; and one intervention directly addressing adult couples, with a dedicated focus on involving fathers in the lives of their children. Notably, all the interventions reported on in this handbook are manualized, and clinicians whose aim is to become skilled in any of these approaches are required to pursue face-to-face training, including follow-up supervision, which can be arranged through direct contact with the authors.

Readers interested in early interventions that aim to help parents of infants and toddlers have much to consider in the first 12 chapters, including home-visiting programs, work with individual parent–child relationships (dyadic work) in the clinic, and therapy that is based on a group or multifamily model. Interestingly, the vast majority of these early interventions include video feedback as a central component of the therapeutic work. There can be no doubt that seeing oneself on film, interacting with one's child, is a deeply evocative experience, ripe with opportunities to consider how one might like to change as a parent.

Readers who are primarily interested in how to help troubled adolescents will want to turn immediately to the four chapters that address this age group (Chapters 17, 18, 19, and 20). Autism is addressed in detail in Chapter 12. Working with parents (and children) who have been exposed to trauma is a common theme across many chapters.

We are grateful to all the contributing authors for their patience with us in the preparation of this volume. We owe a debt of thanks to C. Deborah Laughton, Senior Editor, Developmental Psychology, at The Guilford Press, who has been our main nonintrusive and supportive contact throughout preparation of this handbook. Editor-in-Chief Seymour Weingarten's steady hand in the background, offering support of this volume and all things attachment-wise, is greatly appreciated. Finally, we hope that this volume makes readers more aware of the rich range of attachment-based interventions with a significant and growing evidence base, meaning that the lives of children and adolescents at risk can be dramatically improved with the right investment that will have immediate and long-term benefits—psychologically, socially, and economically—in terms of reduced monies that would otherwise need to be spent on special education, health, legal, and prison costs.

Contents

Video-Feedback Intervention to Promote Positive Parenting and Sensitive Discipline
Development and Meta-Analytic Evidence for Its Effectiveness

FEMMIE JUFFER, MARIAN J. BAKERMANS-KRANENBURG, and MARINUS H. VAN IJZENDOORN

Video-feedback Intervention to promote Positive Parenting and Sensitive Discipline (VIPP-SD; Juffer, Bakermans-Kranenburg, & van IJzendoorn, 2008, 2014, 2017) is an attachment-based intervention aimed at enhancing sensitive parenting and adequate discipline strategies of parents,[1] with the ultimate goal of promoting positive parent–child relationships and reducing behavior problems in children. In this chapter we describe how we developed VIPP and extended the intervention with a module on Sensitive Discipline into the current VIPP-SD program. VIPP is based on attachment theory (Ainsworth, Blehar, Waters, & Wall, 1978; Bowlby, 1982), while the Sensitive Discipline module is inspired by coercion theory (Patterson, 1982). We elaborate on key features of VIPP-SD (e.g., the themes of the program and the video-feedback technique), and present a narrative review of the studies that have implemented and tested VIPP-SD in various samples. We conclude with a meta-analytical approach to compute the effectiveness of the VIPP-SD program in enhancing sensitive parenting and positive child outcomes.

Theoretical and Empirical Background

Attachment and Coercion Theory

According to attachment theory (Ainsworth et al., 1978; Bowlby, 1982, 1988), and confirmed by meta-analytical evidence (De Wolff & van IJzendoorn, 1997;

---

[1]The VIPP-SD program can be implemented in families and in child care settings. In general, we use the word *parent* for both parents and caregivers.

Bakermans-Kranenburg, van IJzendoorn, & Juffer, 2003), parental sensitivity is the key to secure child–parent attachment relationships. Ainsworth defined *parental sensitivity* as the ability to perceive and interpret the child's signals accurately and respond to these signals in an adequate and prompt way (Ainsworth et al., 1978). Secure children have experienced that their parents usually perceive and understand their distress, and that their needs are adequately met. Insecurely attached children tend to have less positive and supportive experiences with their parents. Secure attachment is not only important for children's current well-being, but also for their later development. Three meta-analyses confirmed the importance of attachment security for children's later social competence (Groh et al., 2014), for their externalizing behavior problems (Fearon, Bakermans-Kranenburg, van IJzendoorn, Lapsley, & Roisman, 2010), and internalizing problems (Groh, Roisman, van IJzendoorn, Bakermans-Kranenburg, & Fearon, 2012). These outcomes indicate that securely attached children show more social competence and fewer externalizing and internalizing behavior problems than do insecurely attached children.

VIPP-SD is based on an integration of attachment theory (Ainsworth et al., 1978; Bowlby, 1982) and social learning theory, particularly coercion theory (Patterson, 1982). While sensitivity is the central parenting concept in attachment theory, coercion theory emphasizes how ineffective parental discipline strategies result in increasingly difficult and challenging child behavior ("coercive cycles"; Patterson, 1982). Instead of rewarding negative child reactions—without intending to do so—by giving in to difficult child behavior, parents should reinforce children's positive behaviors and discipline them in adequate ways. For example, in the VIPP-SD program, the parent is encouraged to use "induction," that is, to provide the reason for a prohibition or parental intervention (Hoffman, 2000), thus helping the child to (gradually) understand the parental rules and develop empathy with other people's interests. VIPP-SD can be characterized as an interaction-focused intervention using video feedback to promote sensitive parenting, as well as adequate and sensitive discipline strategies (Juffer, Bakermans-Kranenburg, et al., 2008; Juffer, Bakermans-Kranenburg, et al., 2017; Mesman et al., 2008).

Empirical Background of Attachment-Based Interventions

What do we know about the overall effectiveness of attachment-based interventions? In a comprehensive meta-analysis, we included 70 attachment-based intervention studies, with 88 intervention effects directed at either parental sensitivity or attachment security, or both (Bakermans-Kranenburg et al., 2003). All intervention studies reported *observed* parental sensitivity or children's attachment security, or both, as outcome measures. The intervention studies were not restricted to specific populations. Some samples comprised low-risk families with typically developing infants, but studies with clinical and at-risk populations were included as well.

We found evidence for the parental sensitivity hypothesis formulated in attachment theory. Attachment-based interventions appeared to be able to enhance sensitive parenting and children's attachment security, while the causal role of sensitivity for attachment was confirmed. We found that more successful interventions in terms of enhanced parental sensitivity resulted in larger increases in children's attachment security (Bakermans-Kranenburg et al., 2003). In another meta-analysis, we examined 15 attachment-based intervention studies that reported on children's insecure-disorganized attachment as an outcome measure (Bakermans-Kranenburg, van IJzendoorn, & Juffer, 2005). The five interventions focusing on parental sensitivity were most effective; they were significantly more effective in reducing attachment disorganization than the interventions not focusing on sensitive parenting.

Our series of meta-analyses also contributed to the knowledge of how we should deliver an attachment-based intervention. The title of the meta-analytical review, "Less Is More" (Bakermans-Kranenburg et al., 2003), refers to the meta-analytical outcome that relatively brief interventions—up to 16 sessions—were more effective than longer interventions to enhance parental sensitivity. The meta-analysis also revealed that interventions with video feedback—recording and reviewing parent-child interactions—were more successful in improving sensitive parenting than interventions without this method (Bakermans-Kranenburg et al., 2003).

In summary, our series of meta-analyses resulted in several useful, evidence-based guidelines for the development of attachment-based interventions: Positive parent–child relationships can be supported by promoting sensitive parenting; interventions should be relatively brief; and video feedback is an effective tool to enhance sensitive parenting.

Development and Current Practice

Based on attachment and coercion theory, and convergent with the meta-analytical outcomes of effective attachment-based interventions, we designed the VIPP-SD program. Here we describe how we developed VIPP-SD at the Centre for Child and Family Studies at Leiden University, the Netherlands, and we elaborate on current practice with respect to implementation and training opportunities.

Development

When we started our intervention research in the 1980s, Lambermon and van IJzendoorn (1989) found that providing parents with a videotaped role model—that is, showing videos of an unknown mother interacting in a sensitive way with her child—did not work. Apparently, parents have problems identifying with a parent or child model as portrayed on the video; consequently, they may not feel encouraged to integrate the modeled parenting behavior in their own daily lives. At the same time, we started to use video feedback with parents, and we discovered that these identification problems did not occur. With video feedback, parents are recorded interacting with their own child, and they are shown these videos soon afterward. Video-feedback may serve as a mirror to see and reflect on one's *own* parenting behavior (Juffer & Steele, 2014), supported by an intervener who is providing feedback to the parent on relevant aspects of the parent's *own* parent–child interactions. In VIPP-SD, video feedback is seen as not only an effective method to work with parents but also one of the most essential ingredients of the program.

VIPP was initially implemented and tested with parents and infants in their first year of life: in adoptive families (Juffer, Bakermans-Kranenburg, & van IJzendoorn,

2005; Juffer, van IJzendoorn, & Bakermans-Kranenburg, 2008) and in families with insecure mothers (Bakermans-Kranenburg, Breddels-van Baardewijk, Juffer, Klein Velderman, & van IJzendoorn, 2008). Subsequently, we extended VIPP to other types of families and to child care settings, and to a broader age range of children (currently 0 to 6 years), and we described the intervention in a protocol with home visits, standardized themes, and a fixed structure. To also accommodate the intervention to the demands of parenting a child beyond infancy, we extended VIPP with an extra module on Sensitive Discipline (VIPP-SD; Juffer, Bakermans-Kranenburg, et al., 2008; Mesman et al., 2008). Currently, VIPP without the SD module can be implemented with parents and infants before the first birthday, while VIPP-SD is recommended for use with parents and children after the first birthday. The VIPP part in the VIPP-SD program follows exactly the same protocol as in the VIPP program without the SD module (with only minor changes in videotaped episodes and play material). We therefore use the overall name—the VIPP-SD program—to indicate both VIPP and VIPP-SD.

Implementation

The VIPP-SD program is home based and short term: The interventions are implemented in the home or child care setting in a modest number of visits, usually six sessions. VIPP-SD is implemented in the home or child care setting, because the intervention focuses on recording and reinforcing naturally occurring parent–child interactions in daily situations. Also, parents may find it easier to integrate new behaviors in their daily lives when these behaviors have been practiced in the home, and the home setting usually is a safe place to receive personal feedback (also see Juffer, Struis, Werner, & Bakermans-Kranenburg, 2017). In addition, parents with preschool-age children may find it difficult to travel to health services or clinics, and they may be more likely to cancel visits for these reasons. By offering VIPP-SD at home, we increase the chance that parents complete the entire program. In studies testing VIPP-SD, we found that program attendance is usually high (e.g., in a sample including parents of toddlers with high levels of externalizing problem behavior, all 120 families in the intervention group received all six home visits; Van Zeijl et al., 2006), although lower attendance rates may be expected in high-risk or poverty samples (e.g., Negrão, Pereira, Soares, & Mesman, 2014).

VIPP-SD can be implemented in a broad range of clinical and nonclinical families and in child care settings. Several adaptations have been made for parents or children at risk, for families in special situations, and for child care settings (see below in our narrative review). To date, primarily dyadic parent–child interactions—mostly mother–child interactions—have been targeted, although the first studies on VIPP-SD with fathers (Lawrence, Davies, & Ramchandani, 2013) as well as parent couples are in progress.

It should be noted that the VIPP-SD program, with its modest number of sessions, cannot be a panacea for all parental or family problems. VIPP-SD, with its focus on sensitive parenting and children's problem behavior, has not been developed to address all areas of family malfunctioning, including child maltreatment or a parent's psychiatric problems. For example, specific approaches may be needed to prevent child maltreatment in high-risk families (Euser, Alink, Stoltenborgh,

Bakermans-Kranenburg, & van IJzendoorn, 2015), although even in groups with maltreating parents, the program has shown its effectiveness in enhancing attachment security (Moss et al., 2011, 2014). Dependent on the population to serve, a useful framework is to combine VIPP-SD with another treatment module. For example, in a study of mothers with eating disorders, the mothers received not only VIPP to support parent–child interactions during mealtime but also a guided cognitive-behavioral self-help manual to address their eating problems (Stein et al., 2006; Woolley, Hertzmann, & Stein, 2008). VIPP-SD can therefore be used as the only intervention, or it can be combined with another or a longer treatment. In clinical treatment of psychiatrically disturbed parents, their children often are deprived of the support they need, although they clearly might suffer from their parent's problems. VIPP-SD may be considered such support as a complement to regular treatment.

Training

To become a VIPP-SD intervener, training opportunities are offered on a regular basis at various places in the world, for example in the United Kingdom and the United States, Italy, and the Netherlands (for an actual overview, see *www.vippleiden.com*). During a 4-day workshop, participants are taught the basic principles of the VIPP-SD program (Juffer, Bakermans-Kranenburg, et al., 2008) and start working with the protocol (manual VIPP-SD version 3.0; Juffer, Bakermans-Kranenburg, & van IJzendoorn, 2015). The manual and training workshop are available in several languages (including English, Spanish, Italian, and Dutch). Additional training opportunities are available for specific adaptations, such as VIPP-AUTI for families of children with autism (see also Green, Chapter 12, this volume). Training in the VIPP-SD program is open to a relatively broad range of educational and vocational strata, including (child) psychologists, therapists, social workers, family coaches, and (mental) health professionals. After the training, workshop participants start with a practice case, supervised by a VIPP-SD trainer or supervisor. After having completed this practice case successfully, participants receive the certificate of VIPP-SD intervener. When they start working with the program, new interveners are advised to join a VIPP-SD review group, in which peers learn from each other's experiences. To date (August 2017) we estimate that we have trained over 600 professionals in the use of VIPP or VIPP-SD, from more than 15 countries, including Australia, Belgium, Chile, Colombia, Italy, Netherlands, Peru, Poland, the United Kingdom, Uruguay, and the United States.

Key Features of VIPP-SD

What are the key characteristics of the VIPP-SD program? Here we describe how the theoretical concepts of sensitive parenting and sensitive discipline have been translated into an overall structure and specific themes for the intervention. Above all, building a supporting and empathic relationship between the intervener and parent ("alliance"; Stolk et al., 2008) is a crucial element of the intervention (see also Bowlby, 1988). Other important aspects of the program are that parents are recognized as the "experts" on their children, and that their own behavior is the basis of—and the model for—change. In other words, parents are empowered with (more) positive parenting experiences on which they can rely during (future) daily interactions with their child. Interveners work with video feedback to initiate and consolidate these processes. Video feedback provides a unique opportunity to promote parents' understanding of their child and also enables the reinforcement of positive moments in parent–child interactions.

Structure and Themes in the VIPP-SD Program

Based on attachment theory (Ainsworth et al., 1978; Bowlby, 1982, 1988), themes for sensitive parenting were developed, and based on coercion theory (Patterson, 1982) and Hoffman's (2000) work on empathy, themes for sensitive discipline were formulated. In each intervention session, one sensitive parenting theme and one sensitive discipline theme is highlighted (see Table 1.1).

For *sensitive parenting,* the structure of the VIPP-SD program closely follows the two main components of Ainsworth's definition of sensitivity: (1) accurate perception and interpretation of the child's signals, and (2) prompt and adequate reactions to these signals. In the first and second intervention sessions, parents are encouraged to accurately observe and interpret their child's behavior on the recorded video fragments. During the third and fourth sessions, the video feedback also focuses on the second part of Ainsworth's definition, and parents are supported to respond to their child's behavior and emotions in a sensitive way. The specific order of first addressing child behavior, then parental behavior, is part of the VIPP-SD protocol: The possibly more demanding task of addressing parental behavior is postponed until the parent and the intervener have had time to consolidate a working relationship. Because all parents are curious to see their child on the video recordings, and engage easily with watching the child's behavior, VIPP-SD gives first and primary focus to the child's perspective. In practice, this is realized by recording episodes in which the child plays on his or her own, among episodes of parent and child interacting together, and watching first a fragment of the child alone at the beginning of the initial intervention sessions.

TABLE 1.1. Themes in the VIPP-SD Program

Session	Sensitive parenting	Sensitive discipline
1	Exploration versus attachment behavior	Inductive discipline and distraction
2	Speaking for the child	Positive reinforcement
3	Sensitivity chain	Sensitive time-out
4	Sharing emotions	Empathy for the child
5	Booster session	Booster session
6	Booster session	Booster session

By showing on the video recordings the difference between attachment and exploration behavior (Session 1), parents learn to understand when and how their child needs them: to be a secure base when the child needs their emotional support, and to provide the child with opportunities to discover the world through playing and learning. Through "speaking for the child" (Carter, Osofsky, & Hann, 1991), the parent is invited and encouraged to verbalize the child's behavior on the video recordings (Session 2), thus practicing observational skills. In Session 3, sensitivity chains are used to illustrate moments of positive interactions on the video recordings, that is, a signal of the child (e.g., reaching for a toy), followed by an adequate response of the parent (giving the toy to the child), and the child's reaction (giving the parent a happy smile). The intervener explains that such interactions are important for children, because they contribute to children trusting their parents to attend to their needs and help them if necessary. In Session 4, moments of shared emotions are highlighted, for example, comforting a sad child or sharing joy during play together. When parents share their child's positive and negative emotions, children feel supported to express their feelings openly. During the last two booster sessions, all sensitive parenting themes are repeated and integrated. In these booster sessions, as newly acquired parenting behaviors are reinforced and possible changes may be consolidated, there is room to address possible (new) concerns or questions brought by the parent.

For *sensitive discipline,* several relevant themes are highlighted during the intervention sessions (see Table 1.1). In Session 1, parents are encouraged to use inductive discipline (discussed earlier) by explaining to the child the reason for their commands, thus helping the child to internalize parental rules and develop empathy with other people's interests. In this session, it is also suggested that parents use distraction as a useful technique to support child compliance, for example, by suggesting alternatives or postponing attractive activities to a later moment. In Session 2, parents learn to use more positive reinforcement, for example, by giving compliments for compliant child behavior and ignoring challenging child behaviors. In Session 3, parents get detailed information about a "sensitive time out" as a way of dealing with difficult child behavior, which makes them aware of ways to deescalate temper tantrums sensitively. It is explained that the time-out method should be a last resort and pointed out how to use time-out in a sensitive way, for example, by maintaining contact with the child and remaining available as a secure base (e.g., locating the time-out spot in sight of the parent). Finally, by encouraging parents to share the feelings of their child in difficult moments, parents *show and teach* their child empathy (Session 4), that is, understanding and identifying with the perspective of the other person (Hoffman, 2000). Comparable with the sensitive parenting themes, all sensitive discipline themes are repeated and integrated during the two booster sessions.

Video Feedback

The VIPP-SD program is standardized *and* individualized, which means that interveners work from a standard protocol but attune the guidelines from the protocol to the parent–child dyad, resulting in individualized video feedback. Each intervention visit starts with filming parent–child interaction and continues with video feedback based on the recordings of the previous visit.

Parent and child are videotaped during daily situations at their home—for example, playing together, reading a children's book—during brief episodes of usually about 10 minutes (to a maximum of 30 minutes in case of a mealtime—videotaped once in the intervention process). Parents are encouraged to react to their children the way they normally do. In the period between the home visit and the next intervention session (typically 2 weeks later), the intervener reviews the video recordings on his or her own and prepares feedback on the parent–child interaction as shown on the video. The intervener writes down comments for the feedback, directed by the guidelines of the protocol, and by screening the recordings for suitable moments to connect the information in the guidelines to the video. The resulting "script" is connected to the time codes on the video and serves as a guide for the video feedback in the intervention session. The whole range of minutes of video is covered in the script. For a second opinion or advice, the script can be reviewed in a session with peer interveners or supervisors before the actual intervention takes place. To deliver the intervention as prepared, the intervener has his or her script available during the video feedback.

For example, when the theme of exploration versus attachment behavior (see Table 1.1) is to be discussed in the next intervention visit, the intervener searches for relevant moments on the video. Thus, images of the child making eye contact or seeking physical proximity are used to illustrate the child's attachment behavior, whereas moments of the child's play behavior are used to illustrate exploration. The intervener uses "speaking for the child" (Carter et al., 1991) by providing "subtitles" to the child's emotions, facial expressions, and behavior shown on the video. The intervener also connects specific moments to general messages from the protocol. For example, when showing moments of attachment and exploration behavior, the intervener may explain that these behaviors ask for differential parental reactions: Children's attachment signals should be met with prompt, adequate reactions, whereas parents should adopt a different role during children's play and support the child's activities without being intrusive or interfering. The intervener may also comment that play behavior is important for children, because they learn a lot from play material. At the same time, playing together provides children with an extra dimension compared to playing alone: their overtures are responded to, making them feel understood, and moments of joy can be shared (the intervener could say, "A toy does not smile back, you do!").

During the next visit, the intervener reviews the video of the previous visit together with the parent, showing all recorded episodes and giving feedback on the basis of the comments in the script prepared before the session. Positive interaction moments shown on the video recordings are always emphasized. Focusing on positive interactions serves the goal of showing the mother that she is able to act as a sensitive, competent parent: She should feel empowered by positive feedback instead of being made to feel incompetent by negative feedback. To focus the parent's attention on positive moments, the video recording is stilled frequently, and the parent is shown a picture of a successful interaction or a happy child. By repeating brief fragments of sensitive interactions, positive moments are enlarged and emphasized, while negative moments are counterbalanced. In case of insensitive parental behavior, parents are encouraged to use more sensitive behaviors, preferably behaviors they displayed at other moments on the video, so that they are their own model of competent parenting. These "corrective messages" are, however, postponed to the third and later intervention sessions, so that the intervener and parent have some time to build a working relationship.

Intervention Elements

In conclusion, the content of the VIPP-SD program reflects how the theoretical concepts of parental sensitivity and adequate discipline have been translated into an overall intervention structure and pertinent intervention themes. Separate themes for sensitivity and for discipline were developed. Of paramount importance is a trusting relationship between the parent and intervener, a relationship in which the parent is recognized as an "expert" and empowered with positive parenting experiences.

Video feedback plays an important role in the VIPP-SD program. Video provides a "useful 'looking glass' through which parents can see their child and their own behavior with 'new' eyes and relive shared positive moments" (Juffer & Steele, 2014, p. 313). While reviewing the child's behavior as shown on the video and through "speaking for the child," parents are stimulated to include and consider the child's perspective in their thinking. Moreover, watching videos of themselves during daily interactions with their child may also encourage parents to reflect on their parenting behavior and stimulate reflective functioning (see also Steele et al., 2014). For example, in the VIPP project on mothers with eating disorders, specific moments during the video feedback were seen as turning points in the reframing of the mothers' perceptions of themselves as having a potential influence on their children (Woolley et al., 2008). For example, one mother missed her child's excited response to the food during the live interaction, and during the intervention in the next visit, she appeared to have no memory of this positive exchange. The intervener stilled this moment on video, and together the mother and the intervener watched this episode several times. This proved to be a turning point in the intervention. The mother suddenly realized how important she was for her child, and she later commented that the video still was like a photograph that she was carrying about in her head (Woolley et al., 2008).

A next question is whether VIPP-SD, with these potentially positive intervention ingredients, is effective in reaching its goal of supporting sensitive parenting. We therefore continue with a narrative and meta-analytical review of the available VIPP-SD studies.

Effectiveness of VIPP-SD: A Narrative Review

The effectiveness of VIPP-SD was examined in 13 empirical studies (including 12 randomized controlled trials) in various samples of children at risk, parents at risk or in special situations, and in child care settings (see Table 1.2). Before we analyze the outcomes of these studies meta-analytically, we describe the main findings of the pertinent studies in a narrative review. All studies used the VIPP-SD program or a version of it adapted for a specific group of families, parents, or children, and some studies used the module for Sensitive Discipline.

TABLE 1.2. Studies Using the VIPP-SD Program with Main Intervention Outcomes on Sensitive Parenting and Child Behavior

Design (RCT) in chronological order of publication	Sample (N); VIPP/VIPP-SD program	Child's age at intervention start (no. of sessions)	Positive intervention outcomes on sensitive parenting/caregiving	Positive intervention outcomes on child behavior
Juffer et al. (2005) (RCT)	Mothers with adopted infant (N = 130); VIPP	6 months (three sessions)	Increase in sensitivity	Lower rates of disorganized attachment
Follow-up: Stams et al. (2001)				Follow-up (7 years): Fewer internalizing behavior problems in subsample
Klein Velderman et al. (2006a); Bakermans et al. (2008) (RCT)	Insecure mothers (N = 81); (1) VIPP; (2) VIPP-R: VIPP with representational discussions	7 months (four sessions)	VIPP and VIPP-R: increase in sensitivity (with no difference between VIPP and VIPP-R)	Change in maternal sensitivity affected attachment security more in highly reactive infants
Follow-up: Klein Velderman et al. (2006b)				Follow-up (40 months): VIPP: fewer total and externalizing behavior problems in the clinical range; VIPP-R: n.s.
Stein et al. (2006); Woolley et al. (2008) (RCT)	Mothers with eating disorders (N = 80); adapted VIPP program	4–6 months (13 sessions including seven video-feedback sessions)	Less mealtime conflict; increase in positive parenting (e.g., more facilitation of infant)	Greater autonomy during mealtimes
Van Zeijl et al. (2006) (RCT)	Mothers of children at risk for externalizing behavior problems (N = 237); VIPP-SD	1–3 years (six sessions, including two booster sessions)	Increase in positive parenting; more favorable attitudes toward sensitivity and sensitive discipline	In families with more marital discord and in families with more daily hassles decrease of overactive behavior
Follow-up: Bakermans-Kranenburg, van IJzendoorn, Mesman, et al. (2008); Bakermans-Kranenburg, van IJzendoorn, Pijlman, et al. (2008)				Follow-up (1 year after posttest): Decrease of externalizing behavior problems in intervention children with the *DRD4* 7-repeat allele, particularly when their mothers improved more in sensitive discipline; decrease in daily cortisol production in intervention children with the *DRD4* 7-repeat allele

(continued)

TABLE 1.2. *(continued)*

Design (RCT) in chronological order of publication	Sample (*N*); VIPP/VIPP-SD program	Child's age at intervention start (no. of sessions)	Positive intervention outcomes on sensitive parenting/caregiving	Positive intervention outcomes on child behavior
Kalinauskiene et al. (2009) (RCT)	Insensitive mothers (*N* = 54); VIPP	7 months (five sessions, including one booster session)	Increase in sensitivity	No effects on attachment security
Groeneveld et al. (2011) (RCT)	Caregivers in home-based child care (*N* = 48); VIPP-CC: VIPP-SD adapted to child care	Under the age of 4 years (six sessions)	Increase in global quality of child care; more positive attitude toward caregiving and limit setting	Not reported
Moss et al. (2011) (RCT)	Maltreating families (*N* = 67); program based on VIPP	1–5 years (eight sessions)	Increase in sensitivity	Greater proportion of insecure children became secure; greater proportion of disorganized children became organized; externalizing and internalizing problems decreased in older children
Negrão et al. (2014); Pereira et al. (2014) (RCT)	Highly deprived, high-risk mothers (*N* = 43); VIPP-SD	1–4 years (six sessions including two booster sessions)	Increase in positive parenting, particularly nonintrusiveness; increase in family cohesion; in mothers with high levels of stress: decrease of harsh discipline	Increase in positive child behavior, including child responsiveness and involvement
Poslawsky et al. (2014, 2015) (RCT)	Parents (90% mothers) of children with ASD (*N* = 78); VIPP-AUTI: VIPP and elements of VIPP-SD adapted to children with autism	16–61 months (5 sessions)	Increase in parental nonintrusiveness; increase in parental self-efficacy	At 3-month follow-up: Increase in child-initiated joint attention skills

(continued)

TABLE 1.2. *(continued)*

Design (RCT) in chronological order of publication	Sample (*N*); VIPP/VIPP-SD program	Child's age at intervention start (no. of sessions)	Positive intervention outcomes on sensitive parenting/caregiving	Positive intervention outcomes on child behavior
Yagmur et al. (2014) (RCT)	Turkish minority mothers (*N* = 76); VIPP-TM: VIPP-SD adapted to Turkish minority	20–47 months (six sessions including two booster sessions)	Increase in sensitivity and nonintrusiveness	Not reported
Cassibba et al. (2015) (intervention and matched comparison group)	Secure and insecure mothers (*N* = 32); VIPP-R: VIPP with representational discussions	7 months (five sessions)	Increase in sensitivity in insecure mothers	More attachment security in children of insecure mothers
Green et al. (2015) (RCT)	Families with an infant at familial high risk of autism (*N* = 54); iBASIS-VIPP: VIPP adapted to infants at risk of autism	7–10 months (12 sessions, including six core sessions)	Increase in parental nondirectedness	Increase of infant attentiveness to parent; reduction of autism risk behaviors; improved parent-rated adaptive function
Werner et al. (2016) (RCT)	Caregivers in center-based child care (*N* = 64 from 64 centers); VIPP-CC: VIPP-SD adapted to child care	Under the age of 4 years (six sessions including two booster sessions)	Increase in sensitivity; more positive attitude toward caregiving and limit setting	Not reported

Note. ASD, autism spectrum disorder; RCT, randomized controlled trial; VIPP, Video-Feedback Intervention to promote Positive Parenting; VIPP-SD, Video-Feedback Intervention to promote Positive Parenting and Sensitive Discipline.

Studies with Children at Risk

Adopted Children

In an intervention study involving 130 Dutch families with 6-month-old adopted infants, two attachment-based interventions were tested (Juffer et al., 2005). Two subsamples were combined in this study: a subsample of 90 families with a first adopted child (Juffer, 1993) and a subsample of 40 families with birth children and a first adopted child (Rosenboom, 1994). In the first intervention program, mothers were provided with a personal book, with tips for their adopted child's development, and in the second intervention program mothers received the same book and a first version of VIPP that comprised three home-based sessions of video feedback. The control group received a brochure with general information about adoption. The first program, with the personal book only, did not promote maternal sensitivity and was not able to prevent disorganized attachment in the adopted children. However, the intervention with the personal book and video feedback resulted in enhanced maternal sensitivity and lower rates of disorganized attachment in the children (6 vs. 22% in the control group), and these intervention effects were identical in the two subsamples of adoptive families.

On the basis of these results a new nationwide and state subsidized adoption aftercare service with video feedback was started, and since 2000, Dutch parents can ask for this service for each newly adopted child, including special-needs or older-placed children and sibling placements (Juffer, van IJzendoorn, et al., 2008).

Children at Risk of Externalizing Behavior Problems

VIPP, with the additional Sensitive Discipline module (VIPP-SD), was tested in a study with 237 Dutch families screened for their 1- to 3-year-old children's relatively high scores on externalizing behavior (van Zeijl et al., 2006). VIPP-SD was implemented during six home visits, whereas the control group received a dummy intervention of six telephone calls. VIPP-SD proved to be effective in enhancing maternal positive discipline behaviors and maternal attitudes toward sensitivity and sensitive discipline in the intervention group as compared to the control group. In families with more marital discord, and in families with more daily hassles, the intervention resulted in lower rates of overactive problem behavior in the children.

In a follow-up study about 2 years after the start of the study, parents collected children's saliva samples at home on a typical day, and total daily cortisol production was analyzed at the lab (Bakermans-Kranenburg, van IJzendoorn, Mesman, Alink, & Juffer, 2008). The VIPP-SD program proved to be effective in decreasing daily cortisol production in children *with* the dopamine receptor D4 7-repeat (DRD4-7R) allele, but not in children *without* the DRD4 7-repeat allele. In the same follow-up, the role of genetic differences in explaining variability in intervention effects on children's externalizing behavior was tested, and outcomes revealed a moderating role of the dopamine *DRD4* polymorphism (Bakermans-Kranenburg, van IJzendoorn, Pijlman, Mesman, & Juffer, 2008). VIPP-SD proved to be effective in decreasing externalizing behavior in children with the *DRD4*-7R allele, and these effects were largest in children with the *DRD4*-7R allele whose parents showed the largest increase in the use of positive discipline. These outcomes indicate that the children were differentially susceptible to the VIPP-SD program, dependent on their genetic makeup and on the positive change in their mothers' behaviors. Findings from this study did much to inform the theory of differential susceptibility, which remains a focus for ongoing work (Bakermans-Kranenburg & van IJzendoorn, 2015; Ellis, Boyce, Belsky, Bakermans-Kranenburg, & van IJzendoorn, 2011).

Children with Autism and Infants at Risk of Autism

VIPP-AUTI, adapted to parenting a child with autism spectrum disorder (ASD), consists of five sessions, with the first four sessions each addressing the usual sensitive parenting theme (see Table 1.1) and an additional autism theme in each session (e.g., stereotypical behavior of the child, joint attention), followed by one booster session in which all previous information is reviewed. In VIPP-AUTI, parents are encouraged to verbalize the child's facial expressions and nonverbal cues through "speaking for the child" in order to stimulate parents' recognition of the child's (often subtle) signals and communication patterns (Poslawsky et al., 2014). The sensitive discipline themes of VIPP-SD are reviewed during the third session to teach parents how to manage noncompliant child behavior.

VIPP-AUTI was tested with 78 Dutch primary caregivers and their 16- to 61-month-old children with ASD (86% boys; Poslawsky et al., 2015). Whereas the control group received care as usual, VIPP-AUTI was implemented in the intervention group in five home-based sessions. The program focused on improving parent–child interaction and reducing the child's symptomatology. VIPP-AUTI resulted in reduced parental intrusiveness, and (at 3-month follow-up) increased "child-initiated joint attention," which refers to the child's ability to attract another person's visual attention to communicate, a developmental skill often compromised in young children with ASD (Poslawsky et al., 2014). Parents who received VIPP-AUTI also showed increased feelings of efficacy (Poslawsky et al., 2015).

In a related British study, Green et al. (2015; see Chapter 12, this volume) examined the effectiveness of an adapted version of the VIPP program, iBASIS-VIPP, in 54 families with infants at familial high risk of autism. Siblings of children with autism were screened in the British Autism Study of Infant Siblings (BASIS) at ages 7–10 months (baseline) and randomly assigned to the intervention and control group (with no planned intervention). The iBASIS-VIPP group received six core home-based sessions and six booster sessions. The video feedback aimed at helping the parents understand and adapt to their infant's individual communication style to promote the best possible social and communicative development in the child. The intervention increased the infants' attentiveness to the parent and reduced their autism-risk behaviors. iBASIS-VIPP also resulted in increased parental nondirectiveness (comparable with nonintrusiveness) and parent-reported adaptive functioning of the infant.

Studies with Parents at Risk or in Special Situations

Insecure Parents

VIPP-R, VIPP with additional Representational attachment discussions, was developed to address sensitive parenting and mental attachment representations of insecure parents (Bakermans-Kranenburg, Breddels-van Baardewijk, et al., 2008). To test the VIPP-R program, Dutch mothers were screened for the presence of an insecure attachment representation (measured with the Adult Attachment Interview [AAI]; Main, Goldwyn, & Hesse, 2003), and 81 mothers and their 7-month-old infant were included in the intervention study. Mothers were assigned to one of two intervention groups (VIPP or VIPP-R, both implemented in four sessions) or to the control group. Both VIPP and VIPP-R enhanced maternal sensitivity (Klein Velderman, Bakermans-Kranenburg, Juffer, & van IJzendoorn, 2006a). The intervention was most effective for mothers of highly reactive children (reactivity was measured with a temperament questionnaire). Moreover, the experimentally induced change in maternal sensitivity appeared to impact more strongly on the attachment security of the highly reactive infant group compared to the less reactive infants (Bakermans-Kranenburg, Breddels-van Baardewijk, et al., 2008) irrespective of VIPP versus VIPP-R group status. Finally, a follow-up study revealed that the VIPP program (but not the VIPP-R program) protected children from developing total and externalizing behavior problems in the clinical range at preschool age (Klein Velderman et al., 2006b). Thus, the potential added value of discussing representations of past attachment difficulties is not established by this work.

In a related study, Cassibba, Castoro, Constantino, Sette, and van IJzendoorn (2015) tested the VIPP-R program in a sample of 32 Italian mothers with insecure and secure attachment representations and their 7-month-old infants. Compared to secure parents, insecure parents might be more in need of a preventive intervention. The sample included two groups: an intervention group and a comparison group matched with the intervention group on maternal attachment representation (measured with the AAI). The VIPP-R intervention was implemented in five home-based sessions, whereas the comparison families received two dummy home visits during which some mother–child interaction was recorded (without reviewing the videotape). VIPP-R enhanced the sensitivity of the mothers with insecure attachment representations, but the secure mothers' sensitivity did not improve. Similarly, at the posttest, the children of the insecure intervention mothers were more secure than the children of the insecure comparison mothers, whereas the children of the secure mothers did not profit from the intervention. This exploratory study showed that the effectiveness of the VIPP-R program was moderated by the security of parental attachment representations, underscoring the potential value of discussing representations of childhood attachment experiences when those memories trigger ongoing insecurities.

Parents with Eating Disorders

Stein et al. (2006; Woolley et al., 2008) examined the effectiveness of an adapted version of the VIPP program in the United Kingdom in a sample of 80 mothers with eating disorders and their 4- to 6-month-old infants. The intervention was implemented in 13 home-based sessions, including seven video-feedback sessions, whereas the control group received supportive counseling. Both groups also received guided cognitive-behavioral self-help for eating disorders. For the primary outcome of conflicts during mealtime, the VIPP program appeared to be effective and resulted in reduced mealtime conflicts. Also, compared to the control condition, the VIPP program resulted in greater maternal facilitation of the infant (assisting the infant in an activity) and more appropriate maternal nonverbal responses to infant cues, while the infants showed greater autonomy during mealtimes.

Insensitive Parents

Kalinauskiene et al. (2009) tested the VIPP program in a sample of 54 mothers screened for insensitive parenting (using the Ainsworth Maternal Sensitivity Scale; Ainsworth, Bell, & Stayton, 1974) and their 7-month-old infant. In Lithuania, VIPP was implemented in five home-based sessions, including one booster session. Control mothers were contacted by phone (five times) and asked for information on their child's development. Compared to the control group, VIPP enhanced maternal sensitivity, but there were no intervention effects on children's attachment security.

Maltreating Parents

In Canada, Moss et al. (2011) examined the effectiveness of a program based on VIPP in a sample of 67 primary caregivers reported for maltreatment and their children ages 1–5 years. The intervention was implemented in eight home visits, and both the intervention and control groups received the standard agency services (monthly visit by a child welfare caseworker). The intervention resulted in enhanced parental sensitivity. Also, a greater proportion of insecure children in the intervention group became secure in comparison with the control group, while a greater proportion of disorganized children in the intervention group became organized in comparison with the control group. In addition, child age moderated the influence of the intervention on children's internalizing and externalizing behavior problems, with a larger decrease of behavior problems in older children.

Ethnic-Minority Parents

VIPP-SD was adapted for Turkish minority families, resulting in VIPP-TM (VIPP–Turkish Minority). VIPP-TM was tested in the Netherlands in 76 Turkish minority families with 20- to 47-month-old children with high levels of externalizing behavior problems (Yagmur, Mesman, Malda, Bakermans-Kranenburg, & Ekmekci, 2014). VIPP-TM was implemented in six home-based sessions (including two booster sessions) and parallel to the intervention sessions, the mothers in the control group received six telephone calls in which they were invited to talk about their children's development. Compared to the control condition, VIPP-TM resulted in enhanced maternal sensitivity and "nonintrusiveness," which refers to the parent's ability to follow the child's lead and to wait for optimal opportunities to join the child's activities. Maternal discipline strategies were not affected by the intervention.

Highly Deprived, High-Risk Parents

In Portugal, Negrão et al. (2014) examined the effectiveness of VIPP-SD in 43 poor families of toddlers (mean age 29 months) screened for professionals' concerns about the children's caregiving environment. VIPP-SD was implemented in six home-bases sessions (including two booster sessions), whereas the control group received, parallel in timing, six telephone calls. VIPP-SD resulted in enhanced positive parenting, particularly nonintrusiveness, and an increase in family cohesion (indicating the support and involvement that family members perceive from each other). In addition, VIPP-SD resulted in enhanced positive child behavior during parent–child interaction, indicated by child responsiveness (responding positively to parental initiatives) and child involvement (inviting and engaging the parent in to play). Parental stress appeared to be a moderator of intervention effects: VIPP-SD resulted in a decrease of harsh discipline, but only in mothers with high levels of stress (Pereira, Negrão, Soares, & Mesman, 2014).

Studies in Child Care

To support the sensitivity of caregivers in group settings such as child care centers, VIPP-SD was adapted from a dyadic program including one parent and one child into a program focusing on one caregiver and several children.

Home-Based Child Care

VIPP-SD was adapted for implementation in home-based child care, resulting in VIPP–Child Care (VIPP-CC). VIPP-CC was tested with 48 caregivers in home-based child care in the Netherlands (on a weekly basis taking care of on average seven children under age 4; Groeneveld, Vermeer, van IJzendoorn, & Linting, 2011). VIPP-CC was implemented in six sessions at the home-based child care center (including two booster sessions), whereas the control group received six telephone call with conversations about child development. Compared to the control condition, VIPP-CC enhanced global quality, indicating quality and quantity of stimulation and support available to a child in the home-based child care environment. The caregivers in the intervention group also showed a more positive attitude toward sensitive caregiving and limit setting at the posttest than the caregivers in the control group.

Center-Based Child Care

The effectiveness of VIPP-CC was also examined in the setting of center-based child care (Werner, Vermeer, Linting, & van IJzendoorn, 2016). In The Netherlands, 64 caregivers from 64 child care centers received either the VIPP-CC program or telephone calls (control group). As in the study on home-based child care, VIPP-CC consisted of six sessions, including two booster sessions. VIPP-CC resulted in enhanced caregiver sensitivity (particularly in structured play situations) and a more positive attitude toward sensitive caregiving and limit setting.

Evaluating the VIPP-SD Programs

VIPP-SD was implemented in several samples with children or parents at risk or in special situations. In all studies, positive parenting increased, and several indices of child behavior were positively affected by the intervention as well. Even in samples in which parenting is often compromised, such as families living in poverty

(Mesman, van IJzendoorn, & Bakermans-Kranenburg, 2012), and in samples in which specific child characteristics (e.g., autism) challenge the parent's parenting quality, VIPP-SD appeared to make a difference. The two child care studies showed that the VIPP-CC program adapted for child care has the potential to increase the quality of the caregiving environment in child care, with possible positive implications for the millions of children using child care on a regular base.

In a narrative review, we presented all currently available VIPP-SD studies and their outcomes in some detail, and we elaborated on how VIPP-SD has been tested in various (at-risk) populations and childrearing contexts. We asked: How effective is the VIPP-SD program overall in changing parenting behavior? A meta-analysis can answer this question; we therefore continue with a meta-analytical approach to examine the combined effect sizes of the VIPP-SD program on sensitive parenting and positive child outcomes.

Meta-Analytical Evidence of the Effectiveness of VIPP-SD on Sensitive Parenting and Positive Child Outcomes

We meta-analyzed the results of the 12 randomized controlled trials (including 1,116 parents and caregivers) testing the effectiveness of VIPP-SD on sensitive parenting (for the pertinent studies see Table 1.2 and the preceding narrative review). The studies showed a combined effect size of $d = 0.47$ ($p < .001$; 95% confidence interval [CI] = 0.34–0.60) in a homogeneous set of outcomes. This implies that sensitivity increased by about half a standard deviation as a result of participation in the VIPP-SD program. The individual and combined effect sizes are illustrated in Figure 1.1. Six studies involved samples with parents at risk (e.g., insecure, ethnic-minority, or poverty samples). The combined effect size for these six studies was $d = 0.54$ ($p < .001$; 95% CI = 0.33–0.74). The four studies including children at risk (due to adoption, externalizing behavior, or ASD) showed a combined effect size of $d = 0.41$ ($p < .001$; 95% $CI = 0.23$–0.59). The difference between these two combined effect sizes was not significant, $Q(1) = 0.86$, $p = .35$. We may conclude that the VIPP-SD program is as effective in samples with children at risk for problematic development as it is with parents at risk for insensitive parenting.

The combined effect size for improved child outcomes was $d = 0.37$ ($k = 8$, $N = 721$) in a homogeneous set of outcomes (attachment $d = 0.36$, 4 studies; problem behavior $d = 0.26$, 7 studies) (Juffer, Bakermans-Kranenburg, et al., 2017). Follow-up studies revealed a combined effect size of $d = 0.25$. VIPP-SD thus promoted long-term improvement in child outcomes that are probably related to the effects on positive parenting.

Discussion

Key elements of the current VIPP-SD program are the *standardized* protocol that includes detailed descriptions of the general intervention structure and themes combined with *individualized* video feedback targeted at the parent–child dyad involved. VIPP-SD has matured into an internationally recognized intervention,

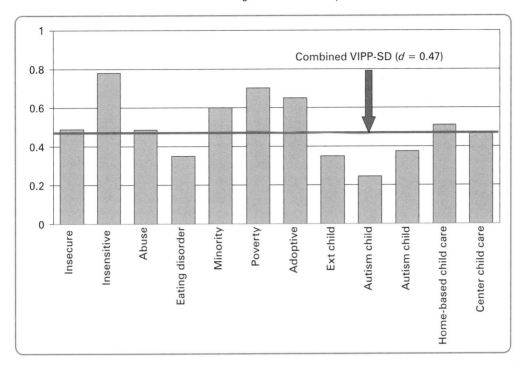

FIGURE 1.1. Individual and combined effect sizes for sensitivity of the 12 VIPP-SD randomized controlled trials (total N = 1,116).

with a manual and training opportunities in several languages, and with a growing databank of research studies on the effectiveness of VIPP-SD. As reported in our narrative review, the program was tested in 13 studies (including 12 randomized controlled trials), resulting in positive outcomes on parent and child behaviors. Our meta-analysis on the 12 randomized controlled trials revealed that sensitive parenting increased by about half a standard deviation as a result of participation in the VIPP-SD program, while VIPP-SD appeared to be as effective in samples with children at risk for problematic development as in samples with parents at risk for insensitive parenting.

A "Less Is More" Intervention

Two important outcomes from the meta-analysis on attachment-based interventions ("Less Is More"; Bakermans-Kranenburg et al., 2003) on how to enhance parental sensitivity are incorporated in the VIPP-SD program: (1) It is a brief intervention (usually six sessions) and, (2) the intervener works with video feedback by recording and reviewing parent–child interactions. Compared to many (therapeutic) programs, VIPP-SD is relatively easy to train and implement because of the availability of a standardized protocol with detailed instructions for the intervention. Moreover, the preparation of an intervention script—containing all messages and feedback for the next session—is helpful and efficient. During the intervention session, the intervener works with this script and does not have to draw on in-the-moment clinical intuition or long years of therapeutic experiences. The possibility of becoming a VIPP-SD intervener is open to a broad range of workers in the field of social work and (mental) health. Finally, VIPP-SD is flexible and can be integrated—as a building block—in a longer or more comprehensive treatment. More than a decade after the claim that "Less Is More" (Bakermans-Kranenburg et al., 2003; van IJzendoorn, Bakermans-Kranenburg, & Juffer, 2005), there is substantially stronger evidence for this claim that offers so much hope for infants at risk and their caregivers.

The Power of Video

Enabled by the common availability of video equipment to date, the use of video feedback in attachment-based interventions has become feasible and attractive (see also Juffer & Steele, 2014). Through video feedback, parents are offered a mirror of their child's behavior and their own parenting behavior, and these images can be examined and reexamined again. Parents learn to recognize and observe even subtle behaviors and expressions of their child, and the videos also show them how their own responses are received by the child. Pictures are more telling than words when showing parents how their own behavior has an influence on their child. Also, feedback connected to relevant video fragments can bring about change in the way parents view and reflect on their own parenting.

From the VIPP-SD studies conducted thus far, it can be concluded that video feedback can be implemented in a wide range of families and in child care settings. Even in populations of poor, low socioeconomic status (SES), maltreating, insensitive, or insecure parents, video feedback has been used and has been effective in promoting more sensitive parenting. The threshold to implement video feedback appears to be quite low, and one of the explanations may be found in the focus of VIPP-SD on the child's perspective. It is their own child who is in the foreground of the video, and "speaking for the child" helps parents to understand and empathize with their child. Parents may—sometimes for the first time—realize how they can and do affect their child's behavior.

Beyond the Mother

Convergent with a similar trend in attachment research with primarily mothers included in the first attachment studies (De Wolff & van IJzendoorn, 1997; van IJzendoorn & De Wolff, 1997), the first focus of VIPP-SD has been on mothers. VIPP-SD was implemented in samples of mothers in varying circumstances (e.g., living in poverty with low resources), in varying cultures (e.g., in a minority group), or with their own specific risks or problems (e.g., eating problems) or their children's (e.g., externalizing problems). VIPP-SD was also adapted for substitute mothers, that is, adoptive and foster mothers and caregivers in child care. The next step is to implement VIPP-SD in samples of fathers (for a first pilot study, see Lawrence et al., 2013) and couples. Future studies may show to what extent the use of the VIPP-SD program can be stretched and when the limits of its effectiveness will be reached. Does VIPP-SD work for difficult-to-train parents (Hodes, Meppelder, Schuengel, & Kef, 2014) or in extremely deprived settings such as orphanages?

Another important question is whether VIPP-SD is equally effective for different types of children and parents.

Differential Susceptibility

The VIPP-SD intervention has been shown to be quite effective in enhancing parental sensitivity, but this "average" effect is not the same for everyone: Some parents and some children profit more from the intervention, whereas others seem to be relatively resistant to change. The term "differential susceptibility" refers to the idea that some individuals, due to their personal characteristics in terms of temperament, biological system, or genetic makeup, are not only more vulnerable to negative experiences and environments but are also more open to the beneficial effects of interventions. Indeed, there is accumulating evidence for differential susceptibility also in the context of interventions (Bakermans-Kranenburg & van IJzendoorn, 2011; Bakermans-Kranenburg & van IJzendoorn, 2015; van IJzendoorn & Bakermans-Kranenburg, 2012). This points to the hidden efficacy of interventions: In subgroups, the intervention is (much) more effective than the overall effect size suggests. For VIPP-SD, the largest effects have been found for children with difficult temperaments and those with a certain variant of the dopamine D4 receptor gene (*DRD4*–7R). These children were most susceptible to changes in their caregiving environment: Temperamentally difficult children showed more secure attachment behavior after a change for the better in their mothers' sensitivity (Klein Velderman et al., 2006a), and children with the *DRD4*–7R allele showed the strongest decrease in externalizing behavior and daily cortisol production after participation of their mothers in the VIPP-SD intervention. Their mothers' increase in the use of sensitive discipline mediated this effect (Bakermans-Kranenburg, van IJzendoorn, Mesman, et al., 2008; Bakermans-Kranenburg, van IJzendoorn, Pijlman, et al., 2008). An important issue for future studies is to examine variation in susceptibility of parents and caregivers who participate in the VIPP-SD programs, and to adapt intervention efforts in a way that provides optimal "susceptibility fit" with the recipients.

Concluding Remarks

Attachment theory is fundamentally eclectic and interdisciplinary. At the core of the theory is an evolutionary perspective, but Bowlby integrated a range of other ideas from a large variety of disciplines into the framework that was labeled "attachment theory." Intervention programs based on such a theory should necessarily be eclectic as well, and not refrain from integrating principles from social learning theory and other sources of inspiration, such as differential susceptibility theory. VIPP-SD is eclectic in at least two ways. It integrates social learning ideas about coercive cycles into its attachment framework, and it also should be considered a module to be included in a variety of interventions and therapies with broader aims than enhancing the quality of parent–child interactions and relationships.

In line with the evolutionary core of attachment theory, there is a growing emphasis on neurobiological foundations and components of attachment relationships and representations (e.g., Riem, Bakermans-Kranenburg, van IJzendoorn, Out, & Rombouts, 2012). A crucial question about the effectiveness of interventions such as the VIPP-SD program is its "embodiment" in parents and children, thus affecting their relationship in not only the short term but also the long term. We found positive changes in cortisol production in our toddlers participating in VIPP-SD even 2 years after the last intervention session. This hormonal change might be a link in a cascade of neurobiological changes as a consequence of the changed parenting. To trace other links in this cascade, from epigenetic changes influencing the expression of genes responsible for neurotransmitters such as oxytocin to changes in neural connectivity in the brain is a major challenge in the search for mechanisms of effective attachment-based interventions.

ACKNOWLEDGMENTS

Femmie Juffer (NWO Meerwaarde grant), Marian Bakermans-Kranenburg (NWO Vici grant), and Marinus Van IJzendoorn (NWO Spinoza Prize) are supported by The Netherlands Organization for Scientific Research (NWO).

REFERENCES

Ainsworth, M. D. S., Bell, S. M., & Stayton, D. J. (1974). Infant–mother attachment and social development: Socialization as a product of reciprocal responsiveness to signals. In M. P. M. Richards (Ed.), *The integration of a child into a social world* (pp. 99–135). London: Cambridge University Press.

Ainsworth, M. D. S., Blehar, M. C., Waters, E., & Wall, S. (1978). *Patterns of attachment: A psychological study of the Strange Situation.* Hillsdale, NJ: Erlbaum.

Bakermans-Kranenburg, M. J., Breddels-van Baardewijk, P., Juffer, F., Klein Velderman, M., & van IJzendoorn, M. H. (2008). Insecure mothers with temperamentally reactive infants: A chance for intervention. In F. Juffer, M. J. Bakermans-Kranenburg, & M. H. van IJzendoorn (Eds.), *Promoting positive parenting: An attachment-based intervention* (pp. 75–90). New York: Taylor & Francis.

Bakermans-Kranenburg, M. J., & van IJzendoorn, M. H. (2011). Differential susceptibility to rearing environment depending on dopamine-related genes: New evidence and a meta-analysis. *Development and Psychopathology, 23,* 39–52.

Bakermans-Kranenburg, M. J., & van IJzendoorn, M. H. (2015). The hidden efficacy of interventions: Gene × environment experiments from a differential susceptibility perspective. *Annual Review of Psychology, 66,* 381–409.

Bakermans-Kranenburg, M. J., van IJzendoorn, M. H., & Juffer, F. (2003). Less is more: Meta-analysis of sensitivity and attachment interventions in early childhood. *Psychological Bulletin, 129,* 195–215.

Bakermans-Kranenburg, M. J., van IJzendoorn, M. H., & Juffer, F. (2005). Disorganized infant attachment and preventive interventions: A review and meta-analysis. *Infant Mental Health Journal, 26,* 191–216.

Bakermans-Kranenburg, M. J., van IJzendoorn, M. H., Mesman, J., Alink, L. R. A., & Juffer, F. (2008). Effects of an attachment-based intervention on daily cortisol moderated by dopamine receptor D4: A randomized control trial on 1- to 3-year-olds screened for externalizing behavior. *Development and Psychopathology, 20,* 805–820.

Bakermans-Kranenburg, M. J., van IJzendoorn, M. H., Pijlman, F. T. A., Mesman, J., & Juffer, F. (2008). Experimental evidence for differential susceptibility: Dopamine D4 receptor polymorphism (DRD4 VNTR) moderates effects on toddlers' externalizing behavior in a randomized controlled trial. *Developmental Psychology, 44*, 293–300.

Bowlby, J. (1982). *Attachment and loss: Vol. 1. Attachment.* New York: Basic Books. (Original work published 1969)

Bowlby, J. (1988). *A secure base: Clinical applications of attachment theory.* London: Routledge.

Carter, S. L., Osofsky, J. D., & Hann, D. M. (1991). Speaking for the baby: A therapeutic intervention with adolescent mothers and their infants. *Infant Mental Health Journal, 12*, 291–301.

Cassibba, R., Castoro, G., Costantino, E., Sette, G., & van IJzendoorn, M. H. (2015). Enhancing maternal sensitivity and infant attachment security with video feedback: An exploratory study in Italy. *Infant Mental Health Journal, 36*(1), 53–61.

De Wolff, M. S., & van IJzendoorn, M. H. (1997). Sensitivity and attachment: A meta-analysis on parental antecedents of infant attachment. *Child Development, 68*(4), 571–591.

Ellis, B. J., Boyce, W. T., Belsky, J., Bakermans-Kranenburg, M. J., & van IJzendoorn, M. H. (2011). Differential susceptibility to the environment: A neurodevelopmental theory. *Development and Psychopathology, 23*, 7–28.

Euser, S., Alink, L. R. A., Stoltenborgh, M., Bakermans-Kranenburg, M. J., & van IJzendoorn, M. H. (2015). A gloomy picture: A meta-analysis of randomized controlled trials reveals disappointing effectiveness of programs aiming at preventing child maltreatment. *BMC Public Health, 15*, 1068.

Fearon, R. P., Bakermans-Kranenburg, M. J., van IJzendoorn, M. H., Lapsley, A. M., & Roisman, G. I. (2010). The significance of insecure attachment and disorganization in the development of children's externalizing behavior: A meta-analytic study. *Child Development, 81*(2), 435–456.

Green, J., Charman, T., Pickles, A., Wan, M. W., Elsabbagh, M., Slonims, V., . . . Johnson, M. H. (2015). Parent-mediated intervention versus no intervention for infants at high risk of autism: A parallel, single-blind, randomised trial. *Lancet, 2*, 133–140.

Groeneveld, M. G., Vermeer, H. J., van IJzendoorn, M. H., & Linting, M. (2011). Enhancing home-based child care quality through video-feedback intervention: A randomized controlled trial. *Journal of Family Psychology, 25*(1), 86–96.

Groh, A. M., Fearon, R. P., Bakermans-Kranenburg, M. J., van IJzendoorn, M. H., Steele, R. D., & Roisman, G. I. (2014). The significance of attachment security for children's social competence with peers: A meta-analytic study. *Attachment and Human Development, 16*(2), 103–136.

Groh, A. M., Roisman, G. I., van IJzendoorn, M. H., Bakermans-Kranenburg, M. J., & Fearon, R. P. (2012). The significance of insecure and disorganized attachment for children's internalizing symptoms: A meta-analytic study. *Child Development, 83*(2), 591–610.

Hodes, M. W., Meppelder, H. M., Schuengel, C., & Kef, S. (2014). Tailoring a video-feedback intervention for sensitive discipline to parents with intellectual disabilities: A process evaluation. *Attachment and Human Development, 16*(4), 387–401.

Hoffman, M. L. (2000). *Empathy and moral development. Implications for caring and justice.* Cambridge, UK: Cambridge University Press.

Juffer, F. (1993). *Verbonden door adoptie. Een experimenteel onderzoek naar hechting en competentie in gezinnen met een adoptiebaby* [Attached through adoption: An experimental study of attachment and competence in families with adopted babies]. Amersfoort, The Netherlands: Academische Uitgeverij.

Juffer, F., Bakermans-Kranenburg, M. J., & van IJzendoorn, M. H. (2005). The importance of parenting in the development of disorganized attachment: Evidence from a preventive intervention study in adoptive families. *Journal of Child Psychology and Psychiatry, 46*, 263–274.

Juffer, F., Bakermans-Kranenburg, M. J., & van IJzendoorn, M. H. (Eds.). (2008). *Promoting positive parenting: An attachment-based intervention*. New York: Taylor & Francis.

Juffer, F., Bakermans-Kranenburg, M. J., & van IJzendoorn, M. H. (2014). Attachment-based interventions: Sensitive parenting is the key to positive parent–child relationships. In P. Holmes & S. Farnfield (Eds.), *The Routledge handbook of attachment: Implications and interventions* (pp. 83–103). London: Routledge.

Juffer, F., Bakermans-Kranenburg, M. J., & van IJzendoorn, M. H. (2015). *Manual Video-Feedback Intervention to promote Positive Parenting and Sensitive Discipline (VIPP-SD)* (version 3.0). Leiden, The Netherlands: Leiden University, Centre for Child and Family Studies.

Juffer, F., Bakermans-Kranenburg, M. J., & van IJzendoorn, M. H. (2017). Pairing attachment theory and social learning theory in video-feedback intervention to promote positive parenting. *Current Opinion in Psychology, 15*, 189–194.

Juffer, F., & Steele, M. (2014). What words cannot say: The telling story of video in attachment-based interventions. *Attachment and Human Development, 16*(4), 307–314.

Juffer, F., Struis, E., Werner, C., & Bakermans-Kranenburg, M. J. (2017). Effective preventive interventions to support parents of young children: Illustrations from the Video-feedback Intervention to promote Positive Parenting and Sensitive Discipline (VIPP-SD). *Journal of Prevention and Intervention in the Community, 45*(3), 202–214.

Juffer, F., van IJzendoorn, M. H., & Bakermans-Kranenburg, M. J. (2008). Supporting adoptive families with video-feedback intervention. In F. Juffer, M. J. Bakermans-Kranenburg, & M. H. van IJzendoorn (Eds.), *Promoting positive parenting: An attachment-based intervention* (pp. 139–153). New York: Taylor & Francis.

Kalinauskiene, L., Cekuoliene, D., van IJzendoorn, M. H., Bakermans-Kranenburg, M. J., Juffer, F., & Kusakovskaja, I. (2009). Supporting insensitive mothers: The Vilnius randomized control trial of video feedback intervention to promote maternal sensitivity and infant attachment. *Child: Care, Health and Development, 35*, 613–623.

Klein Velderman, M. K., Bakermans-Kranenburg, M. J., Juffer, F., & van IJzendoorn, M. H. (2006a). Effects of attachment-based interventions on maternal sensitivity and infant attachment: Differential susceptibility of highly reactive infants. *Journal of Family Psychology, 20*, 266–274.

Klein Velderman, M. K., Bakermans-Kranenburg, M. J., Juffer, F., van IJzendoorn, M. H., Mangelsdorf, S. C., & Zevalkink, J. (2006b). Preventing preschool externalizing behavior problems through video-feedback intervention in infancy. *Infant Mental Health Journal, 27*(5), 466–493.

Lambermon, M. W. E., & van IJzendoorn, M. H. (1989). Influencing mother–infant interaction through videotaped or written instruction: Evaluation of a parent education program. *Early Childhood Research Quarterly, 4*, 449–458.

Lawrence, P. J., Davies, B., & Ramchandani, P. G. (2013). Using video feedback to improve early father–infant interaction: A pilot study. *Clinical Child Psychology and Psychiatry, 18*(1), 61–71.

Main, M., Goldwyn, R., & Hesse, E. (2003). *Adult Attachment Scoring and Classification Systems*. Unpublished manuscript, University of California at Berkeley, Berkeley, CA.

Mesman, J., Stolk, M. N., van Zeijl, J., Alink, L. R. A., Juffer, F., Bakermans-Kranenburg, M. J., . . . Koot, H. M. (2008). Extending the video-feedback intervention to sensitive discipline: The early prevention of antisocial behavior. In F. Juffer, M. J. Bakermans-Kranenburg, & M. H. van IJzendoorn (Eds.), *Promoting positive parenting: An attachment-based intervention* (pp. 171–191). New York: Taylor & Francis.

Mesman, J., van IJzendoorn, M. H., & Bakermans-Kranenburg, M. J. (2012). Unequal in opportunity, equal in process: Parental sensitivity promotes positive child development in ethnic minority families. *Child Development Perspectives, 6*, 239–250.

Moss, E., Dubois-Comtois, K., Cyr, C., Tarabulsy, G. M., St-Laurent, D., & Bernier, A. (2011). Efficacy of a home-visiting intervention aimed at improving maternal sensitivity, child attachment, and behavioral outcomes for maltreated children: A randomized control trial. *Development and Psychopathology, 23*(1), 195–210.

Moss, E., Tarabulsy, G. M., St-Georges, R., Dubois-Comtois, K., Cyr, C., Bernier, A., . . . Lecompte, V. (2014). Video-feedback intervention with maltreating parents and their children: Program implementation and case study. *Attachment and Human Development, 16*(4), 329–342.

Negrão, M., Pereira, M., Soares, I., & Mesman, J. (2014). Enhancing positive parent–child interactions and family functioning in a poverty sample: A randomized control trial. *Attachment and Human Development, 16*(4), 315–328.

Patterson, G. R. (1982). *Coercive family process.* Eugene, OR: Castalia.

Pereira, M., Negrão, M., Soares, I., & Mesman, J. (2014). Decreasing harsh discipline in mothers at risk for maltreatment: A randomized control trial. *Infant Mental Health Journal, 35*(6), 604–613.

Poslawsky, I. E., Naber, F. B. A., Bakermans-Kranenburg, M. J., De Jonge, M. V., van Engeland, H., & van IJzendoorn, M. H. (2014). Development of a Video-Feedback Intervention to promote Positive Parenting for Children with Autism (VIPP-AUTI). *Attachment and Human Development, 16*(4), 343–355.

Poslawsky, I. E., Naber, F. B. A., Bakermans-Kranenburg, M. J., van Daalen, E., van Engeland, H., & van IJzendoorn, M. H. (2015). Video-Feedback Intervention to promote Positive Parenting adapted to Autism (VIPP-AUTI): A randomized controlled trial. *Autism, 19*(5), 588–603.

Riem, M. M. E., Bakermans-Kranenburg, M. J., van IJzendoorn, M. H., Out, D., & Rombouts, S. (2012). Attachment in the brain: Adult attachment representations predict amygdala and behavioral responses to infant crying. *Attachment and Human Development, 14*(6), 533–551.

Rosenboom, L. G. (1994). *Gemengde gezinnen, gemengde gevoelens?: Hechting en competentie van adoptiebaby's in gezinnen met biologisch eigen kinderen* [Mixed families, mixed feelings?: Attachment and competence of adopted babies in families with biological children]. Utrecht, The Netherlands: Utrecht University.

Stams, G. J., Juffer, F., van IJzendoorn, M. H., & Hoksbergen, R. A. C. (2001). Attachment-based intervention in adoptive families in infancy and children's development at age 7: Two follow-up studies. *British Journal of Developmental Psychology, 19*, 159–180.

Steele, M., Steele, H., Bate, J., Knafo, H., Kinsey, M., Bonuck, K., . . . Murphy, A. (2014). Looking from the outside in: The use of video in attachment-based interventions. *Attachment and Human Development, 16*(4), 402–415.

Stein, A., Woolley, H., Senior, R., Hertzmann, L., Lovel, M., Lee, J., . . . Fairburn, C. G. (2006). Treating disturbances in the relationship between mothers with bulimic eating disorders and their infants: A randomized, controlled trial of video feedback. *American Journal of Psychiatry, 163*, 899–906.

Stolk, M. N., Mesman, J., van Zeijl, J., Alink, L. R. A., Bakermans-Kranenburg, M. J., van IJzendoorn, M. H., . . . Koot, H. M. (2008). Early parenting intervention aimed at maternal sensitivity and discipline: A process evaluation. *Journal of Community Psychology, 36*, 780–797.

van IJzendoorn, M. H., & Bakermans-Kranenburg, M. J. (2012). Differential susceptibility experiments: Going beyond correlational evidence: Comment on beyond mental health, differential susceptibility articles. *Developmental Psychology, 48*, 769–774.

van IJzendoorn, M. H., Bakermans-Kranenburg, M. J., & Juffer, F. (2005). Why less is more: From the dodo bird verdict to evidence-based interventions on sensitivity and early attachments. In L. J. Berlin, Y. Ziv, L. Amaya-Jackson, & M. T. Greenberg (Eds.),

Enhancing early attachments: Theory, research, intervention, and policy (pp. 297–312). New York: Guilford Press.

van IJzendoorn, M. H., & De Wolff, M. S. (1997). In search of the absent father: Meta-analyses of infant–father attachment: A rejoinder to our discussants. *Child Development, 68*(4), 604–609.

van Zeijl, J., Mesman, J., van IJzendoorn, M. H., Bakermans-Kranenburg, M. J., Juffer, F., Stolk, M. N., . . . Alink, L. R. (2006). Attachment-based intervention for enhancing sensitive discipline in mothers of one- to three-year-old children at risk for externalizing behavior problems. *Journal of Consulting and Clinical Psychology, 74*(6), 994–1005.

Werner, C., Vermeer, H. J., Linting, M., & van IJzendoorn, M. H. (2016). *Video-feedback intervention in center-based child care: A randomized controlled trial.* Leiden, The Netherlands: Leiden University.

Woolley, H., Hertzmann, L., & Stein, A. (2008). Video-feedback intervention with mothers with postnatal eating disorders and their infants. In F. Juffer, M. J. Bakermans-Kranenburg, & M. H. van IJzendoorn (Eds.), *Promoting positive parenting: An attachment-based intervention* (pp. 111–138). New York: Taylor & Francis.

Yagmur, S., Mesman, J., Malda, M., Bakermans-Kranenburg, M. J., & Ekmekci, H. (2014). Video-feedback intervention increases sensitive parenting in ethnic minority mothers: A randomized control trial. *Attachment and Human Development, 16*(4), 371–386.

CHAPTER 2

Attachment and Biobehavioral Catch-Up

MARY DOZIER, KRISTIN BERNARD, and CAROLINE K. P. ROBEN

Attachment and Biobehavioral Catch-Up (ABC), an intervention for parents of young children who experience early adversity, has been developed and refined over the last 20 years (Dozier, Meade, & Bernard, 2014; Dozier, Lindhiem, & Ackerman, 2005; Dozier, Stovall, & Albus, 1999). Developing the intervention was an iterative process, informed by research (conducted in our own and in other laboratories) and our clinical observations with families. In its first incarnation, the program had only two sessions. At that point, it targeted the first issue that we had identified through our research—helping caregivers not be pushed away by the signals of young children who had experienced adversity. As attachment researchers, we also realized the importance of attending to parents' own issues that might interfere with their providing nurturing care. Thus, we incorporated a brief approach aiming to help parents "override" their own issues and provide nurturing, responsive care. We then conducted psychophysiological research, finding that many children who had experienced adversity were dysregulated physiologically and needed caregivers who could help them develop adequate regulatory capabilities. We added a component to address this issue, by helping parents follow their children's lead. As we moved from implementing our intervention with foster parents to birth parents, we observed high rates of intrusive and frightening behavior. Based on the work of Mary Main, Karlen Lyons-Ruth, Deborah Jacobvitz, and others (e.g., Jacobvitz, Hazen, Zaccagnino, Messina, & Beverung, 2011; Lyons-Ruth, Bronfman, & Parsons, 1999; Main & Solomon, 1990), we realized the importance of helping parents behave in nonfrightening ways and built attention to this into the intervention. In its current form (Dozier & the Infant Caregiver Project, 2013), the ABC intervention consists of 10 sessions delivered in parents' homes to address these three targets: (1) providing nurturance to distress even when children do not elicit it and even when it does not come naturally to parents, (2) following children's lead with delight, and (3) behaving in nonfrightening ways.

The development of the intervention occurred in the context of several randomized clinical trials with foster parents, high-risk birth parents, and internationally adopting parents. As will be described in greater detail later, we found evidence that the intervention is effective in enhancing parents' sensitivity (Bick & Dozier, 2013) and brain activity in response to infant stimuli (Bernard, Simons, & Dozier, in press) and children's attachment quality (Bernard et al., 2012), cortisol production (Bernard, Dozier, Bick, & Gordon, 2014; Bernard, Hostinar, & Dozier, 2015), emotion expression (Lind, Bernard, Ross, & Dozier, 2014), and executive functioning (Lewis-Morrarty, Dozier, Bernard, Terraciano, & Moore, 2012).

Upon finding that the intervention was effective as implemented in randomized clinical trials, we worked to disseminate the intervention to other sites. After facing many challenges familiar to dissemination and implementation researchers (Southham-Gerow, Rodriquez, Chorpita, & Daleiden, 2012), we adopted a number of strategies that have enhanced our effectiveness. Most important is our development of a fidelity assessment measure that guides training and provides a metric for assessing progress over the course of supervision. We are now implementing the intervention in a number of sites around the United States and in some limited sites internationally.

In this chapter, we first describe how past research and theory guided our identification of the three targets of the ABC intervention. Second, we present the approach of the ABC intervention, with an overview of session content, in-the-moment commenting, and video feedback. Third, we consider how the ABC intervention fits within the broader context of attachment theory. Fourth, we discuss the evidence base of the ABC intervention, presenting findings from several randomized clinical trials showing effects on child and parent outcomes. Finally, we conclude with a focus on our dissemination efforts.

Development of the ABC Intervention

The intervention was launched rather precipitously. After studying the role of an adult attachment-oriented state of mind on treatment use among adults with serious psychiatric disorders over the course of a decade, I (M. D.) became haunted by concerns that my research have direct implications for treatment. Looking for attachment-oriented research that would reach this objective, I stumbled on the case of a young child being separated from her foster mother. Being a new parent myself at the time, I expected that forming new attachments on the heels of losing one's primary attachment figure would represent an almost overwhelming challenge for young children.

Developing ABC Target 1: Providing Nurturance to Distress

The first target of the intervention, helping parents respond in nurturing ways when children are distressed, was primarily informed by research in our laboratory concerning how young children form attachments in foster care. Along with graduate student Chase Stovall-McClough and others on the team, we began study-ing how young children coped with forming new attachments after the loss of a primary attachment figure. We set out to look at attachment quality in the Strange Situation, but the literature did not inform us as to how long it would take a child to form a new attachment, or how we would know whether a child had formed a consolidated attachment, or other such critical and rudimentary issues. Thus, it occurred to us that we needed a measure of attachment that we could use daily, so that we could look at children's behaviors that would reflect their turning toward their caregivers as attachment figures. The Strange Situation would not work for this purpose—rather, it could not be used more often than about every 6 months or the context would come to have unintended meaning to the child. Clearly, it could not be used daily. The other alternative of which we were aware, the attachment *Q*-set (Vaughn & Waters, 1990; Waters, 1987), was too demanding for parents to complete daily. Given the lack of tools to assess attachment quality on a daily basis, we developed a diary measure that asked parents to report on children's attach-ment behaviors. Although we shared the concern that many attachment research-ers have regarding the systematic bias associated with parent report of behavior, we considered our measure preferable to most, because we asked parents to report *specific behaviors* (rather than an overall evaluation), and to report on the *most recent* behavior (rather than choosing among all behaviors).

After developing the Parent Attachment Diary (Dozier & Stovall, 1997), we set out to examine the formation of attachment relationships as children transitioned to a new caregiver. Following infants who were newly placed into foster care, we asked foster parents to record children's behaviors at the end of each day, describing the most recent time that the child was frightened, separated from the parent, and hurt. Each day, for each of these three incidents of potential distress, the parent recorded both how the child responded to the incident, and how the parent then responded to the child. We made several observations that surprised us. First, infants younger than about 10 months very quickly showed secure behaviors when placed with moth-ers with autonomous states of mind. Within about 7 days, a stable pattern of secure behaviors characterized their reliance on their new foster parent, as described by the diary data. For example, such children cried and reached for their foster moth-ers when hurt, and quieted when their foster mothers picked them up. We were sur-prised to find such patterns emerge and consolidate quickly—indeed, often within the first 7 days of placement. However, despite the short time frame from an adult's perspective, it occurred to us that 7 days was a very long time from an infant's per-spective. Indeed, Bowlby's (1969/1982) attachment theory drew on the work of evo-lutionary biologists (e.g., Lorenz, 1935; Tinbergen, 1951), and the theory suggests that young infants are evolutionarily prepared to display behaviors that maximize proximity to their caregivers. However, we found that infants who were older than about 12 months of age did not always use these evolutionarily prepared behaviors at times of distress (e.g., crying, following, and clinging) as they should.

Young Children Who Have Experienced Adversity Push Caregivers Away

For infants older than about 12 months of age, what we saw was very different. These infants tended to show avoidant and resistant behaviors over the several months we followed them (Stovall & Dozier, 2000). These behaviors included turning away from caregivers when distressed or failing to be soothed when comforted by their foster parents. Of greatest concern, though, was that foster parents tended to respond "in kind" to children. Contingency analyses revealed that children's behaviors appeared to drive parents' responses (Stovall-McClough & Dozier, 2004); that is, when children behaved in avoidant ways, parents responded as if their children did not need them; when children behaved in resistant ways, parents responded in an irritable or fussy fashion. This finding led to our first intervention target: *Parents need to behave in nurturing ways even when children do not elicit it.*

In order to address this first target, we ask parents to consider the ways that children might behave that make it easy or difficult to provide care. We use a standard set of video clips from the Strange Situation of children showing avoidant or resistant behaviors in order to introduce the idea that children do not always signal their needs clearly. We discuss research, such as a study demonstrating that children classified as avoidant in the Strange Situation (with minimal behavioral signs of distress) still show elevated heart rate activity (Sroufe & Waters, 1977). We also discuss the earlier findings from our own research about children in foster care, suggesting that parents tend to respond "in kind" to children's behaviors. As parents understand that children may fail to signal their needs clearly, we help them consider ways that they can look past these behaviors and provide nurturing care even when it is not elicited. Initially, we planned to have an intervention that had this single component implemented through two sessions. However, we almost immediately recognized the need to include several additional key issues in the intervention.

Caregivers' Own Issues Affect Their Propensity to Nurture Their Distressed Children

Even though infants in foster care tended to "lead the dance" early on in their relationships with new foster parents, caregivers eventually took the lead, with caregiver attachment state of mind predicting children's attachment quality (Dozier, Stovall, Albus, & Bates, 2001). The good news was that foster parents with autonomous states of mind were likely to have infants with secure attachments. And this was indeed good news—despite infants pushing caregivers away initially, foster parents' tendency to be nurturing must have won out, with children being able to develop a trusting relationship. At least in the first 2 years of life (the oldest we studied in this early work), children were able to organize their attachment around the availability of new foster parents, providing that that foster parent was nurturing (or had an autonomous state of mind).

However, the bad news was that children of nonautonomous foster parents were at disproportionately high risk of developing disorganized attachments (Dozier et al., 2001). In contrast, among children from low-risk conditions, dismissing and preoccupied states of mind are associated with insecure but organized attachments (van IJzendoorn, 1995). Finding that dismissing and preoccupied states of mind, as well as an unresolved state of mind, predicted disorganized attachment in our high-risk group of foster children was concerning. Disorganized attachment places children at elevated risk for a number of problematic outcomes, including externalizing problems (Fearon, Bakermans-Kranenburg, van Ijzendoorn, Lapsley, & Roisman, 2010; van IJzendoorn, Schuengel, & Bakermans-Kranenburg, 1999), posttraumatic stress disorder (PTSD) symptoms in middle childhood (MacDonald et al., 2008), and dissociative symptoms in adolescence (Carlson, 1998; Lyons-Ruth & Jacobvitz, 2016). On the basis of these findings, we reasoned that it was critical that caregivers provide nurturing care to children who had experienced early adversity, even if it was difficult for them to do so. Thus, we refined our first intervention target: *Parents need to provide nurturing care even when children fail to elicit it, and even when it does not come naturally to parents.*

Whereas we were able to introduce the idea that children might behave in ways that pushed them away early in the intervention, we became aware that talking with parents about how their own attachment experiences affected their caregiving was a more sensitive subject that required the foundation of a strong relationship with the parent coach. We therefore pushed these two sessions that introduced this concept from Sessions 3 and 4 forward to Sessions 6 and 7, and ultimately to Sessions 7 and 8. We find that it works well to deal explicitly with parents' "voices from the past" in Sessions 7 and 8, because by that point parents have become aware of the issues with which they struggle.

Our intent is to help parents see issues from their past that influence the way that they are predisposed to parent. Parents have characteristic ways of responding that in fact may be automatic for them—that is, it may not occur to them that there are other ways of responding (e.g., when a child falls, the parent says, "Oh you're OK. You don't need to cry"). Often such "automatic" ways of responding are the result of their own attachment experiences. If they can become aware of the influences on their parenting, their responses can become nonautomatic—and then they can choose how to respond. We often talk about these influences as "voices from the past," referring to childhood experiences and messages that shape current parenting. Our conceptualization of voices from the past was informed by Selma Fraiberg's "ghosts in the nursery" (Fraiberg, Adelson, & Shapiro, 1975), and Alicia Lieberman's early interpretation of Fraiberg's work for practice (Lieberman & Pawl, 1988). If parents can access some memories of how they were raised that relate to challenges they are having with nurturance or following the lead, this may help them interrupt what is otherwise an automatic sequence. If they can recognize where their tendencies come from, they can make the automatic nonautomatic, and therefore have control in how they respond—thereby "overriding" their voices from the past. For example, consider a mother who has been observed in early sessions to repeatedly dismiss her child's distress, such as saying, "You're fine," and hushing her child after he falls. In this case, we would aim to help this mother recognize that she is missing opportunities to respond in a nurturing way when her child needs her. We would help her identify "voices from the past" that interfere with providing nurturance—guiding her through such a discussion by asking her to recall how her parents' responded when she was upset as a child and consider possible ideas or messages she received from how her parents responded to her (e.g., picking up her child would spoil him). This discussion is often further informed by using video clips of the parent interacting with her child in ways that are consistent with her voices from the past (e.g., missing an opportunity to provide nurturance) and inconsistent with her voices from the past (e.g., providing nurturance even though it was not automatic). As the parent becomes aware of her voices from the past, she is helped to recognize them in the moment and is supported in overriding them by responding in a way that is different.

Developing ABC Target 2: Following Children's Lead

As we became aware that children who have experienced early adversity are often dysregulated biologically and behaviorally, we developed the second target of the intervention: helping parents follow their children's lead. Seymour Levine, a pioneer in psychoneuroendocrinology, came to the University of Delaware in 1996. At that point, we had developed only the first component of the intervention, emphasizing the child's need for nurturing care. Dr. Levine gave a talk in the psychology department, in which he talked about his early work. In particular, Levine described the effects that separations had on infant squirrel monkeys. One especially noteworthy finding involved the divergence of behavioral and physiological responses to separation observed when infants could or could not hear and smell their mothers in nearby cages (Wiener, Bayart, Faull, & Levine, 1990). Parallels between infants in foster care who experienced separations from caregivers were readily apparent.

At that point, we began collaborative work with Levine, first exploring the effects of foster care and maltreatment on young children's ability to regulate their neuroendocrine systems. As anticipated, there were rich connections to be made between the nonhuman neuroendocrine work and research with human infants. The steroid hormone cortisol plays a role in the stress response and in helping the organism function as a diurnal creature (in the case of diurnal animals). We found that children living with neglecting birth parents showed non-normative diurnal patterns of cortisol production (Bernard, Butzin-Dozier, Rittenhouse, & Dozier, 2010). Compared with children growing up under low-risk conditions, children living with neglecting birth parents showed lower morning values of cortisol and flatter slopes across the day. Children in foster care were intermediate between children living with neglecting birth parents and low-risk children. Other colleagues observed similar disruptions in cortisol regulation among children who experienced neglect, abuse, or disruptions in care (e.g., Bruce, Fisher, Pears, & Levine, 2009).

These findings of physiological dysregulation, combined with findings that children who have experienced adversity are at increased risk for behavioral and emotional dysregulation (e.g., Blair & Raver, 2012; Calkins & Leerkes, 2011; Cicchetti & Toth, 2005; Lewis, Dozier, Ackerman, & Sepulveda-Kozakowski, 2007), led us to think that we needed to develop an intervention component that targeted dysregulation. Whereas developing an intervention for attachment organization was intuitive, developing an intervention targeting regulation was less so. In looking at the literature, we found that in correlational studies, parents who followed their children's lead and were responsive to their signals under nondistress conditions had children with stronger self-regulation capabilities (Raver, 1996; Rocissano, Slade, & Lynch, 1987).

Thus, our second intervention target is that *parents need to follow their children's lead.* We introduce this component specifically in Sessions 3 and 4, but often point out parental behaviors that exemplify the concept in the earliest minutes of the first session, as we describe later. Similar to the first intervention target, we help parents consider the importance of following children's lead by introducing research evidence (in parent-friendly terms) showing that children who experience early adversity are at risk for problems controlling their behavior and regulating their biology. After identifying regulation as a key developmental task for children, we suggest that having a parent who follows the child's lead helps the child develop these capacities to control attention, behavior, and physiology. Thus, we encourage parents to constantly look for opportunities to respond to their children in synchronous ways. When the child hands the parent a toy, the parent can take it. When the child smiles as a block tower falls over, the parent can share in the child's excitement and say, "You noticed it fall over!" When the child bangs a puzzle piece on the table rather than putting it in the correct spot, the parent can join in and also bang a puzzle piece. Following the lead is targeted by providing feedback to parents—not only primarily in the moment, during interactions that occur in session, but also through brief video clips of their interactions. We consider following the lead to be a style of interaction that can occur throughout the session, and therefore capitalize on the many opportunities that occur to highlight and reinforce the behavior, as we describe in detail later.

As we helped parents to follow their children's lead, we noted that some did so in very rote, mechanical ways, whereas others were animated, showing genuine delight in their children. Differences in displays of delight were also evident among foster parents, with parents who voiced more commitment to their children (i.e., evidence of emotional investment, interest in providing long-term care, consideration of the foster child as one's own) showing more delight in their interactions than parents who voiced less commitment (Bernard & Dozier, 2011). We came to see delight as a key variable signaling the parent's appreciation for and enjoyment of the child, an observation that resonates with Bowlby's (1951) statement that the healthy mother–infant relationship is a continuous one from which both experience "satisfaction and enjoyment" (p. 11), and later attachment researchers who emphasized delight as an important element to well-functioning parent–child relationships (Ainsworth, 1967; Britner, Marvin, & Pianta, 2005). We therefore revised the second intervention component somewhat, specifying that *parents need to follow their children's lead with delight.*

Developing ABC Target 3: Providing Nonfrightening Care

In our initial evaluation of the intervention, we aimed to intervene with children wherever they moved. Thus, when children previously in foster care returned to their biological parents, we aimed to provide the intervention to the biological parent. When we moved our intervention from foster parents to birth parents, we observed birth parents showing frightening behaviors that we previously had not often encountered. We observed perhaps intentional frightening behaviors in response to child behaviors that parents considered inappropriate, such as smacking their children's hands, glaring at or speaking to children in a threatening way, or speaking in a harsh and loud tone of voice. We also observed frightening behaviors that were not as clearly tied to disciplinary tactics, but perhaps rather the result of trauma, such as odd/disoriented changes in the parent's voice. We were aware of the findings linking frightening behavior with disorganized attachment (Lyons-Ruth & Jacobvitz, 1999; Madigan, Moran, Schuengel, Pederson, & Otten, 2007; Schuengel, Bakermans-Kranenburg, & van IJzendoorn, 1999), as well as evidence suggesting that children raised in maltreating or multi-risk families were especially at risk of disorganized attachment (Carlson, Cicchetti, Barnett, & Braunwald, 1989; Cyr, Euser, Bakermans-Kranenburg, & van IJzendoorn, 2010). Even if parents became more nurturing and followed their children's leads more, it seemed likely that frightening behavior would undermine children's ability to develop organized attachment relationships and optimal biological and behavioral regulation. Thus, our third intervention component is that *parents need to behave in nonfrightening ways all of the time.*

We introduce this target primarily in Sessions 5 and 6. Building from the focus on the importance of following children's lead in the previous two sessions, we first introduce the idea that intrusive behaviors (e.g., putting a puppet in a child's face, tickling the child despite cues of disengagement) can be overwhelming and overstimulating for children. After discussing these behaviors, we move in Session 6 into a discussion of more overtly frightening behaviors. We help parents to recall times when they were frightened by adults whom they trusted during childhood, and how these experiences influenced those relationships. By showing a brief video clip of a child with a disorganized attachment (who simultaneously cries for the parent as she backs away), we discuss how having a parent who is scary, even once in a while, interferes with a child's ability to depend on that person. Parents are further helped to consider their own behaviors that may be frightening to children, a topic that may be further addressed in remaining sessions as needed.

Description of the ABC Intervention Approach

The ABC intervention is a 10-session parenting program implemented in the home. At minimum, a primary caregiver and the young child are present, but we invite anyone else in the house who is interested, including, for example, a grandmother, a boyfriend, and the child's siblings. We consider it very important to implement the intervention in the home, because we want parents to practice nurturing and following the lead in the environment in which they live, so that they experience challenges typical to their everyday life during sessions.

The intervention is manualized—that is, we have developed a manual that specifies the content of the sessions. Originally the manual was about three times the length of the current manual. We have found, though, that responsible interventionists, whom we call "parent coaches," feel the need to discuss everything in the manual, even though it was our intent to include verbatim text only as examples of what might be said. We describe the manual content below. However, before doing so, we want to emphasize that we consider the use of "in the moment" comments to be the most important part of implementing the intervention. We describe these "in the moment comments" and how they are used, after providing an overview of the manual's content (see Table 2.1).

TABLE 2.1. Overview of ABC Intervention Sessions

Intervention session	Topic
Sessions 1 and 2	Providing nurturance even when children do not elicit it
Sessions 3 and 4	Following the child's lead with delight
Session 5	Reducing intrusive/overstimulating behaviors
Session 6	Reducing frightening behaviors
Sessions 7 and 8	Recognizing and overriding voices from the past
Sessions 9 and 10	Consolidating gains and celebrating progress

Content of ABC Sessions

Sessions 1 and 2

Sessions 1 and 2 focus on our first ABC target: providing nurturance. Before introducing this topic, parent coaches set the tone for the 10 sessions. They describe how sessions will be collaborative, with the parent as the expert on the child and the parent coach bringing the research perspective, and how the sessions focus on the parent–child interaction. The parent coach tells the parent that he or she will comment about his or her observations of the parent and child during the sessions—suggesting that the parent is probably already doing many of the things that will be discussed throughout the 10 sessions—and begins making these comments immediately. The parent coach also presents three myths about parenting (e.g., picking up a baby when it cries will spoil the baby) and asks for the parent's opinions on the myths, while presenting relevant research that supports nurturing and responsive interactions.

Overall, across the two sessions, parent coaches convey that (1) all children need nurturance even if they do not signal their need for it clearly, (2) parents tend to respond "in kind" to children's signals and that their children's behaviors are powerful, and (3) parents can recognize negative feelings and respond with nurturance anyway. Parent coaches show several videos of children during the Strange Situation procedure (Ainsworth et al., 1978), the standard research procedure in the developmental field of attachment, used to assess the quality of attachment by observing how the child responds to brief separations from and reunions with the parent. In one video, the child shows clear cues of distress (e.g., crying, reaching for parent) following the separation, effectively signaling his or her need for nurturance from the parent. In the other videos, children fail to signal clearly; one child turns away (reflecting avoidant attachment) and appears unaffected by the separation, whereas another remains fussy and difficult to soothe when the parent returns (reflecting resistant attachment). These videos guide the discussion of child cues, how a parent would be likely to respond "in kind" to such behaviors, and the challenges of responding to a child who is turning away or a child who accepts nurturing contact but continues to cry and even pushes away.

Sessions 3 and 4

The next two sessions focus on the second target: following the lead with delight. Research supporting the importance of following the lead of the child in terms of the benefits this has for self-regulation, attention, and brain development is discussed with the parent. In Session 3, the parent coach shows the parent sample videos of a parent first following her child's lead, then not following her child's lead (e.g., being overly instructive or "teachy" and directive). The parent is then asked to engage in tasks similar to those shown on the video with his or her own child and is coached through the tasks with in-the-moment comments. Session 4 has a similar structure and focuses on following the child's lead during a challenging task (e.g., making pudding with the child).

Sessions 5 and 6

Sessions 5 and 6 address the third target: frightening behavior. In Session 5, parent coaches discuss behaviors that can be overwhelming and scary to children (e.g., tickling) and normalize how tempting it can be to engage in such behaviors. Parents watch two videos of parents and children interacting with puppets. In one video, the parent is scary with the puppet; in the other, the parent follows the child's lead with the puppets. Parents are then provided with puppets and other toys and are coached to follow the child's lead and engaging in intrusive or overwhelming ways. Session 6 continues this topic but focuses on more frankly frightening behaviors, such as smacking, glaring at, or threatening a child. Parent coaches ask parents to reflect on their own experiences of being frightened and discuss the negative effects of frightening behaviors on the parent–child relationship.

Sessions 7 and 8

Although aspects of the parent's own caregiving history may have been discussed in earlier sessions, in Sessions 7 and 8, the explicit focus is on how one's own experiences being parented can influence one's later parenting. As described earlier, these influences are called "voices from the past." Parent coaches use video feedback to contrast times when parents' voices from the past may have gotten in the way of nurturance, following the lead with delight, or not being frightening and times when parents were able to override those voices and nurture, follow, or *not* behave in a frightening way.

Sessions 9 and 10

In earlier iterations of ABC, we introduced new material in Sessions 9 and 10. We have since decided to reserve these two sessions for review and consolidation. We have found that doing so prevents earlier discussions from being forgotten and provides time for individualized feedback and focus on remaining challenges. In the final session, parent coaches present a montage video of the parents nurturing and following their children with delight.

In-the-Moment Comments

What we consider most important in implementing the intervention is making "in-the-moment comments" regarding parents' behaviors. These comments direct parents' attention to times when they have nurtured or followed their children's lead, or to opportunities for doing so. The comments may contain specific description of the behavior (e.g., "He fell down and you picked him right up"), the intervention target (e.g., "That's such a good example of nurturance"), and/or the outcome for the child (e.g., "That will let him know he can depend on you when he's upset"). At first, incorporating this live coaching or feedback was primarily based on observations during supervision that parent behavior almost immediately changed in response to parent coaches' comments. Since identifying in-the-moment commenting as our key approach for changing behavior, we have evaluated its power through research studies. Indeed, the frequency of in-the-moment comments is associated with parents' change in sensitivity (Meade & Dozier, 2012).

We think that in-the-moment comments are important for several reasons. First, they bring parents' attention to the behaviors of interest and allow them to see exactly what is meant. Without clearly specifying the behavior, parents may assume that the parent coach was referring to something else. Take the following example: A child hands his mother a block, and she takes it and says, "Oh, thanks for the red block, honey"; the parent coach says, "Wonderful." The parent may then start talking about colors, assuming that the parent coach was referring to her labeling of the "red" block. Instead, a comment such as "Wonderful! He handed you the block and you took it and said 'thank you!' is an example of following his lead—you responded to exactly was he was doing." As opposed to the general praise offered by the first comment, requiring the mother to speculate what was "wonderful" about her response, the second, more specific comment makes it very obvious which aspect of the response was consistent with the intervention target. By being very specific, the comments link the mother's behaviors with one of the intervention targets, and hence with the session content.

Second, in-the-moment comments help the parent to see why nurturing and following the child's lead are so important, because the parent coach links these behaviors with important child outcomes. Although these outcomes are also discussed more generally as manual content is presented, linking outcomes very specifically to parent behaviors *as they occur* provides further reinforcement of these concepts. For example, in response to a parent picking up a child when he cries, a parent coach might say, "Look how you picked him up when he cried! When you provide that nurturance, he is learning that he can trust you . . . And just think how important that is as he gets older. He will know that he can come to you when he gets in a fight with his best friend in elementary school, when his girlfriend breaks his heart in high school, and when he becomes a stressed parent with his own babies as an adult!" Hearing the positive outcomes associated with nurturing care (or with following the lead) further supports parents' valuing and motivation to respond in these ways.

Third, in-the-moment comments celebrate what parents are doing well and build on their strengths. The value of the positive nature of comments cannot be overstated. Having someone come into your home to educate you on how to parent can be incredibly threatening not only for birth parents who are at risk of having their children removed from their care but also for foster parents who may already feel like experts given their experiences with many children. Anecdotally, we have observed that in-the-moment comments in early sessions can reduce parents' defensiveness or resistance very quickly. A parent referred by child protective services following allegations of neglect may be used to hearing professionals tell her that what she is doing wrong, how her child is in danger, and how she is in need of parenting classes. Upon starting the ABC intervention, she might expect to receive similar feedback. Instead, entering her home for the first time, an ABC parent coach would try to comment within the first few minutes on what she is doing well; for example, "Did you notice how you just smiled at her when she looked up at you? That is a wonderful example of showing your delight in her! We are going to talk about just that in a couple weeks—how expressing your delight in her can really help build her confidence . . . but you're already doing it! And did you see how her face just lit up?" Now, this is not always easy to do initially, because parents might not be behaving in ways that are consistent with ABC targets. In the first session, parents may ignore the child's distress, or only turn their attention to the child to correct a mistake. But the parent coach works hard to find opportunities. Even in the context of relatively negative or disengaged interactions, parent coaches find brief opportunities to make in-the-moment comments.

Fourth, in-the-moment comments can gently challenge or shape behaviors that are not consistent with the targets. At first, we typically ignore times when parents do not respond in line with the targets. If a parent is insensitive when the child cries, or does not follow the child's lead, we would not comment on it in the first session or two in order to avoid defensiveness and resistance and to build rapport and parent confidence. Beginning around Session 3 or Session 4, once a relationship is established and parents are familiar with the targets, parent coaches may begin to comment in ways that aim to shape parent's behaviors when they are non-nurturing or nonsynchronous. For example, when practicing following the child's lead in Session 3 with a book with pull-out shapes, a parent says, "Put the piece here—the duck goes here . . . push it in." The parent coach might say jokingly, "Oops—who's taking the lead?," gently pointing out that the parent is taking the lead herself. If the parent then follows the child's lead by laughing and saying, "duck on your head!" when the child places the duck shape on his head, the parent coach would immediately offer a positive comment: "There you go! Right back to following his lead. He wanted to put the duck on his head, and you followed right along with his game." Other types of comments that gently challenge parents when they are not nonresponsive to children's signals include taking the blame oneself for the lack of response (e.g., "Here I am talking on and on about this research study and we haven't attended to [child] in several minutes! What could we do to follow his lead right now?") or more directly suggesting to the parent a way to respond (e.g., "That was so nice that you looked at her and noticed that she was upset. . . . I wonder if she might need a little more—Let's see what happens if you pick her up"). Following any such suggestions, the parent coach would praise the parent's response, giving the parent credit for providing nurturance or following the child's lead, even if it was directly suggested by the parent coach.

Finally, and importantly, in-the-moment comments make it clear to the parent that interactions with the child during sessions are much more important than discussion of the manual content with the parent coach. Strong parent coaches constantly interrupt themselves and the parent to offer in-the-moment comments. It may take a parent coach 5 minutes to get out one sentence about a research study because she interrupts herself 10 times to comment on observations in the moment; not only is this digression from manual content OK from our perspective, it is encouraged.

Video Feedback

In Sessions 2–10, parent coaches are encouraged to show the parents clear, brief clips (2–10 seconds) of themselves from the previous session. These clips typically show the parents engaging in nurturance, following the lead with delight, or avoiding frightening behaviors. The clips are shown not only to encourage a clearer understanding of the target behaviors but also to provide positive feedback and motivation to the parents. Video feedback can be particularly useful in Sessions 7 and 8, when the parent coach is trying to help the parents recognize times when their voices from the past interfere with intervention targets. Rather than leaving these discussions open-ended, the parent coach focuses the discussion on "voices" relevant to the behavioral target of interest.

Attachment Base of the ABC Intervention

Our intervention is strongly based in attachment theory. Even though each component is included because of its basis in research findings, each could equally be motivated by the observations of Bowlby, Ainsworth, and Ainsworth's students (e.g., Mary Main) relative to effective parenting and key principles of attachment theory.

Nurturance

In Ainsworth's early studies of mothers and infants in Uganda (Ainsworth, 1967), then in Baltimore (Ainsworth et al., 1978), she carefully observed precursors of children's attachment behaviors. A primary finding was that parents' sensitivity is strongly predictive of infants' patterns of behavior in response to separation and reunion (Ainsworth et al., 1978), with infants of sensitive parents clearly more able to seek comfort and to be soothed than infants of insensitive parents. This emphasis on the parent as a source of comfort or as a "secure base" was indeed consistent with Bowlby's assertion that parental protection in the face of threat is at the root of the developing child's sense of security (Bowlby, 1969/1982). In recent efforts to understand the developmental sequelae of receiving sensitive care to distress (distinctive from responsive care in response to nondistress cues), other attachment researchers continue to find support for nurturance as a predictor of attachment security (e.g., McElwain & Booth-LaForce, 2006). Thus, our first ABC target of helping parents provide nurturance in times of distress is quite consistent with this central tenet of attachment theory.

Following the Lead with Delight

In Ainsworth's original scales for coding maternal behavior, she measured dimensions of sensitivity beyond parents' responsiveness to infants' distress. Specifically, she developed scales for dimensions of Cooperation–Interference, Availability–Ignoring, and Acceptance–Rejection (Ainsworth et al., 1978). Taken together, behaviors coded along these dimensions reflect parents' ability to respond contingently to children's interests, behaviors, and signals; to follow the child's pace; and to delight in the child with genuine affection. By targeting these aspects of responsiveness to nondistress, the ABC intervention is well aligned with these other constructs that Ainsworth believed mattered in predicting the quality of parent–infant relationships.

Nonfrightening Care

Bowlby (1969/1982) emphasized the importance of the attachment figure serving as a source of comfort in the face of threat, suggesting that maintaining proximity to the parent would support the infant's survival. What, then, would happen if the parent, who is supposed to be a source of comfort, is also the source of fear? Although the issue of frightening parental behavior was not explicitly addressed by Bowlby, later work by leading attachment researchers demonstrated that frightening behavior significantly undermined children's ability to seek comfort from their parents. Main and Solomon (1990) introduced the idea that frightening parental behavior leaves children with an unsolvable dilemma ("fright without solution"), leading to disorganized attachment. The third target of ABC, helping to reduce frightening parental behaviors, is well motivated by such observations of the devastating effects of threatening parental behavior.

Parents' Issues

The intergenerational transmission of attachment is a common topic of interest among attachment researchers. One of the best predictors of infant attachment security is parents' attachment state of mind (Pederson, Gleason, Moran, & Bento, 1998; van IJzendoorn, 1995; Verhage et al., 2016). *Attachment state of mind,* coded from the Adult Attachment Interview (AAI; George, Kaplan, & Main, 1996) by applying the rating and classification system (Main, Goldwyn, & Hesse, 2008) refers to how adults conceptualize their own attachment experiences. Adults with *autonomous* states of mind openly and coherently describe their attachment experiences, demonstrating that they value attachment. In contrast, nonautonomous adults are incoherent in their presentation of childhood memories, perhaps minimizing distress, idealizing attachment figures, or claiming to lack memories (*dismissing*) or appearing angry or passive when describing experiences (*preoccupied*). Attachment research showing that state of mind is one of the strongest predictors of attachment security certainly points to the importance of addressing parents' own issues, or "voices from the past," in ABC sessions.

Evidence Base for the ABC Intervention

The ABC intervention has been assessed in four randomized clinical trials, compared to a well-matched control intervention that is also guided by a manual, lasts 10 sessions, and implemented in parents' homes. The four ABC trials include one enrolling infants in foster care, another enrolling infants living with neglectful birth parents, another enrolling toddlers (2- to 3-year-olds) in foster care, and still another enrolling infants adopted internationally. The latter two randomized clinical trials are still not complete, and we have only preliminary data at this point. For the two earlier trials, we have a number of outcomes at least several years following the intervention, and continue to follow the children of neglectful parents through ages 8, 9, and 10. In addition, we have studied the effectiveness of the intervention as administered in other communities through pre- and postintervention designs. The California Clearinghouse has assessed the ABC intervention at the highest level of 1 (California Evidence-Based Clearinghouse, 2014), which is awarded to programs considered "well supported by research evidence." The outcomes of attachment and cortisol production were of primary interest given the identified problems of these children and the intervention targets. Outcomes of emotion expression, executive functioning, and parents' brain activity were seen as logical, but more distal, outcomes associated with the intervention and with the more proximal outcomes of attachment and cortisol production. See Figure 2.1 for overview of hypothesized effects.

As shown in Figure 2.1, we expected that the ABC intervention would lead to changes in parenting behavior (i.e., increased nurturance, increased following the lead [*synchrony*], and reduced frightening behavior), which would in turn support

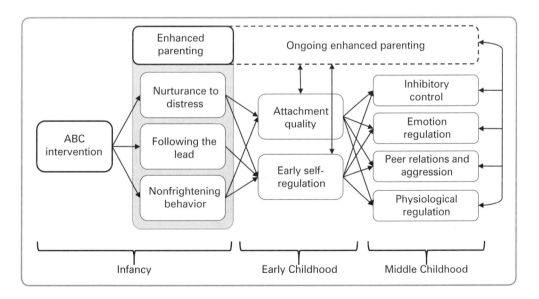

FIGURE 2.1. Hypothesized effects of the ABC intervention. Results on outcomes of enhanced parenting (behavior and brain activity), attachment quality, and early self-regulation (physiology, attention, and emotion) are published. Middle childhood outcomes are being assessed in ongoing randomized clinical trials.

the development of secure attachment and good self-regulation (i.e., normative cortisol rhythms, executive functioning). With the continued support of ongoing sensitive parenting, we expected these short-term competencies to support middle childhood outcomes of improved inhibitory control, emotion regulation, social competence with peers, and healthy physiological regulation.

Child Outcomes

Attachment

In the randomized clinical trial with neglected children living with their parents, significantly more of the children whose parents received the ABC intervention had secure attachments, and fewer had disorganized attachments than children whose parents received a control intervention. Of the children in the ABC group, 32% had disorganized attachments as contrasted with 57% of the children in the control intervention group, reflecting a medium effect size (Cohen's $d = 0.52$) (Bernard et al., 2012).

Cortisol Production

Neglected children are at risk for physiological dysregulation, marked by low morning cortisol levels and a blunted decline across the day (Bernard et al., 2010). In the trial of children reported to be neglected, children in the ABC group showed a more normative diurnal production of cortisol than children from the treatment comparison, within several months of receiving the intervention (Bernard et al., 2014). More specifically, ABC children showed higher morning cortisol levels and a steeper slope across the day than children in the treatment comparison group. These improvements in biological regulation persisted at a preschool follow-up assessment, approximately 3 years after the intervention (Bernard, Hostinar, et al., 2015).

Emotion Expression

Also in the trial of children identified as neglected, we assessed children's emotion expression in the Tool Task (Matas, Arend, & Sroufe, 1978), a series of challenging problem-solving tasks that children were unlikely to be able to complete without the help of their parents. We found that children in the ABC group showed less negative affect, and less anger toward their parents, than children in the control group (Lind et al., 2014).

Executive Functioning

Erin Lewis-Morrarty assessed executive functioning among foster children in her dissertation research. These were children from the trial of infants in foster care, but assessed at follow-up, when the children were between ages 4 and 6 years. She used the Dimensional Change Card Sort developed by Zelazo and colleagues (Zelazo, 2006; Zelazo, Müller, Frye, & Marcovitch, 2003). This task requires children to learn rules to sort cards that vary on two dimensions. First, in "preswitch" trials, children learn to sort the cards based on one dimension (i.e., color). Then, in "postswitch" trials, children are asked to stop following that rule and to sort the cards based on the other dimension (i.e., shape). Children in the ABC group and children in the treatment control group were able to perform the first preswitch task well, with performance not significantly different from that of children in the treatment control group (Lewis-Morrarty et al., 2012). After the dimensional shift, however, children in the ABC group performed the task significantly better than did children from the treatment control group.

Parent Outcomes

Sensitivity

Perhaps the most proximal outcome of the ABC intervention is assessing changes in parenting behavior. In a study of foster parents, Johanna Bick assessed changes in parental sensitivity from preintervention to postintervention follow-up visits. Specifically, parents were observed during play interactions and rated on a 5-point scale based on Ainsworth's definition of *sensitivity* (i.e., appropriately and consistently responding to children's signals). Foster parents who received the ABC intervention showed a more significant increase in sensitivity compared to foster parents who received the control intervention (Bick & Dozier, 2013).

Mothers' Brain Activity

In her dissertation that followed up with mothers from the neglect sample, Kristin Bernard examined whether the ABC intervention affected mothers' brain activity (Bernard, Simons, et al., 2015). Mothers viewed pictures of children with crying, laughing, and neutral facial expressions while we recorded their electroencephalographic (EEG) activity. Mothers who completed the ABC intervention showed larger N170 responses (a brain wave that occurs approximately 170 ms after seeing a stimulus) and larger LPP responses (a brain wave at occurs approximately 300–650 ms after seeing a stimulus) to emotional faces than to neutral faces. In contrast, mothers in the control intervention group did not show larger responses to emotional faces than to neutral faces. ABC mothers' patterns of brain responses were similar to a comparison group of low-risk mothers recruited from the community. Furthermore, the magnitude of brain responses to emotional faces relative to neutral faces was correlated with observed maternal sensitivity.

Dissemination

Having found the ABC intervention effective across a range of outcomes and over a period of time following the intervention, we began to disseminate it to other sites. Several issues suggested as important in the literature emerged as critical to effective dissemination.

We began disseminating the intervention before we had developed a system for quantifying in-the-moment comments. Although we stressed the importance of making such comments as we trained and supervised parent coaches, we found that we were not especially effective in getting parent coaches to make such comments.

We then developed the system for quantifying comments, tracked parent coach comments, and provided parent coaches feedback. Even then, many parent coaches did not make frequent in-the-moment comments, and not nearly at the level that we wanted to see (at least 1 per minute and missing no more than 50% of all opportunities for comments). We then modified our coding system to make it amenable to nonresearchers to code, and trained parent coaches to code their own sessions. We saw a significant increase in parent coach comments (Meade, Dozier, & Bernard, 2014), and parent coaches began to meet expected criteria. Therefore, we see as critical our having developed a quantifiable fidelity assessment tool, for application to videos by the parent coaches themselves, that captures the most important aspect of the intervention's implementation.

A second important issue in disseminating the intervention has been identifying clinicians with the requisite skills for learning the intervention. We have not considered degree (e.g., MSW, PhD) as essential to learning the intervention, because we have observed clinicians with PhDs fail to learn to implement the intervention effectively, and some with BA degrees learn to implement the intervention well. This actually complicated our efforts, because it would have been easier to specify the need for an advanced degree than to find other criteria. We realized that *being able to make in-the-moment comments* and *being nondefensive* were two key qualities we wanted to see in parent coaches. We developed a screening tool that asked potential parent coaches to make in-the-moment comments in response to video-recorded parent–child interactions after observing examples of good in-the-moment comments (to assess the ability to make in-the-moment comments), and to respond to several questions from the AAI (to assess valuing of attachment and nondefensiveness). In particular, we ask each potential trainee for three adjectives that describe his or her childhood relationship with his or her mother and to instantiate each adjective, and for memories of times as a child when he or she was upset, hurt, and sick. This screening tool has been excellent in identifying parent coaches who will be successful at learning the intervention. Almost all (94.6%) parent coaches that we have trained since instituting the criteria have been certified if they have not left the program due to reasons unrelated to parent coaching skills (e.g., promotion at the dissemination site, inadequate site support to support ABC work).

Finally, a third issue critical to success is "buy-in" and support from agencies in which the intervention is being implemented. It is essential that supervisors or agency administration are aware or supportive of the time needed to learn the intervention, attend supervision, and review video-recorded sessions. Without such support, parent coaches are at risk for not investing the time needed to master the intervention.

Training of Parent Coaches

Initial Training

Initial training in ABC takes place in person and lasts for 2–3 days. Training for smaller groups is at the University of Delaware. I (M. D.) and/or Dr. Caroline Roben and University of Delaware staff travel to the training site for larger groups. Training includes theoretical and practical orientation to the intervention, practice with in-the-moment commenting and coding, review of session content, consultation concerning site-specific implementation, and planning for the supervision year. Parallel to our coaching of parents, we train our parent coaches using frequent video examples and live practice of commenting and in-the-moment coding.

Supervision

Supervision is conducted via video conferencing. Trainees have two supervision meetings per week: General Clinical Supervision and In-the-Moment Commenting Supervision. In General Clinical Supervision, trainees meet for 1-hour weekly group supervision conducted in groups of two or three with an experienced clinician who is an expert in ABC. Supervision includes video review each week. In-the-Moment Commenting Supervision is 30 minutes per week, conducted by staff members at the University of Delaware who have been trained to reliability with in-the-moment coding. Trainees review sections of coding of each week's sessions with the University of Delaware staff members, working to become reliable coders and to improve quantity and quality of comments.

Certification

After a year of supervision, parent coaches' adherence and fidelity are evaluated for certification. Adherence is determined by manual content and certain prescribed general factors (e.g., the parent coach has all the materials needed for session) and proscribed factors (e.g., the parent coach reads directly from the manual). Fidelity is determined by examination of the parent coach's 10 most recent in-the-moment commenting coding segments. Commenting is evaluated in terms of both frequency and quality. After 2 years, parent coaches are asked to submit new cases for reevaluation of adherence and fidelity.

Selection of Parent Coaches

As mentioned earlier, we have a screening process for parent coaches. We use the half-hour screening to predict which coaches will be most successful at the intervention. We can conduct the screening remotely through video conferencing with potential coaches, then discuss the scores with the site leader. Those interested in training in ABC should e-mail Dr. Caroline Roben (*croben@psych.udel.edu*) to discuss fit between the dissemination site and the program.

Conclusion

ABC is an evidence-based intervention for young infants who have experienced early adversity. Although the format and structure of the intervention has changed since its inception 20 years ago, the foundation in attachment has remained constant in its present form, which encourages parents to nurture their children even when their children do not elicit nurturance, to follow their children's lead with delight, to refrain from frightening behaviors, and to examine how their own issues may influence parenting. ABC is implemented through discussion of manualized content and video feedback, but more importantly through the use of specific in-the-moment comments about targeted parenting behaviors that occur during session. We find strong evidence for intervention effects across several randomized clinical trials, including some immediate and long-term improvements in factors such as attachment, diurnal cortisol patterns, executive functioning, negative emotion expression, maternal sensitivity, and maternal event-related potential (ERP) patterns. As we continue to explore the effects of the intervention into middle childhood, we also prioritize adherence and fidelity to the model.

REFERENCES

Ainsworth, M. D. S. (1967). *Infancy in Uganda: Infant care and growth of love.* Baltimore: Johns Hopkins University Press.

Ainsworth, M. D. S., Blehar, M. C., Waters, E., & Wall, S. (1978). *Patterns of attachment: A psychological study of the Strange Situation.* Hillsdale, NJ: Erlbaum.

Bernard, K., Butzin-Dozier, Z., Rittenhouse, J., & Dozier, M. (2010). Young children living with neglecting birth parents show more blunted daytime patterns of cortisol production than children in foster care and comparison children. *Archives of Pediatrics and Adolescent Medicine, 164,* 438–443.

Bernard, K., & Dozier, M. (2011). This is my baby: Foster parents' feelings of commitment and displays of delight. *Infant Mental Health Journal, 32,* 251–262.

Bernard, K., Dozier, M., Bick, J., & Gordon, K. M. (2014). Normalizing blunted diurnal cortisol rhythms among children at risk for neglect: The effects of an early intervention. *Development and Psychopathology.* [Epub ahead of print]

Bernard, K., Dozier, M., Bick, J., Lewis-Morrarty, E., Lindhiem, O., & Carlson, E. (2012). Enhancing attachment organization among maltreated infants: Results of a randomized clinical trial. *Child Development, 83,* 623–636.

Bernard, K., Hostinar, C., & Dozier, M. (2015). Intervention effects on diurnal cortisol rhythms of child protective services–referred infants persist into early childhood: Preschool follow-up results of a randomized clinical trial. *JAMA Pediatrics, 169*(2), 112–119.

Bernard, K., Simons, R., & Dozier, M. (2015). Effects of an attachment-based intervention on CPS-referred mothers' event-related potentials to children's emotions. *Child Development, 86*(6), 1673–1684.

Bick, J., & Dozier, M. (2013). The effectiveness of an attachment-based intervention in promoting foster mothers' sensitivity toward foster infants. *Infant Mental Health Journal, 34,* 95–103.

Blair, C., & Raver, C. C. (2012). Child development in the context of adversity: Experiential canalization of brain and behavior. *American Psychologist, 67,* 309–318.

Bowlby, J. (1951). *Maternal care and mental health.* New York: Jason Aronson.

Bowlby, J. (1982). *Attachment and loss: Vol. 1. Attachment.* London: Hogarth Press. (Original work published 1969)

Britner, P. A., Marvin, R. S., & Pianta, R. C. (2005). Development and preliminary validation of the caregiving behavior system: Association with child attachment classification in the preschool Strange Situation. *Attachment and Human Development, 7,* 83–102.

Bruce, J., Fisher, P. A., Pears, K. C., & Levine, S. (2009). Morning cortisol levels in preschool-aged foster children: Differential effects of maltreatment type. *Developmental Psychobiology, 51,* 14–23.

California Evidence-Based Clearinghouse Rating of ABC. (2014, September). Retrieved January 6, 2014, from *www.cebc4cw.org/program/attachment-and-biobehavioral-catch-up*.

Calkins, S. D., & Leerkes, E. M. (2010). Early attachment processes and the development of emotional self-regulation. In K. D. Vohs & R. F. Baumeister (Eds.), *Handbook of self-regulation: Research, theory, and applications* (2nd ed., pp. 355–373). New York: Guilford Press.

Carlson, E. A. (1998). A prospective longitudinal study of attachment disorganization/disorientation. *Child Development, 69,* 1107–1128.

Carlson, V., Cicchetti, D., Barnett, D., & Braunwald, K. (1989). Disorganized/disoriented attachment relationships in maltreated infants. *Developmental Psychology, 25,* 525–531.

Cicchetti, D., & Toth, S. L. (2005). Child maltreatment. *Annual Review of Clinical Psychology, 1,* 409–438.

Cyr, C., Euser, E. M., Bakermans-Kranenburg, M. J., & van IJzendoorn, M. H. (2010). Attachment security and disorganization in maltreating and high-risk families: A series of meta-analyses. *Development and Psychopathology, 22,* 87–108.

Dozier, M., & the Infant Caregiver Project. (2013). *Attachment and biobehavioral catch-up.* Unpublished manuscript, University of Delaware, Newark, DE.

Dozier, M., Lindhiem, O., & Ackerman, J. (2005). Attachment and biobehavioral catch-up. In L. Berlin, Y. Ziv, L. Amaya-Jackson, & M. T. Greenberg (Eds.), *Enhancing early attachments: Theory, research, intervention, and policy* (pp. 178–194). New York: Guilford Press.

Dozier, M., Meade, E. B., & Bernard, K. (2014). Attachment and biobehavioral catch-up: An intervention for parents at risk of maltreating their infants and toddlers. In S. Timmer & A. Urquiza (Eds.), *Evidence-based approaches for the treatment of child maltreatment* (pp. 43–60). New York: Springer.

Dozier, M., & Stovall, K. C. (1997). *Parent Attachment Diary.* Unpublished manuscript, University of Delaware, Newark, DE.

Dozier, M., Stovall, K. C., & Albus, K. (1999). A transactional intervention for foster infants' caregivers. In D. Cicchetti & S. L. Toth (Eds.), *Rochester Symposium on Developmental Psychopathology: Developmental approaches to prevention and intervention* (pp. 195–219). Rochester, NY: University of Rochester Press.

Dozier, M., Stovall, K. C., Albus, K. E., & Bates, B. (2001). Attachment for infants in foster care: The role of caregiver state of mind. *Child Development, 72,* 1467–1477.

Fearon, R. P., Bakermans-Kranenburg, M. J., van IJzendoorn, M. H., Lapsley, A. M., & Roisman, G. I. (2010). The significance of insecure attachment and disorganization in the development of children's externalizing behavior: A meta-analytic study. *Child Development, 81,* 435–456.

Fraiberg, S., Adelson, E., & Shapiro, V. (1975). Ghosts in the nursery: A psychoanalytic approach to the problems of impaired infant–mother relationships. *Journal of the American Academy of Child and Adolescent Psychiatry, 14,* 387–421.

George, C., Kaplan, N., & Main, M. (1996). *Adult Attachment Interview.* Unpublished protocol. Department of Psychology, University of California, Berkeley, Berkeley, CA.

Jacobvitz, D., Hazen, N., Zaccagnino, M., Messina, S., & Beverung, L. (2011). Frightening maternal behavior, infant disorganization, and risks for psychopathology. In D. Cicchetti & G. I. Roisman (Eds.), *The origins and organization of adaptation and maladaptation* (pp. 283–322). Hoboken, NJ: Wiley.

Lewis, E. E., Dozier, M., Ackerman, J., & Sepulveda-Kozakowski, S. (2007). The effect of placement instability on adopted children's inhibitory control abilities and oppositional behavior. *Developmental Psychology, 43*(6), 1415–1427.

Lewis-Morrarty, E., Dozier, M., Bernard, K., Terraciano, S., & Moore, S. (2012). Theory of mind and cognitive flexibility outcomes among adopted children: Early school age follow-up results of a randomized clinical trial. *Journal of Adolescent Health, 51,* 17–22.

Lieberman, A., & Pawl, J. H. (1988). Clinical applications of attachment theory. In J. Belsky & T. Nezworski (Eds.), *Clinical implications of attachment* (pp. 327–351). Hillsdale, NJ: Erlbaum.

Lind, T., Bernard, K., Ross, E., & Dozier, M. (2014). Interaction effects on negative affect of CPS-referred children: Results of a randomized clinical trial. *Child Abuse and Neglect, 38*, 1459–1467.

Lorenz, L. (1935). Der Kumpan in der Umwelt des Vogels [The companion in the environment of the bird]. *Journal of Ornithology, 83*, 137–213.

Lyons-Ruth, K., Bronfman, E., & Parsons, E. (1999). Maternal frightened, frightening, or atypical behavior and disorganized infant attachment patterns. *Monographs of the Society for Research in Child Development, 64*, 67–96.

Lyons-Ruth, K., & Jacobvitz, D. (1999). Attachment disorganization: Unresolved loss, relational violence, and lapses in behavioral and attentional strategies. In J. Cassidy & P. R. Shaver (Eds.), *Handbook of attachment: Theory, research, and clinical applications* (pp. 520–554). New York: Guilford Press.

Lyons-Ruth, K., & Jacobvitz, D. (2016). Attachment disorganization from infancy to adulthood: Neurobiological correlates, parenting contexts, and pathways to disorder. In J. Cassidy & P. R. Shaver (Eds.), *Handbook of attachment: Theory, research, and clinical applications* (3rd ed., pp. 667–695). New York: Guilford Press.

MacDonald, H. Z., Beeghly, M., Grant-Knight, W., Augustyn, M., Woods, R. W., Cabral, H., . . . Frank, D. A. (2008). Longitudinal association between infant disorganized attachment and childhood posttraumatic stress symptoms. *Development and Psychopathology, 20*(2), 493–508.

Madigan, S., Moran, G., Schuengel, C., Pederson, D. R., & Otten, R. (2007). Unresolved maternal attachment representations, disrupted maternal behavior and disorganized attachment in infancy: Links to toddler behavior problems. *Journal of Child Psychology and Psychiatry, 48*, 1042–1050.

Main, M., Goldwyn, R., & Hesse, E. (2008). *Adult Attachment Interview: Scoring and Classification System. Version 8.* Unpublished manuscript, University of California at Berkeley.

Main, M., & Solomon, J. (1990). Procedures for identifying infants as disorganized/disoriented during the Ainsworth Strange Situation. In M. T. Greenberg, D. Cicchetti, & E. M. Cummings (Eds.), *Attachment in the preschool years: Theory, research, and intervention* (pp. 121–160). Chicago: University of Chicago Press.

Matas, L., Arend, R. A., & Sroufe, L. A. (1978). Continuity of adaptation in the second year: The relationship between quality of attachment and later competence. *Child Development, 49*(3), 547–556.

McElwain, N. L., & Booth-LaForce, C. (2006). Maternal sensitivity to infant distress and nondistress as predictors of infant–mother attachment security. *Journal of Family Psychology, 20*, 247–255.

Meade, E., & Dozier, M. (2012). *"In the Moment" commenting: A fidelity measurement and active ingredient in a parent training program.* Unpublished manuscript, University of Delaware, Newark, DE.

Meade, E., Dozier, M., & Bernard, K. (2014). Using video feedback as a tool in training parent coaches: Promising results from a single-subject design. *Attachment and Human Development, 16*, 356–370.

Pederson, D. R., Gleason, K. E., Moran, G., & Bento, S. (1998). Maternal attachment representations, maternal sensitivity, and the infant–mother attachment relationship. *Developmental Psychology, 34*, 925–933.

Raver, C. C. (1996). Relations between social contingency in mother–child interactions and 2-year-olds' social competence. *Developmental Psychology, 32*, 850–859.

Rocissano, L., Slade, A., & Lynch, V. (1987). Dyadic synchrony and toddler compliance. *Developmental Psychology, 23*, 698–704.

Schuengel, C., Bakermans-Kranenburg, M. J., & van IJzendoorn, M. H. (1999). Frightening maternal behavior linking unresolved loss and disorganized infant attachment. *Journal of Consulting and Clinical Psychology, 67*, 54–63.

Southham-Gerow, M. A., Rodriquez, A., Chorpita, B. F., & Daleiden, E. L. (2012). Dissemination and implementation of evidence based treatments for youth: Challenges and recommendations. *Professional Psychology: Research and Practice, 43*, 527–534.

Sroufe, L. A., & Waters, E. (1977). Attachment as an organizational construct. *Child Development, 48*, 1184–1199.

Stovall, K. C., & Dozier, M. (2000). The development of attachment in new relationships: Single subject analyses for 10 foster infants. *Development and Psychopathology, 12*, 133–156.

Stovall-McClough, K. C., & Dozier, M. (2004). Forming attachments in foster care: Infant attachment behaviors during the first two months of placement. *Development and Psychopathology, 16*, 253–271.

Tinbergen, N. (1951). *The study of instinct*. Oxford, UK: Oxford University Press.

van IJzendoorn, M. H. (1995). Adult attachment representations, parental representations, parental responsiveness, and infant attachment: A meta-analysis on the predictive validity of the adult attachment interview. *Psychological Bulletin, 117*, 387–403.

van IJzendoorn, M. H., Schuengel, C., & Bakermans-Kranenburg, M. J. (1999). Disorganized attachment in early childhood: Meta-analysis of precursors, concomitants, and sequelae. *Development and Psychopathology, 11*, 225–249.

Vaughn, B. E., & Waters, E. (1990). Attachment behavior at home and in the laboratory: Q-sort observations and Strange Situation classifications of one-year-olds. *Child Development, 61*, 1965–1973.

Verhage, M. L., Schuengel, C., Madigan, S., Fearon, R. M. P., Oosterman, M., Cassiba, R., . . . van IJzendoorn, M. H. (2016). Narrowing the transmission gap: A synthesis of three decades of research on intergenerational transmission of attachment. *Psychological Bulletin, 142*, 337–266.

Waters, E. (1987). *Attachment Behavior Q-set* (Revision 3.0). Unpublished instrument, State University of New York at Stony Brook, Department of Psychology, Stony Brook, NY.

Wiener, S. G., Bayart, F., Faull, K. F., & Levine, S. (1990). Behavioral and physiological responses to maternal separation in squirrel monkeys (*Saimiri sciureus*). *Behavioral Neuroscience, 104*, 108–115.

Zelazo, P. D. (2006). The Dimensional Change Card Sort (DCCS): A method of assessing executive function in children. *Nature Protocols, 1*(1), 297–301.

Zelazo, P. D., Müller, U., Frye, D., & Marcovitch, S. (2003). The development of executive function in early childhood. *Monographs of the Society for Research in Child Development, 68*, vii–137.

CHAPTER 3

The Circle of Security Intervention
Design, Research, and Implementation

SUSAN S. WOODHOUSE, BERT POWELL, GLEN COOPER,
KENT HOFFMAN, and JUDE CASSIDY

We begin this chapter with an account of the origins of the Circle of Security® (COS) intervention, including the initial collaboration that led to the first evaluation of the COS program, a description of the families for whom it was initially designed, as well as the underlying assumptions and key intervention goals of the COS intervention. Next, we describe the three initial COS protocols, all of which entail personalized diagnostic and treatment plans for individual parents, with accompanying video review of themselves and their child. We then present findings from research examining each of these protocols, including data related to the efficacy of the three initial COS protocols, research on moderators of the efficacy of COS that help to answer questions about "what works for whom," as well as recent research on the psychotherapy process and the intervener–mother relationship within COS. Then, we discuss the ways in which implementation considerations led to the development of a new protocol: COS–Parenting. We end with a call for future research on the COS protocols. Throughout, when we use the term *parent,* we include in this usage all of the many caregivers who are not birth parents.

The COS intervention approach was developed as an early intervention group program lasting 20 weeks for at-risk families enrolled in Head Start and Early Head Start. A University/Head Start Partnership grant led to a research collaboration involving an evaluation of the COS intervention protocol as it began to be implemented with parents participating in Head Start. Three psychotherapists in Spokane, Washington—Glen Cooper, Kent Hoffman, and Bert Powell—initiated design of the clinical intervention and delivered it to the parents; Robert Marvin, from the University of Virginia, led the research component for the project. The principal goal for the project was to create and evaluate a systematic protocol based on attachment theory and designed to reduce the risk of insecure attachment (Hoffman, Marvin, Cooper, & Powell, 2006).

A key moment in the development of COS came several years prior to applying for the University/Head Start Partnership grant, when the Spokane team attended Jude Cassidy's training workshop for the MacArthur Preschool Attachment system (Cassidy, Marvin, & the MacArthur Attachment Working Group, 1992). The Spokane therapists were familiar with attachment theory, but during the training workshop they became intrigued by the degree to which the coding system highlighted children's attachment-related behavioral strategies and by the nuances of behavioral patterns associated with each attachment classification. They were struck by the idea that attachment theory had important implications for clinical intervention. The team began several years of training and reflection to reevaluate, both personally and professionally, the centrality of relationships. When they introduced attachment-related material to other clinicians, many of them reported the same personal and professional reevaluation. This response suggested to the team that learning about attachment could stimulate a process of self-evaluation regarding relationships. It is this process of reflection and reevaluation that guides the COS intervention. The thinking at the time of COS development was: If Head Start parents could be taught the basics of attachment theory, they too would reevaluate their relationships with their children.

The challenge was to teach attachment theory and the fine distinctions of behavioral strategies in a manner that is accessible and engaging for at-risk families. A number of mothers who participated in the project were adolescents who had not completed high school. To maximize the possibility of success, all the materials used in the program had to pass what we called the "16-year-old parent test." Many iterations of the program materials were submitted to the parents for their keen criticism; from this, the COS graphic and other program handouts were born. We are grateful for the feedback that the parents provided us in making COS intuitively understandable, without losing the integrity of the theory. Below we introduce the underlying assumptions and key goals of the COS intervention (shown in Table 3.1).

Underlying Assumptions and Key Intervention Goals of COS

The COS approach is based on three assumptions:

1. At their core, parents bring positive intentionality to childrearing.
2. All parents have well-established strategies to protect themselves from the painful emotions associated with adverse experiences in their own developmental histories. In some cases, these protective strategies exert a sufficiently powerful effect to prevent the parent from seeing and responding to the child's basic attachment cues, and a secure attachment is not created.
3. Given that a child thrives when the parent is relatively responsive to both attachment and exploratory behavior, it is important that the parent consider

what may hinder his or her capacity to respond to particular aspects of the child's behavior.

The key goals of COS (see Table 3.1) are built on these three assumptions. Note that these five key intervention goals are important for not only the original 20-week protocol but also all of the subsequent versions of COS described later in this chapter. First, parents are asked to develop a better understanding of their children's needs (Goal 1). All versions of the COS use the COS graphic to facilitate communication with parents about children's needs. The COS graphic is also useful in helping parents to enhance their observational and inferential skills (Goal 2), by providing a context within which parents practice describing what they see the child doing, then make meaning of those observations. Once parents develop a foundational understanding of children's needs for attachment and exploration, develop awareness of children's signals, and begin to understand how children behave when their signals are not responded to accurately, the next step is for parents to recognize their own cognitive and emotional responses to child behavior (Goal 3), which is supported by use of the *Shark Music* metaphor (described below). Parents also engage in an active, reflective dialogue about how these responses influence their infant. This process of reflective dialogue tends to allow parents to learn to regulate their emotional responses to their children's behavior (Goal 4). Parents learn new ways of responding to their children's signals, while repairing inevitable lapses in sensitive responsiveness (Goal 5). The starting point of the COS intervention is to use attachment theory to create an individualized treatment plan for the parent that is based on observations of parent–child interactional patterns and, if available, on his or her child's attachment classification (i.e., secure, insecure, disorganized); thus, parents are encouraged to meet the goals outlined here in a way that is tailored to the specific relationships they have with their children.

In summary, the central goal of the COS approach is to provide children with a secure attachment by inviting their parents into a process of reflective dialogue that helps them serve as a secure base when the children's exploratory systems are activated, and as a safe haven when the children's attachment systems are activated. The importance of an attachment figure to whom a child can return for comfort

TABLE 3.1. Key Intervention Goals of Circle of Security
The intervention focuses on working with parents to . . .
1. Develop a better understanding of their children's needs
2. Enhance their observational and inferential skills
3. Recognize their own cognitive and emotional responses to their children's behavior and understand how these responses influence their children
4. Learn to regulate their emotional responses to their children's behavior
5. Learn new ways of responding to their children's signals, while repairing inevitable lapses in sensitive responsiveness

when distressed, then use as a secure base from which to safely explore with confidence, is a central idea in attachment theory, referred to as the *secure base phenomenon* (Bowlby, 1988). For Bowlby, the secure base phenomenon was at the heart of attachment theory: "No concept within the attachment framework is more central to developmental psychiatry than that of the secure base" (pp. 163–164). The key intervention goals of the COS approach are the steps through which parents move to attain a clear understanding of what children need to have a secure base (and safe haven), and are provided in a relational environment within which the parent feels safe enough to engage in a reflective dialogue that ultimately leads to better parental regulation and parental provision of a secure base/safe haven.

Key Components of the COS Intervention

Individualized Assessment of the Parent–Child Relationship

The COS intervention begins with an assessment of the parent–child relationship. Parents are interviewed using the COS Interview (COSI; Powell, Cooper, Hoffman, & Marvin, 2014) to allow for assessment of parents' representations of themselves and of their children. For children age 12 months and older, an age-appropriate Strange Situation Procedure (SSP; Ainsworth, Blehar, Waters, & Wall, 1978; Cassidy et al., 1992) provides an assessment of child attachment to the parent. Parents and children enter a room with a box of toys, and the child experiences a series of separations from and reunions with the parent. After the SSP, parents and children complete two additional tasks. First, age-appropriate books are brought into the room, and parents are asked to read a story to their children. Finally, parents and children complete a cleanup task, in which parents are asked to get their children to place all the toys back into a box. For infants below age 12 months, no specific protocol has been developed. Typically, however, there is an analysis of a video of infant–parent interactions, such as face-to-face interaction (gaze, face, orientation, touch, and vocalization) between parent and infant (Beebe & Lachmann, 1994; Beebe, Lachmann, & Jaffe, 1997), or other interactions, such as during free play, after a stressor task (e.g., the infant is seated in child's car seat and his or her arms are gently restrained; Laboratory Temperament Assessment Battery [Lab-TAB]; Goldsmith & Rothbart, 1999), or videotaped interactions in the home. The COS assessment focuses on identifying *the linchpin struggle*, defined as the central interaction that most interferes with the child developing a secure attachment to the parent.

The COS model recognizes that all parents have what John Bowlby (1973) called a *working model of attachment*. This internal template is used to understand current and future relationships, including the parent's current relationship with the child. The parent's representations of self and child are identified from the parent's responses during the semistructured COSI (Powell et al., 2014). This information is used, along with the observational data described earlier, to create a treatment plan that is compatible with the parent's procedural belief system about how intimate relationships work (Powell et al., 2014). Importantly, although the COS intervention was originally designed to be offered to small groups of five to six parents, the intervener creates an individualized treatment plan for each parent–child dyad. A separate, individualized treatment plan is used to guide the work with each parent in the group.

The COS Graphic: A User-Friendly Vocabulary for Talking about Attachment

The initial segments of the COS intervention focus on helping parents feel sufficiently safe to share their thoughts and feelings as they learn basic attachment theory through the use of the COS graphic. Once parents have learned how to use the COS graphic, the group then shifts to a focus on individual parents, one at a time. Each parent has the opportunity to be the focus of three sessions over the course of the 20 weeks. The group members who are not the focus of the session in a given week provide support to the focal parent and learn from the process of observing the focal parent's process of reflection. While viewing videotaped interactions of themselves with their children, focal parents practice creating behavioral descriptions of the interactions (e.g., "He couldn't reach the toy and I gave it to him"; "She is reaching for me to pick her up"). Once an interaction is described, the parents create hypotheses about the principal attachment or exploratory need that is displayed in the clip. This process. called *Seeing and Guessing,* becomes the basic procedure for viewing videotapes throughout the group. The core process in all COS protocols is to reflectively engage parents as they learn the concepts of attachment theory using the COS graphic (see Figure 3.1).

Parents are given a tour of the Circle, beginning with an explanation that parents serve as the *hands on the Circle*; in other words, they are the secure base from which children explore and the safe haven to which children return. Parents are

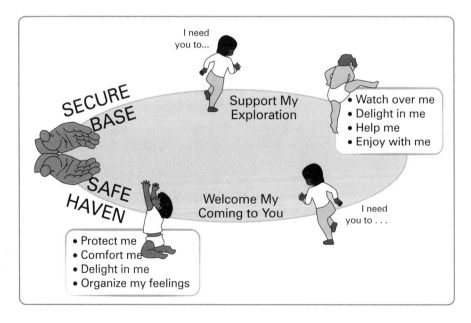

FIGURE 3.1. The Circle of Security: Parent attending to the child's needs. From Powell, Cooper, Hoffman, and Marvin (2014). Copyright © 1998 Glen Cooper, Kent Hoffman, Bob Marvin, and Bert Powell.

then told that when children feel safe and secure, their innate curiosity and desire for mastery is supported. Even when children feel safe, before they begin to explore, they look to their secure base (their parent) for support. This support comes from both having a history of the parent's comfort with separation and receiving a signal in the moment that it is safe to venture out. Children shift between activation of their exploratory and attachment systems rapidly throughout the day, and each system raises a different set of needs. Key to the COS intervention is helping the parent understand that children need their parent as much while exploring as they do when sitting in their parent's lap. When exploring, sometimes children simply need their parent to watch over them. The parent's presence allows the child to maintain the sense of security he or she needs to continue to explore. Sometimes children need help in their exploration. It is the parent's job to scaffold the exploration by offering the child just enough help so that he or she can do it him- or herself. Sometimes children want their parents to enjoy the activity with them by engaging in the exploration. Sometimes they need to experience their parents' delight in them, not for what they are doing but for who they are.

When children have been exploring long enough, their attachment systems inevitably become activated. Children then need to be welcomed by their parent as they approach. As with support for exploration, children need both a history with closeness and a signal indicating that they are welcome in the present moment. Sometimes their attachment systems may be activated by a need for protection from either present or perceived danger. Other times children are distressed by a known cause or event and need comfort. Sometimes children simply need to know that their parents find them delightful, even when they need closeness or care. Often children are distressed and do not have a clear sense of what is causing the feeling. They may well need comfort, but in addition, need help organizing their feelings. Being able to recognize, name, express, and regulate multiple, sometimes conflicting, feelings is an essential skill that is optimally learned within the child–parent relationship.

In addition to learning about the child's needs through the COS graphic, parents are taught a formula for being the hands on the Circle: "Always be bigger, stronger, wiser, and kind. Whenever possible, follow your child's need. Whenever necessary, take charge." Sometimes when parents feel they need to be bigger and stronger, they sacrifice being kind and become mean, perhaps justifying their behavior as "tough love." Parents who act this way often believe they must become aggressive and evoke fear to gain the respect of their children, as if violence deserves respect. Other parents, when they try to be kind, give up being bigger and stronger and become weak, thus requiring children to take charge of the relationship, implicitly asking the child to be the parent. Some parents are so profoundly not available, or *gone*, that the child is left with a significant loss of hands (i.e., parental support) on the Circle. Parents who have a pattern of being "mean, weak, or gone" (as labeled within the protocol terminology) leave the child in a circumstance that is abnormally frightening. It is an ongoing challenge for all parents to be simultaneously bigger, stronger, and kind, and to have the wisdom to understand that a child's need for security rests on the parent's ability to perform this important and multifaceted function.

Reflective Dialogue Regarding the Parent–Child Relationship and Internal Representations of Both the Child and the Self

As mentioned earlier, after the basics of the Circle are presented and parents have built up some experience engaging in dialogue within the group, Phase 1 individual videotape review begins, with the other group members present to provide support to (and learn from) the focal parent. Parents watch edited video clips from their child–parent assessment, while being invited to reflect on what they see their child doing and needing. The COS graphic is used as a model for understanding their child's needs. The use of videos allows the intervention to be tailored to each dyad's specific attachment-caregiving strategy and each parent's specific defensive process. Phase 1 review is focused on video examples of the parent demonstrating success with an underdeveloped parenting capacity (e.g., a parent who is uncomfortable with a child seeking care shares a moment of emotional connection) and a modestly vulnerable struggle (e.g., a parent who avoids taking charge struggles with some success in getting his or her child to cooperate when asked).

Once parents demonstrate competence using the COS graphic to discern children's attachment and exploration needs during the Phase 1 videotape review, they learn the concept of mental representations (*internal working models*), which are the building blocks of parents' responses to the child. Parents are then invited in the Phase 2 review to begin considering their own mental representations and how they may be linked to their own reactions to the child. Parental responsive behavior is likely to reflect multiple representations: an *internal representation of the child* (e.g., a parental representation of "She is a frightened child who seeks comfort" vs. "She's a spoiled child who needs to be toughened up" would likely lead to different parental responses); an *internal representation of the self* (e.g., "I am competent at helping children in distress" vs. "I can't tolerate whining" vs. "I am not tricked by children's tears"); and *an emotional response that ties the representations together* (e.g., empathy, anguish, annoyance). Parents' understanding of how children's needs evoke specific thoughts and feelings within parents lays the foundation for parents to learn skills of *reflective dialogue* and *affect regulation* (i.e., skills of thinking about, talking about, and regulating emotions).

With the combination of the COS graphic as a guide and the video review, parents develop skills to better track, moment by moment, children's attachment needs. In many cases, being able to identify these needs as they occur is enough to enable parents to respond in appropriate ways to meet the needs. In other cases, however, parents may feel so uncomfortable or threatened by those needs that they fail to respond, often without being aware of this struggle. To enhance responsiveness, it is important that parents take the vulnerable step of reflecting on what they do, think, and feel that supports or inhibits their response to particular attachment needs.

When parents are able to reflect on their caregiving, even for a brief moment, a pause is created in their nonconscious procedural caregiving behaviors (*implicit relational knowing*; Lyons-Ruth & the Process of Change Study Group, 1998). This reflective pause increases the likelihood that parents can see their children's perspectives and have empathy for their children's emotional experiences. In addition, the COS intervention invites parents to explore their own mental representations (internal working models), which are a major factor in shaping their responses to their children. Engaging parents in a reflective process aimed at helping them enhance their *reflective functioning* (i.e., the capacity to reflect on one's thoughts, feelings, intentions and behaviors, as well as those of the child) is one of the principal goals for the program, because higher reflective functioning is linked to security of attachment in infancy, and longer term optimal social and emotional child outcomes (Steele & Steele, 2008).

Reflection about Representational and Emotional Influences on Caregiving

To facilitate parental reflection about the parent–child relationship, it is important to provide parents a way to notice and talk about powerful thoughts and feelings that are aroused while parenting. Bowlby (1969/1982) theorized that one's own attachment experiences color both how social information is processed cognitively and how one feels emotionally in relational contexts. He theorized that internal representations stemming from past relationships tend to be carried forward into new relationships. Unfortunately, when negative representations influence parental caregiving, the responsiveness of caregiving can suffer. In other words, there is increased likelihood that parents will fail to meet their children's current, in-the-moment needs for attachment and exploration if parents interpret their children's behavior in terms of unconscious procedural memories or strong emotional reactions rooted in negative aspects of past relationships. Bowlby (1988) theorized that internal representations can change in the context of the therapeutic relationship, within which it is safe to explore these previously unconscious working models of attachment.

Bowlby (1980) argued that the construct of *attachment representations* (i.e., internal working models of self and other) provided a new way of understanding Freud's (1940/1963) ideas about the dynamic unconscious and defenses, such as repression. He argued that attachment representations, as well as the affect associated with early attachment-related experiences, can guide current behavior in problematic ways. For example, Bowlby (1980) described defensive exclusion of attachment-related information as unconscious processing of information so as to keep out of awareness information that would be painful. Defensive exclusion and other such defensive processes can be adaptive in some circumstances but become problematic if they become chronic and no longer match the current environment. Defensive processes can be particularly problematic when they influence parenting, such that parents are unable to clearly perceive and respond to children's signals regarding attachment and exploration needs.

COS uses the construct of *shark music* to provide parents with a vocabulary for talking about the complex idea of defensive processes and to raise awareness about parents' defensive processes that tend to function outside of conscious awareness yet influence parenting. Parents explore the idea that their past experiences in their own relationships with important attachment figures have led certain situations to feel threatening or scary; thus, often without being consciously aware, parents allow those perceptions of threat to drive their parenting behavior.

Parents are introduced to the shark music construct by being shown the same video with two different audio tracks. In the first showing, the background music is the soothing *Canon in D Major* by Johann Pachelbel. When the clip is shown the second time, the background music is the cello solo from the theme of the movie *Jaws*. This juxtaposition of pleasant and foreboding music elicits a powerful visceral response, and illustrates for parents how the same scene can appear quite different depending on the emotions in the background. The contrasting background music becomes a metaphor for the parents' internal working models of attachment that make some of their children's needs on the Circle seem welcome and comfortable, whereas others seem frightening and aversive. The shark music metaphor helps to normalize defensive processes and provides a language for talking about parents' own defensive processes.

Recognizing that an experience "feels scary but is not dangerous" creates a choice point for parents—to continue to protect themselves from the frightening but nonexistent sharks to reduce the immediate discomfort of the fear, or to bear the discomfort, while overriding the defensive behavior and meeting the child's needs. By naming a previously undefined negative affect triggered by a child's need with the words "shark music," parents can momentarily pause a procedural script, name the affect, and create an opening to choose a response based on a more accurate assessment of the child's needs in the current situation. In this way, shark music is a metaphor that makes clear to parents that they, like all parents, are influenced by an emotional soundtrack that is rooted in their history of relationships. Most importantly, parents are helped to experience that when they are able to turn down the volume of the (old) troubling music long enough to allow reflection, it becomes possible for different caregiving choices to emerge. Parents can allow the now non-existent "shark" to become small enough that the child him- or herself can be seen in terms of the child's actual needs.

Once parents learn to identify the specific needs of their children that induce negative feelings (i.e., that "turn on their shark music"), they are in a position to reflect on how these feelings fit or do not fit with what they now know about their child's needs on the Circle. This process helps parents identify thoughts and feelings that inhibit responding to the current situation rather than reacting with emotional responses learned from past experiences. By identifying and modulating shark music responses, parents can more clearly see the genuine needs that they have been unable to see in their child before, and heighten their empathy.

Discussion of Insecure Relational Patterns

When the parent is uncomfortable with separation and responds negatively to the child's desire to explore, sending the message that the child should not have the positive feelings associated with curiosity, mastery, or autonomy, the child may learn to inhibit exploration and instead focus excessively on needing proximity to the parent as a way to maintain connection and diminish worries engendered by the parent's reaction. COS labels this struggle *Limited Top of the Circle* (see Figure 3.1). Over time, this interactional pattern takes on characteristics that appear clinically to be associated with the type of insecure attachment called *ambivalent attachment*.

A parent who is uncomfortable with providing a safe haven—one who communicates that the child should not have the feelings associated with wanting safety, comfort, and closeness—will discourage and dismiss care-seeking behavior in the child, resulting in what is called *Limited Bottom of the Circle*. This interaction patterns appears clinically to share characteristics with the type of insecure attachment called *avoidant attachment*.

A parent who has a pattern of being emotionally dysregulated when the child needs him or her to be *bigger, stronger, wiser, and kind* and defensively manages his or her dysregulation by being *mean, weak, or gone* fosters a relationship in which attachment needs on the Circle are associated with fear. This parent's struggle is called *Limited Hands*. Children of such parents tend clinically to behave in ways similar to those with disorganized attachment.

The shark music construct is central to Phase 2 tape reviews, which focus on helping parents reflectively process the *linchpin* from the preintervention assessment and talk about the shark music that is activated by this specific need on the Circle. The parents are supported in their capacity to do this by viewing and discussing key moments in which they are able to more fully respond to this linchpin need; the therapeutic message is always that parents have the capacity to respond, and it is their defensive (protective) management of shark music that interferes.

After Phase 2 reviews, parents and children are again videotaped, so that any new caregiving capacities may be observed. The focus of Phase 3 is celebrating the positive changes in the child–parent relationship, acknowledging ongoing current struggles, and reflecting on the new choices for responding to children's needs that parents are using. In summary, the COS video review and discussion are designed to help parents to reach the five intervention goals outlined earlier.

Through this systematic process of learning core attachment concepts via the COS graphic, developing observational and inferential skills via watching video to identify children's needs, and building empathy for their children through a greater ability to reflect on and regulate their defensive responses, parents learn to make new choices about their parenting behaviors. These new choices help parents become the competent and confident parental presences their children need them to be, and allow parents to provide care that matches their children's needs. As their children learn to trust these changes, they are able to use their parents as a secure base from which to explore and a safe haven to whom they can return when distressed, and their sense of attachment security is therefore greatly enriched.

The Initial COS Protocols: The Use of Individualized Diagnostic and Treatment Plans with Video Review

COS 20-week Group Protocol

The COS 20-Week Group Protocol (COS-20 week) uses a preintervention relational assessment that begins with an SSP, followed by the parent reading a book to his or her child for 4 minutes, and ends with the parent directing the child to return the toys to the storage box. Approximately six parents meet weekly for 20 weeks in 75-minute sessions to review video-recorded attachment–caregiving interactions between themselves and their children. All the video vignettes reviewed are either from the preintervention assessment or an SSP recorded in Week 15.

The first 2 weeks of the COS protocol focus on helping parents feel safe, valued, and engaged. During the first 2 weeks, the parents learn about the Circle by watching highly edited, successful moments from the preintervention assessment of group members meeting their children's needs on the Circle. Phase 1 videotape reviews begin in Week 3 and continue through Week 8. Each week, edited video clips from one parent's SSP are shown to the group. In Phase 1, parents learn how to participate in the videotape review and most of the vignettes shown are of parents successfully meeting a child's need. One clip in the review is selected to show a struggle that is chosen to help prepare the parent for the more demanding task of reflecting on the linchpin struggle in Phase 2.

In Week 9, shark music and *Limited Circles* (insecure attachment) are introduced. From Weeks 10 through 15, parents participate in Phase 2 videotape reviews. Again, one parent each week is presented with video clips that have been reedited from his or her preintervention assessment, with a focus on that parent's linchpin struggle. Helping parents normalize and identify their linchpin shark music is a central theme for Phase 2. After Phase 2 reviews, the parents are videotaped in a modified SSP from which vignettes are selected for Phase 3 reviews. The focus in Phase 3 is on helping the parent acknowledge current strengths and struggles. Two tape reviews are completed each week during Weeks 16–19.

Week 20 is reserved for the ending and graduation celebration. Each parent receives a copy of his or her videos and a "Certificate of Graduation." Parents are encouraged to discuss their experiences in the group.

COS Perinatal Protocol

The COS Perinatal Protocol (COS-PP; Cooper, Hoffman, & Powell, 2003), a preventive intervention adapted from the original COS protocol, was designed to be part of the Tamar's Children program located in Baltimore, Maryland. Tamar's Children is a jail diversion program designed to address the multiple needs of pregnant, substance-abusing women convicted of nonviolent offenses and their infants (Cassidy et al., 2010). The Tamar's Children program addressed the medical and psychiatric needs of the mothers and the well-being of their infants by creating an integrated network of prenatal and medical care; substance abuse, mental health, and trauma treatment; individual and group psychotherapy; educational enhancement (e.g., general equivalency degree [GED] classes); work skills training; housing assistance; and advocacy. The COS-PP was included to provide parenting education and treatment designed to promote maternal sensitivity and increase the likelihood of secure infant attachment. Mothers met twice weekly for 90-minute group sessions throughout their enrollment in the program. Two therapists, who remained with the group until completion, led each group. The protocol developers trained the therapists and conducted weekly supervision of the groups to ensure fidelity of the protocol.

Video clips of mother–infant interactions were used to facilitate discussion of complex ideas related to attachment theory in user-friendly terms in a safe group setting. While pregnant, mothers were introduced to the basics of mother–infant interaction from the perspective of attachment theory by first watching and discussing 72 stock footage clips of mothers interacting with their babies, edited for this project. These stock footage clips, which included examples of secure, insecure, and disorganized attachment, sensitive and insensitive parenting, as well as "before and after" mother–infant interactions from women who had participated in previous COS groups, allowed mothers to learn the basics of the Circle and to build a foundation of reflection and observational skills before their babies were born.

Starting when their infants reached 2 months of age and continuing for the duration of the intervention, mothers took turns being the focus of a session. For each session, the therapists selected four clips of the target mother interacting with her infant in a variety of activities in the residential treatment center (e.g., feeding, free play, and face-to-face interactions) to view and discuss during the group session. Like the 20-week protocol, this protocol included Phase 1 and Phase 2 tape reviews. Because the mothers were in residential treatment and would be meeting for a year, the Phase 3 review procedure of recording new interactions and using the tape to acknowledge current strengths and struggles was used multiple times over the course of the year.

COS—Home Visiting–4 Intervention

The COS—Home Visiting–4 Intervention (COS-HV4; Cooper, Hoffman, & Powell, 2000) protocol was designed to incorporate the core COS elements into a protocol that could be delivered in a brief, four-session, home-visiting program with individual parents of infants in the first year of life. Each home visit is scheduled with the baby present and rested and (except for the initial session) begins with a review of the previous session. The intervener and mother then watch and discuss clips from videotapes of the mother and her infant that were filmed the previous day (mothers were asked to "go about your normal routine" for a 30-minute session in the home). In addition, mother–infant interactions (both infant cues and maternal responses) are discussed as they occur during each home visit.

Following the central components of the COS approach, each session has a specific focus, as follows. The first session focuses on engaging the mother affectively, forming an intervener–mother alliance, helping the mother understand her importance as a secure base for her infant and successfully providing her infant with a sense of security, and improving the mother's skills at recognizing her baby's signals related to both attachment and exploration. The second visit extends the focus on the importance of maternal sensitive responsiveness to the infant's signals. At the same time, the intervener begins to help the mother identify the infant signals to which she has more difficulty responding. The intervener introduces the idea that all parents are sometimes insensitive, and that such behavior is human, forgivable, and can be reflected on, discussed, and changed.

The focus of the third session is exploration of the psychological factors that at times interfere with the mother's capacities to respond sensitively (a teaching of the concept of defensive processes through the user-friendly metaphor of shark music described earlier). Specifically, the intervener discusses with the mother the ways her behavior is influenced by her cognitive and affective responses to the baby's needs and behaviors. The goal is to increase the mother's reflective capacity, so that she can consider new options when confronted with situations in which she finds sensitive responsiveness to be difficult. Mothers are also provided "homework" between sessions (e.g., explain infant needs on the Circle to a friend; observe infant needs on the Circle during daily interactions). During the fourth visit, the home visitor gives the mother a copy of some of the videos used in the intervention and provides the mother with an opportunity to discuss the intervention and any ongoing parenting topics of interest.

COS Intervention Training and Supervision

In each of the three COS intervention protocols described earlier, the basic training requirement for interveners is the COS 10-day training workshop in assessment and treatment planning. The training is offered several times a year in many parts of the world, including Norway, Italy, Great Britain, Australia, New Zealand, Canada, and the United States. The training is for mental health professionals. Information regarding these trainings can be found on the COS International website (*www. circleofsecurity.com*).

In this training, participants learn to use the SSP to identify parent's strengths and struggles on the Circle. Then, participants must discern the central struggle (linchpin) for each dyad. Participants also learn to appraise internal working models of relationships, core defensive processes, reflective functioning, and capacity for empathy through the COSI (Powell et al., 2014), an interview that taps the parent's representations of self and child. Based on parent–child interactions and the interview-based parental perceptions, participants learn to organize treatment plans.

Participants who wish to receive certification in COS assessment and treatment planning must pass an exam that entails submitting a treatment plan for two parent–child dyads based on videotape of the SSP and the COSI, which the trainers provide. Passing the exam is a prerequisite to receiving supervision. To be considered a COS provider, the facilitator must receive supervision on two 20-week groups or 50 hours of supervision on individual interventions. A detailed implementation manual is provided for the supervisees. All interventions are videotaped, and reviewing these tapes is central to the supervision process. As part of the supervision, trainees also receive technical help in filming the dyads and in editing videotape. To offer the COS model, it is necessary to have facilities and equipment to administer SSPs and/or face-to-face, split-screen interactions. Providing child care during the group helps in recruiting and retaining parents.

Empirical Examination of Initial COS Protocols

Research on the COS 20-Week

Two separate groups of researchers, using independent samples, have examined the COS 20-week. Both studies found that intervention is associated with significant increases in attachment security and significant decreases in disorganization of attachment, as compared to attachment assessed prior to beginning COS (Hoffman et al., 2006; Huber, McMahon, & Sweller, 2015a). Attachment security and attachment disorganization are important variables because they have been linked to an array of important developmental and mental health outcomes (e.g., Fearon, Bakermans-Kranenburg, van IJzendoorn, Lapsley, & Roisman, 2010; Groh, Roisman, van IJzendoorn, Bakermans-Kranenburg, & Fearon, 2012; for a review see Thompson, 2016). Thus, it is notable that two independent studies of the 20-week protocol have provided empirical evidence that COS treatment is associated with shifts toward more optimal child attachment.

Hoffman et al. (2006) focused on a sample of 65 low-income toddlers and pre-schoolers enrolled in Head Start and Early Head Start programs in the United States. Before the COS intervention, only 20% of the children were classified as securely attached; 60% were classified as exhibiting disorganized attachment. Statistically significant shifts in attachment were found from pre- to postintervention. Specifically, Hoffman et al. found that following the COS intervention, the percentage of children who were securely attached increased significantly to 54%; disorganization decreased significantly to 25%. Similarly, Huber et al. (2015a) found significant changes in attachment security and disorganization in an Australian sample of 83 children, ages 13 months to 7 years, who had been referred to a community-based mental health service agency due to existing problems. Those with the least optimal preintervention scores appeared to benefit the most from intervention (Huber et al., 2015a).

Importantly, in addition to finding significant change in attachment outcomes, Huber, McMahon, and Sweller (2015b) found pre–post reductions in both mother-rated internalizing and externalizing symptoms, and teacher-rated externalizing symptoms. These results were exciting because, if replicated in future research, they suggest that the potential benefits of COS could be useful in ameliorating children's existing behavioral health problems, in addition to improving attachment outcomes.

Huber, McMahon, and Sweller (2016) found pre–post changes in maternal emotional function in parents who participated in the COS intervention. These were parents of children who had been referred to the mental health clinic due to behavioral and emotional problems. Huber et al. found pre–post reductions in parenting stress and clinically significant reductions in parent psychological symptoms. Those parents with higher baseline levels of symptoms tended to benefit more than did parents with low levels of symptoms. These results were intriguing because, if replicated, findings suggested that COS could be useful in improving parent mental health, in addition to reducing child behavior problems.

It is important to note that, to date, the only published studies of the 20-week COS protocol (Hoffman et al., 2006; Huber et al., 2015a, 2015b, 2016) used a pre–post design. Additional research using a randomized controlled trial (RCT) design is needed. There are a number of well-known reasons that the RCT design is at the top of the hierarchy of research designs (Gold, 2015). Random assignment to treatment groups and inclusion of a control group allow for both optimal internal validity and inferences about causality. Use of the RCT design allows researchers to infer that the intervention of interest is responsible for the observed outcomes (Kazdin, 2006). It is important to note that although two separate research groups have provided pre–post data showing COS was associated with change in child attachment and child behavioral outcomes, without RCT data, it is impossible to rule out other non-COS explanations for the changes observed.

Research on the COS-PP

The COS-PP was tested in the context of the Tamar's Children jail diversion program, using a pre–post design (Cassidy et al., 2010). The 15-month jail diversion option was offered to women who were identified as being pregnant while in jail or who were pregnant during their sentencing period and were nonviolent offenders. The women in the program had a history of substance abuse, and received extensive wraparound social services in addition to COS-PP, described earlier in this chapter. The program included a phase from pregnancy until the infant was 6 months old, during which time the mother and infant lived on site, followed by a phase in which the mother continued in the program while living in the community, which lasted until the infant was 12 months old. Because there was no control group, attachment outcomes were compared to outcomes identified in other research studies, based on levels of risk. Results for the 20 mothers who completed the full program indicated that program infants showed rates of attachment security and disorganization that were comparable to low-risk, middle-class samples, and better than typical high-risk samples. Specifically, 14 of the 20 infants (70%) were classified by coders blind to sample characteristics as securely attached to mother, and only four infants (20%) were classified as insecure/disorganized. Mothers' sensitivity was similar to that of a community comparison group, and maternal depression improved over time as well. Results of this study suggest that the COS-PP can be used as part of an integrated treatment for extremely high-risk families.

Research on the COS-HV4

Cassidy, Woodhouse, Sherman, Stupica, and Lejuez (2011) conducted an RCT of the COS-HV4 in a sample of 220 economically stressed mothers of irritable infants. Participants in the intervention condition received COS-HV4. Participants in the control condition received three home-visiting sessions that focused on psychoeducational topics relevant for new parents (i.e., infant sleep, feeding, and play) and were given readings on these topics from the popular press. Mother–infant dyads in both the intervention and control groups were videotaped in the home for 30 minutes at the end of each home visit. Because this study by Cassidy et al. used an RCT design, it is possible to make causal attributions about the COS-HV4 intervention. In addition, the study examined two potential moderators of intervention effects: infant temperamental irritability and mothers' own attachment styles. These moderators turned out to be quite important, because the moderators helped not only to shed light on the efficacy of COS-HV4 but also to answer important questions about "what works for whom" in terms of attachment-based interventions.

First, COS-HV4 was found to be efficacious for infants who were at greater risk of insecurity (Cassidy et al., 2011). Specifically, the COS-HV4 significantly improved attachment outcomes only for those infants who were *highly* irritable. These highly irritable infants had levels of irritability that previous research had identified as placing them at risk of insecure attachment in the context of low family income (van den Boom, 1994). In contrast, there was no difference in the percentage of secure infants between the intervention and control groups among the *moderately* irritable infants. The findings of Cassidy et al. (2011) showed that when risk was high, the intervention was efficacious; expanding the definition of irritability to include more infants (i.e., the moderately irritable infants) did not lead to additional infants benefiting from intervention. It may be difficult to lower risk if risk is not already high.

These results highlighted the idea that infants may be differentially susceptible to environmental influence (Belsky & Pluess, 2009) or have biologically based differences in sensitivity to context (Boyce & Ellis, 2005), and that infant temperamental reactivity can serve as a marker of this differential susceptibility. Thus, Cassidy et al. (2011) demonstrated that it could be important to include factors such as observer-rated infant temperament as a potential moderator of treatment effects in order to understand "what works for whom."

Second, Cassidy et al. (2011) found that maternal attachment styles assessed with the Experiences in Close Relationships (ECR; Brennan, Clark, & Shaver, 1998) also moderated the intervention effects, with important implications for questions about what works for whom. The ECR scale assesses attachment style in terms of two dimensions, attachment *anxiety* (i.e., the degree of preoccupation with rejection and abandonment by close others) and attachment *avoidance* (i.e., the degree of discomfort with closeness, and a tendency to avoid relying on others for support or comfort). It is important to note that Cassidy et al. (2011), following Fraley and Shaver (1997; see also Mohr, Gelso, & Hill, 2005), mathematically rotated the ECR dimensions in order to assess attachment in terms of two alternative dimensions of attachment. The *secure-fearful* dimension is characterized at one end as *secure* (i.e., low attachment anxiety and low attachment avoidance) and at the other end as *fearful* (i.e., high attachment anxiety and high attachment avoidance). The *dismissing-preoccupied* dimension is characterized as *dismissing* at one end (i.e., low attachment anxiety and high attachment avoidance) and as *preoccupied* at the other end (i.e., high attachment anxiety and low attachment avoidance).

Moderating effects indicated that when the combination of maternal attachment style and infant temperament put the infant at risk (as indicated by low security rates in the control group), the COS-HV4 intervention was efficacious in reducing insecure attachment. For example, among mothers who were more *secure*, highly irritable infants benefited more than did moderately irritable infants. For more *dismissing* mothers, the study found that highly irritable infants (as compared to moderately irritable infants) were more likely to be secure if they received intervention and less likely to be secure when in the control group. In contrast, for more *preoccupied* mothers, a treatment effect emerged only for moderately irritable infants; highly irritable infants of highly preoccupied mothers were not at increased risk. In summary, when the combination of maternal attachment style and infant temperament put the infant at higher risk, the COS intervention was efficacious in reducing insecure attachment. Such findings might suggest that in the context of scarce resources, it might be best to focus provision of attachment-based interventions on those mother–infant dyads who are at higher risk. If so, then it would be important to continue to investigate factors that place infants at heightened risk of insecurity. The study by Cassidy et al. (2011) is helpful because it showed that mother and infant characteristics can interact in ways that are linked to risk.

Woodhouse, Lauer, Beeney, and Cassidy (2015) examined videotaped intervention sessions from the Cassidy et al. (2011) study in order to study the intervention process and the mother–intervener relationship, and investigate the links between intervention process and outcome. Despite decades of theory and research under-lining the key importance of the therapeutic relationship to outcome in individual psychotherapy (Norcross, 2011), little research has focused on these factors in par-enting interventions (for a review of the few notable examples, see Korfmacher, Green, Spellmann, & Thornburg, 2007). Similarly, despite decades of psycho-therapy research focused on links between the process of psychotherapy and the outcome of treatment (for a review, see Gelo & Manzo, 2015), such factors have been virtually ignored in the context of parenting interventions. Because Bowlby (1988) theorized that the therapist serves as a secure base from which the client can explore, Woodhouse et al. (2015) were particularly interested in therapist contribu-tions to the process that would be likely to influence the degree to which mothers would feel safe to explore with the intervener (e.g., therapist warmth or therapist negative attitudes toward the mother), as well as interveners' direct efforts to sup-port exploration. Similarly, given Bowlby's (1988) focus on client use of the thera-pist as a secure base from which to explore, Woodhouse et al. (2015) were particu-larly interested in mothers' contributions to the process of intervention reflecting mothers' active engagement, participation, and exploration.

O'Malley, Suh, and Strupp (1983) provided a conceptualization of psychother-apy process that meshed well with the goals of examining the process of interven-tion from an attachment perspective, as outlined earlier. O'Malley et al.'s conceptu-alizations can be applied to the COS intervention as follows: Therapists contributed to the process in terms of (1) therapist behaviors that communicate warmth (with higher scores for warmth when that warmth occurred at times that the client was expressing greater vulnerability or affective arousal), (2) therapist behaviors that conveyed a negative attitude toward the mother, and (3) therapist efforts to pro-mote the mother's exploration (e.g., a question asking the mother to consider the meaning of a particular child behavior). Mothers' contributions to process included (1) mothers' behaviors demonstrating active participation and involvement in the session (e.g., talking openly and freely during the session) and (2) mothers' explora-tion of clinically relevant material.

Woodhouse et al. (2015) coded all available videotaped COS-HV4 intervention sessions from the Cassidy et al. (2011) study for these process variables (O'Malley et al., 1983) and found that observer-rated therapist warmth and therapist sup-port for exploration were positively associated with observed maternal participa-tion/involvement and maternal exploration: Mothers tended to explore more when therapists were warmer or supported exploration more. In contrast, observer-rated therapists' negative attitude was inversely related to observed maternal exploration; that is, if the therapist showed a more negative attitude, mothers tended to explore less. Additionally, therapists' contributions to the process were linked to mothers' ratings of their attachment to the therapist. Specifically, observed therapist warmth was linked to higher maternal ratings of secure attachment to the therapist, whereas observed therapist negative attitude was associated with higher maternal ratings of preoccupied-merger attachment to the therapist. Results suggested that examina-tion of the process of intervention and the mother–intervener relationship could shed light on how COS interventions work.

Although not published in the Woodhouse et al. (2015) study, the researchers also examined whether observer-rated psychotherapy process dimensions (i.e., both therapist and mother contributions) could distinguish successful versus unsuccessful outcomes of intervention (i.e., infant attachment security vs. insecurity). Table 3.2 presents the results of the two discriminant analyses examining successful versus unsuccessful outcomes of COS-HV4 (while controlling for maternal SES, maternal attachment anxiety and avoidance, infant sex, and maternal psychological symptoms).

As expected, successful versus unsuccessful cases could be distinguished on the basis of therapist contributions to process (Wilks's λ = .66, χ^2 = 22.67, p = .004, Canonical R^2 = .34; see Table 3.2). The model correctly predicted 83.3% of those with secure infant outcomes and 66.7% of those with insecure infant outcomes. The therapist behavior that contributed most to distinguishing secure versus insecure outcomes was observer-rated therapist warmth. Such findings mesh with Bowlby's (1988) theory that having an understanding, empathic therapist who can serve as a secure base is crucial in psychotherapy. It is possible that therapist warmth may be more important at certain times than others (e.g., perhaps when mothers are openly exploring parenting struggles); future research can examine this question and allow us to better refine supervision.

Also, consistent with expectation, successful versus unsuccessful cases could be distinguished on the basis of mothers' contributions to psychotherapy process

TABLE 3.2. Discriminant Analyses Examining Observer-Rated Psychotherapy Process Dimensions (Therapist and Mother Contributions) That Distinguish Successful versus Unsuccessful Outcomes of COS-HV4

Analysis focusing on therapist behavior			Analysis focusing on mother behavior		
Variables	Standardized function coefficients	Correlations: Variables and discriminant function	Variables	Standardized function coefficients	Correlations: Variables and discriminant function
SES	−.443	−.510	SES	−.442	−.459
Baby sex	−.483	.332	Baby sex	.281	.299
M symptoms	−.733	.149	M symptoms	.949	.134
M attachment anxiety	−1.048	−.360	M attachment anxiety	−1.274	−.324
M attachment avoidance	.416	.131	M attachment avoidance	.516	.118
T warmth and friendliness	.535	.065	M participation	.632	.188
T exploration	−.386	−.011	M exploration	−.072	.092
T negative attitude	.151	.224			

Note. T, therapist; M, mother. Maternal SES, maternal attachment anxiety and avoidance, infant sex, and maternal psychological symptoms were included as control variables in this analysis. This table did not appear in Woodhouse, Lauer, Beeney, and Cassidy (2015), but is based on data from that study.

(Wilks's λ = .61, χ^2 = 27.10, p < .001, Canonical R^2 = .39). The model correctly predicted 83.3% of those with secure infant outcomes and 79.2% of those with insecure infant outcomes. The mother behavior that contributed most to distinguishing secure versus insecure outcomes was observer-rated mother involvement/participation in the therapeutic dialogue. Contrary to expectation, however, observer-rated mother exploration did not appear useful in distinguishing successful from unsuccessful outcomes. In fact, although mother involvement/participation was correlated with mother exploration (35% shared variance), only mother involvement/participation differentiated successful from unsuccessful outcomes. This is an intriguing finding, because it suggests that maternal emotional engagement in dialogue with the intervener, elaboration, and willingness to disclose personal information to the therapist are more important than exploration per se. Thus, a focus on the relationship and on engaging caregivers may be important for outcomes.

Consideration of Mediating Mechanisms

Research examining the COS protocols has yet to examine meditational models that can elucidate mechanism of change. Some empirical attention, however, has been paid to variables that could potentially serve as mediators of treatment effects, and merit additional attention. For example, Huber et al. (2015a) found that caregivers who received the COS-20 week protocol showed significant pre–post changes in caregiver reflective functioning (i.e., awareness of mental states in oneself and others; Fonagy, Gergely, & Target, 2008), as well as significant improvements in caregiver representations of the child and the relationship with the child.

Little attention, however, has been paid to another important potential mediator of treatment effects, quality of parental caregiving. Bowlby (1969/1982) theorized that attachment develops in the context of the child's experiences with the caregiver. In fact, parental sensitivity (i.e., a caregiver's ability to accurately interpret infant needs and to respond promptly and appropriately; Ainsworth, Bell, & Stayton, 1971; National Institute of Child Health and Human Development [NICHD] Early Child Care Research Network, 1999) has been empirically linked via meta-analysis to later child attachment in both mothers (De Wolff & van IJzendoorn, 1997) and fathers (Lucassen et al., 2011). Bakermans-Kranenburg, van IJzendoorn, and Juffer (2003) found that parenting interventions that tended to improve parental sensitivity were those most likely to enhance child attachment. It is important to note, however, that the variance in attachment explained by sensitivity has been found to be smaller than expected, particularly in low-income families (De Wolff & van IJzendoorn, 1997). Woodhouse, Beeney, Doub, and Cassidy (under review) noted that according to the meta-analysis by De Wolff and van IJzendoorn (1997), sensitivity explains only 2% of the variance in attachment in low-income families. Given that interventions are often targeted to low-income families—justifiably so, because attachment security has been found to serve as a protective factor in children's socioemotional development in the context of environmental adversity (e.g., Keller, Spieker, & Gilchrist, 2005)—it would be crucially important to consider how to best assess quality of caregiving across socioeconomic groups. Improvements in assessment of caregiving would enhance the prediction of child attachment and allow for improved testing of mediating mechanisms for intervention effects.

In order to examine caregiving in low-income families, Cassidy et al. (2005) conducted a qualitative study based on mothers drawn from the control group of the RCT testing COS-HV4. Findings revealed that many of the mothers could be viewed as highly insensitive, yet approximately half of the infants were securely attached at 12 months. Cassidy et al. proposed *secure base provision* (i.e., the degree to which a caregiver ultimately meets attachment-related needs [e.g., fully soothing a crying infant] even in the presence of high levels of insensitive behavior) as an alternative to sensitivity. Woodhouse et al. (under review) went on to develop an observational secure base coding system and showed that secure base provision predicted later infant attachment in a low-income sample, whereas sensitivity did not. It will be important to carefully consider how best to assess caregiving in tests of parental caregiving quality as a mediator of treatment results, particularly in low-income families.

Conclusions and Implications for Future Research on the Original COS Protocols

In summary, research on the various forms of COS indicates success in reducing the risk of insecure attachment, but is just beginning. More research is needed, particularly research using RCT designs. It will be important to do research that examines potential mediators and moderators of treatment effects. More research is also needed on the process of intervention and the caregiver–intervener relationship; such research could have important implications for training and supervision. Nevertheless, despite the fact that research on forms of COS is still in its infancy, results suggest that treatment is associated with increased attachment security, decreased attachment disorganization, as well as reduced child symptoms.

COS Parenting: A Move toward Broader Implementation

The COS protocols described earlier all involve filming parent–child interaction during an assessment phase, using the video to identify the primary strengths and struggles, and creating a series of video vignettes to assist the parent in making new choices with that child—and as such, they are labor intensive and difficult to implement in many settings. For example, during the learning phase, trainees dedicate almost 1 day each week to implementing the program. Once they learn the process, clinicians become more efficient, and even then, the protocol requires more time in preparation than in delivery. It has been difficult for agencies and clinicians to find a way to bill for the preparation time. Such challenges made it clear that it would be highly desirable to have a COS protocol that could be implemented more easily in a variety of types of sites.

To facilitate implementation, and thus allow COS to be available to more families, the Spokane team created COS Parenting (COS-P; Cooper, Hoffman, & Powell, 2009). This protocol was created using the same intervention goals as prior COS programs (listed in Table 3.1), with one critical difference: All of the video clips discussed with the parents have been previously created by the developers (currently provided with training on a DVD); as such, each intervention session requires little preparation time.

This shift to archival video clips yields a stable COS intervention protocol that lends itself to a high degree of flexibility in intervention delivery. COS-P can be used widely and used in many formats (e.g., parent groups, home visitation programs, individual and family therapy) and in many contexts (e.g., the home, community centers, clinics). Prior COS protocols emphasized individualized treatment planning using video segments obtained from interactions between each parent and child. The prior protocols can be considered a "first-person" model of treatment and looking at video of his or her own engagement with the child influences the parent: a "watching us" methodology. The first-person approach to video review has many advantages as parents view their relationship directly. COS-P, on the other hand, takes a video modeling approach. The attachment concepts are presented through watching other parents, children, and sometimes actors. Influencing parents by having them observe "third-person" parent–child interactions is a "watching them" methodology (Coyne, Powell, Hoffman, & Cooper, 2012).

COS-P requires parents to take generalized information regarding children's needs and apply it to their interactional and internal struggles. Whether parents can make the needed changes in their internal representations, attributions, and behavior without viewing video of interactions specifically between themselves and their children is an important question that had to be considered in developing this protocol.

To facilitate the internalization of the material and to explicitly focus on individualizing the intervention for the parents participating in the group, parents are invited each session to present descriptions of attachment interactions with their child during the past week. The stories are framed as *Circle Stories* and are used by the intervener to help the group members understand and enhance their secure base/safe haven provision. Each time a parent describes an interaction with his or her own child is an opportunity for the facilitator to individualize the material for that parent. The supportive presence of the intervener creates a secure base from which the parent can explore difficult experiences and feelings (Bowlby, 1988) and therefore reevaluate the meaning of distressful situations in parenting.

The COS-P protocol is divided into eight chapters that may be delivered in eight 90-minute weekly sessions. Often the program is delivered over 10, 12, or more weeks, and sometimes multiple times a week for fewer weeks, depending on the requirements of the situation. The protocol is designed for parents of children from birth to approximately age 6.

The eight chapters of COS-P aim to give parents the same capacities in their relationship with their child that are provided by the original COS interventions. The first two chapters of the program introduce parents to the basic concepts of attachment, the use of the COS graphic as a map for parent–child interaction, and the idea of "exploring our children's needs all the way around the Circle" (Cooper et al., 2009, p. 17). Chapter 3 of COS-P addresses the important concept of *being with* children emotionally. The core of *being with* is providing an emotional safe haven by meeting children in whatever affective state they are experiencing. This emotional meeting allows children both to use their parent as a coregulating other and to build their own parental capacity for emotion regulation. Chapter 4 of COS-P applies this concept specifically to the idea of *being with* infants. The first four chapters parallel the beginning of the original COS protocols by helping parents learn how to identify the needs of their child and develop the ability to use the COS graphic to track these needs and practice *being with*.

The next three chapters of COS-P are analogous to the second half of the original COS. In Chapter 5 of COS-P, the concept of shark music and its role in perpetuating relationship struggles is introduced. Avoidant and ambivalent attachment styles are also introduced as Limited Circles. In these three sessions, parents are introduced to the importance of reflecting on their struggles, which is hypothesized to lead to different responses that support secure relationships.

In Chapter 6 of COS-P, parents are introduced to disorganized attachment through the concept of *limited hands*, wherein the concept of *mean, weak, and gone* is discussed, as described earlier. In Chapter 7 of COS-P, parents are introduced to the importance of *rupture and repair* in relationships. A useful way of defining security is for the child to have the confidence that when the relationship inevitably has a rupture, a repair is likely to follow. Relationship repair supports the long-term development of emotion regulation and successful functioning in relationships. Chapter 8 of COS-P consists of a summary, an opportunity to discuss the group experience, and celebration of the parents' completion of the protocol. Parents are invited to use their expertise to analyze a video of struggling mother–child dyad. Then they view the mother being successful with her child and listen to the mother's experience of the changes she made through COS-P.

Like all COS protocols, the COS-P protocol is strategically presented so that each section builds on the previous one to provide a complex understanding of children's attachment needs. Focusing first on the child's needs for secure attachment leads to the more vulnerable process of focusing on the self and difficulties in responding to these needs. Developing a working knowledge of defensive process through shark music makes it possible for parents to operationalize this learning in their relationship with their children.

The training requirement to be a registered facilitator who is licensed to use the COS-P DVD, manual, and handouts is completion of the 4-day COS-P training workshop. Participation in reflective consultation/supervision, a model widely used in the field of early intervention (Heffron & Murch, 2010), is considered best practice for COS-P registered facilitators while delivering the program. In addition to English, the COS-P is available in Spanish, Norwegian, Swedish, Danish, Italian, Japanese, Chinese (Mandarin), and Romanian. Training is offered multiple times a year in many parts of the world. The training is for mental health professionals, parent educators, home visitors, social workers, nurses, and other professionals involved in providing early intervention and education for parents. More information is available at the COS website (*www.circleofsecurity.com*).

Research examining the new COS-P protocol is in its infancy. To date, there have been only two published quantitative studies investigating changes in parenting associated with participation in a COS-P group. Horton and Murray (2015) used a pre–post design and focused on a sample of 15 mothers who participated in a COS-P group while in residential treatment for substance abuse. Results showed that among the nine mothers who attended the majority of the sessions (i.e., six to nine sessions), a significant number of mothers showed improvement in mother-rated discipline practices on a measure of both lax and overreactive/harsh discipline practices. These mothers also showed improvements, on average, in mother-rated emotion regulation and in parental hostile attributions about the causes of child behavior, although these factors did not have a significant number of participants with improved scores. These data from the Horton and Murray study can only be considered preliminary, because of not only the extremely small sample size but also a number of limitations that affected the internal validity of the study, including lack of an RCT design.

More recently Cassidy et al. (2017), however, published results of a study that used an RCT design to examine treatment effects of COS-P in low-income mothers and their preschool children, who were enrolled in Head Start programs in Baltimore, Maryland. The sample included a total of 141 mothers, with 75 in the COS-P intervention group and 66 in the waiting-list control group. Intent-to-treat analyses (controlling for maternal age and marital status) showed that mothers who received COS-P reported fewer unsupportive responses to preschoolers' distress than did mothers in the control group. It appears, therefore, that COS-P was successful in one of its central goals: that of building parental empathy for child emotional experiences. Reductions in unsupportive responses to child distress are important, because research has shown that parental responses to child distress are linked to later child attachment (e.g., Del Carmen, Pedersen, Huffman, & Bryan, 1993) and child behavioral problems (Leerkes, Blankson, & O'Brien, 2009; see also Spinrad et al., 2007).

In addition to a main effect of COS-P on maternal reports of unsupportive responses to child distress, Cassidy et al. (2017) found a main effect of treatment on one type of child executive functioning (i.e., child inhibitory control, but not cognitive flexibility). Inhibitory control, a form of executive functioning that involves regulation of both attention and behavior, is an important outcome, because higher levels of child inhibitory control are associated with greater school readiness (e.g., Blair & Razza, 2007; Bull, Espy, & Wiebe, 2008) and lower risk for psychopathology (Schachar & Logan, 1990). It is important to note that this main effect was moderated by maternal self-reported attachment style: the difference between the COS-P and control groups on child inhibitory control did not hold if mothers were high on self-reported attachment anxiety (Brennan et al., 1998).

Although the study by Cassidy et al. (2017) found no other main effects of treatment in the outcomes assessed (i.e., child attachment classification as assessed from the Strange Situation, or child behavior problems), results showed that maternal self-reported attachment style and maternal depressive symptoms each served as important moderators of treatment effects with regard to child attachment security, attachment disorganization, and child internalizing (but not externalizing) symptoms. First, for preschool children whose mothers were high (1 standard deviation [SD] above the mean) in self-reported attachment avoidance (Brennan et al., 1998), treatment with COS-P was associated with increased attachment security and reduced attachment disorganization in comparison to wait-list control; for children whose mothers were low (1 SD below the mean) in attachment avoidance, COS-P was associated with decreased attachment security in comparison to wait-list control. Second, maternal attachment anxiety and maternal depressive symptoms each moderated treatment effects on children's internalizing behavior problems, such that treatment group children whose mothers were either low on self-reported attachment anxiety or low on depressive symptoms (1 *SD* below the mean) showed lower levels of internalizing symptoms than did wait-list control children.

This first RCT examining the efficacy of COS-P is promising, and results suggest that it will continue to be important to actively examine "what works for whom." In addition to examining maternal characteristics that may moderate treatment effects, it may also be useful to examine child characteristics and contextual characteristics that may also moderate treatment effects. Given the potential of COS-P to allow for more affordable implementation and wider dissemination of the COS model within existing service systems working with low-income families, it will be important to continue research on COS-P.

There is one RCT of COS-P currently underway that will allow for further empirical examination of the efficacy of COS-P (Vaever, Smith-Nielsen, & Lange, 2016).

Conclusion

The research thus far supports the efficacy of the various COS protocols, although additional research is needed. As mentioned earlier, additional research on COS employing an RCT design would be particularly useful, as would investigation of potential moderators and mediators of COS efficacy. Such research would allow for a better understanding of "what works for whom," as well as why COS works.

In addition to RCT designs, other designs can also be used to answer important questions about COS. As Sexton, Kinser, and Hanes (2008) noted, methodological diversity is important in answering questions that go beyond simple questions about efficacy. For example, process-to-outcome studies examine links between processes occurring within the session and outcomes of intervention. Systematic case studies of COS (e.g., Page & Cain, 2009) can allow for an ideographic description of the clinical process, and might have important implications for generating hypotheses about change mechanisms. Research on the role of the intervener–mother relationship (e.g., Woodhouse et al., 2015) would be helpful in delineating aspects of the relationship that are important to attend to, and could be important for training and supervision. Likewise, case study methodology can be used to examine new populations of children who might benefit from parental participation in COS. For example, Fardoulys and Coyne (2016) examined changes in attachment (pre- and postintervention) for two children diagnosed with autism whose mothers participated in COS. One child remained securely attached throughout, and the other child shifted from insecurely attached at baseline to securely attached postintervention. Such initial findings are promising and suggest that future research in this population may be useful.

Given compelling data that individual therapists vary in effectiveness in terms of psychotherapy outcomes (Kim, Wampold, & Bolt, 2006; Wampold & Bolt, 2006), it will be important for future research on COS to examine whether interveners are differentially effective, and examine factors that might be linked to differential outcomes between therapists. Such research could help to refine selection and training of COS interveners.

In some settings, it may be important for researchers to build community trust for parenting intervention and research. In such cases, partnership-building methods drawn from community-based participatory research models (Israel, Eng, Schutz, & Parker, 2013) may be useful in building community–researcher partnerships and community engagement for research on COS and implementation of COS models more broadly.

COS-P was designed with implementation in mind, and as such, research that examines the process of its implementation in real-world settings (i.e., both barriers and facilitating factors) could have important implications for providing wider access to parenting supports for those who need them most. It may be important to consider what might be the best models for delivery of COS in different community settings. For example, in some contexts, groups may provide an efficient delivery model where there are naturally existing groups or opportunities for meeting. In other cases, home visiting may be a better way to ensure appropriate dosage of intervention (e.g., if there are barriers to regular group meetings). Hoffman, Cooper, Powell, and Benton (2017) recently translated COS ideas into a self-help parenting book that families can access on their own. This delivery format offers yet another option for dissemination of COS tools that may be useful for some parents.

In some contexts it may be beneficial to think systemically about the challenges families with young children are facing. Some communities have complex systemic problems, and it may not be enough to intervene at the individual family level with a parenting intervention. In such cases, COS protocols could be embedded within more systemic approaches (e.g., approaches that consider jobs, economics, danger in the community, toxicity/pollution, education), and in fact, COS has already been integrated into treatment across a variety of settings.

In conclusion, it is important to note that COS provides a user-friendly language with which to talk with parents about important aspects of parenting, as well as a model of intervention has been useful with diverse parents and caregivers. A growing body of research suggests that COS is linked to improvements in child attachment and behavioral health outcomes, as well as improvements in parent outcomes, and that it is a useful intervention approach across a variety of contexts. COS-P was designed with implementation in mind and has the potential for wide application.

REFERENCES

Ainsworth, M., Bell, S., & Stayton, D. (1971). Individual differences in strange situation behavior of one-year-olds. In H. R. Schaffer (Ed.), *The origins of human social relations* (pp. 17–57). London: Academic Press.

Ainsworth, M., Blehar, M., Waters, E., & Wall, S. (1978). *Patterns of attachment*. Hillsdale, NJ: Erlbaum.

Bakermans-Kranenburg, M. J., van IJzendoorn, M. H., & Juffer, F. (2003). Less is more: Meta-analyses of sensitivity and attachment interventions in early childhood. *Psychological Bulletin, 129*(2), 195–215.

Beebe, B., & Lachmann, F. (1994). Representation and internalization in infancy: Three principles of salience. *Psychoanalytic Psychology, 11*(2), 127–165.

Beebe, B., Lachmann, F., & Jaffe, J. (1997). Mother–infant interaction structures and pre-symbolic self and object representations. *Psychoanalytic Dialogues, 7*(2), 133–182.

Belsky, J., & Pluess, M. (2009). Beyond diathesis–stress: Differential susceptibility to environmental influences. *Psychological Bulletin, 135*, 885–908.

Blair, C., & Razza, R. P. (2007). Relating effortful control, executive function, and false belief understanding to emerging math and literacy ability in kindergarten. *Child Development, 78*, 647–663.

Bowlby, J. (1973). *Attachment and loss: Vol. 2. Separation: Anxiety and anger.* New York: Basic Books.

Bowlby, J. (1980). *Attachment and loss: Vol. 3. Loss.* New York: Basic Books.

Bowlby, J. (1982). *Attachment and loss: Vol. 1. Attachment.* New York: Basic Books. (Original work published 1969)

Bowlby, J. (1988). *A secure base.* New York: Basic Books.

Boyce, W. T., & Ellis, B. J. (2005). Biological sensitivity to context: I. An evolutionary-developmental theory of the origins and functions of stress reactivity. *Development and Psychopathology, 17*, 271–301.

Brennan, K. A., Clark, C. L., & Shaver, P. R. (1998). Self-report measurement of adult romantic attachment: An integrative overview. In J. A. Simpson & W. S. Rholes (Eds.), *Attachment theory and close relationships* (pp. 46–76). New York: Guilford Press.

Bull, R., Espy, K. A., & Wiebe, S. A. (2008). Short-term memory, working memory, and executive functioning in preschoolers: Longitudinal predictors of mathematical achievement at age 7 years. *Developmental Neuropsychology, 33*, 205–228.

Cassidy, J., Brett, B. B., Gross, J. T., Stern, J. A., Martin, D. D., Mohr, J. J., Woodhouse, S. S. (2017). Circle of Security—Parenting: A randomized controlled trial in Head Start. *Developmental Psychopathology, 29*, 651–673.

Cassidy, J., Marvin, R. S., & the MacArthur Attachment Working Group. (1992). *Attachment organization in preschool children: Coding guidelines.* Unpublished manuscript, University of Virginia, Charlottesville, VA.

Cassidy, J., Woodhouse, S. S., Cooper, G., Hoffman, K., Powell, B., & Rodenberg, M. (2005). Examination of the precursors of infant attachment security: Implications for early intervention and intervention research. In L. J. Berlin, Y. Ziv, L. Amaya-Jackson, & M. T. Greenberg (Eds.), *Enhancing early attachments: Theory, research, intervention, and policy* (pp. 34–60). New York: Guilford Press.

Cassidy, J., Woodhouse, S., Sherman, L., Stupica, B., & Lejuez, C. (2011). Enhancing infant attachment security: An examination of treatment efficacy and differential susceptibility. *Journal of Development and Psychopathology, 23*, 131–148.

Cassidy, J., Ziv, Y., Stupica, B., Sherman, L. J., Butler, H., Karfgin, A., . . . Powell, B. (2010). Enhancing maternal sensitivity and attachment security in the infants of women in a jail-diversion program [Special issue]. *Attachment and Human Development, 12*, 333–353.

Cooper, G., Hoffman, K., & Powell, B. (2000). *The COS–Home Visiting-4 Intervention* (COS-HV4). Unpublished manuscript. Spokane, WA: COS International.

Cooper, G., Hoffman, K., & Powell, B. (2003). *The COS Perinatal Protocol* (COS-PP). Unpublished manuscript. Spokane, WA: COS International.

Cooper, G., Hoffman, K., & Powell, B. (2009). *COS Parenting: A relationship-based parenting program* (DVD). (More information at *http://circleofsecurity.com*).

Coyne, J., Powell, B., Hoffman, K., & Cooper, G., (2012). *Watching Us–Watching Them: Two forms of video review in the COS Treatment Protocols.* Unpublished manuscript, Queensland University of Technology, Brisbane Queensland, Australia.

De Wolff, M., & van IJzendoorn, M. H. (1997). Sensitivity and attachment: A meta-analysis on parental antecedents of infant attachment. *Child Development, 68*(4), 571–591.

Del Carmen, R., Pedersen, F. A., Huffman, L. C., & Bryan, Y. E. (1993). Dyadic distress management predicts subsequent security of attachment. *Infant Behavior and Development, 16,* 131–147.

Fardoulys, C., & Coyne, J. (2016). Circle of security intervention for parents of children with autism spectrum disorder. *Australian & New Zealand Journal of Family Therapy, 37*(4), 572–584.

Fearon, R. M. P., Bakermans-Kranenburg, M. J., van IJzendoorn, M. H., Lapsley, A.-M., & Roisman, G. I. (2010). The significance of insecure attachment and disorganization in the development of children's externalizing behavior: A meta-analytic study. *Child Development, 81*(2), 435–456.

Fonagy, P., Gergely, G., & Target, M. (2008). Psychoanalytic constructs and attachment theory and research. In J. Cassidy & P. R. Shaver (Eds.), *Handbook of attachment: Theory, research, and clinical applications* (2nd ed., pp. 783–810). New York: Guilford Press.

Fraley, R., & Shaver, P. R. (1997). Adult attachment and the suppression of unwanted thoughts. *Journal of Personality and Social Psychology, 73,* 1080–1091.

Freud, S. (1963). *An outline of psychoanalysis* (J. Strachey, Trans.). New York: Norton. (Original work published 1940)

Gelo, O. C. G., & Manzo, S. (2015). Quantitative approaches to treatment process, change process, and process–outcome research. In O. C. G. Gelo, A. Pritz, & B. Rieken (Eds.), *Psychotherapy research: Foundations, process, and outcome* (pp. 247–277). Vienna: Springer.

Gold, C. (2015). Quantitative psychotherapy outcome research: Methodological issues. In O. C. G. Gelo, A. Pritz, & B. Rieken (Eds.), *Psychotherapy research: Foundations, process, and outcome.* (pp. 537–558). Vienna: Springer.

Goldsmith, H., & Rothbart, M. K. (1999). *Laboratory Temperament Assessment Battery, Prelocomotor Version 3.1.* Unpublished manuscript, University of Wisconsin, Madison, WI.

Groh, A. M., Roisman, G. I., van IJzendoorn, M. H., Bakermans-Kranenburg, M. J., & Fearon, R. M. P. (2012). The significance of insecure and disorganized attachment for children's internalizing symptoms: A meta-analytic study. *Child Development, 83*(2), 591–610.

Heffron, M. C., & Murch, T. (2010). *Reflective supervision and leadership in infant and early childhood programs.* Washington, DC: ZERO TO THREE.

Hoffman, K., Cooper, G., Powell, B., & Benton, C. (2017). *Raising a secure child: How Circle of Security Parenting can help you nurture your child's attachment, emotional resilience, and freedom to explore.* New York: Guilford Press.

Hoffman, K., Marvin, R., Cooper, G., & Powell, B. (2006). Changing toddlers' and preschoolers' attachment classifications: The COS Intervention. *Journal of Consulting and Clinical Psychology, 74,* 1017–1026.

Horton, E., & Murray, C. (2015). A quantitative exploratory evaluation of the COS-parenting program with mothers in residential substance-abuse treatment. *Infant Mental Health Journal, 36*(3), 320–336.

Huber, A., McMahon, C. A., & Sweller, N. (2015a). Efficacy of the 20-week COS Intervention: Changes in caregiver reflective functioning, representations, and child attachment in an Australian clinical sample. *Infant Mental Health Journal, 36*(6), 556–574.

Huber, A., McMahon, C. A., & Sweller, N. (2015b). Improved child behavioural and emotional functioning after COS 20-week intervention. *Attachment and Human Development, 17*(6), 547–569.

Huber, A., McMahon, C., & Sweller, N. (2016). Improved parental emotional functioning after Circle of Security 20-week parent–child relationship intervention. *Journal of Child and Family Studies, 25*(8), 2526–2540.

Israel, B. A., Eng, E., Schulz, A. J., & Parker, E. A. (Eds.). (2013). *Methods for community-based participatory research for health*. San Francisco: Jossey-Bass.

Kazdin, A. E. (2006) Arbitrary metrics: implications for identifying evidence based treatments. *American Psychologist, 61*, 42–49.

Keller, T. E., Spieker, S. J., & Gilchrist, L. (2005). Patterns of risk and trajectories of preschool problem behaviors: A person-oriented analysis of attachment in context. *Development and Psychopathology, 17*(2), 349–384.

Kim, D. M., Wampold, B. E., & Bolt, D. M. (2006). Therapist effects in psychotherapy: A random effects modeling of the National Institute of Mental Health Treatment of Depression Collaborative Research Program data. *Psychotherapy Research, 16*, 161–172.

Korfmacher, J., Green, B., Spellmann, M., & Thornburg, K. R. (2007). The helping relationship and program participation in early childhood home visiting. *Infant Mental Health Journal, 28*, 459–480.

Leerkes, E. M., Blankson, A. N., & O'Brien, M. (2009). Differential effects of maternal sensitivity to infant distress and nondistress on social–emotional functioning. *Child Development, 80*, 762–775.

Lucassen, N., Tharner, A., van IJzendoorn, M. H., Bakermans-Kranenburg, M. J., Volling, B. L., Verhulst, F. C., . . . Tiemeier, H. (2011). The association between paternal sensitivity and infant–father attachment security: A meta-analysis of three decades of research. *Journal of Family Psychology, 25*(6), 986–992.

Lyons-Ruth, K., and the Process of Change Study Group. (1998). Implicit relational knowing: Its role in development and psychoanalytic treatment. *Infant Mental Health Journal, 19*(3), 282–289.

Mohr, J., Gelso, C., & Hill, C. (2005). Client and counselor trainee attachment as predictors of session evaluation and countertransference behavior in first counseling sessions. *Journal of Counseling Psychology, 52*, 298–309.

NICHD Early Child Care Research Network. (1999). Child care and mother–child interaction in the first three years of life. *Developmental Psychology, 35*(6), 1399–1413.

Norcross, J. C. (2011). *Psychotherapy relationships that work: Evidence based responsiveness* (2nd ed.). New York: Oxford University Press.

O'Malley, S. S., Suh, C. S., & Strupp, H. H. (1983). The Vanderbilt Psychotherapy Process Scale: A report on the scale development and a process–outcome study. *Journal of Consulting and Clinical Psychology, 51*, 581–586.

Page, T. F., & Cain, D. S. (2009). "Why don't you just tell me how you feel?": A case study of a young mother in an attachment-based group intervention. *Child Adolescent Social Work Journal, 26*, 333–350.

Powell, B., Cooper, G., Hoffman, K., & Marvin, B. (2014). *The Circle of Security Intervention: Enhancing attachment in early parent–child relationships*. New York: Guilford Press.

Schachar, R., & Logan, G. D. (1990). Impulsivity and inhibitory control in normal development and childhood psychopathology. *Developmental Psychology, 26*, 710–720.

Sexton, T. L., Kinser, J. C., & Hanes, C. W. (2008). Beyond a single standard: Levels of evidence approach for evaluating marriage and family therapy research and practice. *Journal of Family Therapy, 30*(4), 386–398.

Spinrad, T. L., Eisenberg, N., Gaertner, B., Popp, T., Smith, C. L., Kupfer, A., . . . Hofer, C. (2007). Relations of maternal socialization and toddlers' effortful control to children's adjustment and social competence. *Developmental Psychology, 43*, 1170–1186.

Steele, H., & Steele, M. (2008). On the origins of reflective functioning. In F. N. Busch (Ed.), *Mentalization: Theoretical considerations, research findings, and clinical implications* (pp. 133–158). New York: Analytic Press.

Thompson, R. A. (2016). Early attachment and later development: Familiar questions, new answers. In J. Cassidy & P. R. Shaver (Eds.), *Handbook of attachment: Theory, research, and clinical applications* (3rd ed., pp. 330–348). New York: Guilford Press.

Væver, M. S., Smith-Nielsen, J., & Lange, T. (2016). Copenhagen infant mental health project: Study protocol for a randomized controlled trial comparing circle of security–parenting and care as usual as interventions targeting infant mental health risks. *BMC Psychology, 4*(1), 57.

van den Boom, D. C. (1994). The influence of temperament and mothering on attachment and exploration: An experimental manipulation of sensitive responsiveness among lower-class mothers with irritable infants. *Child Development, 65,* 1457–1477.

Wampold, B. E., & Bolt, D. M. (2006). Therapist effects: Clever ways to make them (and everything else) disappear. *Psychotherapy Research, 16,* 184–187.

Woodhouse, S. S., Beeney, J. R. S., Doub, A. E., & Cassidy, J. (under review). *Secure base provision: A new approach to links between maternal caregiving and attachment.*

Woodhouse, S. S., Lauer, M., Beeney, J. R. S., & Cassidy, J. (2015). Psychotherapy process and relationship in the context of a brief attachment-based mother–infant intervention. *Psychotherapy, 52*(1), 145–150.

CHAPTER 4

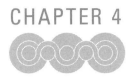

The Nurse–Family Partnership
Theoretical and Empirical Foundations

NANCY DONELAN-McCALL and DAVID OLDS

For the past several decades, Olds and his colleagues have developed and rigorously tested the Nurse–Family Partnership® (NFP), a home-visiting program for high-risk, first-time mothers, through a series of three randomized controlled trials. The nurses implementing the program have three major goals: (1) to improve the outcomes of pregnancy by helping women improve their health-related behaviors; (2) to improve the child's health and development by helping parents provide more competent care; and (3) to improve parents' own personal development by helping them develop a vision for their futures and make constructive decisions about the timing of subsequent births, staying in school, and finding work. The development of the NFP began more than 40 years ago, when the theories that lay the foundation for the model were in their infancy with regard to guiding intervention capable of positively impacting the parent–child relationship and health outcomes in contexts where poverty, young parental age, substance use, mental health problems, and abuse and trauma characterized the history of the new parent.

As pioneers in the field of early childhood prevention and attachment informed interventions, Olds and his colleagues endeavored to bring together theory, epidemiology, and eventually public policy to improve the lives of vulnerable families as early in the lifecycle as possible. Olds's work has been heavily influenced by his experiences as an undergraduate and graduate student working with Mary Ainsworth and Urie Bronfenbrenner, respectively. As an undergraduate, Olds had the privilege to take courses with Mary Ainsworth, who introduced him to attachment theory (Ainsworth, Blehar, Waters, & Wall, 1978), and he worked as a research assistant, coding data from her Baltimore study of infant attachment. After finishing undergraduate school, he worked in an inner-city day care center for low-income children, where he taught a classroom of 4-year-olds and arranged parent groups that met at naptime to address their concerns about their children's needs. He approached this work with the hope that if he provided a more nurturing and cognitively stimulating classroom environment for the children and helped their parents support one another, their children would have better prospects in life. And while the classroom environment was indeed enriching and many parents valued meeting during naptime, it soon became clear that, for many children, a supportive preschool environment was simply too little and too late.

Olds soon realized through his own experiences and the evolving literature on environmental factors that influence prenatal development that a program that begins when children reach preschool could not undo damaging earlier experiences. Moreover, the children he worked with every day were growing up in neighborhoods devastated by drugs, crime, and limited employment opportunities; the children and their parents had almost no personal experiences or models within the community to give them hope for a better life. Olds realized that he knew too little about the multiplicity of influences on children's development, and that he had no power to influence those factors that appeared to shape their lives, so he went to graduate school and studied with Urie Bronfenbrenner (1979), who was just beginning to formulate his theory of human ecology.

These firsthand experiences with children and families living in poverty and his studies with Mary Ainsworth and Urie Bronfenbrenner shaped Olds's career since then and laid the foundation for the development of the NFP. In addition, Olds reasoned that interventions would gain strength if they were able to reduce biological risks for children's compromised neurological development during pregnancy, and if they reduced critical contextual risks affecting child and family functioning. Moreover, he was deeply concerned that any program make sense to parents—that it resonate with their views of the world and their beliefs about what was needed to ensure their children's healthy development, and that the content and approach embodied in the program be assimilable. Moreover, parents would have to find the program sufficiently compelling to find the investment of their time worth the effort.

The NFP has been significantly influenced by attachment theory, with a focus on promoting sensitive and responsive parenting, and a sense of shared joy and regulation in the parent–child relationship. We describe in this chapter the theoretical and empirical foundations on which this program of research was founded; the design of the program itself; and the research designs, methods, and findings from the three randomized controlled trials. We continue with a discussion of policy implications of the findings and describe replication of the program model outside of research contexts, including international replication activities. We end with a discussion of attachment-informed augmentations designed to improve the program in community practice.

A Theory-Driven Model

The NFP is grounded in theories of human ecology (Bronfenbrenner, 1979, 1995), self-efficacy (Bandura, 1977), and attachment (Bowlby, 1969). Together, these theories emphasize the importance of families' social context and individuals' beliefs, motivations, emotions, and internal representations of their experience in explaining the development of behavior. The integration of these theories has shaped the design of the program.

Attachment Theory

Attachment theory posits that infants are biologically predisposed to seek proximity to specific caregivers in times of stress, illness, or fatigue in order to promote survival (Bowlby, 1969). Attachment theory hypothesizes that children's trust in the world and their later capacity for empathy and responsiveness to their own children once they become parents is influenced by the degree to which they formed an attachment with a caring, responsive, and sensitive adult when they were growing up, which affects their internal representations of themselves and their relationships with others (Main, Kaplan, & Cassidy, 1985). Parents with histories of abuse or neglect, intimate partner violence, or failed interpersonal relationships are at particular risk for having difficulty caring competently for their children, because, according to attachment theory, the models of interpersonal relationships they have acquired as a result of their experience lead them to doubt their own value and to be at greater risk for misreading their infants' communicative signals (Main & Cassidy, 1985).

The NFP therefore explicitly promotes sensitive, responsive, and engaged caregiving in the early years of the child's life. In addition, home visitors try to help mothers and other caregivers review their own childrearing histories and make decisions about how they wish to care for their children in light of the way they were cared for as children. Finally, the home visitors seek to develop an empathic and trusting relationship with the mother and other family members, because experience in such a relationship is expected to help women eventually trust others and to promote more sensitive, empathic care of their children. To the extent that the nurse's relationship with parents (primarily the mother) is characterized by deep appreciation for the mother's needs and helps her gain control over a host of challenges that are of concern to her, the nurse will have demonstrated the essence of an effective attachment relationship. In theory, this will make it easier for parents to understand what the program is designed to accomplish with respect to parents' care of their infants.

Attachment theory provides the foundation for understanding the influence the caregiving relationship has on long-term outcomes for children and a framework for understanding parenting behaviors, so that service providers can guide intervention with an understanding of how the client's own childhood experiences and attachment framework influence how she responds to her child. Building on this foundation, as mentioned previously, the NFP is grounded in theories of human attachment, as well as human ecology and self-efficacy. Together, these theories emphasize the importance of sensitive, responsive caregiving within families' social context and individuals' beliefs, motivations, emotions, and internal representations of their experience in explaining the development of behavior.

Human Ecological Theory

The ecological model of human/child development emphasizes that human development is influenced by how parents care for their children, and that in turn is influenced by characteristics of the families, homes, social networks, neighborhoods, communities, and interrelations among them (Bronfenbrenner, 1979). Theoretically and empirically, caregiver–child interactions are influenced by the immediate and more distal environment. The *environment* is often referred to as the stage or setting in which caregiver–child interactions occur (Wachs, 1989).

Factors that create stressful conditions in the household may interfere with parents' ability to care for their children include unemployment, poor housing and household conditions, and isolation from supportive family members and friends. Therefore, to support parents' sensitive caregiving, NFP nurses work to decrease stress and increase economic stability, in part by linking families with community resources such as quality child care, education, and health services. Nurses attempt to enhance the material and social environment of the family by involving other family members, especially fathers, in the home visits, and by linking families with needed health and human services.

Self-Efficacy Theory

Attachment and human ecology are essentially theories of development that help guide our understanding of the mechanisms and possible intervention pathways to support healthy outcomes for children. The inclusion of a theoretical model with a firm basis for how one might reliably bring about changes in women's prenatal health, parenting, or family circumstances was an essential part of the early formation of the program. The program incorporated Bandura's *self-efficacy theory* (Bandura, 1977)—a theory of motivation and behavioral change. Self-efficacy theory provides a useful framework for understanding how women make decisions about their health-related behaviors during pregnancy, their care of their children, and their own personal development. This theory posits that individuals choose those behaviors (1) that they believe will lead to a given outcome, and (2) that they themselves can successfully carry out (Bandura, 1977).

The NFP curriculum is therefore designed first to help women understand what is known about the influence of particular behaviors on their own health, and on the health and development of their babies. The program guidelines are periodically updated to reflect the most recent evidence regarding influence on family and child health. Second, the home visitors help parents establish realistic goals and small, achievable objectives that, once accomplished, increase parents' reservoir of successful experiences. In turn, these successes increase their confidence in taking on larger challenges.

Epidemiological Foundations

Attachment, human ecology, and self-efficacy provided a framework for the development of the NFP program, with emerging developmental and epidemiological research guiding decisions about the families to be served by the NFP and the content of the program.

Focus on Low-Income, Unmarried, and Teen Parents

All trials of the NFP have examined the program's impact on women with no pre-vious live births, and each focused recruitment on low-income, unmarried, and adolescent women. The primary difference among the studies is that in the first trial in Elmira, New York, any woman bearing a first child was allowed to regis-ter, although those who were poor, unmarried, and teens were actively recruited. Women with these characteristics were recruited, because the problems the pro-gram was designed to address (e.g., poor birth outcomes, compromised child health and development, and diminished economic self-sufficiency of parents) are con-centrated in those populations (Elster & McAnarney, 1980; Furstenberg, Brooks-Gunn, & Morgan, 1987; Overpeck, Brenner, Trumble, Trifiletti, & Berendes, 1998).

Program Content

The program seeks to modify specific risk and promote protective factors that are associated with the negative outcomes the program seeks to address: poor birth outcomes, child health and developmental problems, and compromised parental life course. Figure 4.1 summarizes how these influences are thought to reinforce one another over time.

On the far left side of Figure 4.1, we note the three broad domains of proxi-mal risks and protective factors that the program was designed to affect: prena-tal health behaviors; sensitive, competent care of the child; and early parental life course. The middle set of outcomes reflects corresponding child and parent out-comes that the program was designed originally to influence: birth outcomes, child abuse, neglect, and injuries (attachment); child neurodevelopmental impairment; and later parental life course. On the far right, we show child and adolescent out-comes that the program might affect after completion of the program at child age 2, such as decreases in youth antisocial behavior.

Prenatal Health Behaviors

Prenatal exposure to tobacco, alcohol, and illegal drugs are established risks for poor fetal growth (Kramer, 1987) and, to a lesser extent, preterm birth (Kramer, 1987) and neurodevelopmental impairment (e.g., attention deficit disorder or poor cognitive and language development) (Fried, Watkinson, Dillon, & Dulberg, 1987; Milberger, Biederman, Faraone, Chen, & Jones, 1996; Olds, 1997; Olds, Hender-son, & Tatelbaum, 1994a, 1994b; Streissguth, Sampson, Barr, Bookstein, & Olson, 1994). Research indicates that prenatal tobacco exposure is a unique risk for con-duct disorder and youth crime (Brennan, Grekin, & Mednick, 1999; Wakschlag et al., 1997), presumably because it compromises neurological development, increas-ing children's risk for impulsive, distractible behavior. Adverse prenatal influences on fetal neurological development are sometimes exacerbated by adverse postnatal experiences.

In all three trials (Elmira, Memphis, and Denver) the home visitors therefore sought to reduce mothers' use of these substances. The prenatal protocols also

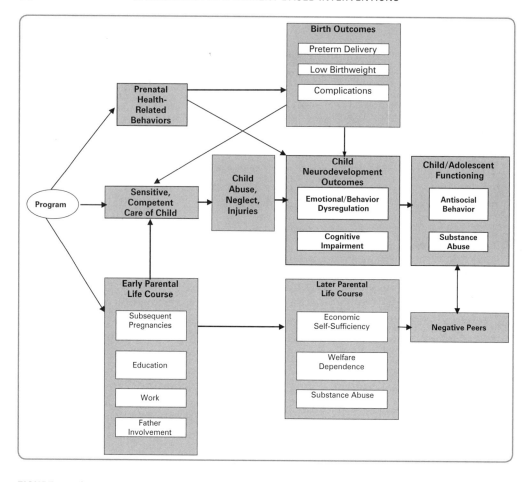

FIGURE 4.1. General conceptual model for program influences on maternal and child health and development.

address other behavioral factors that increase the risk for low-birthweight, preterm delivery and poor child development: inadequate weight gain (Institute of Medicine, 1990), inadequate diet (Institute of Medicine, 1990), inadequate use of office-based prenatal care (Klein & Goldenberg, 1990), and early identification and treatment of obstetric complications such as genitourinary tract infections and hypertensive disorders (high blood pressure) (Klein & Goldenberg, 1990).

Sensitive, Competent Care of the Child

Parents who empathize with their infants and sensitively read and respond to their infants' communicative signals are less likely to abuse or neglect their children, and they are more likely to read their children's developmental competencies accurately, which leads to fewer unintentional injuries (Cole et al., 2004; Peterson & Gable, 1998). Competent early parenting is associated with better child behavioral regulation, language, and cognition (Hart & Risley, 1995). While it makes sense to target these proximal behaviors, it is helpful to understand and address the general sets of influences that affect parents' abilities to care for their children. We have hypothesized that these influences on parenting skills can be moderated with targeted intervention strategies.

Parents' caregiving skills are affected by ontogenetic and contextual factors. Parents who grew up in households with punitive, rejecting, abusive, or neglectful caregiving are more likely to abuse or neglect their own children (Egeland, Jacobvitz, & Sroufe, 1988; Quinton & Rutter, 1984; Rutter, 1989). Parents' psychological immaturity and mental health problems can reduce their ability to care for their infants (Newberger & White, 1989; Sameroff, 1983). Children who have been abused are more likely to develop negative attribution biases that make them more likely to interpret ambiguous behaviors on the part of others as threatening (Dodge, Bates, & Pettit, 1990) and to have internal representations of interpersonal relationships characterized by dysregulated aggression and violence (Buchsbaum, Toth, Clyman, Cicchetti, & Emde, 1992), both of which probably reflect an adaptive neurological response to a threatening world (Teicher, 2000). While it is impossible to change parents' personal histories, and it is very difficult to reduce personal immaturity and mental illness, as indicated below, the program has sought to mitigate the effect of these influences on parents' caregiving. In addition, unemployment (Gil, 1970), poor housing and household conditions (Gil, 1970), marital discord (Belsky, 1981), and isolation from supportive family members and friends (Garbarino, 1981) are all associated with higher rates of abuse and neglect, perhaps because they create stressful conditions in the household that interfere with parents' ability to care well for their children (Bakan, 1971; Kempe, 1973).

Early Parental Life Course

One of the major risks for compromised maternal educational achievement and workforce participation is rapid, successive pregnancies, particularly among unmarried women (Furstenberg et al., 1987). Rapid successive pregnancies may also limit parents' ability to protect their children. Such pregnancies often occur when women have limited visions for their futures in the areas of education and work (Musick, 1993), as well as limited belief in their control over life circumstances, and over their contraceptive practices in particular (Brafford & Beck, 1991; Heinrich, 1993; Levinson, 1986).

To the extent that families improve their economic conditions over time, they are less likely to live in unsafe, crime-ridden neighborhoods where children are exposed to negative peer influences. And even if children are exposed to negative peers, nurse-visited children are less likely to be susceptible to those negative influences, because they have stronger relationships with their parents, which help them develop a stronger moral core (Emde & Buchsbaum, 1990).

Young women in the program consult with nurses as they make these significant life-shaping decisions. In all of this, the nurses help women envision a future consistent with their deepest values and aspirations; evaluate different contraceptive methods, child care options, and career choices; and develop concrete plans for achieving their goals.

Program Design

The program design employed in the Elmira, Memphis, and Denver trials has remained essentially the same in each of the trials and has guided key features of the program and content in community practice.

First-Time Mothers

All three of the trials focused on women who had no previous live births, because it was hypothesized that such women would be more receptive to home-visitation services concerning pregnancy and child rearing than would women who had already given birth. Moreover, as parents learn parenting and other skills through the program, they should be better able to care for subsequent children, and the program should have an even greater positive effect. Finally, if the program helped parents plan subsequent births, then it would be easier for parents to finish their education and find work because of fewer problems with child care (Furstenberg et al., 1987), and the children would benefit from more focused parental nurturance and guidance (Tygart, 1991).

Women bearing first children are particularly receptive to this service given their perceived vulnerability associated with the major life transition they are experiencing. The extent to which they improve their prenatal health, care of their firstborns, and life course, they are likely to apply those skills to care of subsequent children they choose to have.

Frequency of Visitation

The recommended frequency of home visits changes with the phase in the program and is adapted to the parents' needs. When parents are experiencing crises or present with greater needs, the nurses are encouraged to visit more frequently; they reduce visit frequency when mothers and children are doing well. In general, mothers are visited every other week, with more frequent visits around the time of the child's birth and less frequent visits toward the child's second birthday. Each visit lasts approximately 75–90 minutes.

Nurses as Home Visitors

Nurses were selected to be the home visitors because of their formal training in women's and children's health and their competence in managing the complex clinical situations often presented by at-risk families. Nurses' abilities to competently address mothers' and family members' concerns about the complications of pregnancy, labor, and delivery, and the physical health of the infant, are thought to provide nurses with increased credibility and persuasive power in the eyes of family members. In addition, through their ability to teach mothers and family members to identify emerging health problems and to use the health care system, nurses enhance their clinical effect through the early detection and treatment of disorders.

Program Education

During all three trials, nurses participated in a structured education program designed to enhance their knowledge of the theoretical underpinning of the NPF program. The primary objectives of education have been to support nurses' understanding of the theoretical and clinical foundations of the program, principles of forming effective therapeutic relationships, reflective practice, solution-focused therapies, parent–child interaction observation approaches, stages of readiness for change, issues related to ethnic and racial diversity, safety issues related to home visiting, communication and problem-solving skills, and the program content and protocols.

This model of education used in the trials has continued to evolve to meet the needs of nurses and supervisors in community practice, while adhering to the primary objectives specified earlier. Nurses and supervisors receive over 100 hours of education over a 12-month period. Education is provided through self-guided learning modules, as well as classroom, group-based, and Web-based approaches to education. Supervisors receive additional education (40 hours) to support reflective practice, nurse recruitment and retention, site recruitment, administrative responsibilities, and quality implementation.

Supervision and Reflective Practice

During each of the trials, the role of the supervisor was viewed as critical to ensuring quality clinical and programmatic implementation, as well as nurse retention. In addition to structured education, nurses in all three trials received reflective supervision on a weekly basis through one-to-one supervisory meetings, with the purpose of reflecting on the nurses' caseloads, including discussions of alterations to visit frequency and visit content and ensuring quality implementation in alignment with the program model. Nurses and supervisors participated in regularly scheduled team meetings, case conferences, and joint supervisory field visits to support nurses' clinical practice and quality implementation. This supervisory model has been translated to community practice, with one-to-one supervision, and assessment of team meetings and case conferences as important indicators of implementation fidelity.

Program Content

During the home visits, the nurses carried out three major activities: (1) They promoted improvements in women's (and other family members') behaviors thought to affect pregnancy outcomes, the health and development of the child, and parents' life course; (2) they helped women build supportive relationships with family members and friends; and (3) they linked women and their family members with other needed health and human services.

The nurses followed detailed visit-by-visit guidelines whose content reflects the challenges parents are likely to confront during specific stages of pregnancy and the first 2 years of the child's life. Specific assessments were made of maternal, child, and family functioning that corresponded to those stages; and specific activities were recommended to address problems and strengths identified through the assessments.

During pregnancy, the nurses helped women complete 24-hour diet histories on a regular basis and plot weight gain at every visit; they assessed the women's cigarette smoking and use of alcohol and illegal drugs, and facilitated a reduction in the use of these substances through behavioral change strategies. They taught women to identify the signs and symptoms of pregnancy complications, encouraged women to inform the office-based staff about those conditions, and facilitated compliance with treatment. They gave particular attention to urinary tract infections, sexually transmitted diseases, and hypertensive disorders of pregnancy (conditions associated with poor birth outcomes). They coordinated care with physicians and nurses in the office and measured blood pressure when needed.

After delivery, the nurses helped mothers and other caregivers improve the physical and emotional care of their children. They taught parents to observe the signs of illness, to take temperatures, and to communicate with office staff about their children's illnesses before seeking care. Curricula were employed to promote parent–child interaction by facilitating parent's understanding of their infants' and toddlers' communicative signals, enhancing parents' interest in playing with their children in ways that promote emotional and cognitive development, and creating households that are safer for children.

Overview of Research Designs, Methods, and Findings

In each of the three studies, women were randomized to receive either home visitation services or comparison services. While the nature of the home-visitation services was essentially the same in each of the trials as described earlier, the comparison services were slightly different and included transportation to prenatal and well-child visits, health and developmental screenings, and/or referrals. All three studies employed a variety of data sources. The Elmira sample ($N = 400$) was primarily white. The Memphis sample ($N = 1,138$ for pregnancy and 743 for the infancy phase) was primarily black. The Denver trial ($N = 735$) included a large sample of Hispanics (46%) and systematically examined the impact of the program when delivered by paraprofessionals (individuals who shared many of the social characteristics of the families they served) and by nurses.

The paraprofessional visitors produced effects that were roughly half the size of effects produced by nurses and were rarely statistically significant. We therefore have focused the summary of results for the nurse-visited families in the report of the Denver findings. High rates of sample retention in each of the trials increases the validity of the treatment contrasts found in these studies. We looked for consistency in program effects across multiple sources before assigning importance to any one finding.

Assessments of attachment quality (e.g., the Strange Situation) were not employed in any of the three trials. Instead, measures of sensitive, competent care of the child and infant responsiveness to the caregiver based on standardized measures, as well as self-report and administrative data on child maltreatment and injury, were obtained. Following presentation of these results, we present findings related to prenatal health and parental life course given the influence these outcomes have on the caregiver–child relationships, as previously described. Finally, we present findings on long-term child outcomes.

A summary of key findings across all three trials is presented in Table 4.1 and summarized below. Unless otherwise stated, all findings presented in Table 4.1 are significant at $p < .05$; when a trend is noted, significance values are between $p > .05$ and $p < .10$. *Nurse-visited* refers to women visited during pregnancy and the child's infancy, unless otherwise noted.

Sensitive, Competent Care of Child

In general, the findings presented in Table 4.1 demonstrate a general pattern of effects observed across all three trials and provide indirect evidence that the program was helping mothers engage in behaviors that led to more physical contact, improved home environments, higher-quality interactions, more communicative and responsive infants, and maternal views of their children that were more developmentally appropriate compared to those of their counterparts in the control group. These finding were often concentrated in those families at greater risk with regard to their socioeconomic status, age, and/or psychological resources.

Child Abuse, Neglect, and Injuries

As indicated in Table 4.1, the Elmira trial produced a treatment–control difference in the overall rates of substantiated reports of child abuse and neglect (irrespective of risk) 15 years after the birth of the first child and, as a trend, an 80% difference during the first 2 years following the birth of the child for families in which the mothers were low-income and unmarried at registration. Furthermore, the Elmira trial resulted in a reduction in children's health care encounters for injuries and ingestions during the first 4.5 years following the birth of the first child.

Corresponding rates of child maltreatment were too low to serve as a viable outcome in the Memphis and Denver trials. However, program effects on children's health care encounters for serious injuries and ingestions at child age 2 and reductions in childhood mortality from preventable causes at child age 9 in the Memphis trial were consistent with the prevention of abuse and neglect. In the Denver trial, the investigators could not access women's or children's medical records to assess their injury encounters, because the health care delivery system was too complex to reliably abstract all of their health care encounters.

Prenatal Health Behaviors and Pregnancy Outcomes

In both the Elmira and Denver trials, nurse-visited women reduced prenatal tobacco use in comparison to the control group, and in the Memphis trial, nurse-visited women had fewer instances of pregnancy-induced hypertension than those in the comparison group.

TABLE 4.1. Summary of Key NFP Program Findings across Three Randomized Controlled Trials

Elmira	Memphis	Denver
	Sensitive, competent care of the child	

Nurse-visited compared to comparison group mothers:
 	
• At 34 and 46 months of child's life:
   o Home environments were more conducive to their children's emotional and cognitive development and were safer (Olds, Henderson, & Kitzman, 1994)
 	
• Between 25 and 50 months of child's life:
   o Had fewer child behavioral/parental coping problems reported in physician record (Olds, Henderson, & Kitzman, 1994)
 	
Nurse-visited, poor, unmarried teens compared to poor unmarried teens in the comparison group:
 	
• Demonstrated less punishment and restriction of their infants (10 and 22 months)
• Provided more appropriate play materials
• Provided safer, more developmentally conducive, home environments (Olds, Henderson, Chamberlin, & Tatelbaum, 1986)
	Nurse-visited compared to comparison group mothers:
	
	• Attempted breast feeding more frequently
	• By the 24th month of the child's life:
	   o Held fewer beliefs about childrearing associated with child abuse and neglect
	   o Had homes that were rated on the HOME scale as more conducive to children's development (Kitzman et al., 1997)
	
	Infants born to nurse-visited women with low levels of psychological resources[a] compared to similar mothers in the comparison group:
	
	• Were observed to be more communicative and responsive toward their mothers (Kitzman et al., 1997)
		Nurse-visited compared to comparison group mothers:
		
		• During the first 24 months of the child's life:
		   o Interacted more responsively
		   o As a trend, provided home environments that were more supportive of children's early learning (Olds, Robinson, et al., 2002)

(continued)

TABLE 4.1. *(continued)*

Elmira	Memphis	Denver
	Child abuse, neglect, and injury	
Nurse-visited compared to comparison group children: • Had fewer emergency room visits during the first and second year of life. • A difference that was explained in part by a 56% reduction in visits for injuries and ingestions in the second year (Olds, Henderson, Chamberlin, & Tatelbaum, 1986) • Between 25 and 50 months of age, were less likely to visit a physician for injuries and ingestions and as trend, to receive emergency room treatment (Olds, Henderson, & Kitzman, 1994) Nurse-visited versus comparison group mothers: • During the 15-year period after delivery of their first child, mothers were less likely to be identified as perpetrators of child abuse and neglect based on verified reports (Olds et al., 1997) Nurse-visited children born to low-income, unmarried teens compared to low-income, unmarried teens in the comparison group: • As a trend, had 80% fewer verified cases of child abuse and neglect during the first 2 years following first delivery (Olds, Henderson, Tatelbaum, & Chamberlin, 1986)	Nurse-visited compared to comparison group children: • During the first 2 years of life, had 23% fewer health care encounters for injuries and ingestions • Were hospitalized for fewer days with injuries and/or ingestions o Effects that were more pronounced for children born to mothers in the lower half of the sample with respect to their psychological resources (Kitzman et al., 1997) • As a trend, by age 9, were 4.5 times less likely to have died (Olds et al., 2007)	Data not available

91

(continued)

TABLE 4.1. *(continued)*

Elmira	Memphis	Denver
	Prenatal health behaviors and pregnancy outcomes	
Nurse-visited compared to comparison group women: • Women identified as smokers at registration had 75% fewer preterm deliveries • Experienced greater informal social support • Made better use of formal community resources • Had fewer kidney infections at the end of pregnancy (Olds, Henderson, Tatelbaum, & Chamberlin, 1986)	Nurse-visited compared to comparison group women: • Had fewer yeast infections during pregnancy • Had fewer instances of pregnancy-induced hypertension (Kitzman et al., 1997)	Nurse-visited compared to comparison group women (all defined as smokers at intake): • Had greater reductions in urine cotinine from intake to the end of pregnancy (Olds et al., 2002)
	Parental life course	

Nurse-visited compared to comparison group women:
 	
• At 4 years after first delivery
  o Had fewer subsequent pregnancies
  o Longer intervals between births of first and second children
  o Greater participation in the work force (Olds, Henderson, Tatelbaum, & Chamberlin, 1988)
 	
Nurse-visited, poor, unmarried women compared to poor, unmarried women in the comparison group:
 	
• At the 15-year follow-up
  o Averaged fewer subsequent pregnancies
  o Fewer subsequent births
  o Longer intervals between the birth of their first and second children
  o Fewer months on welfare
  o Fewer months receiving food stamps
  o Fewer behavioral problems due to substance abuse
  o Fewer arrests (Olds et al., 1997)
	Nurse-visited compared to comparison group women:
	
	• Reported fewer subsequent pregnancies (2, 4.5, 6, 9 years following first delivery)
	• reported fewer subsequent live births (2, 6, 9 years following first delivery)
	• Longer intervals between the birth of the first and second child (4.5, 6, and 9 years following first delivery)
	• Used fewer government services (welfare, Aid to Families with Dependent Children, food stamps) 2, 4.5, 6, 9, and 12 years following first delivery
	• Reported higher rates of living with a partner and living with the biological father of the child (4.5 years following first delivery)
	• Had partners who had been employed for longer durations (4.5 years following first delivery)
	• Had longer relationships with current partners (6 and 9 years following first delivery)
	• Were more likely to register their children in formal out-of-home care between ages 2 and 4.5 years (Kitzman et al., 1997, 2010; Olds et al., 2004)
		Nurse-visited compared to comparison group women:
		
		• By 24 months after first delivery
		  o Were less likely to have had a subsequent pregnancy and birth
		  o Had longer intervals until the next conception
		  o Were employed longer during the second year following the birth of their first child (Olds, Robinson, et al., 2002)

(continued)

TABLE 4.1. *(continued)*

Elmira	Memphis	Denver
	Child/adolescent development	

Nurse-visited compared to comparison group children:
 	
 • At age 15 years:
   ○ Had fewer arrests and adjudications as Persons in Need of Supervision (PINS)—these effects were greater for children born to mothers who were poor, unmarried at registration.
   ○ As trends, reported fewer sexual partners and fewer convictions and violations of probation (Olds et al., 1997)
 	
 Nurse-visited poor unmarried teens compared to counterparts in the comparison group:
 	
 • Reported that their infants (at 6 months) were less irritable and fussy (Olds, Henderson, Tatelbaum, & Chamberlin, 1986)
 • At 12 and 24 months as trends had higher scores on mental-development tests (Olds, Henderson, Chamberlin, & Tatelbaum, 1986)
	Nurse-visited compared to comparison group children:
	
	 • At age 6 years:
	   ○ Had higher intellectual functioning
	   ○ Had higher receptive vocabulary scores
	   ○ Had fewer behavior problems in the borderline or clinical range (Olds et al., 2004)
	 • At age 12:
	   ○ Reported lower use of substances
	   ○ Had fewer internalizing disorders (depression and anxiety) (Kitzman et al., 2010)
	
	 Nurse-visited children born to mothers with low psychological resources compared to counterparts in the comparison group:
	
	 • At age 6:
	   ○ Had higher arithmetic achievement test scores
	   ○ Expressed less aggression and incoherence in response to story stems (Olds et al., 2004)
	 • At age 9:
	   ○ Had higher grade point averages in reading and math (Olds et al., 2007)
	 • At age 12:
	   ○ Had higher rates of reading and math achievement (Kitzman et al., 2010)
		Nurse-visited compared to comparison group children:
		
		 • At 6 months:
		   ○ Were less likely to exhibit emotional vulnerability in response to fear stimuli
		 • At 21 months:
		   ○ Were less likely to exhibit language delays—an effect concentrated among children born to mothers with low psychological resources
		
		 Nurse-visited children born to mothers with low psychological resources compared to counterparts in the comparison group:
		
		 • At 6 months of age:
		   ○ Were less likely to exhibit emotional vulnerability in response to fear stimuli and those born to women with low psychological resources were less likely to display low emotional vitality in response to joy and anger stimuli (Olds, Robinson, et al., 2002)
		 • At 21 months:
		   ○ Had superior language and mental development (Olds, Robinson, et al., 2002)
		 • At ages 2, 4, and 6:
		   ○ Had more advanced language
		   ○ Had better behavioral adaptation during testing
		   ○ Had superior executive functioning through child age 9
		   ○ Received fewer therapeutic services (Olds et al., 2004, 2014)

Memphis "psychological resources" are defined as intellectual functioning, belief in control over one's own life, and rates of mental health symptoms.

Parental Life Course

In the Elmira trial, there were enduring effects of the program 15 years after birth of the first child on maternal life-course outcomes (e.g., interpregnancy intervals, use of welfare, behavioral problems due to women's use of drugs and alcohol, and arrests among women who were low-income and unmarried at registration). Findings related to interpregnancy intervals, numbers of subsequent pregnancies, and use of government services were replicated in the Memphis and Denver trials, as indicated in Table 4.1.

Child/Adolescent Development Outcomes

As presented in Table 4.1, the Elmira trial produced treatment–control differences in 15-year-olds' arrests, and as a trend, fewer sexual partners. In addition, as trends, the program resulted in higher scores on mental development tests at 12 and 24 months for nurse-visited children born to poor, unmarried teens compared to their counterparts in the control group. Children born to nurse-visited women in the Memphis trial had higher intellectual functioning and receptive language scores at 6 years of age, and 12 year-olds' reported lower use of substances and had fewer internalizing disorders compared to children in the comparison group. Nurse-visited children born to mothers with low psychological resources in Memphis had higher academic achievement at ages 6, 9, and 12 years, and expressed less aggression and incoherence at 6 years of age compared to children in the comparison group. In the Denver trial, children born to nurse-visited women exhibited less language delay (21 months), and those born to women with low psychological resources had superior language and mental development, superior behavioral adaptation during testing, and superior executive functioning, and received fewer therapeutic services compared to comparable children in the comparison group.

Cost Analysis

The Washington State Institute for Public Policy has conducted a thorough economic analysis of prevention programs from the standpoint of their impact on crime, substance abuse, educational outcomes, teen pregnancy, suicide, child abuse and neglect, and domestic violence (Aos, Lieb, Mayfield, Miller, & Pennucci, 2004). While this analysis does not cover all outcomes that have cost implications for the NFP (e.g., subsequent pregnancies or maternal employment), it provides a consistent examination of all programs that have attempted to affect the listed outcomes. This report sums the findings across all three trials of the NFP and estimates that it saves $17,000 per family. This estimate is consistent with a subsequent analysis produced by the RAND Corporation (Karoly, Kilburn, & Cannon, 2005).

Summary of Results, Policy Implications, and Program Replication

Today the program is replicated outside of research contexts in over 581 counties throughout the United States, currently serving 32,692 families. The growth of the program as a credible preventive intervention rests entirely on its having replicated evidence of effectiveness in affecting socially and clinically important outcomes in separate randomized controlled trials, with different populations living in different contexts, and at different points in our country's history. Many of the beneficial effects of the program found in the Elmira trial that were concentrated in higher-risk groups were reproduced in the Memphis and Denver replications. Overall, the Elmira and Memphis trials demonstrate that the nurse home-visitation program achieved two of its most important goals—the reduction in dysfunctional care of children and the improvement of maternal life course. The impact on pregnancy outcomes, however, was equivocal.

Policy Implications

One of the clearest messages that emerged from this program of research is that the functional and economic benefits of the NFP are greatest for families at greater risk. In the Elmira study, it was evident that most married women and those from households with higher socioeconomic levels managed the care of their children without serious problems and were able to avoid lives of welfare dependence, substance abuse, and crime without the assistance of the nurse home visitors. Similarly, on average, their children avoided encounters with the criminal justice system, the use of cigarettes and alcohol, and promiscuous sexual activity. Low-income, unmarried women and their children in the comparison group, on the other hand, were at much greater risk for these problems, and the program was able to avert many of these untoward outcomes for this at-risk population. Cost analyses suggested that the program's cost savings for the government are solely attributable to benefits accruing to this higher-risk group. Among families at lower risk, the financial investment in the program was a loss.

This pattern of results challenges the position that these kinds of intensive programs for targeted at-risk groups ought to be made available on a universal basis. Not only is it likely to be wasteful from an economic standpoint, but it may lead to a dilution of services for those families who need them the most, because of insufficient resources to serve everyone well.

Replication and Scale-Up of the NFP

Even when communities choose to develop programs based on models with good scientific evidence, such programs run the risk of being watered down in the process of being scaled up. So, it was with some apprehension that Olds and his colleagues began to make the program available for public investment in new communities. They established a nonprofit organization in the United States, the Nurse–Family Partnership National Service Office (NFP NSO), to support quality replication of the program. Since 1996, the NFP NSO has helped new communities develop the program outside of traditional research contexts. In 2009, the U.S. federal government passed the Affordable Care Act (health care reform), which included $1.5 billion for states who choose to invest in evidence-based home-visiting programs. The NFP served as the primary evidentiary foundation for that legislation. That legislation has served as a primary foundation for continued expansion of the NFP in the United States during the recent economic downturn.

International Replication

Our approach to international replication of the program is to make no assumptions about its possible benefits in societies that have different health and human service delivery systems and cultures than those in which the program was tested in the United States. Given this, our team has taken the position that the program ought to be adapted and tested in other societies before it is offered for public investment. We currently are working with partners in England, Scotland, Northern Ireland, Holland, Australia, Canada, Norway, and Bulgaria to adapt and test the program with disadvantaged populations. While it is possible that the need and impact of this intervention may be diminished in societies with more extensive health and social welfare systems than are found in the United States, it is possible that the program may have comparable effects for subgroups that do not make good use of those other services and resources that are available to them.

Recent findings from two international replications of the NFP model in England and Holland have produced mixed results. Robling and colleagues conducted a randomized controlled trial ($N = 1,645$) of the Family–Nurse Partnership (FNP) program in England and concluded that, compared with usual care, the FNP had no effects on the study's primary outcomes: prenatal cigarette smoking at the end of pregnancy, subsequent pregnancies, low birthweight, or at least one child emergency encounter or hospital admission at an accident and emergency department (Robling et al., 2016), although NFP-visited children were reported by their mothers to have superior cognitive and language development compared to their counterparts in the control group at 24 months of age. The U.K. FNP implementation has focused on young mothers (< 20 years of age) because their children are at risk of compromised development, and maternal age makes it easy to identify who qualifies. However, young mothers vary substantially in the extent to which they have overlapping challenges, such as financial difficulties, depression, and substance misuse (Olds, 2016). In contrast, positive effects identified in a Dutch trial of 460 disadvantaged women on outcomes such as child maltreatment, children's internalizing behavioral problems, and intimate partner violence might be attributed, at least partly, to its serving highly vulnerable mothers, irrespective of their age (Mejdoubi et al., 2013, 2015). These findings lend further support to the observation that the functional and economic benefits of the NFP are greatest for families at greater risk (Olds, 2016).

Programmatic Improvement

One of the primary concerns in transitioning a program from a controlled research environment to community-based implementation is the degree to which the program is implemented with fidelity to the original model while remaining feasible in a real-world setting. Several programs that have shown significant promise in research settings did not translate well to community practice.

In light of this potential concern, quality monitoring and improvement mechanisms have been developed to ensure quality and implementation integrity of the NFP model at community sites and use of these monitoring systems not just for quality assurance but for programmatic quality improvement. We have developed a framework to guide our understanding of implementation challenges and to address those challenges through rigorous methodologies (Olds et al., 2013). Through this monitoring process, several initiatives have been undertaken to address challenges in program implementation, with the goal of improving NFP implementation. We conclude this chapter by highlighting those programmatic improvements that relate to promotion of attachment.

Improving Nurses' Observation of Caregiver–Child Interaction and Promotion of Parenting

In analyses of program implementation data, we discovered that nurses in community replication sites were not spending as much time during home visits on helping parents care competently for their children as did nurses in the original trials. Because competent parenting is at the core of several of the program goals determining the reasons behind the decreased time spent in this domain, addressing potential program improvements to ameliorate this difference was a critical priority. Through surveys and interviews with nurses and supervisors, we found that the original tool that nurses used to observe qualities of caregiver–child interaction was hard to learn and was not sufficient to guide clinical implementation of the program. To address this issue, Nancy Donelan-McCall and her team at the Prevention Research Center for Family and Child Health at the University of Colorado have developed a new observation tool, the Dyadic Assessment of Naturalistic Caregiver–Child Experiences (DANCE), and clinical pathways called DANCE STEPS (Strategies to Enhance Parenting Skills) that integrate the DANCE into the existing parenting content of the program.

The DANCE measure includes 18 caregiving behaviors that can be observed naturally during a routine home visit. DANCE supports observations of caregiving qualities that are related to the formation of secure attachment relationships, including responsiveness of the caregiver to the child's cues, quality of the caregiver's emotional responses to the child, sensitivity to the child's needs, as well as behaviors that support cognitive (e.g., use of language with child, supportive environments) and socioemotional development (e.g., limit setting). One of the unique aspects of the DANCE tool is both the focus on caregiving behaviors that occur during interactions (e.g., play, feeding) and how caregivers support the child's needs in the space outside of interactions (e.g., children at independent play). We conducted studies to ensure that DANCE had adequate predictive validity, reliability, and superior clinical utility, and that it could be implemented in a cost-effective way relative to the original measure used in the program.

From a clinical perspective, DANCE supports nurses to observe, assess, and target intervention to support caregivers in providing care that fosters children's healthy development. Through the use of DANCE STEPS, nurses are helped in identifying caregivers' strengths and areas for growth, and program resources to support individualized visit planning.

Development of a System for Classifying Families' Risks and Strengths: STAR

Finding the balance between focusing on the promotion of caregiving that will lead to secure attachment and responding to critical contextual pressures facing the family is a challenge that most early preventive interventions for vulnerable families must address. Parents living in poverty and those with multiple stressors must divide their resources between focusing on the emotional needs of their infants and responding to factors external to the parent–child dyad that can interfere with their abilities to care competently for their children (e.g., meeting the next rent payment, paying for diapers, and dealing with interpersonal violence with partners). How programs address this fundamental challenge is crucial. To support nurses regarding prioritization or program content, as well as visitation frequency, we have developed a more rigorous method of classifying families' risks and strengths that provides more explicit guidance to nurses and supervisors in adjusting their frequency of visits, as well as visit content, with the goal of improving program effectiveness and efficiency.

Improving Nurses Resources in Addressing Intimate Partner Violence

In the first trial of the NFP, we found that its impact on state-verified rates of child abuse and neglect through child age 15 was attenuated in households with moderate to high levels of intimate partner violence (IPV; Eckenrode et al., 2000; Olds, 2002). While there was some evidence that NFP reduced IPV in the third trial (Olds, Robinson, Pettitt, Luckey, Holmberg, et al., 2004), that finding has not yet been replicated in the United States. Harriet MacMillan and Susan Jack developed a new intervention for NFP nurses to use in the presence of emerging IPV that is designed to align with NFP's underlying theories and operating procedures; this curriculum is now being tested in a 15-site randomized controlled trial, with funding from the Centers for Disease Control and Prevention (Jack et al., 2012).

Improving Nurses' Resources in Addressing Maternal Depression and Anxiety

Nurses in community settings have requested more support in addressing parents' mental health, so we developed a set of mental health screening tools for NFP nurses to use and pilot tested them in New York City and Los Angeles County. Many nurses felt that they had a better understanding of mental disorders after this training but reported that few mental health services were available in their communities, and even when services were available, their clients used them infrequently. Linda Beeber, from the University of North Carolina School of Nursing, has recently joined our team to develop mental health tools that are consistent with the NFP model, and that can be implemented by nurses with limited burden.

Conclusions

This program of prenatal and infancy home visiting by nurses shows promise for reducing some of the most damaging and widespread problems faced by low-income children and families in our society. The NFP is grounded in epidemiology and theories of development and behavior change, is specified in detailed guidelines, and has produced enduring and replicated effects with different populations, in different contexts, and at different points in time in a series of randomized controlled trials. Since publication of the results from the trials, the demand for the program in local communities, states, and societies outside the United States has been strong. Bringing about reliable, healthful changes in early parental care given varying family contexts, parents' earlier experiences, and genetic makeups, however, continues to be a challenge.

Support for ongoing evaluation and evolution of the NFP and other evidence-based programs to ensure public health impacts is critical. As programs are implemented in community practice, they are likely to serve more diverse populations, in differing economic and historical contexts than originally tested, and with greater diversity in service provider backgrounds and experiences.

In additional to ongoing evaluation, support for research and implementation of program augmentations need to be supported as programs work to address programmatic vulnerabilities and evolve to meet the needs of communities over time. The NFP had developed a model for program augmentation that starts with identifications of program challenges and moves on to formative development, pilot testing of innovations, rigorous testing, then translation into practice (Olds et al., 2013). Application of this model allows evidence-based programs to evolve to meet implementation challenges without compromising program integrity.

ACKNOWLEDGMENTS

The work reported here was made possible by support from many different sources, including the Administration for Children and Families (90PD0215/01 and 90PJ0003), Biomedical Research Support (PHS S7RR05403–25), Bureau of Community Health Services, Maternal and Child Health Research Grants Division (MCR-360403–07–0), the Carnegie Corporation (B-5492), the Colorado Trust (93059), the Commonwealth Fund (10443), the David and Lucile Packard Foundation (95–1842), the Ford Foundation (840–0545, 845–0031, and 875–0559), Maternal and Child Health, Department of Health and Human Services (MCJ-363378–01–0), National Center for Nursing Research (NR01–01691–05), National Institute of Mental Health (1-K05-MH01382–01 and 1-R01-MH49381–01A1), Pew Charitable Trusts (88–0211–000), the Robert Wood Johnson Foundation (179–34, 5263, 6729, 9677, and 35369), U.S. Department of Justice (95-DD-BX-0181), and the W. T. Grant Foundation (80072380, 84072380, 86108086, and 88124688). We thank John Shannon for his support of the program and data gathering through Comprehensive Interdisciplinary Developmental Services, Elmira, New York; Robert Chamberlin for his contributions to the early phases of this research; Jackie Roberts, Liz Chilson, Lyn Scazafabo, Georgie McGrady, and Diane Farr for their home-visitation work with the Elmira families; Geraldine Smith, for her supervision of the nurses in Memphis; Jann Belton and Carol Ballard, for integrating the program into the Memphis/Shelby County Health Department; Kim Sidora and Jane Powers, for their work on the Elmira and Memphis trials; the many other home-visiting nurses in Memphis and Denver; and the participating families who have made this program of research possible.

REFERENCES

Ainsworth, M. D. S., Blehar, M. C., Waters, E., & Wall, S. (1978). *Patterns of attachment: A psychological study of the strange situation*. Hillsdale, NJ: Erlbaum.

Aos, S., Lieb, R., Mayfield, J., Miller, M., & Pennucci, A. (2004). *Benefits and costs of prevention and early intervention programs for youth.* Olympia: Washington State Institute for Public Policy.

Bakan, D. (1971). *Slaughter of the innocents: A study of the battered child phenomenon.* San Francisco: Jossey-Bass.

Bandura, A. (1977). Self-efficacy: Toward a untifing theory of behavioral change. *Psychological Review, 84*(2), 191–215.

Belsky, J. (1981). Early human experience: A family perspective. *Developmental Psychology, 17*, 3–23.

Bowlby, J. (1969). *Attachment and loss: Vol. 1. Attachment.* New York: Basic Books.

Brafford, L. J., & Beck, K. H. (1991). Development and validation of a condom self-efficacy scale for college students. *Journal of American College Health, 39*(5), 219–225.

Brennan, P., Grekin, E., & Mednick, S. (1999). Maternal smoking during pregnancy and adult male criminal outcomes. *Archives of General Psychiatry, 56*, 215–219.

Bronfenbrenner, U. (1979). *The ecology of human development: Experiments in nature and design.* Cambridge, MA: Harvard University Press.

Bronfenbrenner, U. (1995). Developmental ecology through space and time: A future perspective. In P. Moen, G. H. Elder, Jr., & K. Luscher (Eds.), *Examining lives in context* (pp. 619–647). Washington, DC: American Psychological Association.

Buchsbaum, H. K., Toth, S. L., Clyman, R. B., Cicchetti, D., & Emde, R. N. (1992). The use of a narrative story stem technique with maltreated children: Implications for theory and practice. *Development and Psychopathology, 4*, 603–625.

Cole, R., Henderson, C. R. J., Kitzman, H., Anson, E., Eckenrode, J., & Sidora, K. (2004). *Long-term effects of nurse home visitation on maternal employment.* Unpublished manuscript, University of Rochester, Rochester, NY.

Dodge, K. A., Bates, J. E., & Pettit, G. S. (1990). Mechanisms in the cycle of violence. *Science, 250*(4988), 1678–1683.

Eckenrode, J., Ganzel, B., Henderson, C. R., Jr., Smith, E., Olds, D. L., Powers, J., . . . Sidora, K. (2000). Preventing child abuse and neglect with a program of nurse home visitation: The limiting effects of domestic violence. *Journal of the American Medical Association, 284*(11), 1385–1391.

Egeland, B., Jacobvitz, D., & Sroufe, A. (1988). Breaking the cycle of abuse. *Child Development, 59*, 1080–1088.

Elster, A. B., & McAnarney, E. R. (1980). Medical and psychosocial risks of pregnancy and childbearing during adolescence. *Pediatric Annals, 9*(3), 89–94.

Emde, R. N., & Buchsbaum, H. K. (1990). "Didn't you hear my mommy?": Autonomy with connectedness in moral self-emergence. In D. Cicchetti & M. Beeghley (Eds.), *The self in transition: Infancy to childhood* (pp. 35–60). Chicago: University of Chicago Press.

Fried, P., Watkinson, B., Dillon, R., & Dulberg, C. (1987). Neonatal neurological status in a low risk population after prenatal exposure to cigarettes, marijuana, and alcohol. *Developmental and Behavioral Pediatrics, 8*(6), 318–326.

Furstenberg, F. F., Brooks-Gunn, J., & Morgan, S. P. (1987). *Adolescent mothers in later life.* New York: Cambridge University Press.

Garbarino, J. (1981). An ecological perspective on child maltreatment. In L. Pelton (Ed.), *The social context of child abuse and neglect* (pp. 228–267). New York: Human Sciences Press.

Gil, D. (1970). *Violence against children: Physical child abuse in the United States.* Cambridge, MA: Harvard University Press.

Hart, B., & Risley, T. R. (1995). *Meaningful differences in the everyday experience ofr young American children.* Baltimore: Brookes.

Heinrich, L. B. (1993). Contraceptive self-efficacy in college women. *Journal of Adolescent Health, 14*(4), 269–276.

Institute of Medicine. (1990). *Nutrition during pregnancy*. Washington, DC: National Academy Press.

Jack, S. M., Ford-Gilboe, M., Wathen, C. N., Davidov, D. M., McNaughton, D. B., Coben, J. H., . . . NFP IVP Research Team. (2012). Development of a nurse home visitation intervention for intimate partner violence. *BMC Health Services Research, 12*, 50.

Karoly, L. A., Kilburn, M. R., & Cannon, J. S. (2005). *Early childhood interventions: Proven results, future promise*. Santa Monica, CA: RAND Corporation.

Kempe, C. H. (1973). A practical approach to the protection of the abused child and rehabilitation of the abusing parent. *Pediatrics, 51*(Suppl. 4), 804–812.

Kitzman, H. J., Olds, D. L., Cole, R. E., Hanks, C. A., Anson, E. A., Arcoleo, K. J., . . . Barnard, K. (2010). Enduring effects of prenatal and infancy home visiting by nurses on children: Follow-up of a randomized trial among children at age 12 years. *Archives of Pediatrics and Adolescent Medicine, 164*(5), 412–418.

Kitzman, H., Olds, D. L., Henderson, C. R., Jr., Hanks, C., Cole, R., Tatelbaum, R., . . . Holmberg, J. R. (1997). Effect of prenatal and infancy home visitation by nurses on pregnancy outcomes, childhood injuries, and repeated childbearing: A randomized controlled trial. *Journal of the American Medical Association, 278*(8), 644–652.

Kitzman, H., Olds, D. L., Sidora, K., Henderson, C. R., Jr., Hanks, C., Cole, R., . . . Glazner, J. (2000). Enduring effects of nurse home visitation on maternal life course: A 3-year follow-up of a randomized trial. *Journal of the American Medical Association, 283*(15), 1983–1989.

Klein, L., & Goldenberg, R. L. (1990). Prenatal care and its effect on preterm birth and low birthweight. In I. R. Merkatz & J. E. Thompson (Eds.), *New perspectives on prenatal care* (pp. 501–529). New York: Elsevier.

Kramer, M. S. (1987). Intrauterine growth and gestational duration determinants. *Pediatrics, 80*(4), 502–511.

Levinson, R. A. (1986). Contraceptive self-efficacy: A perspective on teenage girls' contraceptive behavior. *Journal of Sex Research, 22*, 347–369.

Main, D. (1985). No decrease in prematurity. *Clinical Aspects of High-Risk Pregnancy, 3*, 1–2.

Main, M. K., & Cassidy, J. (1985). Security in infancy, childhood, and adulthood: A move to the level of representation. In I. W. Bretherton (Ed.), *Growing points of attachment theory and research: Monographs of the Society for Research in Child Development*. (Vol. 50, pp. 66–104). New York: Wiley.

Main, M., Kaplan, N., & Cassidy, J. (1985). Security in infancy, childhood, and adulthood: A move to the level of representation. *Monographs of the Society for Research in Child Development, 50*(1–2, Serial No. 209), 66–104.

Mejdoubi, J., van den Heijkant, S., van Leerdam, F., Heymans, M., Crijnen, A., & Hirasing, R. (2015). The effect of VoorZorg, the Dutch nurse–family partnership, on child maltreatment and development: A randomized controlled trial. *PLOS ONE, 10*, e0120182.

Mejdoubi, J., van den Heijkant, S., van Leerdam, F., Heymans, M., Hirasing, R., & Crijnen, A. (2013). Effect of nurse-home visits vs. usual care on reducing intimate partner violence in young high-risk pregnant women: A randomized controlled trial. *PLOS One, 8*, e78185.

Milberger, S., Biederman, J., Faraone, S., Chen, L., & Jones, J. (1996). Is maternal smoking during pregnancy a risk factor for attention deficit hyperactivity disorder in children? *American Journal of Psychiatry, 153*(9), 1138–1142.

Musick, J. S. (1993). *Young, poor and pregnant*. New Haven, CT: Yale University Press.

Newberger, C. M., & White, K. M. (1989). Cognitive foundations for parental care. In D. Cicchetti & V. Carlson (Eds.), *Child maltreatment:Theory and research on the causes and consequences of child abuse and neglect* (pp. 302–316). Cambridge, UK: Cambridge University Press.

Olds, D. (2016). Building evidence to improve child and family health. *Lancet, 387*(10014), 105–107.

Olds, D., Donelan-McCall, N., O'Brien, R., MacMillan, H., Jack, S., Jenkins, T., . . . Beeber, L. (2013). Improving the nurse–family partnership in community practice. *Pediatrics, 132*(Suppl. 2), S110–S117.

Olds, D., Eckenrode, J., Henderson, C., Kitzman, H., Powers, J., Cole, R., . . . Luckey, D. (1997). Long-term effects of home visitation on maternal life course and child abuse and neglect: A 15-year follow-up of a randomized trial. *Journal of the American Medical Association, 278*(8), 637–643.

Olds, D., Kitzman, H., Cole, R., Robinson, J., Sidora, K., Luckey, D., . . . Holmberg, J. (2004). Effects of nurse home visiting on maternal life-course and child development: Age-six follow-up of a randomized trial. *Pediatrics, 114*, 1550–1559.

Olds, D. L. (1997). Tobacco exposure and impaired development: A review of the evidence. *Mental Retardation and Developmental Disabilities Research Reviews, 3*, 257–269.

Olds, D. L. (2002). Prenatal and infancy home visiting by nurses: From randomized trials to community replication. *Prevention Science, 3*(3), 153–172.

Olds, D. L. (2016). Building evidence to improve maternal and child health. *The Lancet, 387*, 105–107.

Olds, D. L., Henderson, C. R., Jr., Chamberlin, R., & Tatelbaum, R. (1986). Preventing child abuse and neglect: A randomized trial of nurse home visitation. *Pediatrics, 78*(1), 65–78.

Olds, D. L., Henderson, C. R., Jr., & Kitzman, H. (1994). Does prenatal and infancy nurse home visitation have enduring effects on qualities of parental caregiving and child health at 25 to 50 months of life? *Pediatrics, 93*(1), 89–98.

Olds, D. L., Henderson, C. R., Jr., & Tatelbaum, R. (1994a). Intellectual impairment in children of women who smoke cigarettes during pregnancy. *Pediatrics, 93*(2), 221–227.

Olds, D. L., Henderson, C. R., Jr., & Tatelbaum, R. (1994b). Prevention of intellectual impairment in children of women who smoke cigarettes during pregnancy. [Erratum in *Pediatrics* 1994 6(1), 973]. *Pediatrics, 93*(2), 228–233.

Olds, D. L., Henderson, C. R., Jr., Tatelbaum, R., & Chamberlin, R. (1986). Improving the delivery of prenatal care and outcomes of pregnancy: A randomized trial of nurse home visitation. *Pediatrics, 77*(1), 16–28.

Olds, D. L., Henderson, C. R., Jr., Tatelbaum, R., & Chamberlin, R. (1988). Improving the life-course development of socially disadvantaged mothers: A randomized trial of nurse home visitation. *American Journal of Public Health, 78*(11), 1436–1445.

Olds, D. L., Holmberg, J. R., Donelan-McCall, N., Luckey, D. W., Knudtson, M. D., & Robinson, J. (2014). Effects of home visits by paraprofessionals and by nurses on children: Follow-up of a randomized trial at ages 6 and 9 years. *JAMA Pediatrics, 168*(2), 114–121.

Olds, D. L., Kitzman, H., Hanks, C., Cole, R., Anson, E., Sidora-Arcoleo, K., . . . Bondy, J. (2007). Effects of nurse home visiting on maternal and child functioning: Age-9 follow-up of a randomized trial. *Pediatrics, 120*(4), e832–e845.

Olds, D. L., Robinson, J., O'Brien, R., Luckey, D. W., Pettitt, L. M., Henderson, C. R., Jr., . . . Talmi, A. (2002). Home visiting by paraprofessionals and by nurses: A randomized, controlled trial. *Pediatrics, 110*(3), 486–496.

Olds, D. L., Robinson, J., Pettitt, L., Luckey, D. W., Holmberg, J., Ng, R. K., . . . Sheff, K. (2004). Effects of home visits by paraprofessionals and by nurses: Age-4 follow-up of a randomized trial. *Pediatrics, 114*, 1560–1568.

Overpeck, M., Brenner, R., Trumble, A., Trifiletti, L., & Berendes, H. (1998). Risk factors for infant homicide in the United States. *New England Journal of Medicine, 339*(17), 1211–1216.

Peterson, L., & Gable, S. (1998). Holistic injury prevention. In J. R. Lutzker (Ed.), *Handbook of child abuse research and treatment* (pp. 291–318). New York: Plenum Press.

Quinton, D., & Rutter, M. (1984). Parents with children in care–II. Intergenerational continuities. *Journal of Child Psychology and Psychiatry, 25*(2), 231–250.

Robling, M., Bekkers, M.-J., Bell, K., Butler, C., Cannings-John, R., Channon, S., . . . Torgerson, D. (2016). Effectiveness of a nurse-led intensive home-visiting programme for first-time teenage mothers (Building Blocks): A pragmatic randomised controlled trial. *Lancet, 387*(10014), 146–155.

Rutter, M. (1989). Intergenerational continuities and discontinuities in serious parenting difficulties. In D. Cicchetti & V. Carlson (Eds.), *Child maltreatment: Theory and research on the causes and consequences of child abuse and neglect* (pp. 317–348). Cambridge, UK: Cambridge University Press.

Sameroff, A. J. (1983). Parental views of child development. In R. A. Hoekelman (Ed.), *A round-table on minimizing high-risk parenting* (pp. 31–45). Media, PA: Harwal.

Streissguth, A. P., Sampson, P. D., Barr, H. M., Bookstein, F. L., & Olson, H. C. (1994). The effects of prenatal exposure to alcohol and tobacco: Contributions from the Seattle longitudinal prospective study and implications for public policy. In H. L. Needleman & D. Bellinger (Eds.), *Prenatal exposure to toxicants: Developmental consequences* (pp. 148–183). Baltimore: Johns Hopkins University Press.

Teicher, M. H. (2000). Wounds that time won't heal: The neurobiology of child abuse. *Cerebrum, 2*(4), 50–67.

Tygart, C. E. (1991). Juvenile delinquency and number of children in a family: Some empirical and theoretical updates. *Youth and Society, 22*(4), 525–536.

Wachs, T. D. (1989). The nature of the physical microenvironment: An expanded classification system. *Merrill–Palmer Quarterly, 35*(4), 399–419.

Wakschlag, L. S., Lahey, B. B., Loeger, R., Green, S. M., Gordon, R. A., & Leventhal, B. L. (1997). Maternal smoking during pregnancy and the risk of conduct disorder in boys. *Archives of General Psychiatry, 54*(7), 670–676.

CHAPTER 5

Steps Toward Effective, Enjoyable Parenting

Lessons from 30 Years of Implementation, Adaptation, and Evaluation

GERHARD J. SUESS, MARTHA FARRELL ERICKSON,
BYRON EGELAND, HERMANN SCHEUERER-ENGLISCH,
and HANS-PETER HARTMANN

Lucy (not her real name) was pregnant with a baby fathered by an occasional customer at the bar where she worked. After going out with the man a few times, Lucy realized he was disturbed and violent, so she wanted no further involvement with him, even though he was the father of her baby. She proclaimed that she and her baby would do fine on their own. Lucy reported having distant relationships with her parents, who lived in a neighboring state. She described in a flat, unemotional tone repeated childhood episodes of physical and sexual abuse by her father and chronic rejection by her mother. She dismissed her childhood experience by saying brusquely, "That was then, this is now." Within hours after giving birth to a healthy baby girl, Lucy began talking about how her tiny daughter would need to "learn to be tough," so she didn't want to coddle her too much.

Although every family is unique, the multiple issues Lucy and her baby face are not unusual: poverty; lack of marketable job skills to help parent and child move out of poverty; a weak support system (i.e., either isolation or a social network that is not supportive of health, well-being and positive parenting approaches); parent's dismissive state of mind about past relationships, as well as about baby's needs for comfort and security as the foundation for real strength rather than "toughness." It is these issues that the STEEP™ Program (Steps Toward Effective, Enjoyable Parenting) was developed to address through an individualized, relationship-based model of service grounded in attachment theory and research, and guided by longitudinal findings on the risk and protective factors that shape the quality of parent–infant attachment and other aspects of positive parenting, including parents' healthy life choices throughout the child's growing-up years (Sroufe, Egeland, Carlson, & Collins, 2005).

Martha Farrell Erickson and Byron Egeland developed STEEP in 1986, at the University of Minnesota and, with funding from the National Institute of Mental Health (NIMII), implemented the program for the first time as part of a randomized controlled study of the program's effectiveness (Egeland & Erickson, 1993). The focus and overall program design of STEEP was guided by findings from the ongoing Minnesota Longitudinal Study of Risk and Adaptation, particularly the factors shown to predict parental sensitivity and responsiveness, secure parent–infant attachment, and positive parent–child interactions at later stages of childhood. Thus, the program aimed to promote (1) parental knowledge and understanding of infant and child development, with an emphasis on understanding the developmental meaning and significance of key behaviors such as separation anxiety or toddler negativism; (2) parental perspective taking with regard to child behavior, the ability to "see through the eyes of the child"; (3) sensitivity and responsiveness to infant cues and signals; (4) parental recognition of how past relationships, particularly childhood experiences, influence the way parents interpret and respond to their child; (5) life choices that are in the best interest of the child (e.g., relationship decisions, educational pursuits, financial management, health-related behaviors); and (6) support networks that encourage healthy, responsible behavior and positive parenting (Erickson, Korfmacher, & Egeland, 1992; Egeland & Erickson, 2004). Consultation with experienced frontline workers in public health, obstetrics, pediatrics, and social services informed practical components of the STEEP program, including strategies and timing for optimal engagement of participants, effective approaches and incentives for group participation, and logistical issues related to schedules, transportation, communication, and equipment needs.

We describe in this chapter the original STEEP program and the longitudinal research that informed it, original outcome findings from an evaluation of a 1-year version of the program, and highlights of dissemination, implementation, and adaptation of STEEP in various locations and contexts in the United States and Canada. We then provide an account of STEEP practice, research, and training in Germany that dates from 2005, concluding with a discussion of lessons learned from the collective body of more than 30 years of STEEP work.

STEEP Program Description

STEEP (Erickson, Egeland, Simon, & Rose, 2002) was designed from the beginning to be a relationship-based program, guided by research findings that resilience and positive shifts in the course of an individual's development often come about through experience with a caring, responsive person who offers a new way of being in relationship (Sroufe et al., 2005). In other words, relationships change relationships. Thus, the STEEP facilitator who will be working with the family is, whenever possible, the person who first approaches the expectant mother (ideally during the second trimester of pregnancy) to offer her the opportunity to participate in the voluntary program, to describe what the program involves, and to answer any questions the woman has. The general approach is to explain to the potential participant that STEEP is a way for first-time moms to get the support and information they need for themselves and their babies as they embark on what often is the greatest joy and the greatest challenge a person faces—parenthood.

Recruitment usually is done through obstetric clinics, with nurses identifying women who meet eligibility criteria and asking their permission for a STEEP facilitator to talk with them about the program. (Note that as mentioned in later sections of this chapter, there have been necessary variations in recruitment strategies when STEEP has been implemented in different settings and with special populations.)

Home Visits

Biweekly home visits begin as soon as a woman is enrolled in STEEP and continue throughout the program (until the child's first birthday in the original NIMH-funded study, but until the child's second birthday in most subsequent implementations of the program). Home visits typically are 1–2 hours in length and are individualized to address the unique strengths and needs of each family, always with a focus on how the baby is growing and learning, how the parent–child relationship is developing, and how the health, well-being and life circumstances of the parents are (or are not) supporting good parent–child relationships and optimal child development.

There is great value in meeting with the family in the home environment; however, a home visit also may include going outside for a walk with parent and child or visiting a coffee shop or park in the neighborhood, which are especially healthy options when a mother is depressed and/or isolated. Walking side by side sometimes makes it easier for parents to let down their defenses and talk more candidly about their feelings and experiences, gradually building a relationship of trust with their facilitator. Although the mother is the point of entry into the family's participation in STEEP and is a primary focus of the program, fathers or father figures and other adults in the household also are engaged in home visiting when possible. For example, fathers often participate in the Seeing Is Believing® video strategy, described below.

Seeing Is Believing

A core strategy for working with parents during home visits is Seeing Is Believing, a part of the STEEP program from its conceptualization in 1985–1986, but later formalized and trademarked as a strategy that has been integrated into many different home-visiting and parent education program models, with training and support from STEEP trainers (Erickson, 2005). Seeing Is Believing involves video-recording a few minutes of parent–infant interaction (e.g., routine child care tasks such as feeding, dressing, or bathing; interactive floor-play with age-appropriate toys; or a favorite activity suggested by the parent). Then, the STEEP facilitator views the video with the parent, using primarily open-ended questions to help the parent discover how the baby is feeling, how the baby uses cues and signals to tell the parent what he or she needs or wants, and how the parent's responses to baby's cues are teaching the baby what to expect and how to count on the parent. Questions might move from a very broad "What did you notice in this video?" to more specific questions, such as "What do you think your baby was telling you here?" or "What did your baby seem to enjoy most during this activity?"

Sometimes the baby becomes fussy or signals in other ways that this is not what he or she wants to do right now—or perhaps a parent tries too hard to direct the baby's play rather than follow the baby's lead. Then it can be effective to say, "Let's try something different. How about playing 'follow the leader' and letting your baby take the lead. I'll record for just a couple of minutes and we can see how that works." This captures the spirit of shared discovery that is central to the Seeing Is Believing strategy and the STEEP program as a whole.

Ideally, the STEEP facilitator reviews the video with the parent(s) right after recording. However, sometimes the baby's need or a parent's schedule makes that difficult or impossible. In these situations, the facilitator may choose to wait and review the video with the parent during the next home visit. Sometimes the video review process may take only 5 or 10 minutes. But often, what happens between parent and child on video may trigger a deeper discussion of emotionally sensitive issues that require more time. Because Seeing Is Believing is not a scripted curriculum, but a tool for helping parents reflect on their baby's needs and their own strengths and challenges in meeting those needs, STEEP facilitators follow the lead of both baby and parent in the video review process, using it as effectively as possible to help the parent learn and grow.

One of the most important reasons for using Seeing Is Believing during all or most home visits is that it is a very concrete way of keeping the baby—and the parent–infant relationship—front and center. So many other life events and crises (e.g., family conflicts, financial problems, difficulties with job or school) can become the focus of a home visit, just as those challenges can interfere with a parent's emotional availability and responsiveness to the baby's needs. So, no matter what else is going on in the household, using Seeing Is Believing is a very practical and literal way to answer the question, "What about the baby?" Viewing the video together affords an opportunity to explore with the parent(s) how they are managing to stay attuned to their baby even in the midst of challenges and difficult life events they are facing. (As described in a later section of this chapter, one of the positive findings of our initial STEEP evaluation was that participation in the program appeared to serve as a buffer between stressful life events and parental sensitivity [Egeland & Erickson, 2004].)

Mother–Infant Groups

STEEP facilitators recruit participants to form groups of eight to 10 families with due dates within a few weeks of each other. Initially after enrollment (during pregnancy), the facilitator gets to know each participating woman and her family through home visits. During that time, the facilitator sends brief informal newsletters to the participants, including helpful information about labor and delivery, preparing for the arrival of the baby, and ways to stay comfortable during the final days of pregnancy and after childbirth. These newsletters, which may be sent by mail or e-mail, depending on families' preferences and access to technology, also are a way to begin to establish a sense of group belonging even before the participants meet each other. With permission of the individual moms, the facilitator includes in the newsletter a bit of information about each mom—her favorite activities, baby names she's considering, good deals she found on baby equipment, or her plans to return to school or work after her maternity leave.

Then, when some or all of the babies have arrived, the facilitator convenes the first mother–infant group session, with groups continuing to meet biweekly throughout the program. Each session begins with mother–infant interaction time, with activities structured around the developmental issues that are common for babies of the ages in the group. Structure is flexible to allow facilitators to capitalize on teachable moments in their observations of what the babies are doing.

Following interaction time, moms and babies share a healthy meal together—an enjoyable time of relationship building and also a situation rich with teachable moments. After the meal, mothers go with their facilitator into another room for "mom-talk" time while their babies are cared for and engaged in age-appropriate activities by STEEP early childhood staff. The STEEP facilitator's guide (Erickson et al., 2002; Erickson & Egeland, 2006) includes many possible activities to use both for mother–infant interaction time and for "mom-talk" time. But, in general, "mom-talk" is a time for mutual support and discussion of the mothers' own issues, including balancing baby's needs and adult needs, building or maintaining healthy relationships with partners and others, pursuing educational and work goals, and reflecting on how past relationship experiences shape the way mothers understand and respond to their children's needs. There are "aha moments" when mothers discover common feelings and experiences. And, because the same facilitator who

---

TABLE 5.1. Activities and Principles of STEEP Program

Activities

- Home visits
  - Prenatal: biweekly
  - 0–2: biweekly
- Seeing Is Believing: monthly or more
- Mother–infant group: biweekly
- Family nights: occasional (two to three per year)

Principles

- Relationship-based—change happens within a relationship of respect, authenticity, shared discovery, and problem solving
- Reflective—through reflection, knowledge is more easily integrated and applied, and life choices are viewed through a new lens
- Strengths-focused—each child and parent has strengths on which to build; leading with strengths eases the way to facing challenges
- Individualized—each person's history, experience, and life circumstances are unique and need to be addressed as such
- Ecological—the community, culture, and larger society of each family need to be taken into account, with a focus on both opportunity and challenge

is leading the group will be visiting each mother in the next week or so, there are opportunities for personal follow-up and integration of group themes into the individualized work with each parent and child.

Family Nights

To more fully engage fathers of babies, grandparents, and other significant adults in the families of participants, the STEEP program also offers occasional family nights (typically two or three times a year), with each mother deciding whom she would like to invite. These are celebratory events that may be held indoors or outdoors, with a casual meal or refreshments, craft activities or games, or perhaps at a place for taking family photos and providing an opportunity for extended family members to view parent–child videos made during home visits. This can be a good time to give each family a book to read with baby, a CD of songs you have sung with moms and babies during group sessions, or simple tip sheets on parenting, such as how to make bedtime go smoothly, or helpful ways to handle separation anxiety.

Summary of Findings from Initial Research

We have described elsewhere the findings from the original implementation and evaluation of STEEP (Erickson et al., 1992; Egeland & Erickson, 1995, 2004). We summarize those early findings very briefly here, which allows us to focus more on recent findings (particularly from the ongoing research on STEEP in Germany) and on the practical lessons and lingering questions from the many applications and adaptations of STEEP. The initial implementation and evaluation was conducted on 154 low-income, English-speaking women age 17 years and older (range = 17–25, mean = 20.4) who were pregnant with their first child, had no more than a high school education (less in many cases), and were not known to have a diagnosis of a major mental health disorder or cognitive disability. Although marital status was not a selection criterion, 92% of participants were unmarried at the time of enrollment. As more information about the participants emerged during the implementation and evaluation of the program, it became clear that these young women had many other risk factors in their lives, most notably, a very high incidence of abuse and neglect in childhood, abuse by romantic partners, and significant symptoms of depression and other mental health problems (Egeland, Erickson, Butcher, & Ben-Porath, 1991).

The original study evaluated only a 1-year version of the STEEP program, and that evaluation was conducted on the first implementation of the program, without an opportunity to run a pilot intervention before launching the randomized study. Nonetheless, the study showed positive results of the program in promoting protective factors and reducing risks among participants. But results with regard to quality of parent–infant attachment, particularly at 1 year, were disappointing and complicated (Egeland & Erickson, 1995).

Compared to families in the control group ($n = 80$), mother–infant pairs participating in the STEEP program ($n = 74$) were no more likely to be classified as having a secure attachment at infant age 1, when the intervention ended. In fact, infants in the intervention group exhibited more disorganized attachment behavior than the controls in the 1-year end-of-treatment assessments. However, in a second assessment of attachment at 19 months of age (7 months posttreatment), that no longer was the case, and there was a substantial drop in the percentage of control pairs (from 67 to 48%) who were classified as securely attached, which was not true of mothers and children in the intervention group.

In various other ways, intervention families were doing better than control families at the end of the intervention when their babies were 1 year old. Intervention mothers demonstrated better knowledge and understanding of child development. They had more appropriately organized home environments and were more responsive to their babies' needs during in-home assessments. Intervention mothers used better life management skills in their daily lives and more active coping strategies at times of duress. They also reported fewer depressive symptoms than did mothers in the control group. Intervention mothers also were less likely to have another baby within 2 years after the birth of their first child. Interestingly, while high levels of life stress were associated with maternal insensitivity in the control group, that was not true within the intervention group. Thus, it appeared that participating in the STEEP intervention had a buffering effect that allowed mothers in the intervention group to provide to their infants sensitive care even when facing difficult life circumstances.

Both positive and negative findings from the original implementation and evaluation have shaped the way the program—and the training and ongoing support and supervision of staff—have been refined and improved over the years. In a later section of this chapter, we discuss both challenges and successes of those 30 years of STEEP work and implications for practice and future research.

Examples of Subsequent Applications and Adaptations

Soon after the initial STEEP implementation and evaluation study summarized above, several agencies began working with the developers of STEEP to apply or adapt the program in different contexts with specific high-risk populations. What follows are brief descriptions of a small sample of those efforts.

St. David's Center for Child and Family Development

A large, multiservice agency with a focus on early childhood education, mental health and family support services, St. David's Center for Child and Family Development (SDC), in Minnetonka, Minnesota, implemented the full STEEP program, serving families identified by clinics as high risk for child abuse, from pregnancy until children were 3 years old. Families then were encouraged to use other services provided by the agency, including early childhood education for their children, and many did. Internal evaluations showed high participant satisfaction and good progress on measures of parental knowledge, understanding, and parenting behavior.

Adaptations for Substance-Abusing Families

With state funding aimed at substance-abusing families, two medical clinics, Community University Health Care Center (CUHCC) in Minneapolis and Healthstart in St. Paul, implemented the STEEP program with mothers who tested positive for drugs during pregnancy. The dynamics of building relationships with these mothers were especially challenging because of defensiveness and anger that they had been "caught." Many of the participants in the CUHCC program were Native Americans and, despite the many challenges they faced, they responded well to an effort to incorporate traditions and symbols from their native culture into the program, choosing to call their program "Circle of Women." For many, their babies became the motivators in their attempt to become alcohol- and drug-free.

Baby's Space Partnership

Building on the success of "Circle of Women"—and responding to the influx of many young mothers into the workforce due to welfare reform in the 1990s—Amos Deinard, Medical Director of CUHCC, and psychologist Terrie Rose developed the Baby's Space model, which integrated STEEP services and therapeutic child care for high-risk infants and toddlers. With funding from the Irving B. Harris Foundation, the University of Minnesota's Irving B. Harris Center (now merged with the Center for Early Education and Development) expanded the Baby's Space model to multiple urban child care centers in Minneapolis.

Parenting Partnership at Mary Bridge Children's Hospital

At Mary Bridge Children's Hospital in Tacoma, Washington, the STEEP model is used to serve families of premature, medically fragile babies who have spent time in the neonatal intensive care unit (NICU). Babies are at risk for developmental delays, and about 45% face long-term medical issues. On intake questionnaires, all parents in the program endorse having a childhood history of abuse. Families also experience many psychosocial stressors, including poverty, social isolation, and unstable housing, and more than 40% of mothers report domestic violence in their current relationships.

Toward Better Beginnings, Allina Health

Several urban obstetric clinics in Minneapolis and St. Paul implemented a brief (3–4 months) nurse home-visiting program that used STEEP principles and the Seeing Is Believing video strategy with high-risk mothers. Since the program was so brief, to maximize its impact, they also trained clinic staff members to deliver consistent messages about the importance of parental sensitivity and attachment. Compared to a control group of similarly high-risk mothers who gave birth before the program was launched, intervention mothers demonstrated better knowledge of child development and were observed to be more responsive to their infants and to provide more appropriate play materials (Guthrie, Gaziano, & Gaziano, 2009).

STEEP Principles and Strategies in Public Health Nursing

Working with health departments in several states and counties or provinces across the United States and Canada, STEEP developers and approved trainers have provided training and ongoing reflective consultation to public health nurses in how to integrate STEEP principles and the Seeing Is Believing video approach into their home-based work with high-risk mothers and babies. Nurses and administrators indicate that Seeing is Believing helps them focus more carefully on parent–child interaction, helps parents interpret and respond appropriately to infant cues, and provides a useful framework for exploring issues that sometimes hinder parental sensitivity. Also, as in other STEEP programs, mothers and fathers have responded enthusiastically to the use of video. For example, in Ontario, Canada, the Niagara Region Public Health began using Seeing Is Believing in their nurse home-visiting program in 2000. Based on monitoring of nearly 300 participating families from 2010 through 2016, the agency reports that parents say they learn, "when my baby needs me; how to get my baby talking; and how to talk and play differently" (Biscaro & Hicks, 2017, pp. 5–6).

STEEP in Germany

In Germany, prior to 2000, interventions to help young mothers like Lucy, the mother described in the case opening this chapter, were scarce. Generally, support was available for children age 3 or older, but not for infants and parents. However, conferences for researchers and practitioners were beginning to spread knowledge about attachment theory and raise awareness of the importance of early intervention (e.g., Papousek, Schieche, & Wurmser, 2004, 2007; Suess & Pfeifer, 1999; Suess, Scheuerer-Englisch, & Pfeifer, 2001;Scheuerer-Englisch, Suess, & Pfeifer, 2003; Brisch, Grossmann, Grossmann, & Köhler, 2002).

It was at one of those conferences in Munich, in July 2000 (see Brisch et al., 2002), that Martha Erickson, Byron Egeland, and Gerhard Suess met and began to build a collaboration to implement and evaluate the STEEP model with high-risk parents and infants in Germany. From 2001 on, annual workshops with Martha Erickson were carried out in Hamburg for interested professionals, with the aim of bringing STEEP to Germany and designing an evaluation study to test the program's effectiveness empirically with German families. In 2005, with a first grant from the German Ministry of Education and Research (BMBF), the German evaluation project began at the Hamburg University of Applied Sciences and soon extended to other cities.[1] At that time, important cases of fatal child abuse led

---

[1]Initially this expansion began in cooperation with an evaluation project at the University of Applied Sciences in Potsdam (Christiane Ludwig-Koerner). Later STEEP was extended to Frankfurt and Offenburg with additional partners (e.g., Ruediger Kissgen, M. Frumentia Maier, Gabi Mankau) and grants from BHF-Bank-Foundation, National Center for Early Prevention (NZFH), the Thomas Gottschalk Foundation, and the Rotary-Club Offenburg-Ortenau, important milestones in importing STEEP. Most of all, the successful expansion relied on the dedicated STEEP facilitators and competent, committed research assistants, Uta Bohlen and Agnes Mali, and H. Theresita Hettich and M. Frumentia Maier, who contributed enormously to the growth of the German STEEP Project.

to the establishment of the National Center of Early Intervention (NZFH; 2009), which significantly advanced the proliferation of early intervention programs in Germany and the evaluation of STEEP (Renner & Heimeshoff, 2011; Cierpka & Evers, 2015).

Questions and Challenges Confronting the German STEEP Project

The introduction of STEEP in Germany raised the frequently asked question of whether an American program could be effective in Germany. Cultural differences raised skepticism among researchers, who questioned whether the worries and troubles of mothers like Lucy, who exist in both countries, are comparable in Germany and the United States. Would it be feasible and appropriate to formulate comparable intervention goals for these German mothers, and would STEEP provide the path toward those goals? Initially, we asked practitioners. We introduced STEEP facilitators from Minneapolis to German social workers in Hamburg. These personal meetings, which usually included viewing and discussing video recordings together, are deeply rooted in the tradition of attachment theory and research. However, this is not the only reason we emphasized reciprocal visits and personal encounters as part of the transatlantic exchange and the implementation of STEEP. Relationship-based programs such as STEEP are best passed on in personal encounters, with careful reflection on the experience of the babies, the parents, and the service providers—all considered within the broader social and cultural context in which the families live. Last, but not least, this personal approach highly values the experience of the STEEP facilitators in Minnesota, who have accumulated their knowledge over many years of practical involvement in the program. So, building on case examples and video recordings of mother–child pairs from Minnesota and Hamburg, we brought STEEP to Germany. In these meetings, practitioners soon agreed that clienteles in the two countries were comparable, an observation that was confirmed in the later transatlantic exchange.

Evaluation of the adaptability of STEEP in Germany also can be based on the developmental mechanisms on which the program focuses (e.g., parental sensitivity and the significance of the different attachment models in childhood and adulthood, as well as their effects throughout life). These were similar on both sides of the Atlantic, as the attachment research team of Klaus and Karin Grossmann first showed within the German culture (Grossmann, Grossmann, Spangler, Suess, & Unzner, 1985; Suess, Grossmann, & Sroufe, 1992; Grossmann, Grossmann, & Kindler, 2005; Grossmann, Grossmann, Fremmer-Bombik, Kindler, Scheuerer-Englisch, & Zimmermann, 2002). Attachment is a universality (see van IJzendoorn, & Kroonenberg, 1988; De Wolff & van IJzendoorn, 1997) and is suitable worldwide as a basis for intervention and parent programs, as studies by Bakermans-Kranenburg, van IJzendoorn, and Juffer (2003, 2008) have shown.

Another challenge facing the German STEEP project was that practitioners were skeptical about our demand to test the effectiveness of STEEP empirically—an issue not unique to Germany, as we learned during the transatlantic exchange. Practice-oriented research and the translation of the findings from attachment research in a practical context create arcs of tension, which need to be addressed carefully (Cicchetti & Hinshaw, 2002; Coie, Miller-Johnson, & Bagwell, 2000). John

Bowlby (1988) summarized common differences in thinking and interests between scientists and practitioners: "As practitioners we deal in complexity; as scientists we strive to simplify. As practitioners we use theory as a guide; as scientists we challenge that same theory. As practitioners we accept restricted modes of enquiry; as scientists we enlist every method we can" (p. 43). However, this does not mean that practitioners are merely optimists and scientists are hopeless skeptics. Scientists possess enormous faith, according to Bowlby, "faith that in the long run the best route to reliable knowledge is the application of scientific method" (p. 42), something practitioners often doubt.

Attachment theory and research are advantageous, though, in helping practitioners move through their skepticism and uneasiness with empirical evaluation of their work. This is because attachment theory was developed by a practitioner (Bowlby) to improve practice, and in many aspects integrates clinical understanding and empirical testing approaches. Especially the ethological approach that underlies attachment theory (Hinde, 1976; Grossmann, 1988) encourages an understanding through theory-guided observation, which is similar to clinical case understanding, and is the core of STEEP training and practice. As practitioners have become more experienced in theory-guided observation, they generally have become more comfortable and accepting of the value of empirical evaluation of the program.

STEEP Training in Germany

Leaders of the German STEEP project worked closely with their U.S. colleagues to develop a systematic training for STEEP facilitators that was suited to the culture and practices of Germany and its mental health and social services systems. The development of the training program was greatly advanced by the translation, adaptation, and publication in Germany of the *STEEP Facilitators' Guide* (Erickson et al., 2002). That volume includes specific home-visit and group activities and strategies, as well as a practice-friendly summary of the attachment theory and research that frames the STEEP program.

We selected STEEP trainers who had extensive practical experience as mental health professionals and also were scientist-practitioners who had conducted attachment research. We expected that people with that combination of experience would best be able to address the arcs of tension in carrying out both the STEEP intervention and the necessary research procedures, as mentioned before.

The training was structured in 10 two-day modules, beginning with an introduction of the basic principles of attachment theory and the most important results from longitudinal studies of attachment, particularly those at the University of Minnesota in the United States and the University of Regensburg, Germany. Trainees gain insights into the different attachment models in infants and toddlers (Ainsworth, Blehar, Waters, & Wall, 1978; Main & Solomon, 1990), attachment models in adulthood (Steele & Steele, 2008), the mechanisms responsible for continuities and changes in the lifespan, as well as an understanding of the role of early experiences in shaping lifelong relational attitudes and behavior (Sroufe et al., 2005; Grossmann, Grossmann, & Waters, 2005).

Our goal is to provide STEEP facilitators with as deep an understanding of attachment theory as possible, including attachment-based reflections about their own biographies (elaborated later in this chapter). In an individualized program such as STEEP, decisions often present themselves in new shapes and forms, and are not predetermined. But solid theory informs and guides thoughtful decisions across the many individual situations.

Another core focus area within attachment theory and research is Ainsworth's sensitivity concept and its application. In group supervision, which is integrated throughout the initial STEEP training and also in four all-day follow-up sessions, trainees rate video recordings of mother–child pairs on the Ainsworth Sensitivity Scale (*www.psychology.sunysb.edu/attachment/measures/measures_index.html*), achieving reliability in assessing maternal sensitivity. Longitudinal studies of the effects of sensitivity are used to provide an empirically based description of the guiding principle of "good enough parenting" (Grossmann et al., 1985; De Wolff & van IJzendoorn, 1997). Especially during video work, there is a danger of trying to optimize the mother's interaction with her child beyond what is necessary, which may produce undesired effects in high-risk parents. For instance, a level of sensitivity that is "too high" may not be sustainable over the day, the week, and so forth, and may put pressure on the attachment figures. In this way, STEEP mothers who are at risk of trying to be the perfect parent may resign themselves more readily, or, when they experience failure, may withdraw from what they perceive to be the source of this feeling of failure. It is for these reasons that the concept of "good enough" parenting is emphasized in the work with high-risk parents; meanwhile, research on long-term effects of sensitivity allows discussion of "good enough parenting," with the assistance of video clips.

During training and also during follow-up reflective supervision, the STEEP trainees have repeatedly described the quality of the observed interaction; we pay attention to participants' use Ainsworth's terminology from the sensitivity scale in order to encourage an internationally available professional language. So far, the focus on sensitivity has proven to be valuable, as longitudinal studies have repeatedly shown effects of the sensitivity scores on the life course, whether at age 14 or age 32, whether within the parent–child relationship or in new relationships, peer friendships or romantic relationships (Raby, Roisman, Fraley, & Simpson, 2015; Beijersbergen, Juffer, Bakermans-Kranenburg, & van IJzendoorn 2012; Grossmann et al., 2002, 2005).

The intervention focus on "sensitivity" also has proven to be effective, as studies on attachment-based intervention focusing on sensitivity have shown (for a summary, see Juffer, Bakermans-Kranenburg, & van IJzendoorn, 2014). However, interventions regularly show how sensitive parenting is hindered at different times and in different everyday situations. Parents may not react to their children's signals out of fear of spoiling their child, and may profit from information and knowledge that is provided by a psychoeducational approach. Other parents may not even be aware of their insensitivity and may even believe that they are extremely sensitive. The more insensitivity is linked to long-existing and deep-rooted automatic processes, the less a purely behavioral intervention to promote attachment security is sufficient. Hence, trainees learn to encourage parents to reflect critically on their day-to-day behavior toward the child. And they learn to help parents address the various factors that support or hinder them from providing sufficiently sensitive care.

To that last point, interventions can be framed within five different levels:

1. Level of parent–infant interaction.
2. Level of representation.
3. Level of "therapeutic" relationship, including practical help and problem solving.
4. Level of providing information and building knowledge.
5. Level of support (both providing support directly and also helping parents build or strengthen their natural support system).

Cutting across all five levels of intervention is the importance of enjoyment (the second E in STEEP), both in the relationship between the STEEP facilitator and the parents and the relationship between the parent and the child. STEEP developer Erickson has spent a great deal of time with STEEP trainers and facilitators in Germany and often has felt compelled to remind us to keep the second E in STEEP.

When parents do not find joy in the interaction with their child, sensitivity will not be long-lasting, especially for highly burdened young mothers. The Minnesota Longitudinal Study on Risk and Adaptation (Sroufe et al., 2005) observed that a change of attachment status from secure to insecure during the second year of life occurred more often in mothers who were less able to enjoy their time with their child. This was shown by video analyses of their interactions during the first year of life. Sroufe et al. took from these findings that Ainsworth's sensitivity scale tends to measure the technical part and the attainment of attachment security, while the joy in the interaction with the child measures emotional and motivational aspects that ensure sensitivity is sustained.

Interactions between a STEEP facilitator and parent often cut across all five levels of intervention, also embracing the concept of enjoyment. For example, when a facilitator observes during a video intervention that the mother has ignored her baby's cries (Level 1), she can can ask gently about the mother's own childhood memories about how caregivers responded to her cries (Level 2), while reflecting sensitivity toward the mother's desire to figure out the best way to deal with her baby's crying (Level 3). The facilitator also can share information about the importance of sensitivity and responsiveness to help the baby build the security that is the foundation of healthy child development (Level 4). And she can offer emotional support that acknowledges how exhausting it can be to care for a crying baby, encouraging the mother to reach out for help and support from other friends and family members (Level 5). And, of course, the facilitator can make sure to focus the mom's attention on those times (and video images) in which she and her baby share a feel-good moment in a smile or a cuddle or a laugh.

In addition to teaching STEEP trainees the theory and research on attachment patterns and the important role of parental sensitivity as a pathway to attachment security, we also address directly the trainees' attachment representations or states of mind and self-reflective functioning. At the start of training, we use the Adult Attachment Projective Picture System (George & West, 2012)[2] to assess

---

[2]Recently we switched to administering the Adult Attachment Interview (AAI; Main, Hesse, & Goldwyn, 2002; for use of the AAI in clinical settings, see Steele & Steele, 2008).

and then discuss attachment representations with each trainee. In a subsequent module focused on the inner self of the facilitators, we explore the special dynamic that arises from the encounter of different attachment models and examine both the beneficial and potentially negative effects on intervention outcomes. After initial concerns that working with the trainees' own attachment models may be too intimate and personal, we have learned that this part of the training is viewed by participants and trainers as one of the most important components of training. It lays the foundation for the ongoing self-reflection that is central to follow-up supervision and to STEEP work in general. (We say more about the self-reflection of workers in our discussion of the German research results that follow.)

Finally, as noted in the original STEEP research in Minnesota and as we also have found in Germany, mothers in the program often have a history of significant trauma, which they have not resolved, and they often present with symptoms of mental illness. Consequently, we also integrated general mental health competency into our training to prepare STEEP facilitators to recognize and address symptoms of mental illness, trauma, and potential threats to the child's welfare. The intent was not to train facilitators to do therapy but to prepare them to respond appropriately, to stay within the limits of their professional competence and support program participants in accessing psychological or psychiatric evaluation and treatment when needed.

Evaluation of STEEP in Germany

In three cities across Germany—Hamburg in the north, Frankfurt in the center, and Offenburg in the Black Forest in the south—STEEP was implemented by cooperating organizations whose employees successfully completed STEEP training (see Table 5.2), and the intervention was evaluated within a quasi-experimental design. A randomized controlled group design was not possible due to a lack of acceptance in practice. This acceptance was important to us because effective, careful implementation of both the intervention and the evaluation research rests on full acceptance and cooperation, a factor sometimes disregarded by researchers when they study interventions in the field. Thus, our study used a control group of mothers recruited when their babies were 12 months of age from welfare agencies other than those conducting STEEP interventions. Using different agencies prevented spillover effects of STEEP principles and strategies. Our data demonstrated that the 112 mothers who were recruited for the STEEP group across the three cities presented with significantly elevated risk levels compared to the 29 mothers in the control group.

Control-group mothers received treatment as usual within the German Child Welfare System (GCWS) and no STEEP intervention. Since youth services in Germany are of reasonably good quality nationwide, this was a good first test of STEEP in Germany. A better outcome in the intervention group would more readily be explained as a specific intervention effect than if the control group had received no support. As the study spanned 2 years, we ensured that differential attrition would not lead to biased interpretations of differences (for more information, see Suess, Bohlen, Carlson, Spangler, & Frumentia Maier, 2016; Suess, Bohlen, Mali, & Frumentia Maier, 2010).

At infant age one, 3.1 times more mother–child pairs of the STEEP group showed organized (71.8%) secure mother–child attachment in Ainsworth's Strange

TABLE 5.2. STEEP and Seeing Is Believing Training

I. Theoretical and research foundations of STEEP and Seeing Is Believing

   A. Attachment theory and research as a framework for relationship-based work with infants and families (including findings from the Minnesota Longitudinal Study of Risk and Adaptation, the concept of resilience, and the translational approach of STEEP).

   B. Patterns of attachment: antecedents and developmental consequences

   C. Parental sensitivity (Ainsworth Sensitivity Construct) and underlying factors

      1. Realistic expectations of parenthood

      2. Knowledge and understanding of child development

      3. Support for parents

      4. Guided look at history ("state of mind" about remembered attachment)

II. Seeing Is Believing: Using video recording to support and enhance parental sensitivity

   A. Presenting the idea

   B. Recording videos respectfully and effectively

   C. Viewing the video with parents. Using video and open-ended questioning to enhance parental understanding of infant behavior and development and sensitivity to baby's cues and needs

   D. Seeing Is Believing as a springboard for addressing broader issues

   E. Opportunities to practice the Seeing Is Believing approach

III. Prenatal visits: Expectations, preparation, and relationship building

   A. Recruiting participants

   B. Getting to know the family

   C. Gathering critical information: assets and challenges

   D. Preparing physically and emotionally for parenthood

IV. The group component of STEEP

   A. Engaging the group

   B. Establishing trust, ground rules, and confidentiality

   C. Format and activities

   D. Stages of group development

V. Digging deep: Integrating group and home visits to build family strengths and confront challenges

   A. Relationship as a vehicle for change

      1. How parent's relationship history and attachment state of mind shape their interactions with facilitator

      2. How facilitator's relationship history and attachment state of mind shape their interactions with families[a]

   B. Challenging parental state of mind

   C. Support and stress: An ecological approach

   D. Keeping the parent–child relationship center-stage

VI. Confronting issues of trauma, abuse (both domestic violence and child maltreatment), and mental health problems

VII. Opportunities to practice (practice dilemmas for discussion and role play)

[a]STEEP training in Germany has expanded this part of the training to administering the AAI to assess the attachment background and state of mind of trainees. Trainers then work individually with trainees to consider the results of the assessment and reflect on how relationship history and state of mind influence the trainee's perceptions and interactions, both professionally and personally.

Situation, which was significantly higher than in the GCWS control group. With 45.5% secure attachments, the GCWS control group demonstrates a result that is respectable for high-risk groups—especially in Germany, where there is a traditionally high percentage of insecure attachments (Grossmann et al., 1985; Rauh, 2000)—and highlights the significantly better results of the intervention group as a STEEP effect, which had to stand the test against an average quality youth service. A trend toward a positive effect was measured again after completion of the intervention, at age 24 months, this time using Waters's Attachment Q-Sort (AQS), which demonstrated a trend toward higher attachment security in the STEEP group. There also were significant differences between the intervention and control groups with respect to attachment disorganization/disorientation when infants were 12 and 24 months of age, using Main and Solomon's dimensional 9-point rating scale, with higher D scores for the GCWS control group. The same was true only for the 24-month-old infants when using the categorical D coding (Main & Solomon, 1990). Consider that STEEP was not evaluated under laboratory conditions, but in a real-world intervention practice setting. The STEEP intervention had to stand the test against a well-cared for GCWS control group, which had lower initial risk levels. Unfortunately, we were not able to recruit more participants for the control group. As a result, the sample size of the control group ($n = 29$) made it more difficult to consistently reach statistically significant results.

In addition to the attachment measures, we also compared the two groups (STEEP and GCWS control) with regard to parental stress (Parental Stress Index [PSI]), childrearing attitudes (Adult–Adolescent Parenting Inventory [AAPI]), and depression (Edinburgh Postnatal Depression Scale [EPDS]) after 1 year and at the end of the intervention study. In line with the higher risk levels at the start of the study, the mothers in the STEEP group still showed significantly higher stress levels compared to the GCWS control group after 1 year of intervention. However, these differences had disappeared at the 2-year assessment. Regarding the depression measures, there were no significant differences at either time. However, mothers in both groups showed a high risk of depression (EPDS), which indicates substantial strain on these parents. Based on the AAPI (Bavolek, 1989) scale for parental childrearing scores, we compared both groups on the extent to which mothers fell within the clinical risk range. While there was no group difference at age 12 months, STEEP intervention mothers received significantly lower scores on AAPI risk score at age 24 months. Post hoc tests reveal significantly superior scores of the STEEP intervention group on two out of five subscales: They demonstrated significantly more empathy (AAPI-S2) and they value their children more for expressing their views and making good decisions (AAPO-S5). All these differences were in the predicted direction and can be interpreted coherently (for more information, see Suess et al., 2016).

Earlier, we reported that we assessed the attachment background of the participating social workers, using the Adult Attachment Projective (AAP; George & West, 2012), as part of our STEEP training. Based on Bowlby's (1988) conviction about the effects of attachment background on the effectiveness of attachment-based intervention, we reexamined the effectiveness of the STEEP intervention of the STEEP facilitators, who were involved at one of the three study sites mentioned earlier, in relation to their attachment background (Suess et al., 2015). In order to minimize errors, we coded the AAP of the STEEP facilitators twice independently, and in case of a disagreement, the AAP was coded a third time and the mode was used. Professionals with insecure and secure attachment backgrounds did not differ in the effectiveness of their STEEP intervention (i.e., both had similar numbers of parent–child pairs with secure attachment in their STEEP groups). However, when we observed professionals who presented with an unresolved attachment status (i.e., had not sufficiently processed a trauma or separation) and compared them to the rest of the professionals, significantly fewer parent–child pairs of the unresolved professionals showed a secure attachment quality at age 12 months (Suess et al., 2015). This effect of the professionals' unresolved status was not found at 24 months. Although this result is not very strong, we are convinced of the impact of the professional's own attachment status in attachment-based intervention. Our conviction is founded in our experiences in supervision and training settings, as well as evidence from other research (Dozier, Cue, & Barnett, 1994; Stovall-McClough, & Dozier, 2004; Dozier, Albus, Fisher, & Sepulveda, 2002; Schuengel, Kef, Damen, & Worm, 2012). The issue warrants further study with larger sample sizes.

In studies with a larger sample size, which are more tightly controlled, the effect of match between intervention providers' and mothers' different internal working models and the effects of different combinations of deactivating and hyperactivating attachment strategies could be examined more closely in relation to the intervention process. There are indicators suggesting that taking into account "differential susceptibility" and different phases of the intervention process could lead to a more complex transactional model in this area (Mallinckrodt, 2010; Velderman, Bakermans-Kranenburg, Juffer, & van IJzendoorn, 2006).

Further Developments in Germany: STEEP-Based Counseling

The experiences from more than 10 years of implementing STEEP as a training and intervention program within the German youth welfare system have led us to believe that limiting its scope to the first 2 years of a child's life is not sufficient in face of the broad demands of the practical work. Hence, youth service and health professionals who work with families and children beyond age 2 or 3 now participate in STEEP training seminars and are eager to utilize attachment knowledge successfully in their work.

Currently, we are developing additional, specific training modules addressing STEEP-based counseling beyond the second year of the child's life. This work is facilitated by instruments that focus on the attachment representation of the child, such as the Attachment Story-Completion Task for preschoolers (Bretherton, Ridgeway & Cassidy,1990) and the Late Childhood Attachment Interview (LCAI; Zimmermann & Scheuerer-Englisch, 2001), as well as applying an attachment framework to observations of family interaction, and to observations of how children approach and engage peers, teachers and other important adults. How children perform on social perception tasks with respect to pictorial stimuli of conflicts, as well as their attributional style with respect to intentions, are important cornerstones of extending STEEP to the preschool years (Suess et al., 1992; Suess & Sroufe, 2005) and beyond.

Throughout the preschool years, the focus of the intervention is to strengthen secure base use and support within important relationships. Significant questions include the following: Does the child communicate his or her worries? Does he or she seek comfort and support from adults when stressed? Can parents identify how the child feels, and is the child confident that the parents can effectively support him or her (Zimmermann, 1999; Scheuerer-Englisch, 2012).

We also have begun to apply STEEP-based strategies and approaches in inpatient and outpatient treatment of mothers with peripartum depression, with severe personality disorders combined with traumatic experiences, and even with psychotic mothers and their infants. This, of course, is challenging but very worthwhile work if it helps to bring about an early shift from the emergence of disorganized attachment patterns toward organized relationship patterns (Hartmann, 2012).

Lessons Learned from 30 Years of Implementing STEEP

With more than 30 years of implementing STEEP in the United States and more than 10 years in Germany—and with many opportunities for sharing ideas and reflections through our ongoing transatlantic exchange—we have gained insights, drawn cautious conclusions, and grappled with ongoing questions related to future practice and research. First, we have seen repeatedly that, for parents, the greatest challenge lies in the space between what they know and what they do. It is relatively easy to help parents build knowledge, but support (or the lack thereof) for shifts in parental states of mind are more difficult to achieve yet important to promote given the powerful influences of these states of mind on how parents apply what they know on a daily basis (Verhage et al., 2016). So a core challenge in this kind of work is finding ways to motivate parents to become mindful, to observe themselves and their children, and to develop the courage to question old patterns and try new ways of behaving—in other words, to apply the knowledge they have gained. Creating an atmosphere open to mistakes is fundamental. This is most likely to happen when parents feel secure with us rather than feeling devalued, exposed, criticized, or meeting with impatience. And it is most likely to develop when, as professionals, we step off the pedestal and allow parents to see us as vulnerable, imperfect people who also sometimes struggle to apply what we know on a daily basis. This self-revelation runs counter to what many of us learned in our own professional training, but we are convinced that this approach enhances the effectiveness of preventive intervention with high-risk parents and children.

That leads directly to the related issue, or principle, that relationships change relationships. Doing relationship-based work is a new approach for many experienced professionals who are used to working from an expert model (e.g., traditional education or health services). Knowledge alone is not enough for a facilitator to be able to provide the secure base that enables a client to explore new ways of being. Rather, the professional's own reflective capacity is often the engine of change. An intervention without continuous self-reflection on the part of the professional may lead to a standstill for the client, resulting in repetition of old, dysfunctional patterns, resignation, emotional withdrawal, or even dropping out of the program.

Secure facilitators provide support and encouragement to families and also are able to let go when necessary. They can serve as models of self-reflection.

As we have learned through both research and practice, parents' and workers' states of mind intersect in important ways. In an ideal scenario, the professional would bring a secure or "earned secure" state of mind that can complement and gently challenge insecure models or states of mind in parents and in parent–child relationships. But this very often is not the case, with many professionals having insecure or unresolved states of mind. The pulls and draws of inner working models (of both worker and client) create a sometimes invisible but powerful scaffold or framework for the processes of intervention. As we described earlier in this chapter, these forces need to be addressed in training and ongoing reflective supervision, an essential component of a responsible STEEP practice, so that the STEEP facilitator does not become a pawn of these forces and does not lose perspective during the intervention. Here, it is necessary to sensitively challenge trainees or supervisees at certain points, especially when they present with an insecure or unresolved attachment background.

We have never considered excluding candidates from training because of an insecure attachment background, although colleagues have raised the question; however, we challenge and support trainees to do what Erickson and Egeland have called "looking back, moving forward" in order to reflect on and understand their own attachment background and how their history shapes the way they perceive and respond to clients, especially during times of duress. This process of self-reflection parallels the "looking back, moving forward" in which facilitators are expected to engage STEEP parents. We have seen that authentic self-reflection of workers who are supported by sensitive, reflective trainers, and supervisors can bring about change in a worker's state of mind and, in turn, increase the likelihood of that same change process for parents served by the worker.

Without that self-reflection, workers may mirror and inadvertently reinforce a client's ineffective patterns. For example, when a facilitator presents with a dismissive state of mind and interacts with dismissive clients, intervention may remain superficial and be oriented toward enforcing the child's strict adherence to parental rules and limits, interpreting the behavior of the child as inappropriate rather than as a signal. This prevents the parents from developing a clear understanding of attachment needs and motives, and reinforces their dismissal of the child's emotional needs.

A similar process occurs when a facilitator shows a preoccupied—or even more, an unresolved—state of mind regarding his or her own attachment history and is confronted with a similar model in a client. The result may be overreaction on the part of the professional (e.g., a premature emotionally triggered recommendation that the child be removed from the home), overidentification with the aggrieved mother (agreeing without question that the violent partner/father must have his rights terminated), loss of professional boundaries (e.g., lending a client money in a moment of apparent financial crisis), or other enabling actions (jumping in to solve a problem for a parent rather than helping the parent strategize about solutions).

The implementation and evaluation of STEEP in Germany has included a more systematic approach than earlier studies in addressing the attachment representations of the professionals working in the program, and the results have been encouraging. As described elsewhere, the German study has shown that insecure states of mind of professionals can improve through reflective supervision (Suess et al., 2015). These findings affirm our philosophy not to consider excluding facilitators with insecure attachment models, but to aim for an accepting attitude that nevertheless strives for change. We have observed that professionals with an "earned secure" status often develop a particularly deep understanding of insecure attachment processes, enhancing their ability to join with a client to discover new ways of being in relationship and understanding attachment needs in oneself and one's children.

Within the STEEP trainings and service programs in Germany, we continue to dig more deeply into the intersection of different attachment models or states of mind. For example, we are just beginning to empirically map the dyadic processes during the encounter with different attachment models and examine these processes in terms of their effects on the intervention process and also group processes (both among mothers in the STEEP groups and among STEEP facilitators working together). In a training context, we continue to experience the different deactivating and hyperactivating forces, both constructive and obstructive. Our aim in training and in ongoing supervision is to increase awareness and sensitivity regarding these forces and, using attachment theory, create a language that allows us to exchange thoughts about them and shape them in a positive way. Through the interplay of practice and research, perhaps in the future we will find not only developmentally meaningful dimensions and mechanisms but also better ways to help children and parents. This interaction of clinical understanding and empirical science is the very legacy of Bowlby and Ainsworth, as well as the now retiring first generation of attachment researchers.

While there has been a deepening of emphasis on the level of representation throughout the years of implementing and adapting STEEP, we still consider the focus on the here and now as an invaluable part of STEEP. The here-and-now behavioral component of STEEP is especially apparent in the Seeing Is Believing video strategy. Babies need good-enough parenting right now and may not be able to wait for parents to change their state of mind. Knowing this, the support of the parents through STEEP always includes concrete, routine-oriented, practical intervention strategies rooted in a strong learning alliance between the STEEP facilitator and parents. As partners in discovery, parents and their STEEP facilitator not only focus on the child's development but also look toward the future of the parents and other family members. We are convinced that building positive parenting behaviors (e.g., reading a baby's cues, responding sensitively and appropriately) and then seeing oneself on video using those behaviors can bring about change in a parent's self-view. We are not yet sure exactly how that relates to eventual changes in a parent's state of mind, but we believe it does. And we believe that the competence and confidence parents develop in interacting with their baby become a foundation for building other skills and making healthy choices for the well-being of their families and themselves.

We would be remiss if we did not include in our discussion of lessons learned the importance of the second E in STEEP: Enjoyable! Working with high-risk parents and infants is serious and difficult. But just as good parent–child relationships involve a great deal of joy and playfulness, so should the work with families—another important example of parallel process. In a beautiful video made by STEEP facilitators in Hamburg, one of the STEEP groups (moms and toddlers) took a very special weekend trip to "Kalifornien" (not the one in the United States, but a beach in Northern Germany), where they stayed overnight in small cabins and spent a great deal of time romping and playing outdoors together. When we bring active, exuberant play and exploration into our work with families, parents learn firsthand about the importance of play to their children's learning. They hear the delight in their children's laughter and experience the joy of laughing with them. And, for too many moms, they begin learning to play for the first time themselves. It doesn't need to be a trip to California; 10 minutes of dancing to one's favorite music or splashing in buckets of water outside on a hot day work just fine.

Honoring the second E also includes building some fun and playful activities into Momtalk time during STEEP group sessions, just for moms—a lesson in the value of self-care and replenishment in the midst of all the demanding tasks of parenthood. Continuing the theme of parallel process, STEEP workers also deserve some breaks and fun along the way; by caring for each other and themselves, they are more able to care for the families they serve. But it is up to STEEP facilitators and supervisors to be sure that enjoyment is not squeezed out by the many grave and difficult issues they face in their work.

So, what is most important in this work with challenged families? Or phrased another way, what is the most valuable thing a STEEP facilitator brings to families in the program? It is oneself, one's eyes, feelings, thoughts, and honest reflections on one's own experience. The interpersonal encounters and the supportive sharing of observations and insights are cornerstones of the work, so the STEEP facilitator brings his or her whole self to that relationship. When mothers in the program begin to understand that no one's life is perfect, that sometimes we all are tired, sad, or frustrated, and that we all do things we know are not good, then growth and learning can happen. The challenges, sadness, and missteps are all part of the human journey or what the Greek Alexis Zorba in the classic movie called "the full catastrophe" (Kabat-Zinn, 2013). There is great joy and satisfaction for a parent who makes gains in navigating that challenging human journey. And there is great joy and satisfaction for the thoughtful, dedicated worker who has the privilege of supporting the parent in making those gains.

REFERENCES

Ainsworth, M. S., Blehar, M. C., Waters, E., & Wall, S. (1978). *Patterns of attachment: A psychological study of the Strange Situation*. Oxford, UK: Erlbaum.

Bakermans-Kranenburg, M. J., van IJzendoorn, M. H., & Juffer, F. (2003). Less is more: Meta-analysis of sensitivity and attachment interventions in early childhood. *Psychological Bulletin, 129*, 195–215.

Bakermans-Kranenburg, M. J., van IJzendoorn, M. H., & Juffer, F. (2008). Less is more: Meta-analytic arguments for the use of sensitivity-focused interventions. In F. Juffer, M. J. Bakermans, & M. H. van IJzendoorn (Eds.), *Promoting positive parenting: An attachment-based intervention* (pp. 59–74). New York: Taylor & Francis.

Bavolek, S. J. (1989). Assessing and treating high-risk parenting attitudes [Special issue]. *Early Child Development and Care, 42*, 99–112.

Beijersbergen, M. D., Juffer, F., Bakermans-Kranenburg, M. J., & van IJzendoorn, M. H. (2012). Remaining or becoming secure: Parental sensitive support predicts attachment continuity from infancy to adolescence in a longitudinal adoption study. *Developmental Psychology, 48,* 1277–1282.

Biscaro, A., & Hicks, A. (2017). *A brief history of seeing is believing in Niagara: Report to the early childhood community.* Thorold, ON: Niagara Region Public Health.

Bowlby, J. (1988). *A secure base.* London: Basic Books.

Bretherton, I., Ridgeway, D., & Cassidy, J. (1990). Assessing internal working models of the attachment relationship. In M. T. Greenberg, D. Cicchetti, & E. M. Cummings (Eds.), *Attachment in the preschool years: Theory, research and intervention* (pp. 273–299). Chicago: University of Chicago Press.

Brisch, K. H., Grossmann, K., Grossmann, K. E., & Köhler, K. (Eds.). (2002). *Bindung und seelische Entwicklungswege: Grundlagen, Prävention und klinische Praxis* [Attachment and mental pathways: Foundations, prevention and clinical practice]. Stuttgart: Klett-Cotta.

Cicchetti, D., & Hinshaw, S. P. (2002). Editorial: Prevention and intervention science: Contributions to developmental theory. *Development and Psychopathology, 14,* 667–671.

Cierpka, M., & Evers, O. (2015). Implementation and efficacy of early-childhood interventions in German-speaking countries. *Mental Health and Prevention, 3,* 67–68.

Coie, J. D., Miller-Johnson, S., & Bagwell, C. (2000). Prevention science. In A. J. Sameroff, M. Lewis, & S. M. Miller (Eds.), *Handbook of developmental psychopathology* (pp. 93–112). Berlin: Springer.

De Wolff, M. S., & van IJzendoorn, M. H. (1997). Sensitivity and attachment a meta-analysis on parental antecedents of infant attachment. *Child Development, 68*(4), 571–591.

Dozier, M., Albus, K. E., Fisher, P. A., & Sepulveda, S. (2002). Interventions for foster parents: Implications for developmental theory. *Development and Psychopathology, 14,* 843–860.

Dozier, M., Cue, K. L., & Barnett, L. (1994). Clinicians as caregivers: Role of attachment organization in treatment. *Journal of Consulting and Clinical Psychology, 62*(4), 793–800.

Egeland, B., & Erickson, M. F. (1993). *An evaluation of STEEP: A program for high-risk mothers* (Grant No. MH41879). Rockville, MD: U.S. Department of Health and Human Services, Public Health Service, National Institute of Mental Health.

Egeland, B., & Erickson, M. F. (1995). Attachment theory and findings: Implications for prevention and intervention. In S. Kramer & H. Parens (Eds.), *Prevention in mental health: Now, tomorrow, ever?* (pp. 21–50). Northvale, NJ: Jason Aronson.

Egeland, B., & Erickson, M. F. (2004). Lessons from STEEP™: Linking theory, research and practice for the well-being of infants and parents. In A. Sameroff, S. McDonough, & K. Rosenblum (Eds.), *Treating parent–infant relationship problems: Strategies for intervention* (pp. 213–242). New York: Guilford Press.

Egeland, B., Erickson, M. F., Butcher, J. N., & Ben-Porath, Y. S. (1991). MMPI-2 profiles of women at risk for child abuse. *Journal of Personality Assessment, 57*(2), 254–263.

Erickson, M. F. (2005). *Seeing is Believing® Training Videos* (DVD). Minneapolis: Irving B. Harris Training Programs, University of Minnesota. [To order, see *www.cehd.umn.edu/ceed/publications/manuals*]

Erickson, M. F., & Egeland, B. (2006). *Die Stärkung der Eltern-Kind-Bindung* [Strengthening the parent–child attachment] (2nd ed.). Stuttgart, Germany: Klett-Cotta.

Erickson, M. F., Egeland, B., Simon, J., & Rose, T. (2002). *STEEP™ Facilitator's Guide.* Minneapolis: Irving B. Harris Training Center, University of Minnesota. [To order, see *www.cehd.umn.edu/ceed/publications/manuals*]

Erickson, M. F., Korfmacher, J., & Egeland, B. (1992). Attachments past and present: Implications for therapeutic intervention with mother–infant dyads. *Development and Psychopathology, 4,* 495–507.

George, C., & West, M. L. (2012). *The Adult Attachment Projective Picture System: Attachment theory and assessment in adults.* New York: Guilford Press.

Grossmann, K., Grossmann, K. E., Fremmer-Bombik, E., Kindler, H., Scheuerer-Englisch, H., & Zimmermann, P. (2002). The uniqueness of the child–father attachment relationship: Fathers´ sensitive and challenging play as the pivotal variable in a 16-year longitudinal study. *Social Development, 11,* 307–331.

Grossmann, K., Grossmann, K. E., & Kindler, H. (2005). *Early care and the roots of attachment and partnership representations: The Bielefeld and Regensburg longitudinal studies.* In K. E. Grossmann, K. Grossmann, & E. Waters (Eds.), *Attachment from infancy to adulthood: The major longitudinal studies* (pp. 98–136). New York: Guilford Press.

Grossmann, K., Grossmann, K. E., Spangler, G., Suess, G., & Unzner, L. (1985). Maternal sensitivity and newborns orientation responses as related to quality of attachment in northern Germany. *Monographs of the Society for Research in Child Development, 50*(1–2), 233–256.

Grossmann, K. E. (1988). Longitudinal and systemic approaches in the study of biological high- and low-risk groups. In M. Rutter (Ed.), *Studies of psychosocial risk–the power of longitudinal data.* New York: Cambridge University Press.

Grossmann, K. E., Grossmann, K., & Waters, E. (Eds.). (2005). *Attachment from infancy to adulthood: The major longitudinal studies.* New York: Guilford Press.

Guthrie, K. F., Gaziano, C., & Gaziano, E. P. (2009). Toward better beginnings: Enhancing healthy child development and parent–child relationships in a high-risk population. *Home Health Care Management and Practice, 21*(2), 99–108.

Hartmann, H.-P. (2012). Mutter-Kind-Behandlung unter bindungstheoretischer und psychoanalytischer Perspektive [Mother–infant psychotherapy from an attachment and psychoanalytic perspective.]. In S. Wortmann-Fleischer, R. von Einsiedel, & G. Downing (Eds.), *Stationäre Eltern-Kind-Behandlung* [Inpatient parent–child treatment] (pp. 73–85). Stuttgart, Germany: Kohlhammer.

Hinde, R. A. (1976). On describing relationships. *Journal of Child Psychology and Psychiatry, 17*(1), 1–19.

Juffer, F., Bakermans-Kranenburg, M. J., & van IJzendoorn, M. H. (2014). Attachment-based interventions: Sensitive parenting is the key to positive parent–child relationships. In P. Holmes & S. Farnfield (Eds.), *Attachment: The guidebook to attachment theory and interventions* (pp. 83–104). London: Taylor & Francis.

Kabat-Zinn, J. (2013). *Full catastrophe living: Using wisdom of your body and mind to face stress, pain, and illness* (rev. ed.). New York: Bantam Books.

Main, M., Hesse, E., & Goldwyn, R. (2008). *Adult Attachment Scoring and Classification Systems, Version. 7.1.* Unpublished manuscript, University of California at Berkeley, Berkeley, CA.

Main, M., & Solomon, J. (1990). Procedures for identifying infants as disorganized/disoriented during the Ainsworth Strange Situation. In M. T. Greenberg, D. Cicchetti, & M. Cummings (Eds.), *Attachment in the preschool years: Theory, research, and intervention* (pp. 121–160). Chicago: University of Chicago Press.

Mallinckrodt, B. (2010). The psychotherapy relationship as attachment: Evidence and implications. *Journal of Social and Personal Relationships, 27*(2), 262–270.

Nationales Zentrum Frühe Hilfen (NZFH). (2009). *Early childhood intervention pilot projects in the German federal states* (English language edition). Bundeszentrale für gesundheitliche Aufklärung (BZgA), Cologne, Germany.

Papousek, M., Schieche, M., & Wurmser, H. (Eds.). (2004). *Regulationsstörungen der frühen Kindheit. Frühe Risiken und Hilfen im Entwicklungskontext der Eltern-Kind-Beziehungen* [Regulatory disorders of early childhood: Early risks and aids in the developmental context of parent–child relationships]. Bern: Huber.

Papousek, M., Schieche, M., & Wurmser, H. (2007). *Disorders of behavioral and emotional regulation in the first years of life: Early risk and intervention in the developing parent–infant relationship*. Washington, DC: Zero To Three.

Raby, K. L., Roisman, G. I., Fraley, R. C., & Simpson, J. A. (2015). The enduring predictive significance of early sensitivity: Social and academic competence through age 32 years. *Child Development, 86*, 695–708.

Rauh, H. (Ed.). (2000). Bindung: Themen-Doppelheft [Attachment]. *Psychologie in Erziehung und Unterricht, 47*.

Renner, I., & Heimeshoff, V. (2011). *Pilot projects in the German federal states: Summary of results*. Köln, Germany: National Centre on Early Prevention (NZFH).

Scheuerer-Englisch, H. (2012). Die innere Welt des Kindes: Das Bindungsinterview für die späte Kindheit (BISK) in Beratung und Therapie [The inner world of the child: Attachment interview for late childhood (BISK) in counseling and therapy]. In H. Scheuerer-Englisch, G. J. Suess, & W.-K. Pfeifer (Eds.), *Wege zur Sicherheit: Bindungswissen in Diagnostik und Intervention* [Pathways to security: Attachment knowledge in diagnostics and intervention] (2nd ed., pp. 277–312). Giessen, Germany: Psychosozial Verlag.

Scheuerer-Englisch, H., Suess, G. J., & Pfeifer, W.-K. P. (Eds.). (2003). *Wege zur Sicherheit: Bindungswissen in Diagnostik und Intervention* [Pathways to security: Attachment knowledge in diagnostics and intervention]. Giessen, Germany: Psychosozial Verlag.

Schuengel, C., Kef, S., Damen, S., & Worm, M. (2012). Attachment representations and response to video-feedback intervention for professional caregivers. *Attachment and Human Development, 14*(2), 83–99.

Sroufe, L. A., Egeland, B., Carlson, E. A., & Collins, W. A. (2005). *The development of the person: The Minnesota Study of Risk and Adaptation from Birth to Adulthood*. New York: Guilford Press.

Steele, H., & Steele, M. (Eds.). (2008). *Clinical application of the Adult Attachment Interview*. New York: Guilford Press.

Stovall-McClough, K. C., & Dozier, M. (2004). Forming attachments in foster care: Infant attachment behaviors during the first 2 months of placement. *Development and Psychopathology, 16*, 253–271.

Suess, G. J., Bohlen, U., Carlson, E. A., Spangler, G., & Frumentia Maier, M. (2016). Effectiveness of attachment based STEEP™ intervention in a German high-risk sample. *Attachment and Human Development, 18*(5), 443–460.

Suess, G. J., Bohlen, U., Mali, A., & Frumentia Maier, M. (2010). Erste Ergebnisse zur Wirksamkeit Früher Hilfen aus dem STEEP-Praxisforschungsprojekt "WiEge." *Bundesgesundheitsblatt, 53*, 1143–1149.

Suess, G. J., Grossmann, K. E., & Sroufe, L. A. (1992). Effects of infant attachment to mother and father on quality of adaptation in preschool: From dyadic to individual organization of self. *International Journal of Behavioral Development, 15*, 43–66.

Suess, G. J., Mali, A., Reiner, I., Fremmer-Bombik, E., Schieche, M., & Suess, E. S. (2015). Attachment representations of professionals—influence on intervention and implications for clinical training and supervision. *Mental Health and Prevention, 3*, 129–134.

Suess, G. J., & Pfeifer, W.-K. P. (1999). *Frühe Hilfen: Die Anwendung von Bindungs- und Kleinkindforschung in Erziehung, Beratung, Therapie und Vorbeugung* [Early intervention. Applying attachment and infancy research in parenting, counseling, therapy and prevention]. Giessen, Germany: Psychosozial Verlag.

Suess, G. J., Scheuerer-Englisch, H., & Pfeifer, W.-K. P. (2001). *Bindungstheorie und Familiendynamik: Anwendung der Bindungstheorie in Beratung und Therapie* [Attachment theory and family dynamics: Application of the attachment theory in counseling and therapy]. Giessen, Germany: Psychosozial Verlag.

Suess, G. J., & Sroufe, J. (2005). Clinical implications of the development of the person. *Attachment and Human Development, 7*(4), 381–392.

van IJzendoorn, M. H., & Kroonenberg, P. M. (1988). Cross-cultural patterns of attachment: A meta-analysis of the strange situation. *Child Development, 69*, 147–156.

Velderman, M. K., Bakermans-Kranenburg, M. J., Juffer, F., & van IJzendoorn, M. H. (2006). Effects of attachment-based interventions on maternal sensitivity and infant attachment: Differential susceptibility of highly reactive infants. *Journal of Family Psychology, 20*(2), 266–274.

Verhage, M. L., Schuengel, C., Madigan, S., Fearon, R. M., Oosterman, M., Cassiba, R., . . . van IJzendoorn, M. H. (2016). Narrowing the transmission gap: A synthesis of three decades of research on intergenerational transmission of attachment. *Psychological Bulletin, 142*(4), 337–366.

Zimmermann, P. (1999). Structure and functioning of internal working models of attachment and their role during emotion regulation. *Attachment and Human Development, 1*, 291–307.

Zimmermann, P., & Scheuerer-Englisch, H. (2001). *LCAI: Late Childhood Attachment Interview* (BISK: Bindungsinterview für die späte Kindheit). Unpublished manual, University of Wuppertal, Wuppertal, Germany.

Zimmermann, P., & Scheuerer-Englisch, H. (2012). Das Bindungsinterview für die Späte Kindheit (BISK): Leitfragen und Skalenauswertung [Late Childhood Attachment Interview]. In H. Scheuerer-Englisch, G. J. Suess, & W.-K. Pfeifer (Eds.), *Wege zur Sicherheit: Bindungswissen in Diagnostik und Intervention* [Pathways toward security: Attachment knowledge in diagnostics and intervention] (2nd ed., pp. 241–276). Giessen, Germany: Psychosozial Verlag.

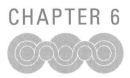

CHAPTER 6

The UCLA Family Development Project
Promoting Healthy Relationships from Within

JESSICA L. BORELLI, DAVID KYLE BOND, KAREN DUDLEY,
VICTORIA PONCE, and CATHERINE MOGIL

Originally delineated by John Bowlby (e.g., 1946, 1958; Bowlby, Robertson, & Rosenbluth, 1952) and later expanded upon by Mary Ainsworth (e.g., Ainsworth & Bell, 1970), attachment theory provides a powerful framework for understanding the parent–infant relationship and its influence throughout the lifespan. Indeed, decades of attachment research support the importance of critical early relationships with caregivers in promoting the health and well-being of children (e.g., Sroufe, 2005). The central tenet of attachment theory is that infants come into this world ready and highly motivated to form attachments with caregivers, and that the quality of these relationships lays the groundwork for the child's ability to relate to others and regulate emotion (Bowlby, 1980). In other words, the parent–infant relationship is of tremendous importance in charting a child's developmental trajectory. This chapter is structured as follows—following a brief introduction to Heinicke's early work, we provide an overview of the intervention program, describing its underlying theoretical premise, participant eligibility criteria, modality of treatment, and therapeutic goals. We then provide a synthesis of the outcomes of Heinicke's intervention, including a review of both mothers' and children's responses to the intervention, as well as areas in which the intervention did not effect change. Finally, we examine the ways in which Heinicke's influential framework is currently applied and extended to novel treatment contexts and populations.

Christoph Heinicke's pioneering work on parent–child relationships was influential in the development of the theory and the measurement of attachment. In his groundbreaking study examining differences between children in residential and day nursery settings, Heinicke (1956) studied the impact of parent–child separations on young children, finding that, in general, separation was associated with deleterious regression behaviors and the presence of internalizing and external-izing symptoms (e.g., hostility). Notably, Heinicke observed that these behaviors were alleviated by the reintroduction of the parent or parent figure. Heinicke's early work led him to respect the fundamental importance of the parent–child relationship in engendering the child with a sense that the world can be emotionally manageable and safe. In observing patterns in parent–child contact, Heinicke remarked that his wish was for readers to "think of the parents' presence as of great importance in maintaining the balance between the two-year-old's impulses and his power to organize and control these impulses in relation to the external world" (p. 172). This wish foreshadowed Heinicke's future work, which focused on pro-viding direct psychoanalytic support to parents of at-risk children (e.g., Heinicke, 1976), culminating in a focus on the most empirically sound ways of providing early family intervention (e.g., Heinicke, 1990).

In light of his initial work on the importance of the parent–child bond (e.g., Heinicke, 1956; Heinicke & Westheimer, 1965), Heinicke set out to craft an interven-tion for at-risk families based on empirically validated methods aimed at promot-ing lasting change in the functioning of the parent–child relationship. Heinicke's UCLA Family Development Project arose in direct response to the need for clear, theoretically informed clinical interventions aimed at meeting the needs of women on the path to becoming mothers with limited financial, psychosocial, and emo-tional resources. Heinicke fashioned the UCLA Family Development Project in accord with his review of long-term interventions aimed at enhancing parent–child relationship quality. Heinicke and his colleagues (Heinicke, Recchia, Berlin, & James, 1993) concluded that there were three critically important socioemotional infant–mother transactions within the first year of life on which an appropriate intervention could focus: first, the way in which the parent responds to the infant's needs as a function of his or her own attachment security; second, the way in which the parent fosters infant autonomy as a function of his or her own autonomy; and third, the way in which the parent fosters infant task engagement as a function of his or her own task orientation (Heinicke et al., 1999).

With intervention strategies focused on each of these three transactional pro-cesses, Heinicke designed the initial 2-year UCLA Family Development Project with the goal of fostering a relationship between a home-visitor and the mother. Heinicke intended for this relationship to be emotionally positive and functionally supportive, and ultimately for the mother's experiences in this relationship to facili-tate improvement of her responsiveness to the needs of her infant, which in turn ought to promote the likelihood of secure infant attachment (Heinicke, Beckwith, & Thompson, 1988). In the sections that follow we present a brief, yet comprehen-sive, summary of the intervention, followed by a close examination of the findings that emerged.

The UCLA Family Development Project Intervention

Eligibility and Overall Premise

In order to be eligible to participate in the intervention, a mother receiving prena-tal care had to meet the following eight inclusion criteria: (1) currently pregnant with her first child, (2) no member of the family suffers from serious health complications, (3) does not currently meet criteria for a DSM-IV Axis I diagnosis, (4) is not currently using drugs, (5) speaks English, (6) lives within a 20-minute drive of the UCLA hospital, (7) is 17 years or older, and, (8) is identified as at-risk by a social history interview (Heinicke et al., 1999, p. 354). To be identified as at risk via the social history interview, the mother had to manifest four or more of the following at-risk conditions: (1) The mother is poor and receiving public aid; (2) the mother lacks social support from partner, family, or friends; (3) the pregnancy is unwanted; (4) the mother was a victim of childhood physical abuse; (5) childhood sexual abuse; (6) childhood emotional abuse; (7) childhood rape, and/or (8) childhood violence; (9) the mother has experienced suicidal thoughts in the past, (10) has been previously referred for mental health counseling, or (11) previously was treated for drug or alcohol addiction, and/or (12) is currently homeless. The resulting sample of all mothers manifested two salient characteristics: They lacked financial and social resources.

Heinicke developed his intervention based on the tenets held by dominant clinical theory at the time with regard to the development of positive relationships— both at the therapeutic level (consistent with intervention delivery best practices) and the personal level (consistent with a fundamental understanding of how the family of origin, the mother's partner, and the infant all fit together; see Table 6.1; Heinicke, 2000). To these ends, Heinicke's intervention underscored the importance of the formation of a mutually positive and trusting relationship between intervener and client, the rationale for which was heavily based on attachment theory, family systems theory, and object relations theory. The central goal of the intervention was for the relationship between intervener and client to launch an iterative therapeutic process that could be utilized as the basis for the resolution of internal and external issues throughout the social network (Bandura, 1986; Egeland & Erikson, 1990; Heinicke et al., 1999; Lieberman, Weston, & Paul, 1991). Through the holding environment built between the intervener and the mother, Heinicke's intervention aimed to help the mothers address issues related to autonomy and dependence within the family of origin, resolve issues between mother and partner regarding the need for individuality, and create a secure emotional base upon which the mother could feel comfortable meeting her infants' needs and

---

TABLE 6.1. Principles of the UCLA Family Development Program

- *Principle 1*: In order for a therapy to effect change, creating a trusting relationship between intervener and parent is necessary.

- *Principle 2*: An effective parent–child intervention for an at-risk population must include assisting the parent in handling practical issues related to social relationships and functioning.

- *Principle 3*: An effective intervention for the parent–child relationship involves observation of interactions between parents and children and assistance in mentalizing for both members of the dyad and reconceiving of conflicts between them.

- *Principle 4*: An effective parent–child intervention entails supporting the parent in his or her attempts to change aspects of the parent–child relationship.

through which the infant would likewise experience having his or her needs met (Heinicke, 2000; Heinicke et al., 1999). It is important to note that these processes were conceptualized as being mutually and reciprocally interactive, existing not in a vacuum, but within an interconnected web of relationships demanding intervention attention.

The UCLA Family Development Project design was based on an in-depth analysis of previous family-oriented interventions (Heinicke, 1990), which led Heinicke to emphasize the importance of three factors that he believed were essential for a treatment to work. First, he discussed the importance of ensuring that clients are acquiescent to the requirements of the intervention. Second, he argued that the duration and intensity of the intervention must be consistent (e.g., including weekly visits) in order to effect lasting change. Third, he felt that the intervention must be comprehensive enough to effect change at multiple levels within a participant's social world (Heinicke, 2000). In the summary of the intervention process that follows below, it is important to keep in mind that the main goal of the intervention is to "offer the mother the experience of a stable trustworthy relationship that conveys understanding of her situation, and that promotes her sense of self-efficacy through a variety of specific interventions" (Heinicke et al., 1999, p. 356).

Modality of Intervention

Two cohorts received the intervention—the first pilot consisting of 46 families (e.g., Heinicke et al., 2000), and the second consisting of 57 families. In this chapter we present data primarily from this second cohort given the limited published data available from the first. Although insights from the first cohort were utilized to formulate hypotheses for the second, the treatment provided was qualitatively the same. Upon study entry, mothers were randomly assigned to one of two groups: "home-visited" (n = 31 families) or "pediatric follow-up," which served as a control condition (n = 33 families). Those participants in the home-visiting condition began weekly 60-minute visits with the intervener in late pregnancy, and these visits continued through the child's first year of life. Once the child turned age 1, 60-minute intervener visits occurred every other week, continuing until the child turned 2. At this point, the frequency of contact shifted again to regular telephone/follow-up contact for Years 3 and 4 of the child's life (Heinicke, 2000). During month 3 to month 15 of the infant's life, mothers were given the option to attend a weekly support group with their infants, in addition to their regularly scheduled individual sessions with the intervener. When possible, sessions with the intervener focused on topics related to the mother and her immediate and principal social network (e.g., discussing marital conflicts with the mother), including the father, immediate family, and friends. By comparison, those in the pediatric follow-up group received only developmental assessments at four time points (1, 6, 12, and 24 months old), with accompanying feedback and referral to other relevant services when necessary; this participant subset was not subject to the home-visiting intervention or sustained face-to-face contact (Heinicke et al., 1999). What follows is a brief overview of the intervention itself, as received only by the randomly assigned "home-visit" group.

In order to accomplish the project's main goal of promoting mother–child relational health, Heinicke articulated specific target goals[1]—areas in which Heinicke wanted to see improvement in the mothers—and alongside these goals, he identified behavioral strategies[2] that interveners could use to meet the stated goals (Heinicke, 2000). Heinicke articulated the following therapeutic goals: consolidation of the helping, working relationship (Goal 1); enhancement of the mother's communication and personal adaptation (Goal 2); provision of alternate approaches to her relationship to her child (Goal 3); and provision of direct affirmation and support (Goal 4; see Table 6.2). These treatment goals are woven throughout the intervention process, beginning in the first few weeks. First, the research team conducts an initial evaluation of family functioning, which gives the intervener a sense of where the mother stands in terms of these desired outcomes before treatment begins. Specifically, the assessment provides the team with a picture of the mother's general psychosocial adaptation, her confidence related to motherhood, the level of partner support and nonromantic support (friends, immediate and extended family, and other relationships) she experiences, and her general ability to respond behaviorally to her infant. After the research team conducts this assessment, they form an initial treatment plan.

Then, during the initial visits with the mother, which occur during the last 2 months of the pregnancy, the intervener seeks to express the understanding of the mother's fears about her ability to love and care for her infant, that the transition to parenthood and becoming a new parent can be exceptionally difficult, and that certain issues are important to consider in the infant's first weeks of life—including differentiation of the infant's cries and reflection on the meaning conveyed in certain infant behaviors. From there, the intervener addresses each of the intervention's target goals, as tentatively planned after the initial assessment. For each of the goals, Heinicke (2000) delineates subgoals in the project's intervention manual (see Table 6.1). We turn to those now, and describe them in the order in which they appear in the manual.

Therapeutic Goal 1: Consolidation of the Helping, Working Relationship

The first therapeutic goal centers around two main targets within the context of the unique experience of first-time parenthood: the parent's awareness about what specific relational processes are operating, and explanations about the nature of the relationships within which these processes operate. In an effort to consolidate the helping, working relationship between the intervener and the mother, the intervener first seeks to make clear what the intervention entails by explaining the nature of the intervener–client relationship and how it functions in the context of the intervention. From there, the intervener and mother share enjoyment, mostly regarding the infant, but also related to other topics; this is enacted with the end

---

[1] Heinicke actually referred to these as "intervention roles." To facilitate interpretation, throughout this chapter we use the term *therapeutic goals* to refer to the targeted outcomes of treatment.

[2] Heinicke referred to the behavioral strategies enacted by the intervener to achieve therapeutic goals as "roles" and "subroles." We preserve his terminology in this chapter but remind readers that *roles/ subroles* refer to therapeutic techniques of the intervener.

TABLE 6.2. Targeted Treatment Intervention Goals and Intervener Roles

Goal 1: Consolidation of the helping, working relationship	Goal 2: Enhancing communication and personal adaptation	Goal 3: Enhancing alternative approaches to parent–child interaction	Goal 4: Providing direct affirmation and support
1. Awareness of relational processes 2. Awareness of nature of specific relationships (e.g., parent–child)	1. Increasing mother's ability to adapt and cope with social, functional, and childrearing concerns	1. Using behavioral observation methodologies to assist the mother in becoming more attuned to her child	1. Delivering pointed, direct advice and support in response to concerns
Subroles[a]	Subroles[a]	Subroles[a]	Subroles[a]
1. Intervener explains what the project entails and what it offers mother	1. Intervener listens to mother's concerns 1a. Reflects back mother's greatest concerns 1b. Empathizes and expresses understanding of concerns 1c. Checks to see if reflected and processed concerns match the mother's understanding	1. Intervener listens to mother's concerns	1. Intervener positively reinforces parent's adaptation and parenting
2. Intervener and mother build a positive relationship 2a. Share enjoyment in infant or other things (e.g., food) 2b. Take time to be together by continuing meetings and lengthening contact 2c. Express feelings about the relationships (positive or negative)	2. Intervener clarifies the antecedents, corollaries, and consequences of mother's perceived difficulties	2. Intervener clarifies the antecedents, corollaries, and consequences of mother's perceived difficulties 2a. Asks about mother's experience with observed interactions and related concerns 2b. Asks about mother's feelings as she interacts with the baby	2. Intervener positively reinforces specific responses to the child
3. Intervener directly observes the behavioral sequence	3. Intervener articulates alternative perceptions of the difficulties	3. Intervener directly advocates that specific instrumental steps be taken in dealing with concerns	
4. Intervener articulates alternative solutions to the difficulties	4. Intervener articulates alternative perceptions of the difficulties	4. Intervener provides direct assistance in pursuing the mother's goals	
5. Intervener helps mother evaluate the consequences of attempted solutions	5. Intervener provides developmental information relevant to concerns		

(continued)

TABLE 6.2. *(continued)*

Goal 1: Consolidation of the helping, working relationship	Goal 2: Enhancing communication and personal adaptation	Goal 3: Enhancing alternative approaches to parent–child interaction	Goal 4: Providing direct affirmation and support
6. Intervener empathically reflects on/clarifies mother's feelings and thoughts 6a. Clarifies feelings/thoughts 6b. Directs attention to conflicting feelings/thoughtsQW	6. Intervener offers alternative solutions to the observed difficulties 6a. Encourages alternative/additional ways of responding to infant needs 6b. Offers guidance in how to provide optimal stimulation to the infant 6c. Helps the parent enhance the infant's autonomy and sense of self		
7. Intervener interprets causal connections between feeling and thoughts 7a. Links current feelings, thoughts, and conflicts to other feelings, thoughts, and conflicts 7b. Links current feelings, thoughts, and conflicts to past feelings, thoughts, and conflicts 7c. Interprets mother's resistance–defense	7. Intervener models alternative solutions to difficulty		
8. Intervener assists mother in evaluating consequences of attempted solutions			
9. Intervener empathically reflects on/clarifies mother's feelings and thoughts with regard to child			
10. Intervener interprets causal connections between feeling and thoughts with regard to the child			

Note. Language used in the table taken in most cases directly from the intervention manual (Heinicke, 2000).

[a]Subroles indicate specific steps taken on the part of the intervener toward the end of accomplishing the stated targeted therapeutic outcome.

goal of building and maintaining a positive relationship overall, which can then serve as a foundation for trust. The intervener bolsters the relationship with the client by regular continuance of meeting times (including rescheduling without judgment when necessary) and the lengthening of sessions when appropriate—typically, when the mother is apprehensive of the intervention itself. Finally, the intervention manual suggests that the intervener and the mother should express their feelings about the intervener–client relationship—either positive or negative—in addition to appreciating the relationship and the affirmation provided by the other.

The intervener evaluates the relationship consolidation after each visit along three continuous dimensions (connection, trust, and work) using a 6-point scale ranging from 0 to 5. Heinicke defined a *positive connection* as the quality of the relationship between the mother and intervener, focusing on expressions of the wish to be with each other and maintain contact over time. The *trusting relationship* dimension is based on three factors—the mother's feelings that the intervener can be counted on for help, that the intervener will respect the mother's autonomy, and that the intervener will create a safe and secure emotional space for the sharing of intimate relational details. Finally, according to Heinicke, *work* refers to the mother's ability to confront issues, describe the issues in sufficient detail, understand the issues after working through them, and create an actionable plan on how to deal with the issues.

For Heinicke, *transference* (the carrying over of relational patterns from unresolved past or current relationships) between the mother and the intervener was a particularly important dynamic within the intervener–mother relationship. Based on the Freudian concept (Freud, 1915, 1937), its association with attachment theory (e.g., Brumbaugh & Fraley, 2006, 2007), and the Bandurian (1986) understanding that relational expectations play into the intervener–parent relationship, the intervention manual accounts for the fact that maternal expectations, as based on previous patterns, may manifest themselves positively, idealistically, or negatively. A central tenet of the intervention project required that the intervener note and explicitly address the mother's transference through discussion and interpretation.

Therapeutic Goal 2: Enhancing Communication and Personal Adaptation[3]

After the working relationship is established, the second therapeutic goal focuses more directly on the mother's childrearing, social, and functional concerns, and is targeted toward growing the mother's ability to adapt and cope with them. In order to achieve the goal of enhancing the mother's communication and personal adaptation, the intervener reflects and clarifies the mother's relationship concerns within her social circle, as applicable (e.g., significant other, family). Furthermore, the intervener demonstrates openness to discussing the intervener–client relationship, encouraging conflict resolution within that relationship as a way of facilitating learning about open communication. Heinicke (2000) further deconstructed the intervener's task in helping the mother achieve this goal by breaking down the

---

[3]Heinicke referred to this therapeutic goal (or "role," in his original terminology), as "Enhancing Communication and Personal Adaptation," though "interpersonal adaptation" may more clearly describe what he meant by this goal.

intervener's role into seven *subroles*. In brief, the first five subroles pertain to assisting the mother to adapt personally, and include listening with the goal of helping the mother formulate her concerns about relationships (Subrole 1); clarifying the antecedents, corollaries, and consequences of these concerns (Subrole 2); presenting alternate perceptions of the concerns (Subrole 3); articulating alternative solutions to the concerns (Subrole 4); and evaluating the consequences of the solutions the mother has adopted to address her relational concerns (Subrole 5). The final two *subroles* of the intervener involve reflection and interpretation of the mother's mental states, and include empathic reflection and/or clarification of feelings and thoughts (Subrole 6), and interpretations of causal connections of feelings and thoughts (Subrole 7). The end goal of this intervention role, writ large, is to assist the mother in organizing, expressing, making sense of, and working through her concerns in the context of a shared, safe space. This aspect of Heinicke's intervention bears a strong resemblance to programs that focus on enhancing *mentalization,* the act of thinking reflectively to understand that thoughts come to bear on, and influence, actions (e.g., Fonagy & Target, 1997; Fonagy, Gergely, Jurist, & Target, 2002; Sadler et al., 2013; Suchman, DeCoste, Leigh, & Borelli, 2010).

Therapeutic Goal 3: Enhancing Alternative Approaches to Parent–Child Interaction[4]

An additional goal of the intervention is the promotion of parenting sensitivity; while this goal uses similar techniques as the previous one, it adds direct behavioral methodology to assist the mother in becoming more sensitive to the needs of her child. Using extant attachment research as his guide (e.g., Main, Kaplan, & Cassidy, 1985), Heinicke assumed that enhancing parenting sensitivity was the most effective way to increase the likelihood of secure attachment in the child, and ultimately, of improved socioemotional development (Heinicke, 2000). Heinicke articulated 10 ways in which the intervener was expected to enact change in mother–child interactions in the larger context of the intervention. These 10 *roles,* as he termed them, mirrored the personal adaptation roles, with one critical difference—these roles involve observation of parent–infant interactions. Prior to observing mother–infant interactions, the intervener listens to the mother to formulate and understand her concerns about her relationship with her child (Role 1). The intervener also articulates the antecedents, corollaries, and consequences of the difficulties she encounters in parenting (Role 2). Then the intervener seeks to observe mother–infant interactions in the hopes of witnessing the behavioral sequence and assisting the mother to recognize the behavioral sequences in real-time (Role 3). The intervener then articulates alternative perceptions of the difficulties (Role 4), providing developmental information in relation to expressed concerns (Role 5), and articulates alternate solutions to the difficulties (e.g., encouraging more efficient responses to infant needs, providing strategies to appropriately stimulate the infant, or helping the mother to better allow for appropriate infant autonomy; Role 6). The intervener would also model alternative behavioral solutions to the difficulties (Role

---

[4]Heinicke referred to this therapeutic goal (or "role," in his original terminology), as "Enhancing Alternative Approaches to Parent–Child Interaction," though "enhancing maternal sensitivity" may more clearly describe what he meant by this goal.

7), evaluating the consequences of such solutions (Role 8). An integral part of this process is that the intervener must adopt empathic reflection (Role 9) and clarify the mother's feelings and thoughts in regard to the child, as well as her interpretation of causal connections of feelings and thoughts in regard to the child (Role 10). The empathic, nonjudgmental stance of the intervener is essential in preserving the trusting bond between the intervener and the mother; without this, Heinicke argued, the intervener would risk alienating the mother and forfeiting potential therapeutic gains (Heinicke, 2000).

Therapeutic Goal 4: Provision of Direct Affirmation and Support

The fourth therapeutic goal, provision of direct affirmation and support, differs from the preceding three in that it involves more direct and pointed advice in response to mother concerns. According to Heinicke's treatment manual (2000), this direct intervener support or affirmation generally assumes one or more of four *subroles*: general positive reinforcement of the parent's adaptation and parenting (Subrole 1); positive reinforcement of specific parenting behaviors (immediately after a collective evaluation of some occurrence; Subrole 2); advocacy of specific instrumental steps (e.g., assisting the mother to be planful while providing support in accomplishing individual goals as necessary; Subrole 3); and direct assistance in pursuing a goal (e.g., accompanying a parent to an important meeting; Subrole 4). Heinicke felt that the provision of tangible support by the intervener was essential in order for the other therapeutic goals to be met (Heinicke, 2000; Polansky, 1981).

Additional Considerations

The four therapeutic goals described earlier must be considered in light of the project's general time line—that is, the tapering of the visits over the first 2 years, and the transition into follow-ups in the third and fourth years of the child's life. Heinicke (2000) recommended that the intervener demystify the gradual termination of the home visits by initiating discussions with the mother about the visit-reduction and the eventual cessation of intervener contact. Consistent with the overall goals of the intervention, Heinicke suggested that during this process of tapering, the intervener express missing more frequent contact with the mother, if and when this is felt by the intervener. Given that one of the dominant goals of the intervention is consistent, professional support and the formation of a trusting bond between intervener and mother, Heinicke felt that direct discussion regarding intervention termination was essential in preventing or diminishing the sense of loss experienced by the mother during this critical time.

Mothers' Response to the Intervention

As a supplement to his careful recommendations for intervener behavior, Heinicke (2000) also delineated ways in which the mother's use of the intervention can vary across six dimensions, ranging from least adaptive to most adaptive, as based on previous research (e.g., Fonagy, Steele, Steele, Moran, & Higgitt, 1991). In general,

Heinicke (2000) noted anecdotally that mothers differed in how they made use of the intervener in the context of the overall intervention, with the measured dimensions clustering around two main poles—interpersonal factors and concrete, logistical factors. In terms of the former, mothers differed in regard to their tendency to express negative emotions, to seek affirmation from, or share personal social stories with the intervener. In terms of the latter, mothers differed in the degree to which they asked for concrete assistance, sought solutions to problems by taking an alternative viewpoint or otherwise adapting to the situation, and engaged in self-reflective behaviors in the therapeutic context.

Assessment of Change

At the end of each visit, the intervener provided quantitative and qualitative ratings of the mother's behavior during the session in terms of how it compared to her behavior during the previous sessions. Quantitative evaluations centered on measuring not only the extent to which behaviors or qualities were observed (frequency) but also the extent to which something had occurred (quality). For example, in the case of transference, it may be easier to quantify the strength of the transference rather than the number of discrete instances in which transference was evident. After the intervener rated the whole session, he or she ranked behaviors according to their relative importance in the session. The intervener also recorded change in behaviors from previous sessions on a 5-point scale from –2 to 2 (score of 0 = no change, score < 0 = negative change, score > 0 = positive change). Additionally, interveners provided narrative qualitative evaluations regarding the content covered during the home visit, the interventions used, a description of the working relationship, how the contact between the intervener and the principal figures (mother, friends, family, etc.) was utilized, and any changes noticed in the principal figures in the mother's life.

Heinicke (2000) described five types of change; interveners rated the mother on the degree to which she demonstrated behaviors falling into each of these five categories. The first, change in subjective state, encapsulates increases or decreases in both anxiety and depressive symptoms (Change 1). The second, alternative perception of the situation, indicates that a previously held felt belief about a situation has changed over time, in either a positive or a negative direction (Change 2). The third, alternative adaptation to the situation, refers to whether the mother has implemented a new strategy and whether this has resulted in a positive or negative outcome (Change 3). The fourth, change in self-evaluation, is subdivided into four further categories (Change 4): degree to which the mother expresses feeling effective in solving an issue (Change 4a), expresses a sense of felt support (Change 4b), expresses affirmation about achieving her goals (Change 4c), and expresses feeling physically attractive (Change 4d). The last type of change is the broadest and relates to the extent to which the mother negatively or positively comments on the intervention or the intervener him- or herself (Change 5).

Within this intervention program, an intervener evaluates the mother on these five change categories across three different intervals of time—pregnancy to 6-months, 6–12 months, and 12–24 months. Researchers also assessed families in the control group using the same assessment tools at these time points; taken together, these shared data points serve as the basis for evaluating the efficacy of the intervention, an area we turn to now.

Outcomes:
An Argument for the Efficacy of the UCLA Development Project

In this section we present the results Heinicke obtained from his program. In general, they converge to suggest that mothers participating in the intervention became better parents, and their children evidenced more optimal developmental outcomes, as compared to control group mothers. We organize the specific results from the intervention trial into two main sections: parent outcomes and child outcomes. Each section also contains a brief discussion of additional variables associated with the outcome measures. It is important to note that although we chose to separate the results by parents and children, their influence on each other cannot be understated. In his work, Heinicke typically examined two sets of research questions related to his intervention: group differences between the intervention and control (pediatric follow-up) groups, and factors that predicted response to treatment. Despite the fact that two cohorts completed the program, most of the reported results came from the second cohort; the subsequent literature reviewed here is weighted more heavily toward the larger cohort for simplicity. Published results related to the first cohort were reported in Heinicke et al. (2000), and are noted below in parallel to those relating to the second. Results summarized below are also noted briefly in Table 6.3, with separate columns for mother, child, and parenting outcomes.

Treatment Outcomes for Mothers

Overwhelmingly, mothers participating in the intervention benefited directly from it in terms of myriad indicators, as compared to mothers participating in only the pediatric follow-up protocols (control group). One area of particular effect was maternal social support. Given the intervention's focus on mothers' social support circles, and its dual focus on promoting mothers' relationships with their partners, it is perhaps not surprising that at the end of the first year, mothers in the intervention group reported experiencing more partner support, whereas mothers in the control group reported a decreasing amount of partner support (Heinicke et al., 1999; see Table 6.3). Furthermore, within the intervention group, only one participant lost contact with her significant other over the first year of the child's life, whereas in the control group, 10 individuals lost contact with their partners during the same amount of time. Likewise, after controlling for baseline measures of family support, mothers in the intervention group reported greater family support at the 1-year mark than their counterparts in the control group (Heinicke et al., 1999); these trends for both family and partner support continued through the second year, with significant differences holding over time (Heinicke, Fineman, Ponce, & Guthrie, 2001). In summary, the intervention increased mothers' perceived social support.

TABLE 6.3. Summary of Significant Outcomes

Publication and assessment time	Intervention group: Mother outcomes	Intervention group: Child outcomes	Intervention group: Parenting outcomes
Heinicke et al. (1999) (end of first year of child's life)	• Greater perceived partner support • Lesser likelihood of losing contact with significant other • Greater perceived family support	• Significantly more likely to be classified as secure in Strange Situation Procedure	• Greater maternal responsiveness to children • Greater displays of positive maternal affect during mother–child interactions • More frequent maternal encouragement of child autonomy • Less frequent maternal use of restriction and punishment as forms of control
Heinicke et al. (2000) (end of first year of child's life)			• More secure response to separation (among children of mothers with high partner support) • Higher expectation of being cared for (among children of mothers with high partner support)

(continued)

TABLE 6.3. *(continued)*

Publication and assessment time	Intervention group: Mother outcomes	Intervention group: Child outcomes	Intervention group: Parenting outcomes
Heinicke et al. (2001) (end of second year of child's life)	• Greater perceived family support	• Displayed more positive affect when interacting with mothers in free-play task	• Mothers used more appropriate controls
			• Children responded more positively to mothers' controls
			• Mothers of boys had significantly lesser difficulty controlling their children
		• Greater sense of separate self	• Greater maternal responsiveness to children
			• Greater displays of positive maternal affect during mother–child interactions
		• Higher involvement in tasks completed with the mother	• More frequent maternal encouragement of child autonomy
		• More compliant in tasks completed with mother	• Less frequent maternal use of restriction and punishment as forms of control
		• Boys displayed higher externalization of control	• During free play session, mothers are more engaged, more synchronized, and less intrusive with children
		• Boys reacted less negatively to control attempts by both mother and home visitor	• Mothers provided more encouragement of their children's engagement with a task
		• More positive responses to maternal control	• Mothers provided more affectionate reunion responses postseparation

Furthermore, social support measured at the end of the child's first year of life appeared to be an important factor in predicting longer-term outcomes in both treatment groups. For mothers in the control group, greater family and friend support at Year 1 predicted their use of more appropriate control at the end of Year 2, whereas mothers in the intervention group used increasingly appropriate control regardless of their level of support at Year 1 (Heinicke et al., 2001; see Table 6.3). Similarly, for mothers in the intervention group, the quality of the mother's perceived partner support at 6 months predicted both her child's secure response to separation and expectation of being cared for at the end of Year 1, as measured by the Bayley Scales of Infant Development and a short mother–child separation (Bayley, 1969; Erickson & Egeland, 1992; Heinicke et al., 2000). The intervention's focus on the support system within the family and tangential network appeared well aimed.

Another significant focus of the UCLA Development Project was improved parenting, and data collected from the first and second years suggest that the intervention succeeded in this area as well. At Year 1, mothers who participated in the program were more responsive to their children, displayed more positive affect during free-play sessions, utilized restriction and punishment as forms of control less frequently, and encouraged child autonomy more than their counterparts in the control group (Heinicke et al., 1999, 2001; see Table 6.3). These same patterns in parenting behavior again held at the end of Year 2 (Heinicke et al., 2001). In addition, mothers in the intervention group demonstrated more affectionate responses upon reunion with their child after a brief separation (Heinicke et al., 2001). Furthermore, during a free-play session, intervention group mothers were less intrusive, more engaged, and more synchronized with their children (Heinicke et al., 2001). These mothers were also rated as providing more encouragement of their children's engagement with a task (Heinicke et al., 2001). Heinicke interpreted the finding related to synchrony as evidence that the mentalization component of the intervention worked, as mothers must cooperate with their children and reflect on the child's mental states in order to display such synchronization (Heinicke et al., 2001).

Heinicke also looked at specific variations within the intervention group early on (within the first year) that predicted response to treatment. Not surprisingly, the degree of positive connection between the intervener and mother correlated positively with the mother's investment in the intervention work during the first year (Heinicke et al., 2000). The mother's attachment classification, as measured via the Adult Attachment Interview (AAI; Main, Goldwyn, & Hesse, 2003) also predicted her level of involvement in the intervention, such that mothers who were given a primary classification of unresolved/disorganized with respect to loss or trauma *and* secondarily classified as secure (U/d/F) were most involved (Heinicke et al., 2006; Heinicke & Levine, 2008). Similarly, intervention group mothers rated as having a primary or secondary secure attachment classification (i.e., were classified as Autonomous or Unresolved/Autonomous) on the AAI (George, Kaplan, & Main, 1985) increased their involvement over time, and had more positive outcomes as a result of the intervention when compared to mothers classified as any other form of insecure attachment (Heinicke et al., 2006; Heinicke & Levine, 2008). Digging into the details, Heinicke identified that Secure mothers and Unresolved/

Disorganized-Autonomous mothers attended significantly more sessions during months 7–12 of the child's life than the mothers with other attachment classifications. Interestingly, both the mother's level of involvement and her attachment classification independently and uniquely predicted scores on outcome measures related to the intervention (e.g., child's expectation of being cared for, mother's responsiveness to child needs, encouragement of child autonomy, and use of positive and verbal controls); furthermore, analysis revealed that it was the therapeutic work done in months 7–12 that really impacted the efficacy of the program overall, as that factor predicted the outcome measures above and beyond attachment classification (Heinicke & Levine, 2008). In turn, the mother's ability to work with the intervener during the second half of the first year (months 7–12) predicted her responsiveness to the needs of her baby at the end of the first year (Heinicke et al., 2000). One of Heinicke's chief aims in creating the UCLA Family Development Project was to create a supportive, collaborative environment through which the mothers would be motivated to stick with the program and enact lasting change (e.g., Heinicke et al., 1988; Heinicke et al., 1993). The results we reviewed earlier suggest that Heinicke's instinct was correct: Dedication to the treatment program clearly augmented positive outcomes.

Treatment Outcomes for Children

One of the central goals of this treatment program was to improve the likelihood of secure attachment in the child. Indeed, children of mothers in the intervention group were significantly more likely to be classified as having secure attachment in the Strange Situation Procedure aaat 1 year of age (Heinicke et al., 1999; see Table 6.3). Furthermore, at age 2, children of intervention group mothers displayed more positive affect overall when interacting with their mothers in a free-play task (Heinicke et al., 2001). Also at age 2, children of intervention group mothers had a greater sense of separate self (as measured by the Bayley Scales testing situation), were more involved in tasks, and were more compliant than children in the control group. Furthermore, Heinicke's analyses revealed that boys in the control group displayed lower externalization of control, received less appropriate maternal control, and reacted more negatively to control attempts by both the mother and the home visitor compared to children of mothers in the intervention group (Heinicke et al., 2001). Likewise, compared to control group children, children of intervention group mothers were more positive in their responses to maternal control by the end of Year 2 (Heinicke et al., 2001).

Salient Exceptions

Despite the successes documented through the program and corresponding literature, there were two areas in which the program appeared to have little effect for those participating. The first, that of child cognitive functioning, appeared unmoved by use of the intervention: There were no significant differences between groups at Years 1 and 2 (Heinicke et al., 1999, 2001). Heinicke and colleagues (1999) made sense of this through the admission that relationship-based interventions often do not impact cognitive functioning, further explaining that changes in measurement between Years 1 and 2 may have been to blame for a washed out effect, as data collected at the end of the second year used the Revised Version of the Bayley Scales of Infant Development rather than the Mental Development Index and the Performance Development Index (Heinicke et al., 1999, 2001). While previous research has indicated that cognitive functioning could be improved through similar interventions when environments were previously lacking in resources or richness (e.g., Heinicke & Ponce, 1999), the lack of growth or group differences here may be due to the fact that the intervention did not focus explicitly on fostering cognitive development.

Similarly, at both 1-year and 2-year data points, there were no between-groups differences on anxiety and depression scores, and the hypothesized reduction in anxiety and depression scores among mothers receiving the intervention was not observed (Heinicke et al., 1999, 2001). At Year 1, Heinicke et al. (1999) suggested that changes in anxiety and depression levels would emerge in the second year, as the ongoing nature of the program altered the mother's relationship to her support network, her child, and her adaptation to life more generally. In response to the fact that this pattern did not emerge in Year 2 (Heinicke et al., 2001), the authors suggested that it was the limited mode of self-report survey assessment (e.g., the Spielberger Anxiety and Beck Depression Inventories) that prevented differences from being measured accurately. Heinicke suggested that future work involving the intervention ought to include semistructured interview measurements of anxiety and depression—an important consideration for practitioners wishing to use the UCLA Family Development Project Development protocols in their upcoming work.

Ongoing Studies Involving the UCLA Family Development Framework

Ongoing research has involved extending Heinicke's intervention to novel treatment contexts and applying the intervention in varying doses. After years of research determining the evidence base for the original intervention, the current UCLA Family Development Program now also operates as a service delivery platform for new parents and their young children. The program has two primary implementation aims: embedding care in medical clinics, where families are most likely to receive services, and adopting a public health model for delivery of the intervention. These two areas of implementation growth mutually inform one another, and we describe them in turn below. Although the program is currently still collecting outcome data on these modifications of the traditional Family Development Program, anecdotal evidence thus far has been encouraging. In the paragraphs that follow, we discuss the ways in which the program has been extended in recent years.

By embedding the program within medical clinics, interveners from the Family Development Program maintain close ties with family medical providers who are often the first line of screening and referral for parents and their children. The Family Development Program has been embedded in departments of obstetrics and gynecology (Ob/Gyn) and most recently in a neonatal intensive care unit (NICU), to date providing services to over 300 families. When working in these contexts, interveners attend regular rounds within the medical department on a daily, weekly, or monthly basis, depending on the specific needs of the medical team. Interveners are able to update physicians regarding ongoing vulnerabilities and current progress that families have made in their work together, as well as provide consultation to the physicians regarding the types of parent–child interactions that would be concerning to attachment-informed interventionists. In addition, initial appointments and consultations with the mothers often take place within the primary care setting, with subsequent weekly home visits taking place over the first year of the child's life. When requested by the mother, visits can also take place in the medical office to coincide with the family's routine or specialty medical visits. Preliminary observations suggest that the interveners have been successful in educating medical staff about the needs of new parents, and in providing them with strategies to support healthy attachment relationships for the infant. Furthermore, introducing the program in the primary care context has served as a bridge for the introduction of mental health services to at-risk families, allowing the Family Development Program to gain access to families who may not otherwise seek its services.

Adopting a public health framework for service delivery has helped the program to better serve families who may not need or want a full 2 years of intervention. In today's context, families (and providers) are often interested in shorter-term intervention. Previously, many families expressed interest in the Family Development Program but were unable or unwilling to commit to 2 years of home visiting. Historically, and consistent with Heinicke's belief that the effective treatment relies, at least in part, on the client's ability to acquiesce to the requirements of the intervention (Heinicke, 1990), these families often declined services or prematurely terminated their treatment. Furthermore, in the current climate of intervention delivery, with a focus on shorter-term evidence-based approaches, a 2-year model may not be fully sustainable and relevant to many family contexts. The program has been adapted to meet the shifting needs of families and now offers a wider variety of prevention and intervention modalities that are consistent with the current psychological health continuum of care (National Research Council, Institute of Medicine, 1994, 2009). Using a "suite of services" approach, the program now offers services such as provider education, parent consultation, and a yearlong intervention. This approach has been used successfully by other family-level preventive interventions (Beardslee, Ayoub, Avery, Watts, & O'Carroll, 2010; Beardslee et al., 2011; Lester et al., 2011; Mogil et al., 2010). Education of community providers and medical professionals supports the broader systems of care in which families reside (Bronfenbrenner, 1977, 1986). Parent consultations may take the form of a single session and focus on one specific piece of developmental guidance or may take place across multiple sessions, during which the intervener provides education and teaches specific skills or strategies to address the parent's primary concern. Families selecting the full intervention receive weekly home visits for up to 14 months. The intervener can also meet the parent and child in the medical office, if requested by the mother, as described earlier. For example, for infants requiring a NICU admission, the parent may choose to have the "home visit" start at the bedside while the child remains hospitalized. This allows for the intervener to observe firsthand how the parent–child relationship is developing in the context of intensive medical care, which can be quite challenging for the infant–parent relationship. NICU visits may occur anywhere from a few days to several months.

Conclusion

In each of the published articles documenting the impact of the UCLA Family Development Project, the overarching theme presented by Heinicke is one of optimism, as well as deep respect for mothers. Given the underprivileged profile of the families selected to participate, and Heinicke's strongly held belief in the efficacy of early intervention, it is no wonder that the goals of the project—namely, to improve the lives of parents and children in the fullest sense—were generally met. Most notably, the targets of the intervention were those who were most at risk, directly underscoring the importance of the project to those whose lives appear changed for the better because of it. From the beginning of his career, Dr. Heinicke was committed to creating an intervention solidly grounded in theory and extant research on attachment relationships. After completing his doctorate at Harvard University, courtesy of a Commonwealth Fund Fellowship, he continued his training in London, where we worked with John Bowlby at his Tavistock Psychiatric Research Unit, whom he had met when Bowlby visited Harvard. While in London, he completed a study on the impact of brief separations on children. The results of his work, which involved extensive, careful observations of children experiencing differing degrees of separation (Heinicke, 1956), suggested that children experiencing more extreme separations (those in residential care) showed greater disturbance than those experiencing less extreme separations (those in day nurseries). The results of this study and Heinicke's subsequent observational work helped Bowlby respond to a criticism of his work, namely, that there was a lack of evidence that long separations of children and parents were harmful. While in London, Heinicke also completed psychoanalytic training at the Anna Freud Centre, becoming the first psychoanalyst without medical training. He would later wed this early child psychoanalytic training to an appreciation for the entire ecosystem surrounding the parent–child relationship, incorporating and citing Bronfenbrenner's bioecological systems model and concurrent push for family- rather than individual-based intervention protocols (e.g., Bronfenbrenner, 1974). Later, in summarizing dominant empirical bases for what makes an intervention more likely to succeed (see Heinicke, 1990, for a review), Heinicke all but outlined what he saw as the most effective way to pursue long-term positive change within families, culminating in the UCLA Family Development Project. One gets the sense that this intervention program was, and truly remained, his masterpiece.

In describing the results of the intervention, Heinicke was always the first to suggest further ways in which the process could be refined and made better, implying that the ultimate goal was for the project to continue to evolve in such a way that others would benefit long after the initial cohort had completed its involvement. To that end, it is our great hope that the Heinicke's legacy be furthered through continuing practice and ongoing refinements to the intervention as new directions emerge in the study of parent–child and family relationships. In that spirit, those wishing to learn more about the intervention are encouraged to reach out to Dr. Catherine Mogil, Director of the UCLA Family Development Program, for additional information regarding the implementation of the intervention.

ACKNOWLEDGMENTS

This chapter is dedicated with heartfelt respect and love to the late Dr. Christoph Heinicke, who spent his life in dogged pursuit of finding ways to help at-risk families. Furthermore, we extend gratitude to the mothers and infants who participated in previous and ongoing studies of the Family Development Project—you were Heinicke's inspiration.

REFERENCES

Ainsworth, M. D., & Bell, S. M. (1970). Attachment, exploration, and separation: Illustrated by the behavior of one-year-olds in a Strange Situation. *Child Development, 41*(1), 49–67.

Bandura, A. (1986). *Social foundations of thought and action: A social cognitive theory.* Englewood Cliffs, NJ: Prentice-Hall.

Bayley, N. (1969). *Manual for the Bayley Scales of Infant Development.* New York: Psychological Corporation.

Beardslee, W. R., Ayoub, C., Avery, M. W., Watts, C. L., O'Carroll, K. L. (2010). Family connections: An approach for strengthening early care systems in facing depression and adversity. *American Journal of Orthopsychiatry, 80*, 482–495.

Beardslee, W. R., Lester, P., Klosinski, L., Saltzman, W., Woodward, K., Nash, W., . . . Leskin, G. (2011). Family-centered preventive intervention for military families: Implications for implementation science. *Prevention Science, 12*(4), 339–348.

Bowlby, J. (1944). Forty-four juvenile thieves: Their characters and home life. *International Journal of Psychoanalysis, 25*, 19–53.

Bowlby, J. (1958). The nature of the child's tie to his mother. *International Journal of Psychoanalysis, 39*, 350–373.

Bowlby, J. (1980). *Attachment and loss: Vol. 3. Loss.* New York: Basic Books.

Bowlby, J., Robertson, J., & Rosenbluth, D. (1952). A two-year-old goes to the hospital. *Psychoanalytic Study of the Child, 7*, 82–94.

Bronfenbrenner, U. (1974). Is early intervention effective? *Early Childhood Education Journal, 2*(2), 14–18.

Bronfenbrenner, U. (1977). Toward an experimental ecology of human development. *American Psychologist, 32*(7), 513–531.

Bronfenbrenner, U. (1986). Ecology of the family as a context for human development. *Developmental Psychology, 22*(6), 723–742.

Brumbaugh, C. C., & Fraley, R. C. (2006). Transference and attachment: How do attachment patterns get carried forward from one relationship to the next? *Personality and Social Psychology Bulletin, 32*, 552–560.

Brumbaugh, C. C., & Fraley, R. C. (2007). Transference of attachment patterns: How important relationships influence feelings toward novel people. *Personal Relationships, 14*, 513–530.

Egeland, B., & Erikson, M. F. (1990). Rising above the past: Strategies for helping new mothers break the cycle of abuse and neglect. *ZERO TO THREE, 11*(2), 29–35.

Erickson, M., & Egeland, B. (1992). *Project STEEP: Free play interaction scales.* Unpublished manuscript, University of Minnesota, Minneapolis, Minnesota.

Fonagy, P., Gergely, G., Jurist, E., & Target, M. (2002). *Affect regulation, mentalisation, and the development of the self.* New York: Other Press.

Fonagy, P., Steele, M., Steele, H., Moran, G. S., & Higgitt, A. C. (1991). The capacity for understanding mental states: The reflective self in parent and child and its significance for security of attachment. *Infant Mental Health Journal, 13*(3), 200–217.

Fonagy, P., & Target, M. (1997). Attachment and reflective function: Their role in self-organization. *Development and Psychopathology, 9*, 679–700.

Freud, S. (1915). Observations on transference-love. In S. J. Ellman (Ed.), *Freud's technique papers: A contemporary perspective* (pp. 65–80). Northvale, NJ: Jason Aronson.

Freud, S. (1937). Analysis terminable and interminable. *International Journal of Psychoanalysis, 18*, 373–405.

George, C., Kaplan, N., & Main, M. (1985). *Adult Attachment Interview.* Unpublished manuscript, University of California, Berkeley, Berkeley, California.

Heinicke, C. M. (1956). Some effects of separating two-year-old children from their parents: A comparative study. *Human Relations, 9*, 105–176.

Heinicke, C. M. (1976). Aiding "at risk" children through psychoanalytic social work with parents. *American Journal of Orthopsychiatry, 46*(1), 89–103.

Heinicke, C. M. (1990). Toward generic principles of treating parents and children: Integrating psychotherapy with the school-aged child and early family intervention. *Journal of Consulting and Clinical Psychology, 6*, 713–719.

Heinicke, C. M. (2000). *The UCLA Development Project: Definition of initial contacts, methods of interventions, use made by the family, and changes seen.* Unpublished manuscript available from the Neuropsychiatric Institute, University of California at Los Angeles, Los Angeles, CA 90024.

Heinicke, C. M., Beckwith, L., & Thompson, A. (1988). Early intervention in the family system: A framework and review. *Infant Mental Health Journal, 9*(2), 111–141.

Heinicke, C. M., Fineman, N. R., Ponce, V. A., & Guthrie, D. (2001). Relation-based intervention with at-risk mothers: Outcome in the second year of life. *Infant Mental Health Journal, 22*(4), 431–462.

Heinicke, C. M., Fineman, N. R., Ruth, G. G., Recchia, S. L., Guthrie, D. D., & Rodning, C. C. (1999). Relationship-based intervention with at-risk mothers: Outcome in the first year of life. *Infant Mental Health Journal, 20*(4), 349–374.

Heinicke, C. M., Goorsky, M., Levine, M., Ponce, V., Ruth, G., Silverman, M., & Sotelo, C. (2006). Pre- and postnatal antecedents of a home-visiting intervention and family developmental outcome. *Infant Mental Health Journal, 27*(1), 91–119.

Heinicke, C. M., Goorsky, M. M., Moscov, S. S., Dudley, K. K., Gordon, J. J., Schneider, C. C., & Guthrie, D. D. (2000). Relationship-based intervention with at-risk mothers: Factors affecting variations in outcome. *Infant Mental Health Journal, 21*(3), 133–155.

Heinicke, C. M., & Levine, M. (2008). The AAI anticipates the outcome of a relation-based early intervention. In H. Steele & M. Steele (Eds.), *Clinical applications of the Adult Attachment Interview* (pp. 99–125). New York: Guilford Press.

Heinicke, C. M., & Ponce, V. A. (1999). Relation-based early family intervention. In D. Cicchetti & S. L. Toth (Eds.), *Rochester Symposium on Developmental Psychopathology* (Vol. 9, pp. 153–194). Rochester, NY: University of Rochester Press.

Heinicke, C. M., Recchia, S., Berlin, P., & James, C. (1993). *Manual for coding global child and parent–child ratings.* Unpublished manuscript, available from the Department of Psychiatry, University of California at Los Angeles.

Heinicke, C. M., & Westheimer, I. (1965). *Brief separations.* New York: International Universities Press.

Lester, P., Mogil, C., Saltzman, W., Woodward, K., Nash, W., Leskin, G., . . . Beardslee, W. (2011). FOCUS (Families OverComing Under Stress): Implementing family-centered prevention for military families facing wartime deployments and combat operational stress. *Military Medicine, 176*(1), 19–25.

Lieberman, A. F., Weston, D. R., & Paul, J. H. (1991). Preventive intervention and outcome with anxiously attached dyads. *Child Development, 62*, 199–209.

Main, M., Goldwyn, R., & Hesse, E. (2003). *Adult attachment scoring and classification systems* (Manual in draft: Version 7.2). Unpublished manuscript, Department of Psychology, University of California, Berkeley, Berkeley, California.

Main, M., Kaplan, N., & Cassidy, J. (1985). Security in infancy, childhood and adulthood: A move to the level of representation. *Monographs of the Society for Research in Child Development, 50*(1-2, Serial No. 209), 66–104.

Mogil, C., Paley, B., Doud, T., Havens, L., Moore-Tyson, J., Beardslee, W., & Lester, P. (2010). Families OverComing Under Stress (FOCUS) for Early Childhood: Building resilience for young children in high stress families. *ZERO TO THREE, 31*(1), 10–16.

National Research Council, Institute of Medicine. (1994). *Preventing mental, emotional, and behavioral disorders among young people: Progress and possibilities.* Washington, DC: National Academies Press.

National Research Council, Institute of Medicine. (2009). *Preventing mental, emotional, and behavioral disorders among young people: Progress and possibilities.* Washington, DC: National Academies Press.

Polansky, N. A. (1981). *Damaged parents.* Chicago: University of Chicago Press.

Sadler, L. S., Slade, A., Close, N., Webb, D. L., Simpson, T., Fennie, K., & Mayes, L. C. (2013). Minding the baby: Enhancing reflectiveness to improve early health and relationship outcomes in an interdisciplinary home visiting program. *Infant Mental Health Journal, 34*(5), 391–405.

Sroufe, L. A. (2005). Attachment and development: A prospective, longitudinal study from birth to adulthood. *Attachment and Human Development, 7*(4), 349–367.

Suchman, N. E., DeCoste, C., Leigh, D., & Borelli, J. (2010). Reflective functioning in mothers with drug use disorders: Implications for dyadic interactions with infants and toddlers. *Attachment and Human Development, 12*(6), 567–585.

CHAPTER 7

Minding the Baby
Complex Trauma
and Attachment-Based Home Intervention

ARIETTA SLADE, TANIKA EAVES SIMPSON, DENISE WEBB,
JESSICA GORKIN ALBERTSON, NANCY CLOSE,
and LOIS SADLER

Although *attachment-based intervention* is a relatively new term (Berlin, Ziv, Amaya-Jackson, & Greenberg, 2005), interventions aimed at helping parents promote secure attachment in their infants have been around for a long time. In the classic article "Ghosts in the Nursery: A Psychoanalytic Approach to the Problems of Impaired Mother–Infant Relationships," Selma Fraiberg and her colleagues (Fraiberg, Adelson, & Shapiro, 1975) described the first ever "infant–parent psychotherapy"; this approach was more fully described 5 years later in the pioneering *Clinical Studies in Infant Mental Health* (Fraiberg, 1980). Although Fraiberg did not frame the work in attachment terms, she and her colleagues were in every way guided by the idea that a loving, reciprocal relationship provides the child both with a sense of essential connection to others and willingness to explore and know the larger world. The intervention introduced a way of working that is now common to many attachment-based interventions: Sessions were carried out in the home, not the office, and the "patients" were infants and their mothers, with whom the clinicians worked in a dyadic way. Every effort was made to enlist even the most challenging and resistant families in the intervention, with the explicit recognition that the most frightened, angry, or hard-to-reach mothers were often those most desperately in need. These were highly traumatized families who had long histories with the social care system and were understandably highly suspicious of anyone who approached them to "help."

Fraiberg and her colleagues were not deterred by the fact that the families they were seeing had significant trauma exposure; indeed, one of their explicit goals was to interrupt the intergenerational transmission of trauma by supporting the development of healthy, reciprocal mother–child relationships and promote secure, safe attachments. Alicia Lieberman, who worked alongside Fraiberg as the infant mental health movement was born, has since then provided an evidence base for infant–parent psychotherapy (Lieberman, Weston, & Pawl, 1991), as well as its modern day iteration "child–parent psychotherapy" (Lieberman, Ghosh Ippen, & Van Horn, 2015; Toth, Michl-Petzing, Guild, & Lieberman, Chapter 13, this volume), and established the core principles and approaches of trauma-informed early intervention (Lieberman & Van Horn, 2008).

Attachment and trauma are inextricably linked. A history of trauma in the mother (and thus a likely insecure or unresolved attachment classification) powerfully increases the likelihood of insecure or disorganized attachment in the child (Carlson, 1998; Lyons-Ruth, Bronfman, & Parsons, 1999; Lyons-Ruth, Yellin, Melnick, & Atwood, 2005; Main & Hesse, 1990; Schuengel, Bakermans-Kranenburg, & van IJzendoorn, 1999). Thus, one of the primary goals of attachment-based interventions with high risk or vulnerable families is to support the development of flexible, loving, secure attachment relationships. These relationships protect the child from the impact of stressful and destructive environments and, we hope, decrease substantially the likelihood of adverse experiences in the child's own early life. In this, they are key to resilience and an openness to the world.

In this chapter, we explore the impact of trauma-related psychopathology in mothers, and in particular complex or developmental trauma (Courtois, 2004; Herman, 1992; van der Kolk, 2014), on attachment-based intervention. Clinical and research data from Minding the Baby® (MTB), our interdisciplinary, intensive home-visiting program for young families, provide the foundation for this discussion. We begin with a description of complex developmental trauma, then turn to the MTB intervention itself. We describe our work with one mother and child, Genevieve and Jimmy, in order to take a deeper look at the challenges of working with complex trauma disorders, as well as the benefits of an interdisciplinary approach in overcoming some of these challenges. We then summarize the results of our pilot randomized controlled trial (RCT) (Sadler et al., 2013). Finally, we describe mechanisms for training in and dissemination of MTB.

Developmental or Complex Trauma

Developmental or complex trauma disorder was first defined by Herman (1992) and later developed fully by van der Kolk and his colleagues (van der Kolk, 1994, 2014; van der Kolk, Roth, Pelcovitz, Sunday, & Spinazzola, 2005). This work formed the essential framework for what is today a considerable literature on trauma study and treatment (for overviews, see Courtois, 2004; van der Kolk, 2014).

Trauma has a profound impact on the body, both the corpus itself *and* the brain. As van der Kolk (1994, 2014) so poignantly notes, "the body keeps the score"; devastating and often unspeakable traumas are stored in the body, in the primitive, precortical parts of the brain, or the limbic system. Memories and affects that cannot be processed consciously live on, manifest in disruptions in consciousness, sensation, and impulse control. In these circumstances, arousal overrides reflection and mentalization again and again. Compelling evidence for the link between trauma and the body has also been provided by results of the Adverse Childhood Experiences studies (*acestudy.org*; Felitti et al., 1998), which document the lifelong and profound impact of trauma on physical health and mental health. Shonkoff (2012) and his colleagues' work on "toxic stress" adds extreme poverty, racism, and familial and community violence to those factors that profoundly disrupt self-regulation. Both the Adverse Childhood Experiences studies and Shonkoff and his colleagues' work on toxic stress implicate the early disruption of the stress regulation and autoimmune systems in the development of a range of health and mental health disturbances. Garner (2013) notes that home visiting provides a particularly direct and important means of ameliorating the impact of toxic stress and adversity on the child's development.

The symptoms of complex trauma are thought to be distinct from "simple" posttraumatic stress disorder (PTSD), which is typically defined as a response to an acute trauma or series of linked traumatic events. Single or short-lived traumatic incidents are unlikely to have nearly the devastating impact on one's fundamental relationship to the body, to others, and to the world as do those that are chronic and repeated, wearing away at the stress regulation system hour by hour, day by day, week by week, and month by month. Ongoing, chronic trauma profoundly affects the development of a sense of a coherent self, a felt body, regulated, tolerable affects, and the capacity to establish close, safe, and loving relationships. In a review article published in 2004, Courtois defined *complex trauma* as "a type of trauma that occurs repeatedly and cumulatively, usually over a period of time and within specific relationships and contexts. [The term] extends to all forms of domestic violence and attachment trauma occurring in the context of family and other intimate relationships. These forms of intimate/domestic abuse often occur over extended time periods during which the victim is entrapped and conditioned in a variety of ways" (p. 412). Thus, "individuals exposed to trauma over a variety of time spans and developmental periods suffered from a variety of psychological problems not included in the diagnosis of PTSD, including depression, anxiety, self-hatred, dissociation, substance abuse, self-destructive and risk-taking behaviors, revictimization, problems with interpersonal and intimate relationships (*including parenting*), medical and somatic concerns, and despair" (p. 413, emphasis added). In other words, many of the symptoms reported by individuals who have high levels of sustained trauma exposure are best viewed as *proxies* for an underlying complex trauma disorder. Thus, signs or symptoms of depression or anxiety cannot be taken at face value, but must be identified *and treated* as they relate to the diagnosis of complex trauma.

Courtois (2004) notes that these symptoms of complex trauma are best seen as "essential elements of complicated posttraumatic adaptations" (p. 414), rather than as symptoms of a range of comorbid disorders. These posttraumatic adaptations include (1) alterations in the regulation of affective impulses (anger and self-destructiveness, self-harming, addictive behavior), (2) alterations in attention and consciousness (amnesia, dissociation, and depersonalization), (3) alterations in self-perception (extreme guilt, shame, and self-hatred), (4) alterations in perceptions of the perpetrator (incorporating the belief system of the abusive caretaker), (5) alterations in relationship to others, *including parenting* (inability to trust), (6) somatic/medical complaints (including all body systems), and (7) alterations in systems of meaning (hopelessness and despair about ever being able to recover from psychic anguish) (see Herman, 1992; Courtois, 2004).

van der Kolk (2014), Courtois (2004), and others suggest that best practice in working with complex trauma involves a combined approach to alliance building on the one hand and stress and distress regulation on the other. As van der Kolk (2014) puts it, interventions must combine "top-down approaches (to activate social engagement) with bottom-up methods (to calm physical tensions in the body)" (p. 86). Both an atmosphere of safety *and* quieting the body (and thus regulating the stress response system in a variety of ways) are crucial to the emergence of thinking, remembering, and mentalizing (i.e., cortical processing).

Alliance building refers to the establishment of a safe clinician–patient relationship, and a focus on rupture and repair. Courtois (2004) describes this as proceeding in stages, with a lengthy first stage of relationship building as crucial in *preparing* patients for the more common treatment for trauma symptoms, namely, psychotherapy and medication. The failure to focus on safety and the relationship, and moving in too quickly on trauma processing, hardens defensiveness and precludes the development of the capacity to reflect on one's own experience without fear and dysregulation. Thus, a stage "devoted to the development of the treatment alliance, affect regulation, education, safety, and skill-building" (p. 418), as well as self-care and self-compassion, is essential. "The middle stage, generally undertaken when the client has enough life stability and has learned adequate affect modulation and coping skills, is directed toward the processing of traumatic material in enough detail and to a degree of completion and resolution to allow the individual to function with less posttraumatic impairment" (p. 418). Courtois notes that many patients do not disclose their traumatic experiences for a very long time; in some instances—despite a good relationship with the clinician—specific working through of trauma may not occur at all. However, the capacities for connection and regulation that are ideally outgrowths of the pretreatment stage may be adequate for functioning to stabilize.

The second, equally important aspect of trauma treatment is direct attention to the body and bodily sensation (van der Kolk, 2014). Techniques include mindfulness meditation, yoga, breathing exercises, sensorimotor therapy (Ogden, Minton, & Pain, 2006), neurofeedback, eye movement desensitization and reprocessing (EMDR), music, dance, and the like. These techniques are meant to increase the awareness and tolerance of emotion, and calm the sympathetic nervous system. These provide, to use van der Kolk's poetic phrase, "limbic system therapy" (2014), and serve to short-circuit fight, flight, and freezing responses, natural defenses in the face of danger (Porges, 2011).

Both approaches pave the way toward meaningful dynamic work (i.e., remembering, feeling, and understanding the roots of one's suffering, or making sense of family relationships), making sense of a child's emotions, or benefiting from psychoeducation; that is, this work develops the skills and capacities necessary for the emergence of mentalization and other forms of reflection and working through. Addressing trauma without these crucial supports in place is to expose the patient to unnecessary harm and the potential for retraumatization. As we describe in the following sections, attention to the relationship and to quieting the body are key to our approach in MTB.

Minding the Baby

....

The Intervention

MTB is a voluntary, preventive, home-visiting intervention that is delivered over the 27-month period from the third trimester of pregnancy through to the child's second birthday (Sadler et al., 2013). First-time mothers are recruited at community health centers during routine prenatal visits toward the latter end of the second trimester of pregnancy, and are seen weekly until the child is age 1, and then biweekly until the child is age 2. Fathers and other family members (grandparents and other siblings) are invited to participate as well, and implementation is flexible and responsive to the family members' needs. MTB was developed in 2002, in a collaboration between Yale Child Study Center and the Yale School of Nursing, and the Fair Haven Community Health Center (FHCHC) in New Haven, Connecticut (Sadler et al., 2013; Sadler, Slade, & Mayes, 2006; Slade & Sadler, 2013; Slade, Sadler, & Mayes, 2005; Slade et al., 2016). MTB has been tested in a federally and privately supported RCT (Sadler et al., 2013), and in 2014 was granted status by the U.S. Health Resources and Services Administration as an "evidence-based" home-visiting model.

The program is delivered by a team that includes a master's level nurse and a social worker, both of whom see the mother regularly on an alternating basis. This interdisciplinary model brings together the strengths of two prominent home-visiting models: the nurse home visiting-model developed by David Olds and Harriet Kitzman, the Nurse–Family Partnership (NFP; Olds, 2002; Donelan-McCall & Olds, Chapter 4, this volume), and the infant–parent psychotherapy model pioneered by Fraiberg, Lieberman, and their colleagues. NFP, the most widely implemented and tested home-visiting intervention in the United States, is delivered by public health nurses and provides sustained attention to the health care needs of vulnerable families. While the nurse home-visiting model effectively addresses health concerns, nurses often struggle to meet the complex *mental health* needs of traumatized mothers and their infants, particularly with "low psychological resource" mothers (Olds et al., 2010). The infant–parent psychotherapy model was designed specifically to address these issues and to remedy their impact on the mother–child relationship and the child. And so in MTB, these two disciplines work closely together, engaging families as a team, and meeting multiple and overlapping needs in a collaborative way. This approach also allows team members to support each other in the inherent challenges of the work, and to share together in its triumphs and successes. This model also removes some of the stigma of mental health treatment, as families are often more open to accepting help from nurses than from mental health workers. As exemplified in one MTB mother's description of a childhood game in which she and her siblings would play "here comes the social worker," social workers are often (correctly) associated with child protective services and terrifying childhood losses. Embedded within the framework of an interdisciplinary intervention, however, the threat of mental health intervention is greatly reduced.

The roles of the nurse and social worker are both distinct and overlapping. On the one hand, each clinician delivers services unique to his or her discipline. The nurse attends to a number of aspects of the infant and mother's health, providing support for labor and delivery, breast feeding, birth control, nutrition, smoking cessation, mindfulness-based stress reduction, pediatric well-baby care, and triage with the community health center when mothers or babies are ill. In addition, the nurse provides pediatric anticipatory guidance, helping mothers to be prepared for and thus able to scaffold their infants' and toddlers' development. The social worker uses a range infant mental health approaches to help mothers "see" and "hear" their babies, in addition to offering crisis intervention, individual counseling and couple therapy, as indicated. The social worker also provides a range case management services, linking mothers with housing, education, and other social services.

The clinicians' roles also overlap in a variety of ways, and indeed, the intervention often relies on a subtle meshing of roles, with one clinician picking up where the other has left off. Both home visitors work to support the mother–child relationship, positive interactions, and the development of secure attachment in the child. More generally, they promote the child's development (e.g., by encouraging the mother to read to the child) as well as positive goals and life course outcomes in mothers and their families. Both also provide a range of concrete supports for mothers, including diapers from a local diaper bank, donated books and toys, and, when necessary, emergency food.

MTB's relationship-based approach builds the alliances that Courtois (2004), van der Kolk (2014) and others (Lieberman & van Horn, 2008) see as foundational to helping them become more regulated and organized, and thus able to begin to live their lives outside of the devastating effects of trauma. As Courtois notes, the alliance-building stage can last for a long time, and may or may not lead to specific processing of trauma-related material. What it does is build the skills that are necessary for higher level functioning and openness to one's internal experience. A number of our mothers were ready to accept referrals for psychotherapy at the end of their time in MTB, although—as anyone who works with disadvantaged populations knows—finding suitable placements can be very difficult.

In addition to alliance building, much of the work of MTB involves the "bottom-up" physical approaches deemed so important by van der Kolk (2014). Both clinicians encourage pleasurable bodily contact between mother and baby from birth onward, helping mothers to rock, soothe, and breast-feed their babies. They also encourage singing to the baby, and joining the baby in pleasurable cycles of engagement. Trauma often robs its victim of the capacity to find pleasure in the body, but the simple contentment of holding a baby close, of feeling a baby calm to one's voice, of smiling, cooing, and laughing together, provide poignant opportunities for comforting and calming physical intimacy, with mother and baby adjusting to each other's heartbeats and breath. When these exchanges go well, when they are pleasurable and relaxing, they provide a kind of "limbic system therapy" for mothers, calming agitation, tension, and anxiety. Indeed, Selma Fraiberg referred to having the baby in the room with the mother as akin to having "God on your side" (Fraiberg, 1980). Perhaps part of what she meant was that the simple acts of touching, smiling, *of engaging with each others' bodies,* can be powerful and transforming for those mothers whose bodies have been sources of great pain and shame.

In addition, much of what the nurses do with mothers is geared specifically toward enhancing an awareness of the body and of bodily sensations well before the baby is born. For example, the nurse helps mothers create a labor plan weeks before the baby is born (Simkin, 1992); together, the mother and nurse review the birth process, starting with the first contractions. Mothers are encouraged to think through what will make them feel most comfortable and safe during the delivery—who they want to have present, when and whether they want to be medicated for pain, and what they anticipate it will be like putting their legs in stirrups (a highly triggering event for sexual abuse victims), and so forth. Many of our mothers are quite naive about both conception and birth, and need a lot of support to listen to their bodies in the most basic ways. They need help recognizing basic cues in their babies, and in establishing regular routines around sleep and eating. Nurses also work directly to support breast feeding and help mothers decide when they feel physically ready to resume sexual relations with their partners. Both nurses and social workers integrate mindfulness practices, breath work, deep relaxation, and yoga into home visits.

These two approaches are essential to moving mothers out of fight, flight, or freeze modes, out of states of dysregulation, and into more reflective and mentalizing modes. Developing a relationship and quieting the body go hand in hand, and out of both evolves the capacity for reflection and mentalization. Without connecting to the home visitors and calming their physiological dysregulation, mothers often cannot turn their attention to the baby.

MTB is also mentalization-based, in that both nurses and mental health clinicians (typically social workers) work to promote and support mothers' capacity to *reflect* on their own and their babies' experience: to accurately envision what their infants and toddlers might be thinking and feeling, to recognize and respond to the intent of attachment behaviors and signals, and to make meaning of what they themselves are feeling as parents, and as individuals (Fonagy et al., 1995). This approach is distinct from a behavioral approach, in which the focus of treatment is changing behavior; mentalization-based approaches assume that behavior change follows from the capacity to understand underlying mental states. A mother's capacity for mentalization, or reflective functioning (RF), is linked to secure attachment in mothers and babies (Slade, 2005; Slade, Grienenberger, Bernbach, Levy, & Locker, 2005), to the relative absence of disrupted affective communication in mother–infant dyads, and lower rates of disorganized attachment in infants (Grienenberger, Kelly, & Slade, 2005).

Because working with highly stressed and vulnerable families is challenging and potentially activating for clinicians (Slade et al., 2016), and because clinicians' capacity for RF is what promotes these same capacities in mothers, MTB provides a deep and wide network of support for clinicians. Both in our local MTB program, which includes three part-time supervisors and four staff members, as well as in our replications, the clinicians receive 1 hour of weekly disciplinary and another hour of interdisciplinary reflective, clinical, and administrative supervision from senior clinicians, and remain in close, continuous contact with their clinical partner through phone calls, texts, e-mails, and in person check-ins. We think of supervision using the "nested mentalization" model (Slade et al., 2016) to describe the layers of "holding" built into the infrastructure of the program: The supervisors hold the team in mind, the team members hold each other *as well as* mother and baby in mind, so that she can hold the baby in mind (see Figure 7.1). Supervisors

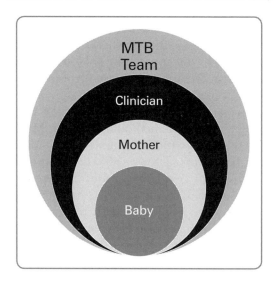

FIGURE 7.1. Nested mentalization.

and administrators also maintain essential parameters around work–life boundaries and self-care, and ensure protected and regularly scheduled time for clinicians to have space to think more deeply about their work and the feelings, thoughts, and fears these very delicate, complicated relationships trigger. This fortifies the clinicians to keep returning to their work in the face of the trauma, pain, and suffering to which they must bear witness (Weatherston & Barron, 2009), and helps them remain reflective. Table 7.1 depicts the MTB model.

The Families

First-time pregnant women between ages 14 and 25 who were receiving their prenatal care at two health care centers in New Haven were invited to join the study during their second trimester. Mothers were eligible for the study unless they were psychotic, abused drugs or alcohol, or had a terminal or life-threatening illness. Mothers were evaluated along a number of dimensions at the time of recruitment into the study, and mother and baby were then evaluated when the child was 4 months, 12 months, and 24 months of age (see Sadler et al., 2013). They were assigned to the treatment or control condition based on the research condition to which their prenatal group had been assigned. Control mothers and babies received routine prenatal, postnatal, pediatric, and medical care at the FHCHC from which they had been recruited. Mothers in the pilot RCT sample were predominantly Latina (66%) and African American/Caribbean (28%), and the mean age of subjects was 19. Nearly 70% of the mothers recruited were teen parents. The average level of education attained was 11 years, 4 months. All of the families seen were on some form of public assistance, and most reported significant trauma exposure in childhood.

Assessing trauma within the framework of a voluntary intervention that is aimed at enhancing the mother–child relationship is complex. Mothers did not (consciously) join the intervention seeking treatment or evaluation, and while some reported trauma or trauma symptoms at intake, others denied or avoided discussing traumatic experiences, even when these had been documented in their medical or social service records, and even when they seemed to trust and rely on us. But it was made clear to the mothers from the beginning of the intervention that we were open to hearing their challenges and their stories, however difficult these might be. Clinicians followed their judgment about whether to press mothers or to wait for the story to unfold over time. Sometimes talking about trauma was a way to

TABLE 7.1. The MTB Model

Service/delivery	MTB
Modality	Home visits with mother, child, and available family members (fathers, grandmothers)
Population	First-time mothers between ages 14 and 25 without severe illness or active drug use
Delivered by	Advanced practice nurse and licensed social worker team. Clinicians alternate visits; joint visits as necessary
Frequency	Weekly visits from third trimester of pregnancy to 12 months; biweekly visits until child is 2
Length	27 months
Characteristics	
Risk	Moderate- to high-risk populations
Age range	Prenatal to 24 months
Intervention	
Theory base	Attachment/mentalization theory Trauma theory Social ecology/self-efficacy theories
Principles of treatment	Clinician–parent relationships provide the basis for stress and distress regulation. Strengthening family relationships by promoting secure base behavior and sensitivity in parents, as well as secure attachment in children. Enhancing RF: mother's attention to own and child's mental and physical states allows her to see child more clearly and promote attachment, health, and development.
Target client	Most visits are conducted with parent and child together, although this can vary to include individual parent visits, couple counseling, and so forth.
Focus of treatment	Clinician–parent relationship, stress regulation to ameliorate dysregulation. Enhancing parental RF so that mother can sensitively respond to child's attachment and physical needs/mother's life course, health, and mental health
Assessment protocols/procedures	Health outcomes relationship/attachment/RF Maternal mental health
Manualized?	Yes

build the relationship, as mothers discovered that we could, in fact, hear what they had to tell us, without judgment, and with compassion. Our curiosity gave them permission to examine the unspoken, and was essential to their feeling safe and known. Sometimes we provided a framework for understanding their reactions to traumatic experiences (i.e., numbness and dissociation is "normal" in the context of certain traumatic experiences). Consistent with Courtois's description of the staged nature of work with complex trauma sufferers, it was sometimes the case that mothers disclosed trauma only at the very end of the intervention, and sometimes only to the research assistant collecting outcome data. Mothers with trauma histories also tended to deny or minimize psychiatric symptoms, and there were no discernible differences between intervention and control mothers on measures of depression or PTSD (Sadler et al., 2013). These empirical findings were quite inconsistent with our clinical experience with mothers, and indeed measures of depression, anxiety, and PTSD seemed inadequate to describing their level of suffering.

Given these measurement challenges, we planned more sensitive trauma assessments for subsequent studies. In addition, we asked clinician teams to jointly complete the Adverse Childhood Experiences (ACE) Questionnaire for mothers they had followed for the full 27 months of the intervention. They did so on the basis of their clinical experience with the mothers and their knowledge of their social history. Analysis of the ACE scores for 29 mothers revealed a mean score of 5.5 in the sample, and a median score of 6. Seventy-two percent of the mothers in this sample had ACE scores of 4 or above (Albertson, 2016). ACE scores of 4 or above have been linked to a range of negative health and mental health outcomes across the lifespan (Felitti et al., 1998).

In addition to experimenting with other ways of assessing trauma, we also spent a good deal of time educating our clinician teams about complex trauma and its manifestations. As their understanding grew, clinicians became more and more sensitive to manifestations of trauma, and estimated that 20–25% of mothers they were seeing showed signs of some form of complex trauma disorder. These mothers had histories of prolonged trauma exposure across their childhood and early adulthood, and manifested many if not all of the posttraumatic adaptations intrinsic to complex trauma (Herman, 1992). They struggled with dysregulation, in the form of both over and underarousal and were unable to rally more cortical functions and reflection in the face of significant levels of bodily disruption (tension; difficulties regulating the breath; heart rate variability; symptoms of fight, flight, and freezing; along with other physical concerns). They were prone to dissociation and other alterations in consciousness, suffered from extreme shame and self-hatred, and readily took on their abusers' negative images of them. Many had significant relationship problems (including the relationship with their child), as well as distorted relationships to their bodies, and to the bodies of their babies, as manifest in problems of eating, sleeping, and feeding. And many despaired of things ever changing.

Naturally, these defensive adaptations—well honed over a lifetime—made it difficult for mothers to engage with the home visitors in meaningful ways. With few, if any, experiences of being held and understood by another, they found it difficult to trust home visitors, and establish either physical calm or a calm, safe relationship. Engagement sometimes took months and months, with frequent setbacks and backsliding. In some instances, as in our work with Genevieve, described below, we were able to engage for months at a time, whereas other mothers used us primarily for help with housing, food, diapers, welfare benefits, and basic health needs. Sometimes periods of engagement would be short-lived, followed by long periods of disengagement, with mothers canceling home visits, ignoring texts and phone calls, and in one way or another "disappearing." Rarely would mothers tell us they wished to withdraw from the program; rather, they allowed us occasional contact, organized primarily around concrete needs and services. This was the level of closeness they could tolerate.

Case Illustration: Genevieve

The following description of our work with Genevieve and her son, Jimmy, highlights the delicate balance between relationship building, bodily approaches, and the uneven but steady emergence of mentalizing—specifically, the capacity to keep the baby *and the self* in mind—over the 27 months of the intervention.

Background

Genevieve joined MTB when she was in her third trimester of pregnancy. She and her husband, Jared, were both in their early 20s. After several months of prenatal work with us, Genevieve gave birth to a baby boy, Jimmy. Genevieve had been a full-time undergraduate student in community college prior to becoming pregnant but had withdrawn from school upon learning that she was going to have a baby. Jared was employed when we met the couple, but later lost his job. Genevieve's parents were in her life on a daily basis.

Genevieve's complex family history was a mosaic of poverty, trauma, physical and emotional abuse and neglect, alcoholism, and violence. She was the firstborn of two children. Her father was a severe alcoholic, and her mother Estelle beat her frequently as a child, although her sister Janet, who was mentally ill and prone to violent outbursts, bore the worst of her mother's wrath. Genevieve often had to intervene in physical fights between her parents and protect her sister, though this too was dangerous. When Genevieve was 13, after years of violence and conflict, her mother left the two girls in the care of their father to embark on a new romantic relationship; Genevieve became de facto head of household. Genevieve's father could not guide or protect his children following their mother's abandonment; indeed, he often bought the girls alcohol and encouraged them to party with him.

Neither parent was in any sense able to meet Genevieve's needs, either as a child, an adolescent, or a young parent. Her father was in all but the physical sense absent, and her mother was manipulative and controlling at best, and cruel at worst. Throughout Genevieve's childhood, Estelle's willingness to help her daughter in any way was contingent on Genevieve's ceding to her control. When Genevieve decided to marry Jared despite her mother's protests, her mother told her, "Well you are stupid and you are gonna' get exactly what you deserve cause he's a bum."

Although capable of verbalizing traumatic incidents from her childhood, Genevieve idealized her parents, and could not acknowledge their role in or contribution to her childhood of deprivation and hardship. This idealization rarely wavered, despite chilling disappointments, and she connected her self-worth to how much she could please them. She would blandly insist: "My parents provided a home and I had what I needed," and she struggled to please everyone. She was the "good daughter" to her parents, and the "good wife" to her husband. Unsurprisingly, her inability to say "no" or to put her own needs first often left her feeling overwhelmed and depleted.

The Treatment

Although Genevieve had wanted to have a baby, Jared was not ready for father-hood and expressed a great deal of ambivalence about becoming a parent. There were many marital ups and downs during the pregnancy; Jared abused alcohol, and both domestic violence and infidelity were suspected by the team. Genevieve suffered from severe anemia during pregnancy, but refused iron pills, and eventually needed intravenous iron several times during the last months of the pregnancy. This added a layer of medical complexity to what was already a very stressful time in this young woman's life.

Following a smooth, healthy labor and delivery and a positive birth experience, both parents found themselves smitten with their beautiful baby boy. Although a successful breast-feeding relationship was established between mother and baby, pediatric well-baby checks 6–8 weeks postpartum revealed diminished growth and weight gain. Despite efforts to increase milk production and protect the breast-feeding relationship, Genevieve became discouraged and gave in to family pressure to switch to formula feeding.

Genevieve relished the fantasy of having a traditional, nuclear family. Unfortunately, however, the euphoric feelings between the couple did not last. During the early months of Jimmy's life, marital tensions mounted, and both Genevieve and Jared felt that their needs were unmet. Jared insisted that they resume their social life and sexual relationship despite Genevieve's repeated declarations of feeling tired, sore, and not at all ready for sexual intercourse. Couple counseling sessions with the MTB social worker focused on creating space for increasing healthy communication, and exploring how the demands of parenthood impacted the relationship and each spouse's expectations of the other. The team also offered to link Jared with services for anger management and alcohol treatment. Nevertheless, physical confrontations between the couple escalated. Jared's drinking increased and he cheated on Genevieve. Her feelings of rage, betrayal, shame, and powerlessness undermined her sense of competence as a wife and mother, and she described feeling intensely sad and fatigued, unable to take pleasure in the daily activities that she previously enjoyed. At this point, Genevieve met criteria for postpartum depression and was placed on a selective serotonin reuptake inhibitor (SSRI). In addition, she presented with various somatic complaints. Nevertheless, she had difficulty making and keeping health appointments for herself.

Genevieve did, however, maintain Jimmy's schedule of pediatric visits reasonably well. Jimmy's temperament was social, low-key, and content for much of the first 6 months of his life. His "easygoing" disposition proved to be adaptive given the volatile family system into which he was born. By 8 months of age, however,

Jimmy appeared to have poor eye contact and low energy. He was still having difficulty sitting on his own and had not tried to roll over. Assessment with the Ages and Stages Questionnaire revealed gross motor development concerns and warranted a referral to early intervention services. The team members shared their concerns with Genevieve about Jimmy's development, yet she was unable to prioritize her son given her own depression and rumination over her failing marriage.

Contact between the MTB team and Genevieve grew increasingly sporadic as Jimmy approached his first birthday, but she found her way back to MTB after a terrifying incident with Jared. The couple had agreed to separate after she learned of another of Jared's affairs, and she decided once and for all that her marriage was over. However, Jared's reaction to her beginning divorce proceedings was brutally violent. After a particularly frightening incident in which she feared for her life, he was arrested. With the help of the clinical team, Genevieve pressed charges, obtained a restraining order, and filed a motion in court that Jared only be allowed access to their son through supervised visitation.

After the incident, Genevieve explained that she had been out of contact for months because she had felt too embarrassed to tell the clinicians what had been going on, worried that they would be disappointed in her and judge her for her current circumstances. The team reassured her of their nonjudgmental support (starkly contrasting her own mother's response), and Genevieve reengaged with MTB, and agreed to increase the frequency of home visits with the nurse and social worker. She had double the usual number of visits during her second year in the program. Her treatment involved a layering of interventions designed to address her needs for safety and support, more peaceful sleep, better nutrition and an exercise plan for weight loss and management, education regarding safer sex, and access to long-term contraception, increased opportunities for pleasurable moments with her baby, and a safe space to explore her feelings about her role as a mother and how her life and relationships had changed. The clinicians also encouraged her to spend more time outside with the baby. Genevieve finally consented to a developmental assessment for Jimmy, who began physical therapy with an early intervention program soon afterwards and began making steady progress.

The second year of the MTB intervention revealed that the explosive confrontations between Jared and Genevieve had deeply affected Jimmy. The clinical team began to suspect that the child had seen his father pushing and hitting his mother on more than one occasion. Jimmy's first word was *angry* and he learned the word *scared* soon after that. The social worker explored the impact on Jimmy of witnessing the violence between his parents, and helped draw some parallels between Genevieve's own early childhood narrative and Jimmy's plight. This work fueled Genevieve's motivation to obtain a long-term protective order against her husband, follow through with the divorce, and continue fighting for supervised visitation as the only means of contact between Jared and Jimmy. It also helped her to think more deeply about how she could regulate her own feelings and learn to communicate in more assertive, modulated ways. She was also able to finally acknowledge that some of her early experiences with her parents had, in fact, been traumatic, letting go of some of her idealizations of her childhood. Supporting Genevieve in putting her experiences into words in a safe, nonjudgmental context eventually led to recommendations and referrals for both Genevieve and Jimmy for more intensive therapeutic intervention. Genevieve's trauma as a domestic violence survivor and her need to control her own anger required more specialized care, as did Jimmy's need to have developmentally appropriate, relationship-based play therapy to recover from his own traumatic experiences.

Over time, Genevieve evolved into a mother engaged in caring for her child's needs. Jimmy's developmental progress and his increasing ability to communicate verbally and interact with his mother helped Genevieve feel more competent and confident. This newfound give-and-take in the attachment relationship enabled Genevieve to become more emotionally available for her child. Jimmy's attachment to his mother was secure in the Strange Situation (Ainsworth, Blehar, Waters, & Wall, 1978) at 14 months.

As graduation drew near, Genevieve was acutely aware that it would soon be time to say good-bye to the MTB team. Although this was difficult, she for the first time had the experience that relationships can end in a positive caring way. She was also able to see the end of her work with MTB as the mark of a new beginning for her as the mother of a healthy, playful, inquisitive toddler. Genevieve noted that she emerged from the past 2 years "stronger," and with a clearer focus as she worked to build a better future for herself and her son. She returned to school full time.

The Diagnosis of Complex Trauma Disorder

Diagnostically, this young mother really didn't "fit" most DSM criteria for PTSD, nor did she consistently meet criteria for an anxiety or mood disorder. Instead, she presented with multiple symptoms of depression, anxiety, and interpersonal problems throughout the first 12–18 months of the intervention, with symptoms shifting and manifesting in different ways over time. She did, however, meet many of the criteria for complex or developmental trauma disorder, specifically, poor self-regulation, minimal tolerance for negative affect, poor impulse control, dissociative tendencies, and a tendency to abuse substances, particularly alcohol. The chaotic nature of her daily life, which included family *and* community violence, the role she adopted in her family as "pleaser" combined with her intimate interpersonal relationship struggles, and her overall internal dysregulation also supported this diagnosis. It is useful, in this regard, to consider Genevieve's clinical presentation in light of the seven essential posttraumatic adaptations of complex trauma, and to describe the clinical strategies used to address them.

1. *Alterations in the regulation of affective impulse (i.e., anger and self-destructiveness).* Genevieve's depressive, immobilized affect masked a simmering rage. At the end of her first year with MTB, it became evident that she was drinking more heavily when she was not with her baby, and inviting random partners into her life. Genevieve also shamefully admitted to an incident in which she broke into her then-separated husband's new apartment and assaulted him upon learning of his latest sexual indiscretion. She was arrested and spent the night in jail. Genevieve described this incident as the "lowest of her lows" and struggled with reconciling this image of herself with the image she aspired to project to the outside world and

most importantly to her son. She worked diligently with the MTB team in mindfulness exercises, learning the difference between aggressive and assertive behavior, and pausing before taking action to think through other ways of responding.

2. *Alterations in attention and consciousness (i.e., amnesia, dissociative episodes).* We saw many instances of dissociation in our work with Genevieve. She reported that when she attacked Jared, she felt as though she were outside of her own body watching herself hit and punch him. And when she saw Jared in court after he attacked her, she became paralyzed with fear and began to panic; her breathing rate increased and she tearfully complained of chest pains and heart palpitations. The MTB team looked to Genevieve's mother, sitting right beside her daughter, to offer comfort and regulation, but she gazed forward with a blank stare, apparently in a dissociative state herself. She showed no awareness of her daughter's distress and offered no comfort or reassurance. Both clinicians, present in the courtroom, stepped in to offer soothing touch, words, and deep breathing to bring Genevieve down from her escalating panic, so that she could approach the witness stand to testify against Jared. She was able to describe the incident calmly and clearly, which resulted in court-ordered supervised visitation time between Jared and Jimmy.

3. *Alterations in self-perception (i.e., chronic guilt and ongoing feelings of shame and low self-worth).* After Genevieve's return to MTB, we learned that her months-long "disappearance" was driven by her own shame and humiliation. Her persona as "the good one" became tarnished following her repeated makeups with Jared, her final assault and arrest. "I was just too ashamed to see you guys," she said. "You both think I am so smart and good, and look at what I have done, I spent a night in jail for doing something so stupid. I wasn't even thinking about Jimmy. I was just so angry and Jared isn't even worth it. I was supposed to finish college, be more educated, and have a good life. What happened to me? How could I sink so low?" Reframing Genevieve's actions and helping her understand the feelings that drove them was key in helping her separate what she had done from who she was, and who she had the potential to become. Making mistakes did not make her "bad" or "unworthy." This was an important parallel for Genevieve, who, as a mother, would need to contain the growing pains and mistakes of her own son.

4. *Alterations in perception of perpetrator.* Genevieve's perceptions of Jared changed almost daily. He was a "monster," a "drunk," "irresponsible," and "useless," yet he was also the father of her child, the man she loved, and the husband with whom she so desperately wanted to craft a marriage and family life. Genevieve vacillated between wanting to make it work and knowing she could not stay in the marriage. Our work was grounded in allowing Genevieve safe space to explore these highly conflicted feelings without judgment, to bring her back to her baby whenever possible (i.e., wondering with her how Jimmy felt when he saw his parents fighting, being curious about how Jimmy made sense of his dad's absence and the new visiting arrangement), and to gently challenge the disconnect between the sense of self-worth she aspired to and how self-destructive she was in relation to Jared. It is important to note that Jared was not the only perpetrator in Genevieve's life, although it was much harder for her to see the depth and breadth of her parents' neglect and emotional abuse.

5. *Alterations in relationships to others, including parenting (i.e., trust and intimacy issues)*. Genevieve endured a great deal of what appeared to be manipulation, coercion, and violation in her marriage before filing for divorce, a pattern of revictimization that mirrored her childhood experience with her parents. She resumed sexual activity during the earliest postpartum weeks to appease Jared, and continued to engage in an intimate relationship with him after they had separated, knowing that he was unfaithful and promiscuous. Genevieve was desperate to believe that if only she could keep the family together, Jimmy's childhood could be happy and carefree. When gently challenged with alternative views of how a home riddled with verbal and physical conflict could impact a child's well-being and development, Genevieve would react defensively, change the subject, or simply shut down and disengage. When the MTB team gently observed her resistance to exploring this territory, Genevieve finally admitted that she could not tolerate the idea of her child being frightened or unhappy, despite knowing deep down that at times this was a reality. She desperately needed to believe that Jimmy was OK, because admitting otherwise would be a reflection and confirmation of her shortcomings as a mother. Her high hopes for herself mirrored the hopes the team held for her, and the sense of promise unfulfilled permeated the therapeutic relationship. The team created a "holding space" (Lieberman & Van Horn, 2008) for Genevieve to forgive herself and strive to be a more responsive, nurturing mother.

6. *Somatization and/or medical problems*. Although a very attractive young woman, Genevieve became obese following her pregnancy and struggled with sleep deprivation, depressed mood, and anxiety. She was aware that she was not herself and rarely felt healthy or energetic, yet she simply could not manage her own medical needs. She was able to articulate concerns about being depressed and feeling a lack of energy or pleasure in her life, but when the MTB team coordinated appointments for her to see her medical provider Genevieve would deny any symptoms or problems. The MTB team literally had to take Genevieve by the hand and accompany her to her appointment with a list of concerns, and to "speak for Genevieve," giving her the words and language she needed to describe what was ailing her. Following a physical exam, insertion of a long-term intrauterine contraceptive device, and prescription of medication for her depressive mood and sleep deprivation, Genevieve began an exercise routine and changed her eating habits. By the time Jimmy reached his second birthday, Genevieve was reporting better quality of sleep and improved mood. The change in her confidence and overall well-being radiated in her smile and the delight she could now express in being with her son.

7. *Alterations in systems of meaning (i.e., hopelessness, despair of the future)*. When Genevieve began her relationship with MTB, she was an ambitious young woman determined to complete her college education and develop a meaningful career. When she lost sight of her goals and her sense of competence, feelings of hopelessness and despair became intense. Genevieve felt low, like a failure, and a poor example for her son. She was desperate not to end up like the women in her community who had multiple children with different men and relied on the government for support; she saw herself and the life she and Jimmy would have differently. As MTB prepared for graduation and a healthier, more emotionally stable Genevieve

emerged, she decided that if she could survive the past 2 years she could certainly complete school. She registered herself for the spring semester following her graduation from MTB.

Stages of the Work

As described earlier, working with trauma often requires a long period of attention to relationship building, as well as self and bodily regulation before the processing of trauma can occur (Courtois, 2004; van der Kolk, 2014). We would add to this that when working with traumatized women *who are also parents*, this "pretreatment" stage is essential for the mother to be able to provide a secure base for her child, and for her developing capacity to reflect on her child's experience. That is, "keeping the child in mind" (Slade, 2002) is impossible until the mother feels safe in the therapeutic relationship and in her body. Our work with Genevieve very much followed this pattern. For nearly the entire intervention, we worked on establishing and maintaining the alliance, providing a secure base for Genevieve to make sense of her emotional life, regulate her intense negative affects, and think about life beyond the chaos of the moment. At the same time, mindfulness, breathing exercises, and body scans were used to build self-regulation skills and assist her in stabilizing herself emotionally when she became distressed. A range of supports for self-care included nutritional counseling, birth control, linkages to her medical home, and so forth. As her body became less alien to her, Genevieve began to settle. Only then could she attend to Jimmy's very real developmental and emotional needs, and the child began to thrive.

As Courtois (2004) has noted, some complex trauma survivors will not be able to move beyond the pretreatment stage during the lifespan of a typical therapeutic relationship. Nevertheless, this stage greatly improves the trauma survivor's quality of life and functioning. In Genevieve's case, the treatment phase only began as she was ending her relationship with MTB, and it was only her recent traumatic experiences with Jared that she could process. She was never really able to work through her own traumatic family history, name her feelings about these experiences, or identify how they might have been connected to her current circumstances as a young adult. At best, she was able to draw some basic parallels between witnessing violence between her parents as a child and Jimmy's witnessing his parents' violent marriage.

The Clinicians' Experience

The constant need to shift focus and contain many of Genevieve's intense feelings left an indelible imprint on the psyches of the clinicians, who at times found themselves in the same grip of rage, helplessness, and hopelessness that plagued Genevieve. The personal strengths that the team saw early on, namely, intelligence, insight, thoughtfulness, curiosity, and a willingness to learn new things, gave them high hopes for her development both as a young woman and as a mother. And the feelings of disappointment that ensued left the clinical team feeling unpleasantly surprised and depleted. This "hazard of caring" for a young mother and baby who had such great potential for better outcomes, yet remained in such peril both physically and psychologically, put each clinician at risk for burnout and vicarious trauma (Pearlman & Caringi, 2009).

The term *vicarious trauma* is used to describe the feelings of despair and hopelessness that may set in when clinicians are unable to remedy or protect their patients from the effects of their traumatic experiences. They may overextend themselves to "save" a family, or they may become focused on minute, concrete details, because these are more easily managed than the more complicated feelings stirred up by relentless confrontation with the residua of trauma. Vicarious trauma can alter a clinician's perceptions of the world and lead to cynicism or bitterness where there was once hope and faith, and can affect the culture of an organization, as well as the personal relationships of the clinician. It can also manifest unsustainable work–life boundaries, unrealistic expectations, feelings of anger, annoyance, or disappointment toward mothers: "What was she thinking?" or "How could she be so irresponsible?" Likewise clinicians can feel guilt, an increased sense of anxiety, preoccupation with a particular parent, a devaluing of the client's true strengths and capacities, and somatic symptoms. These can significantly compromise the therapeutic relationship (Pearlman & Caringi, 2009).

Our team at times showed signs of vicarious trauma and found the work with Genevieve intersecting their personal and professional life in complex ways. Both the nurse and social worker experienced physical symptoms such as chest-tightening or headache prior to a scheduled home visit, as well as feelings of extreme fatigue at the conclusion of the home visit. Both found themselves intensely worried about Genevieve's and Jimmy's safety, listening more intently to local news broadcasts, and feeling a rising sense of panic whenever a story aired about a domestic dispute or murder in Genevieve's violent community. There were also moments of conflation of Genevieve's experiences with what the clinicians were experiencing personally, which likewise altered the way the team members perceived their expectations and hopes for Genevieve, as well as their own sense of competence as helpers and healers in her life.

During these times, the clinicians used clinical and reflective supervision to make meaning of the feelings triggered by their relationship with Genevieve, and to plan next steps and strategies for intervention. When the team members felt that they were failing or were unable to make repairs in the therapeutic relationship, the supervisory relationship provided containment for the clinicians in a way that paralleled the accepting, affirming, nonjudgmental holding space the clinicians provided for Genevieve. The supervisors validated the clinicians' fears for Genevieve's safety and their feelings of helplessness when she temporarily disengaged from the program. The supervisors also reminded the clinicians of how important they had been to Genevieve, in the same way the clinicians underscored the significance of Genevieve in Jimmy's life.

Pilot Study RCT Outcomes

We now briefly review the findings from our pilot study RCT. Sixty intervention and 45 control families were followed for the 27 months of the intervention (for a full report, including detailed descriptions of the sampling methods, sample, data

TABLE 7.2. Results of MTB Pilot Study Attachment: Reflective Functioning

Outcome measure	Stage	Intervention	Control	Significance
AMBIANCE/face-to-face interaction	4 months	60% disrupted interactions; teens: 66% disrupted	75% disrupted interactions; teens: 93.3% disrupted	NS $p = .05$
Strange Situation infant attachment	12 months	64.4% Secure; 26% Disorganized	48.4 Insecure; 43% Disorganized	$p = .028$ $p = .049$
Parental RF[a]	Pregnancy – 24 months	0.5 change	0.7 change	NS
	< 12th-grade education	0.5 change	No change	$p = .09$
	RF < 3 at baseline	1.6 change	0.2 change	$p = .007$

Note. See Sadler et al. (2013) for details. AMBIANCE, Atypical Maternal Behavior Instrument for Assessment and Classification.
[a]Parental RF scored on a 9 point scale from "absent" (1) to "exceptional" (9).

analysis, etc., see Sadler et al., 2013). Analysis of data from this study included a range of positive outcomes. Prominent health outcomes included significantly higher rates of on-time pediatric immunization and lower rates of rapid subsequent childbearing in intervention families. Lower rates of child protective service referrals were reported as well, at the trend (.07) level. Mother–child interaction outcomes included significantly lower rates of disrupted, atypical mother–infant interactions at 4 months in teen mothers, higher rates of secure attachment, and lower rates of disorganized attachment in intervention children compared to the control group. Over the course of the 27 months of the intervention, both intervention and control mothers' levels of RF increased, although there was—compared to control group mothers—a significant increase in RF in those MTB mothers who entered the study with very low levels of RF, or who had an 11th-grade education or less. The attachment and RF findings are summarized in Table 7.2. In a small follow-up study, significantly lower rates of maternally reported externalizing disorders were found in intervention children (Ordway et al., 2014). Recent analyses of data on 158 dyads indicate that MTB children had lower rates of obesity and were more likely to be of normal weight than children in the control group (Ordway, Sadler, Holland, Slade, Close, & Mayes, 2017).

Discussion

As noted earlier, many of the families we worked with were struggling with multiple levels of adversity, chief among them severe poverty and the many toxic stressors that accompany its intrinsic isolation and profound disadvantage (Shonkoff, 2012), as well as high levels of trauma exposure in childhood and/or ongoing relational violence. We came to see some of our success in working with these families as a reflection of (1) our increasing understanding of mothers' trauma-related psychopathology, and particularly symptoms of developmental or complex trauma disorders, and (2) our increasing sensitivity to the clinical needs arising from these difficulties. In particular, the literature on developmental or complex trauma was very helpful in understanding the challenges faced by some of our families and the clinical challenges we encountered in working with them.

All of the attachment-based interventions described in this volume are aimed at laying the foundation for the development and maintenance of secure attachments, using a two-generational approach to help parents provide a haven of safety and reflection for their infants. This is the essence of the MTB approach. Yet, as we hope we have demonstrated here, a truly "trauma-informed" treatment must address the specific disruptions that flow from posttraumatic adaptations in order to promote deep and sustaining attachments. These include attention to the establishment and maintenance of a safe therapeutic relationship, and to self and bodily regulation first in the mother and then in the child. These components are essential to the development of RF, to the ability to make use of psychoeducation, and to the capacity to meaningfully work through trauma. The MTB interdisciplinary model—with its unique emphasis on health and the body on the one hand, and mental health and the emotional life on the other—seems particularly suited to providing both the physical and emotional safety and regulation necessary for both parent and child development to proceed.

Unfortunately, with interveners facing very real economic and logistical constraints on program development, the pressure to create cost-effective (short-term, group, etc.) treatments is great. But when the participants in these programs are severely traumatized, and have lived lives in which "toxic stress" does not begin to describe their day-to-day reality, these treatment approaches cannot help but be limited in their effectiveness. Only when we work on the body and mind together, and incorporate a deep understanding of developmental trauma into treatment and supervision protocols, can we have any hope of achieving the long-term effects so essential for real success in parenting and in life. RCTs of short-term behavioral interventions have not been fully tested on the kinds of populations we see in MTB, and approaches that emphasize psychoeducation, or that ignore the very real challenges of developmental trauma, are unlikely to be effective over time. The level of adverse childhood experiences seen in families living in urban (as well as rural) poverty require us to guard against simplistic diagnostic formulations and treatment approaches, and to instead to think about diagnosis and intervention in a developmentally sophisticated, complex, and nuanced way.

Training and Dissemination

MTB has served nearly 150 families since we saw our first pregnant teenager in 2002. We are in the final stages of data analysis for our efficacy-testing RCT, which was initiated in 2009. We continue to recruit families into MTB through community health centers, although we are now accepting direct referrals as well. Thus, while the program is still entirely voluntary, we are accepting referrals when there are specific clinical concerns and an abundance of risk factors. With our recent designation as an evidence-based home-visiting program, we are looking toward wider implementation in the coming years. We have since 2006 been working closely with the Florida State University Young Parents Program to develop interdisciplinary reflective programs for teen mothers in the juvenile justice system in Tallahassee and Miami, Florida. This group recently received funds to implement a full MTB program in Miami–Dade County. In 2010, we began collaborating with the National Society for the Prevention of Cruelty to Children (NSPCC) in the United Kingdom; in 2011, we established intervention sites in England and Scotland, and in 2014 we began an RCT at all NSPCC MTB sites. In 2016, we began a full-scale replication in Denmark.

In 2009, we held our first MTB Training Institute. This 3-day training focuses on the theoretical and clinical bases for the program, the core elements of our treatment approach, and the specific requirements for supervision and ongoing training. This training is required of all sites wishing to fully replicate MTB, along with intensive distance clinical and administrative supervision over the duration of the intervention, a 2-day train-the-trainer session, a 2-day site visit at 1 year, and continued collaboration on a number of aspects of program implementation. We have developed a treatment manual designed to guide clinicians through all phases of the intervention, a quick-reference guide for clinicians, as well as a replication manual for researchers. These are all available as part of the MTB training package (*mtb.yale.edu*).

REFERENCES

Ainsworth, M. D. S., Blehar, M. C., Waters, E., & Wall, S. (1978). *Patterns of attachment: Psychological study of the Strange Situation*. Hillsdale, NJ: Erlbaum.

Albertson, J. G. (2016). *Minding the Baby®: Maternal adverse childhood experiences and treatment outcomes in a mother–infant home visiting program*. Unpublished doctoral dissertation, City University of New York, New York, NY.

Berlin, L., Ziv, Y., Amaya-Jackson, L., & Greenberg, M. (2005). *Enhancing early attachments: Theory, research, intervention, and policy*. New York: Guilford Press.

Carlson, E. A. (1998). A prospective longitudinal study of disorganized/disoriented attachment. *Child Development, 69*, 1107–1128.

Courtois, C. (2004). Complex trauma, complex reactions: Assessment and treatment. *Psychotherapy: Theory, Research, Practice, Training, 41*, 412–425.

Felitti, V., Anda, R., Nordenberg, D., Williamson, D. F., Spitz, A. M., Edwards, B., . . . Marks, J. S. (1998). Relationships of childhood abuse and household dysfunction to many of the leading causes of death in adults: The Adverse Childhood Experiences Study. *American Journal of Preventive Medicine, 14*, 245–258.

Fonagy, P., Steele, M., Steele, H., Leigh, T., Kennedy, R., Mattoon, G., & Target, M. (1995). Attachment, the reflective self, and borderline states: The predictive specificity of the Adult Attachment Interview and pathological emotional development. In S. Goldberg, R. Muir, & J. Kerr (Eds.), *Attachment theory: Social, developmental and clinical perspectives* (pp. 233–278). New York: Analytic Press.

Fraiberg, S. (1980). *Clinical studies in infant mental health*. New York: Harcourt Brace.

Fraiberg, S., Adelson, E., & Shapiro, V. (1975). Ghosts in the nursery: A psychoanalytic approach to the problems of impaired infant–mother relationships. *Journal of the American Academy of Child Psychiatry, 14*, 387–421.

Garner, A. S. (2013). Home visiting and the biology of toxic stress: Opportunities to address early childhood adversity. *Pediatrics, 132*(Suppl. 2), S65–S73.

Grienenberger, J., Kelly, K., & Slade, A. (2005). Maternal reflective functioning, mother–infant affective communication, and infant attachment: Exploring the link between mental states and observed caregiving. *Attachment and Human Development, 7,* 299–311.

Herman, J. (1992). *Trauma and recovery.* New York: Basic Books.

Lieberman, A. F., Ghosh Ippen, C., & Van Horn, P. (2015). *Don't hit my mommy!: A manual for child–parent psychotherapy with young witnesses of family violence* (2nd ed.). Washington, DC: ZERO TO THREE.

Lieberman, A. F., & Van Horn, P. (2008). *Psychotherapy with infants and young children: Repairing the effects of stress and trauma on early attachment.* New York: Guilford Press.

Lieberman, A. F., Weston, D., & Pawl, J. (1991). Preventative intervention and outcome with anxiously attached dyads. *Child Development, 62,* 199–209.

Lyons-Ruth, K., Bronfman, E., & Parsons, E. (1999). Maternal frightened, frightening, and atypical behavior and disorganized infant attachment strategies. *Monographs of the Society for Research in Child Development, 64*(3, Serial No. 258), 67–96.

Lyons-Ruth, K., Yellin, C., Melnick, S., & Atwood, G. (2005). Expanding the concept of unresolved mental states: Hostile/helpless states of mind on the Adult Attachment Interview are associated with disrupted mother–infant communication and infant disorganization. *Development and Psychopathology, 17*(1), 1–23.

Main, M., & Hesse, E. (1990). Lack of mourning in adulthood and its relationship to infant disorganization: Some speculations regarding causal mechanisms. In M. Greenberg, D. Cicchetti, & M. Cummings (Eds.), *Attachment in the preschool years: Theory, research, and intervention* (pp. 161–182). Chicago: University of Chicago Press.

Ogden, P., Minton, K., & Pain, C. (2004). *Trauma and the body: A sensorimotor approach to psychotherapy.* New York: Norton.

Olds, D. L. (2002). Prenatal and infancy home visiting by nurses: From randomized trials to community replication. *Prevention Science, 3,* 153–172.

Olds, D. L., Kitzman, H. J., Cole, R. E., Hanks, C. A., Arcoleo, K. J., Anson, E. A., . . . Stevenson, A. J. (2010). Enduring effects of prenatal and infancy home visiting by nurses on maternal life course and government spending: Follow-up of a randomized trial among children at age 12 years. *Archives of Pediatrics and Adolescent Medicine, 164*(5), 419–424.

Ordway, M., Sadler, L., Dixon, J., Close, N., & Mayes, L., & Slade, A. (2014). Lasting effects of an interdisciplinary home visiting program on child behavior: Preliminary follow-up results of a randomized trial. *Journal of Pediatric Nursing, 29,* 3–13.

Ordway, M., Sadler, L., Holland, M., Slade, A., Close, N., & Mayes, L. (2017). *Reducing obesity early in life via a home visiting parenting program: A randomized trial.* Manuscript under review.

Pearlman, L. A., & Caringi, J. C. (2009). Living and working self-reflectively to address vicarious trauma. In C. A. Courtois & J. D. Ford (Eds.), *Treating complex traumatic stress disorders (adults): An evidence-based guide* (pp. 202–224). New York: Guilford Press.

Porges, S. P. (2011). *The polyvagal theory: Neurophysiological foundations of emotions, attachment, communication, and self-regulation.* New York: Norton.

Sadler, L. S., Slade, A., Close, N., Webb, D. L., Simpson, T., Fennie, K., & Mayes, L. C. (2013). Minding the Baby: Enhancing reflectiveness to improve early health and relationship outcomes in an interdisciplinary home visiting program. *Infant Mental Health Journal, 34,* 391–405.

Sadler, L. S., Slade, A., & Mayes, L. C. (2006). Minding the Baby: A mentalization based parenting program. In J. G. Allen & P. Fonagy (Eds.), *Handbook of mentalization-based treatment* (pp. 271–288). Chichester, UK: Wiley.

Schuengel, C., Bakermans-Kranenburg, M. J., & van IJzendoorn, M. H. (1999). Frightening maternal behavior linking unresolved loss and disorganized infant attachment. *Journal of Consulting and Clinical Psychology, 67*(1), 54–63.

Shonkoff, J. P. (2012). Leveraging the biology of adversity to address the roots ofdisparities in health and development. *Proceedings of the National Academy of Sciences USA, 109*(Suppl. 2), 17302–17307.

Simkin, P. (1992). Overcoming the legacy of childhood sexual abuse: The role of caregivers and childbirth educators. *Birth, 19,* 224–225.

Slade, A. (2002, June/July). Keeping the baby in mind: A critical factor in perinatal mental health. In A. Slade, L. Mayes, & N. Epperson (Eds.), *Special issue on perinatal mental health* (pp. 10–16). Washington, DC: ZERO TO THREE.

Slade, A. (2005). Parental reflective functioning: An introduction. *Attachment and Human Development, 7,* 269–281.

Slade, A., Grienenberger, J., Bernbach, E., Levy, D., & Locker, A. (2005). Maternal reflective functioning and attachment: Considering the transmission gap. *Attachment and Human Development, 7,* 283–292.

Slade, A., & Sadler, L. S. (2013). Minding the Baby: Complex trauma and home visiting. *International Journal of Birth and Parenting Education, 1,* 50–53.

Slade, A., Sadler, L., Close, N., Fitzpatrick, S., Simpson, T., & Webb, D. (2016). *Minding the Baby*®: The impact of threat on the mother–baby and mother–clinician relationship. In S. Gojman-de-Millan, C. Herreman, & L. A. Sroufe (Eds.), *Attachment across clinical and cultural perspectives: A relational psychoanalytic approach* (pp. 182–204). London: Routledge.

Slade, A., Sadler, L., & Mayes, L. C. (2005). Maternal reflective functioning: Enhancing parental reflective functioning in a nursing/mental health home visiting program. In L. Berlin, Y. Ziv, L. Amaya-Jackson, & M. Greenberg (Eds.), *Enhancing early attachments: Theory, research, intervention, and policy* (pp. 152–177). New York: Guilford Press.

van der Kolk, B. (1994). The body keeps the score: Memory and the evolving psychobiology of posttraumatic stress. *Harvard Review of Psychiatry, 1,* 253–265.

van der Kolk, B. (2014). *The body keeps the score.* New York: Penguin Books.

van der Kolk, B. A., Roth, S., Pelcovitz, D., Sunday, S., & Spinazzola, J. (2005). Disorders of extreme stress: The empirical foundation of complex adaptation to trauma. *Journal of Traumatic Stress, 18,* 389–399.

Weatherston, D., & Barron, C. (2009). What does a reflective supervisory relationship look like? In S. Heller & L. Gilkerson (Eds.), *Practical guide to reflective supervision* (pp. 61–80). Washington, DC: ZERO TO THREE.

CHAPTER 8

New Beginnings
A Time-Limited Group Intervention
for High-Risk Infants and Mothers

TESSA BARADON, MICHELLE SLEED,
REBECCA ATKINS, CHLOE CAMPBELL, ABEL FAGIN,
RACHEL VAN SCHAICK, and PETER FONAGY

New Beginnings (NB) is a structured, manualized program that addresses the mother–baby relationship within a group format. The program, developed at the Anna Freud Centre (Baradon, 2009, 2013), works with the nuanced, cross-modal emotional interactions between mother and infant, tracking attunement and communication errors and emphasizing interactive repair. To this purpose, open (nondefended) and genuine transactions are privileged, confounding intergenerational transference expectancies of rejection and shaming by a "bad" world in which the individual is not seen as a worthwhile person. NB aims to increase mentalization in relation to self, baby, and the relationship between them (Baradon, with Biseo, Broughton, James, & Joyce, 2016). This takes place via the content of sessions, group processes (between the adults, adults and babies, and the baby-group) and personalization of the program. A reopening of *epistemic trust*—trust in the authenticity and personal relevance of interpersonally transmitted knowledge (Fonagy, Luyten, & Allison, 2015)—is seen as the product of the above, and the vehicle for the socialization of the babies into a more benign social context. We begin this chapter by setting out the basic structure and aims of the program (see Table 8.1), before going on to explain how the program was developed, how the program runs, and its theoretical foundations in attachment and mentalizing. We then describe how NB has thus far been evaluated, and finish with a more detailed account of the implementation of the program.

TABLE 8.1. Structure of the NB Program

Activity	Timing	Participants/location
Social worker referrals to the next group are invited	6–8 weeks before program starts	Facilitators e-mail the relevant service workforce and join team meetings to discuss the program and potential referrals, held at the Children's Social Services base
Selection of six dyads out of the total referred by the	1–2 months before program starts	Facilitators and social workers
First interview with dyad to explain program and assess interest and commitment	1–3 weeks before program starts	Both facilitators with mother–infant dyad, in home visit
Research measures (pre)	1–3 weeks before program starts	Each facilitator administers the measures with a different dyad, in a home visit
Program	12 consecutive weekly sessions	Both facilitators, whole group
Midway dyadic feedback session to discuss progress and remaining challenges	5–7 weeks into program	Both facilitators with mother–infant dyad, in home visit
Midway report feedback to social worker	Following meeting with dyad	Both facilitators, written report
Administration of postintervention evaluation measures	2–3 weeks after end of program	Each facilitator administers the measures with a different dyad, in home visit
Three follow-up sessions	Monthly, after end of program	Group and facilitators at Local Children's Centre

NB is delivered by two facilitators, and the groups comprise up to six mother–infant dyads. The program consists of 18 sessions in total, spanning approximately 4 months. The 1.5-hour NB group is embedded in a full morning activity program, involving an informal play session before the group (with facilitators, and including interested fathers) and lunch together afterwards. These activities complement the aims of the program and scaffold the emotionally intense content and processes of the group sessions.

Mothers and babies attend together. Participants are asked to attend sessions regularly with their babies, and to stay in the session. The first two sessions are made up of individual meetings between group facilitators and potential group members to engage the parents' interest in the program, to create a personal relationship, and to administer initial evaluation measures.

The following 12 sessions are group sessions run on consecutive weeks. Each session is structured around a topic. The topics were selected on the basis of evidence for their potential to activate the attachment relationship. The subjects cover the history of the pregnancy, the family tree of the baby, the mother's representations of her own childhood experiences, her aspirations for herself and her baby, and separations. The sequence of session topics has been planned sensitively, beginning with topics that are often easier for mothers to tolerate and reflect on—for example, "How does my baby learn about his or her world?"—progressing to more emotionally painful topics, such as relationships with fathers.

Midway through the program there is an individual session with mother and baby to reflect on progress and remaining difficulties, and to review feedback to the family's social worker (and thereby to the commissioners). At the end of the 12-week program there is another individual meeting between mother and baby and facilitators to bring personal closure, and to administer the evaluation measures. Three monthly follow-up sessions are held in a local Children's Centre. These sessions mediate the transition from the intensive support offered by the closed NB group to use of local service resources.

The central aims of the program are

1. To extend mothers' capacity to think about their babies' intersubjective and attachment needs as separate from their own.
2. To mobilize genuine emotional interest between mother and baby.
3. To broaden the adults' contingent responsivity to their babies' communications.
4. To encourage the parents' ability to trigger epistemic trust in their child, which would manifest in the babies as showing preference for interactions with the mother, using the mother as a safe base for exploration and demonstrating age-appropriate pleasure, ability to be stimulated and soothed, and explorative curiosity.

The clinical process tools used to enhance these capacities are *observation* of individual, dyadic, and group behaviors, communications, transactions, and states of mind; *group discussion between all the adults of attachment-related topics,* presented in the formal content of the program and linked reflective discussions about the observations; and *p*sychoeducational handouts.

Development of the NB Intervention

NB is rooted in the parent–infant psychotherapy model developed at the Anna Freud Centre (Baradon et al., 2005, 2016). The program was originally developed for incarcerated mothers residing with their babies in Mother–Baby Units (MBUs). Imprisoned mothers constitute a high-risk group in terms of past and current trauma (Borelli, Goshin, Joestl, Clark, & Byrne, 2010; Prison Reform Trust, 2012; Zlotnick, 1997). At the time NB was being developed, high turnover in the MBUs necessitated a relatively short and focused program. The result was an 8-week intervention consisting of intensive weekly sessions for 6 weeks, which were bookended by administration of the evaluation measures (Baradon & Target, 2010). Following a pilot in two Her Majesty's (HM) Prison MBUs in 2000–2005, the program was rolled out to four major MBUs in a cluster randomized trial in 2006–2009.

NB was subsequently replicated and evaluated in hostels for HIV-positive, homeless mothers, and babies in a deprived urban area in South Africa (Bain, 2014).[1]

NB in the Community

In 2012, NB was adapted for implementation in nonresidential settings by locally employed staff (Baradon, 2013). It is a model that seeks to disseminate knowledge, so that local staff are skilled and resources are therefore built up within community statutory services.

As with mothers and babies in prison, the community-based program (NB-C) is designed to intervene at a point in time when the authorities are placing active demands on the family system. The families targeted in the community are often characterized by intergenerational relational trauma, a broken attachment history (many have experienced the fostering system), economic and educational deprivation, and multiple current stresses. Their babies are selected for the program because they are within the Child Protection system, often at a point where separation of mother and child is being considered. Many families have previously had children removed from their care; this is a juncture of great pressure for the parents, but one that can also motivate them to try the program. It is also a point of pressure for the professionals and organization, since the legal and protection issues in the service are paramount and evoke enormous anxiety. The facilitators— social workers and psychologists employed by the Social Care services—are experienced in working with families and infants but do not necessarily have a specialist infant mental health background.

The NB-C Program

Referral and Engagement

The referred families are often characterized by chaotic lifestyles that seem predicated on sensitized stress-response mechanisms and impulsive "flight responses" (e.g., into crises, substance abuse, or sexual activity) to avoid overwhelming negative emotions. Thus, the NB-C groups are subject to the widely acknowledged difficulties in engaging and sustaining the attendance of families who already tend not to maintain participation in parenting programs (Brown, Khan, & Parsonage, 2012). Supporting the mothers to engage in the program is seen as an ongoing process, to be continuously addressed and reinforced. This is done on a practical level by providing transport for mothers and babies to the program, through building the group itself as an attachment object (James, 2016), and personalizing the program by making it meaningful to each dyad.

---

[1]In a collaboration between the Anna Freud Centre, University of Witwatersrand, and Ububele—a local nongovernmental organization (NGO), funded by the Carnegie Foundation.

A Typical Session

The mothers and babies start the NB day with an informal "stay-and-play" session. It is a time when mothers can make the step from their often chaotic and stressful lives toward forming relationships, scaffolded play, and calm reflection. It provides an informal way of checking in with each other and enables the facilitators to spend focused time with each parent and infant.

At an allotted time, they then move to the NB room. The sessions take place on the floor: Parents and facilitators sit on large cushions, with the babies placed on baby mats at the parents' feet, forming a little congregation in the center. Time is given to come together as a group, settle the babies, and settle in with each other.

The facilitators then introduce the topic of the day and the rationale for it. Simply worded illustrated handouts, which summarize research findings and give psychoeducational information, are read together and thought about in terms of the mothers' own experience and that of their babies. The facilitators alternate leading the activity in order to model collaborative working. Interactive group activities follow. For example, three consecutive sessions directly address aspects of separation and loss from the mothers' and babies' perspectives. These start with reading, in the group, an illustrated book *Owl Babies;* (Waddell, 1994) that poetically describes the experiences of three small owl siblings whose owl-mother has gone (to fetch food). The mothers are invited to explore their identifications with the owl babies or mother, and may back these up with their own experiences. The topic can be emotionally stirring; some mothers may recount very painful personal memories, while others may defend against them, and working through a book (i.e., in displacement) aids with engagement with the topic. The facilitators pace their engagement in accordance with the evolving dyadic and group process, and maintain a stance of warm inquiry and reflectiveness. The weekly topics assist parents in sharing their experiences and noticing similarities in others. The parents are often interested in the ways in which others have negotiated their struggles and begin to share ideas with and take inspiration from each other. This appears to reduce their fear of being negatively judged. Sharing experiences may also consolidate narratives of survival and aid the group in accepting vulnerabilities. Facilitators assess how the participants are making use of the group and intervene to regulate high levels of emotional arousal.

The facilitators are guided in their training and in the program structure to work directly with the individual infant and the infant "group." Thus, significant program time is devoted to more spontaneous observation and reflection about the babies, and this may, at times, cut across the more adult conversations and activities. The focus therefore moves between adult and infant, individual dyad and group. At first, this direct engagement with the babies—voicing the apprehended feeling states, talking in "motherese," playing even with very small babies—can be puzzling and somewhat embarrassing to the mothers. However, they soon notice their babies' reactions, and their curiosity about their babies increases.

A second informal session ends the morning with the mothers, babies, and facilitators eating lunch together. This serves as a powerful connecting activity and facilitates the development of a sense of community.

Building Up the Group as an Attachment Object

Many of the participants have experienced criticism, social isolation, and bullying, and come to the group apprehensively. The facilitators urge the participants to co-construct a group in which listening, acknowledging, and respecting each other confound transference expectations of rejection. As the group coheres, the mothers increasingly recruit each other into more authentic sharing and reflective exchanges, and some parents can begin to sensitively challenge the rigid representations held by others in a way that may be too threatening if done by a facilitator. This mother-to-mother interaction, while sometimes uncomfortable, can significantly strengthen the individual's sense of worth in relation to others in the group.

The group element is also of crucial importance for the babies. A "baby group" is created in its own right as the infants explore and respond to one another and form connections. The facilitators help mothers to view the babies as separate social beings, and this is further reinforced by ongoing observations of the other infants. Discussions about the babies' group processes can foster mothers' greater awareness of the babies' responses to their actions, evoking surprise, pride, and pleasure. Mothers can visibly take on aspects of attuned and sensitive care demonstrated by other members of the group and/or modeled by facilitators.

Moreover, the facilitators are careful to be explicit in their mentalizing stance—talking in a direct, emotionally genuine way, providing explanations for what they are doing at each step of the program, making their thinking available to the participants ("I am saying this because I noticed a few times that . . ."). The facilitators acknowledge the women's experience of them and behaviors in themselves that may have contributed to bad feelings, and consider with the group how they may work together toward reestablishing trust when it has been peturbed. For many of the women, a readiness on the part of the facilitators to recognize their own contributions to an interaction will come as a surprise. The process of *interactive repair* (Tronick & Weinberg, 1997), whereby mismatches or misunderstanding are recognized, acknowledged, and addressed, mirrors the kind of work mothers and babies need to do together to repair mismatches between them.

Personalizing the Program for the Dyad

NB is built to foster the unfolding relational–developmental story of each infant–mother dyad in parallel to the group process. As trust and safety build between group members and facilitators, facilitators are able to become increasingly explicit in comments and actions aimed at intervening in the relationship between mother and baby, in the expectation that these can be benignly held at a group level.

The individual sessions at the midway point (5–6 weeks into the 12-week program), as well as constituting a report to the responsible social worker (see Table 8.1), open a dialogue about the mother's experience in the group, her own and the facilitators' perceptions of her baby's experiences, and the facilitators' thoughts on the mother's progress. These sessions also enable the co-creation of plans for addressing specific areas in the mother–infant relationship that would benefit from further, focused intervention. By this point, there has often been sufficient relationship building to enable the mother to experience discussion around issues of concern as supportive rather than critical. The feedback process is repeated at the end of the group, providing an opportunity to consolidate progress and highlight areas on which to build.

The Role of Attachment Thinking in NB

NB is designed to work with mothers and babies who are at the higher end of risk of attachment disorders (Sleed, Baradon, & Fonagy, 2013) and with mothers who are parenting within nonmentalizing cultures linked with chaotic lifestyles, often involving substance misuse and domestic violence. The program addresses conscious, nonconscious (procedural), and unconscious (psychologically defended against) elements of the attachment relationship between mother and infant, and this continuously informs the stance taken by facilitators, as manifest in the here-and-now transactions and narratives shared among facilitators, mothers, and their infants.

In their microanalytic study of mother–infant dyads, developmental researchers have demonstrated the extent to which attachment and the emergence of the internal working model is a highly nuanced conversation; when an affectively genuine and personally meaningful dialogue is irregular or absent, the unfolding attachment pathway of the infant can be affected (Feldman, 2007; Tronick & Weinberg, 1997). In a study of the intricate "action dialogue" that takes place between mothers and their babies as young as 4 months, Beebe and colleagues (Beebe, 2013; Beebe, Lachmann, Markese, & Bahrick, 2012; Beebe & Lachmann, 2014) have shown that the emergence of the disorganized internal working model is associated with incongruences in the dialogic conversation. They examine the temporal, cross-modal interactional mechanisms through which the infant's "range, flexibility, and *coherence* of experience" (Beebe, 2013) of becoming known to and getting to know their mothers takes place. NB draws on this body of research and clinical work regarding parent–infant bidirectional behaviors and infant development. The notions of coherence, midrange monitoring and contingency, and the nuances of attunement and repair are woven into facilitator interventions.

Intergenerational transmission of patterns of attachment and their psychoanalytic counterpart in parent–infant psychotherapy—"ghosts in the nursery" (Fraiberg, Adelson, & Shapiro, 1975; Fonagy, Steele, Moran, Steele, & Higgitt, 1993)—informs the content of the sessions, as described earlier. Revisiting the past—to the extent that this happens in the program—is contextualized by the mother's conscious wish to provide her infant with different relational experiences. Through a careful focus on the mentalizing processes taking place in the sessions, the intervention supports the mothers' reflective capacities and seeks to make them more robust in the face of heightened affect. *Mentalizing*—the ability to understand actions of both others and the self in terms of thoughts, beliefs, wishes, and desires (Fonagy, Gergely, Jurist, & Target, 2002; Slade, Grienenberger, Bernbach, Levy, & Locker, 2005)—underpins humanity's unique capacity for social complexity and nuance. Research has demonstrated the central role of mentalizing in the intergenerational transmission of attachment patterns and in the quality of parent–child relationships (Fonagy, Steele, Steele, Moran, & Higgitt, 1991; Slade et al., 2005).

These ideas lie at the core of the verbal and nonverbal reflective processes in NB. The program attempts to direct the mother—through observation, focused attention, modeling, and group discussion—to become more aware of the infant's signals and the moments when her response (or lack of it) needs to be reconsidered. This would include, for example, alternative dialogic frameworks, that is, mentalizing different possibilites, to reframe negative maternal explanations or attributions ("My baby cries to get under my skin") and encourage a broader range of possible ways of understanding her infant. It would also involve reflecting on incongruencies in verbal and nonverbal maternal communication ("You called him over, but when he tried to crawl into your lap, it seems that perhaps you were pulling away from him") that address the communication errors noted by Beebe (2013) in mothers' interactions with their 4-month olds, and highlighted by Lyons-Ruth and colleagues in vulnerable mothers and their older infants/children (Bronfman, Parsons, & Lyons-Ruth, 1999; Lyons-Ruth, 2002). In mirroring and marking the infant's communications, the facilitators offer the infants' experiences of being recognized and "known," which are pivotal to the infant's core sense of safety (Beebe, 2013; Stern et al., 1998; Stern, Hofer, Haft, & Dore, 1985). Moreover, attachment relationships, in which attachment figures are interested in the child's mind and the child is safe to explore the mind of the attachment figure (Fonagy, Lorenzini, Campbell, & Luyten, 2014), allow the infant to explore other subjectivities, including that of his or her caregiver. Finding him- or herself accurately represented in the mind of the caregiver as a thinking and feeling, intentional being is necessary for the infant's own capacities for mentalizing to develop (Fonagy et al., 2002).

Recent elaborations have extended this thinking about the role of attachment as the communication system by which the infant learns to mentalize, with a focus on the significance of how social knowledge and understanding are more broadly conveyed to the child. Building on the model of Csibra and Gergely (2006, 2009, 2011), we suggested that contingent responding and mentalization have a crucial place in establishing *epistemic trust,* that is, trust in the authenticity and personal relevance of interpersonally transmitted specific pieces of knowledge (Fonagy & Allison, 2014; Fonagy et al., 2015). The biological predisposition to learn and abstract what is personally relevant and generalizable from communications is conditioned by the capacity of the communicator to establish epistemic trust by independently recognizing the agency (personhood) of the learner. Secure attachment is obviously one way that epistemic trust is—in most normative experience—conveyed across infant development. This is a transactional process. The predisposition to recognize that others are recognizing one's agency and selfhood is essential in making one's mind accessible to learning, and this predisposition is facilitated by secure attachment. In the context of NB, the facilitators were trained to provide the recognition of agency that underpins participants' willingness to adopt for themselves messages concerning child care. At the same time, we hope that these modifications to caregiving enhanced the capacity of the infant to learn through the parents' increased ability to demonstrate their recognition of his or her personal agency.

For example, an observation of an ordinary, brief, in-the-moment sequence between mother and baby may be used to engage the whole group in thinking about the meaning of what has just happened for the dyad and each partner in it, and to be meaningful to others in the group.

The facilitator observes, "He fretted, you offered him the breast, he looked at you, into your face, but did not latch on. I wonder why he didn't latch right on?"

The group offers different thoughts—some thinking sympathetically about the mother, others curious about baby, and still others holding to concrete ideas about feeding.

The facilitator addresses the baby, summarizing and slightly extending the group's suggestions: "We think that Mummy wants to feed you when you are hungry so your tummy doesn't hurt and you grow big and strong . . ." (validating the mother's positive intentions, acknowledging midrange contingency in that the mother is seen to recognize her baby's cues, rather than intrude or ignore). " . . . But perhaps you felt mummy's tension when she offered you her breast, because her nipple is very cracked . . ." (personalized group construct recognizing baby's embodied experience). "And maybe you need to see Mummy's face reassure you that it is OK to hurt her if you are hungry and you will both be OK" (emphasizing authentic communication between the members of the dyad, disruption and repair).

An infant whose channels for learning about the social world have been disrupted—in other words, whose social experiences with caregivers have caused a breakdown in epistemic trust—is naturally left in a position of mistrust in the authenticity of interactions with his or her caregiver and others. In this state, social communications may be rejected, their meanings confused or distorted, or misinterpreted as having hostile intent. Such *epistemic disruption* or *freezing* can render an individual therapeutically "hard to reach" (a very familiar description to those working in Social Services) (Fonagy & Allison, 2014; Fonagy et al., 2015). Many of the women in NB will have been inadequately mentalized as infants and children in precisely a way that generates the epistemic freezing that can make them so hard to help through conventional services. The accumulating effects of social adversity and alienation from the institutions they encounter and the culture they inhabit will have made such epistemic closure a highly understandable adaptation.

Through the content of the program, as elaborated and interactively personalized in the sessions, NB implicitly provides the parents with a meaningful model of mind and an understanding of their own and their babies' singular development, as well as an idea of the process of change. The work of NB is to create an environment in which epistemic trust can be reopened in the parents. At a group level, there is a transactional and gradual development of a culture whereby the parents entrust the practitioner, and each other, with aspects of their vulnerability and helplessness, and the facilitator reliably helps to hold painful emotions and create meaning out of experience (Sleed et al., 2013). For this critical sense of "genuineness" to pervade the group, the facilitators need to model their own authentic mentalizing processes—observing, listening, and reflecting—and their capacity to be open to their own thoughts and responses, consistently inquiring in a nonjudgmental way about the difficulties and uncertainties that are intrinsic to mentalization. In their facial expressions, tone of voice, and body cues, as much as in what each person says, the facilitators communicate their attitudes. This mental–affective–behavioral stance is linked to the growing understanding across therapeutic modalities about the quality of the practitioner's presence and the co-constructed encounter between client(s) and practitioner as a potentially transformative attachment experience (Bollas, 1987; Broughton, 2016; Fonagy, 1999; Loewald, 1979; Stern, 2004).

At a dyadic level, the work is to attempt to follow and feed back to the mother the complexities of the dyadic interaction in a way that allows the mother to personalize the mentalizing approach of both herself in relation to her infant, and of the infant in relation to her. This process of personalization is so significant because it reveals the relevance of the model to the parents. According to the theory of epistemic trust, the parents' recognition of the personal relevance and validity of the approach is the critical first stage in reopening epistemic trust: the emergence of a state of mind that allows the parents to benefit from more positive social interactions and experiences, reinforcing reflective abilities and becoming open to mentalizing their own relationships. We would suggest that the proverbial "hard-to-reach" parents are those whose emotional and social experiences have generated high levels of epistemic mistrust. The highly mentalizing and personalizing aspects of NB serve to reawaken epistemic openness that social adversity has shut down. The parents' experiences of being "known" translate into greater awareness of their babies' psychological experiences. In parallel, the facilitators' direct work with the babies, in which they consider the babies' communications about how they are feeling, make the infants' mental states more accessible. The most frequent feedback from the participants has been "I understand my baby better" and "I realize that he or she has his own feelings from the beginning."

Evaluation of NB

Outcomes of NB from Previous Studies

The NB intervention in prison MBUs was evaluated first as a pilot outcome study (Baradon, Fonagy, Bland, Lénárd, & Sleed, 2008) and subsequently as a cluster randomized controlled trial (Sleed et al., 2013); see Table 8.2.

The pilot study made use of the Parent Development Interview (PDI; Slade, Aber, Berger, Bresgi, & Kaplan, 2004) to capture qualitative elements of the mothers' representations of their babies, themselves as mothers, and their relationship with their babies, as well as their capacity for reflective functioning (RF; Slade, Bernbach, Grienenberger, Levy, & Locker, 2004). The interview was conducted with 27 mothers, before and after the intervention. The results of this study demonstrated an overall increase in maternal RF from pre- to postintervention. Furthermore, after the intervention, the mothers' representations were found to be less idealized, more nuanced, and more focused on the child as a separate person with his or her own thoughts and feelings (Baradon et al., 2008).

In the cluster randomized controlled trial (Sleed et al., 2013), parent and infant outcomes were evaluated for 88 mother–infant dyads participating in the NB intervention and 75 mothers and infants in prisons where the intervention did not take place. The measures used in this trial were parental RF on the PDI (Slade, Bernbach, et al., 2004), the quality of parent–infant interactions as rated by the Coding Interactive Behavior scales (CIB; Feldman, 1998), maternal depression as measured by the Center for Epidemiologic Studies Depression Scale (CES-D; Radloff, 1977), and mothers' reports of their representations of the babies on the Mother Object Relations Scale (MORS; Oates & Gervai, 2003). The findings confirmed the

TABLE 8.2. Summary of Outcomes of New Beginnings

Study	Population	*N*	Design	Measures	Positive treatment outcomes	No treatment effects found
Baradon et al. (2008)	Mothers and babies in prison, England	27 intervention	Pilot cohort study	• PDI (RF ratings and qualitative analysis)	• Parental reflective functioning (RF) • More adaptive representations of baby	
Sleed et al. (2013)	Mothers and babies in prison, England	88 intervention vs. 75 control	Cluster RCT	• PDI (RF) • CIB • CES-D • MORS	• Parental reflective functioning (RF) • Parent–infant interaction (CIB dyadic attunement)	• Maternal depression (CES-D) • Infant interactive behavior (CIB) • Maternal representations (MORS)
Bain (2014)	Mothers and babies in homeless shelters, South Africa	16 intervention vs. 6 control	Cohort study with small control group	• PDI (RF) • EAS • GSMD	• Parent–infant interaction (EAS maternal structuring) • Infant speech development (GSMD)	• Parental RF • Maternal sensitivity and infant interactive behavior (EAS) • Infant personal–social development (GSMD)

Note. PDI, Parent Development Interview; RF, reflective functioning; CES-D, Center for Epidemiologic Studies Depression Scale; CIB, Coding Interactive Behavior; EAS, Emotional Availability Scales; MORS, Mother Object Relations Scale; GSMD, Griffiths Scales of Mental Development.

beneficial outcomes seen in the pilot study with regard to maternal RF; mothers taking part in the NB program demonstrated significantly better levels of mentalizing over time relative to those in the control prisons. Similarly, there were significantly better mother–infant interactions in the intervention group over time relative to the control dyads. There were no significant group effects over time for the CES-D or the MORS.

A third evaluation of NB was carried out with 16 mothers and babies in homeless shelters in South Africa who participated in the program and a comparison group of six mother–baby dyads not in the program (Bain, 2014). In this study, contrary to the findings in the prison population, the mothers' capacities for RF did not improve significantly. However, significant shifts were found in the infants' speech abilities and in the mothers' abilities to structure interactions with their infants. The number of sessions attended by the dyads correlated with improvements made by the mothers and their infants, suggesting a dosage effect.

The findings of both the pilot qualitative study and the larger randomized controlled trial in the prisons point to the effectiveness of the intervention in improving maternal mentalizing capacity. The capacity for mothers to be curious about their infants' and their own internal psychological worlds, and to make sense of the impact that each person's mental states can have on others has been identified as a crucial component of attachment security (Slade et al., 2005), nondisrupted maternal behavior (Grienenberger, Kelly, & Slade, 2005), and infant social and emotional development (Fonagy, Gergely, & Target, 2007). The content of the intervention is highly focused on drawing the mothers' attention to their babies' internal world, and the evaluation findings indicate that the program appears to be effective in meeting this aim. These findings were not replicated in the South African evaluation (Bain, 2014); no changes in RF were found for this sample. Cultural factors may have played a part in this discrepancy, or there may have been more rigid mentalizing difficulties in this group that made it harder to achieve a shift in this domain. What did shift positively for this group were the more obvious parenting behaviors. The intervention appears to have been successful in helping the mothers to provide playful and appropriate structure to their interactions with their babies. These improvements were seen alongside, and probably directly translated into, improvements in the babies' language development. The prison evaluation also showed improvements in the behavioral quality of parent–infant interaction. Thus, across both contexts, there was evidence that NB was successful in improving the mothers' genuine interest in and responsivity to their infants.

The prison evaluation provided some insight into the appropriateness of certain measures in high-risk parent–infant dyads. High levels of idealization were found on the mother-report questionnaires; mothers tended to report very low levels of depressive symptomatology and had extremely positive representations of their relationships with their babies as measured by the MORS at baseline. There was a ceiling effect on these measures and no further room for "improvement" at the follow-up. Thus, measurement insensitivity may have resulted in bias in assessing clinically meaningful change for this sample. Given that the qualitative analysis of the PDI in the pilot study demonstrated a reduction in idealized maternal representations of the parent–infant relationship following the intervention, it might be argued that a positive outcome in this sample would have been a reduction in overly positive representations on parent-report questionnaires. In fact, defensive idealization has been recognized by many attachment theorists to be indicative of less optimal attachment relationships and the intergenerational transmission of psychopathology (George & Solomon, 2008; Kernberg, 1983; Lerner & Van-Der Keshet, 1995; Lyons-Ruth, 2002). Thus, in planning evaluations with similar high-risk parenting populations, data should be collated from multiple sources and should not rely solely on parent-report questionnaires.

Taken together, the evidence for the effectiveness of the program is promising. The differential outcomes found in different settings highlight the importance of ongoing evaluations that can add to the knowledge base in various contexts.

Evaluation of NB-C

A service evaluation has been incorporated into the implementation of NB-C. The planning of this ongoing evaluation has been informed by the experience gained from evaluating the program in prisons, as well as the local policies and practices relating specifically to the social work unit setting. Data are collected by the course facilitators themselves, and the measures have been selected as instruments that can serve the dual purpose of providing research data and clinically meaningful information. The underlying principle of the evaluation is that routine outcome monitoring not only provides information about the outcomes of treatment but can also serve to improve outcomes (Bickman, Kelley, Breda, de Andrade, & Riemer, 2011; Lambert et al., 2006). The evaluation data are collected during the facilitators' initial and final home visits to each family. It is therefore important to ensure that evaluation data collection does not impinge on the important processes of engagement and ending.

The measures employed in this evaluation include the PDI, which is coded for maternal RF, and video-recorded parent–infant interactions, which is coded for maternal sensitivity. Both of these measures demonstrated beneficial outcomes for the NB program in prisons and the aim is to ascertain whether similar outcomes can be observed from the community-based program. In addition to these externally rated measures, two parent-report questionnaires are being used in this evaluation: The Parenting Stress Index–Short Form (PSI-SF; Abidin, 1995) and the Clinical Outcomes in Routine Evaluation Scale (CORE; (Evans et al., 2000). These are widely used measures, and normative data from multiple sources provide meaningful comparison data in the absence of a control group in this evaluation. Parent-report questionnaires were not found to be appropriate measures in the prison sample due to defensive responding. It is possible that similar socially desirable biases will be observed in the community program with families in the child protection system, although this will only be ascertained through the collection of these data.

The context of the NB-C program has enabled use of a further source of data collection for the purposes of triangulation. Each family in the program is supported by a case-holding member of the social work team who is independent of the intervention. The case-holding social workers are also asked to provide ratings of the quality of parent–infant relationships for each of the participating dyads on the Parent–Infant Relationship Global Assessment Scale (PIR-GAS; Zero-to-Three/National Center for Clinical Infant Programs, 1994, 2005). This rating is provided at the start and at the end of the intervention and provides an independent clinical assessment of the dyads' functioning over time.

The final set of outcomes being measured relate to the public health priorities of the setting in which the program is being carried out. A service-use inventory is used to record the families' engagement in specialized supportive services such as smoking cessation, breast feeding, and healthy eating support programs, as well as universal health and social care services. The child's status on the child protection register is also recorded pre- and postintervention. The aim of this is to determine whether families are more likely to engage with services as they develop more trusting relationships with professionals, and whether there are any changes in the use of more costly services such as hospital emergency visits after the NB-C program.

As sufficient numbers of mothers and babies move through the program and evaluation, the results of these outcomes will become available.

Impact of Training and Implementation of NB-C on Social Worker Practice

In addition to the outcomes for parents and babies in the NB-C program, a qualitative study was carried out to assess the impact of the course on the facilitators' professional practice. The facilitators of the first group were interviewed by the research team about their experiences of running these groups, and a thematic analysis of the interviews was carried out. The analysis revealed six broad themes from these interviews.

A PRIVILEGED EXPERIENCE

A recurring theme from all of the facilitators was that they felt the NB program enabled them and the families to develop an intimate and privileged relationship.

This experience was markedly different from their usual way of working. For example, one of the facilitators spoke of her frustration working in a system that was very stretched for resources to support families, but spoke of the NB experience being very different:

> "You might have very strong opinions about what you want for a baby and a mother, but there just are not the resources or the system to support that, so it just, yeah, feels a bit hopeless sometimes. [Interviewer: "Did that come up with the New Beginnings families you worked with?"] Less, that was a really great thing about the New Beginnings, it felt like you were providing something to the mums, that was so, so, like nurturing and, and they had so much support for that time that they'd never had before."

Another facilitator spoke of the shift in how the families perceived them, and how that might be carried into other aspects of their work:

> "They feel persecuted by social services anyway, so I'm kind of, I'm interested in how to try to shift that, cause it can, that was part of the feedback that we got from the group, that they didn't feel like it was a social services intervention, it felt like something very special and separate. . . . I'm looking at how that could be implemented in different services, social services."

DIFFICULTY WITH ENDING

Given the sense of intimacy that the facilitators felt they had developed with the families, it is probably not surprising that they found ending the group very difficult.

> "It felt really hard when it ended. Because we knew that what was left was a really, really stretched social work system. . . . It felt really hard to end the group, and to think about what, what would sort of become of those dyads."

ASSESSING PARENT–INFANT RELATIONSHIPS

All of the facilitators talked about how the experience of training and implementing the program had increased their knowledge of what to look out for when carrying out assessments, a large component of their usual work.

"I think that I'm better equipped now to spot where are, to identify when the sort of needs of baby are not being met. . . . There's a whole other dimension that I kind of didn't understand as well, which I think I understand much more now, which is the relationship, and the bond, and all the kind of nuances within that, that are more kind of complex . . . really subtle signs."

INTERVENTIONS WITH PARENT AND INFANTS

The team members also spoke of the practical intervention skills they felt they gained from the course, which would be carried forward in their future practice and which had transformed their overall practice with clients.

"The way in which I would support a parent to communicate with their babies, it's very, very different than what I would have done before. I would have talked to the baby before, but now I'm much more comfortable with talking from the baby's position, so being able to verbalize how baby might be experiencing the world in that moment, what it might be like for them to, for a mum to walk away and make a cup of tea, how they might experience that, verbalize that for the baby."

PROFESSIONAL COMPETENCE

A strong theme throughout the interviews was the overall sense of confidence that the facilitators all felt they had gained from the experience, particularly in relation to working with babies.

"Now there is a whole new client group that I feel able to work with."

EFFECTIVE INTERVENTION

The facilitators were unambiguous in their belief that the program was one that could make a positive difference for parents and babies. They all spoke of the observable improvements they noticed in the mothers and babies over the duration of the intervention.

"For example, constantly talking to baby, and explaining to baby: 'Mommy is going over there, she's making a drink, you can see her.' Even just kind of talking to them. And at the beginning the mothers thought we were bonkers. They didn't understand the reasoning behind it, and whether they understood fully the reasoning behind it at the end of the group, I don't know, but they were all implementing it, so I think that they could see how the baby benefited from that, and how the baby responded to that."

The training and supervised experience of running the program in this context appears to have been a positive experience for the facilitators and for the families with whom they worked. Importantly, the facilitators felt that they had gained new skills and more experience working therapeutically with parents and babies, which informs their practice in other aspects of their work. Thus, the program appears to have met a further aim: to embed the NB principles into the broader professional culture. This could have far-reaching implications for all families in contact with the service, not just those in the NB-C groups.

Implementation of the Intervention

The emphasis on the importance of epistemic reopening in the NB program is also applied within the professional and organizational setting from which clients are referred, and in which the program is delivered. In the following section we describe how we approached the need to maintain this focus in the implementation of the program.

Review and Planning for Delivery of NB-C

The changes made for delivery in the community were carefully planned to ensure that there was no drift from the core manualized and evidenced program while addressing the challenges of a new model of delivery. A number of principles guided the process.

Partnership Planning

The starting point was a process of consultation: Focus groups and individual meetings were held with the program facilitators, commissioners, and service users to review the program, learn from experience, and plan for sensitive local delivery.

Each of these groups made important contributions. For example, mothers who had participated in the program recommended adaptations to make certain elements of the program more user-friendly. These were endorsed by the facilitators, who also fed back those aspects of the program that worked well, in their view, as well as those aspects that were not sufficiently sensitive to the mothers' states of mind or group dynamics. The commissioners were invested in the use of NB as an intervention that could inform their decision-making process regarding their most worrying families. To accommodate their agenda, we built in formal but transparent procedures for feedback to professionals while preserving boundaries of participants' confidentiality. The focus groups with potential service users, which were held with local mothers of babies, placed particular emphasis on engagement and supporting participants to complete the program. They brought to the discussion both the realistic difficulties (e.g., transport and finances) and the personal narratives of discouragement and disengagement due to shame, a feeling of being judged, and of being targeted, and had ideas about how these might be addressed in implementing the program. On the basis of discussions with them, we increased the emphasis on increased flexibility in building the relationships with each mother and baby (e.g., telephone calls and messages, home visits when necessary) to accommodate their histories of disrupted attachments and difficulties in sustaining ongoing investment in a group in which attachments are the focus of attention.

Embedding the Program in the Local Services

Whereas NB had previously been delivered in the prisons by the Anna Freud Centre as an external body, with the complexities and advantages this brought (Tomas-Merrills & Chakraborty, 2010), we aimed to embed the community program within local services. This was considered advantageous for a number of reasons. At the level of planning and implementation, the local statutory services were involved in decisions about key areas: staffing, facilities and budget, evaluation design, defining the inclusion criteria, recruitment and engagement processes, feedback model, and management of risk. On the level of public policy it was felt that with the statutory providers taking ownership of the program, infant mental health would become a locally endorsed priority.

The training of the service staff contributed to skills transfer from specialist to generic settings—from the Anna Freud Centre to local services. Within the broader upskilling of the professional workforce employed by the local authority, training and supervising of selected social workers and psychologists as NB facilitators (below), created more specialized core members who, in time, took over infant mental health trainings within the service.

Embedding NB Principles in the Local Services

A central tenet of all mentalization-based approaches is that reflectiveness within the broad professional network is critical to making an impact at the individual level; in other words, mentalizing cannot occur in isolation (Bevington, Fuggle, Fonagy, Target, & Asen, 2013; Midgley & Vrouva, 2013). This was deemed to be of particular importance in the context of the Social Service system, where child protection requirements predominate. For this reason, an initial phase of training was provided to a broad cross-section of the staff group working with these families. The aim of this training was to raise awareness of relational development and difficulties in infancy, and to promote a more knowledgeable and thoughtful approach to work with parents and infants. Thus, the main principles were embedded into the organizational culture, an important element of the model, since all families in the NB-C groups are referred and supported by the broader staff alongside the program.

Selection and Training of Facilitators

Facilitators are clinically trained professional (psychologists, social workers) chosen on the basis of interest and experience in parent–infant work and with groups, ability to assimilate a clinical–therapeutic focus in their work, and ability to work collaboratively in facilitating the program. The personal stance of the facilitator in imbuing a sense of interest, safety, and sensitivity is critical. Facilitators who offer a sense of authenticity and commitment construct a stronger foundation for change to occur.

The training program comprises 10 sessions on infant mental health and the parent–infant relationship (shared with the broader staff group), and working with mothers and infants in a group, and 10 sessions addressing the content and process of the program, maintaining fidelity, and conducting the evaluation measures. The facilitators are expected to model an open, trusting relationship between collaborating adults for the mothers and babies, where domestic friction is a common occurrence. Therefore, their working relationship is central to the program and is attended to by them and in supervision.

Implementation as an Iterative Process

The local service management was highly invested in maximizing the contributions of the program in the execution of their legal responsibilities. Therefore, regular reviews were held with them to monitor delivery in relation to local client and organizational culture. These meetings were helpful to the Anna Freud Centre in refining the program, and to the local authority in terms of reliability of input to their care processes. Similar processes took place with professional and client focus groups.

Clinical Supervision

Weekly supervision is provided to the facilitators during the course of the program as a reflective space to maintain safety, therapeutic efficacy, and adherence to the NB program. Central in this is the need to process highly arousing experiences generated by the individual histories of the mothers and babies and the group dynamics. Supervision also helps facilitators to monitor unconscious attempts by the parents to recruit the facilitators into a worldview that may be indicative of split-off and defensive processes and to maintain awareness of how these are acted upon, sometimes in the facilitator relationship. Supervision is a forum to formulate ways to manage such processes in the group, and to consider how this might influence systemic and risk factors. Tension between facilitators—whether interpersonal or due to group processes (e.g., one of them being less experienced in working with dyads)—is also addressed within supervision.

Challenges in the Implementation of the NB-C Program

The process of embedding NB-C within the statutory authority at a cultural level was one of the issues that required monitoring and reflection (see Table 8.3). Traditionally, work in Child Protective Services requires transparency and sharing of information within the professional network. To this end, in an innovative model of work, social work units work therapeutically alongside clinical services, with clinical hypotheses shared in an ongoing dialogue. The feedback processes for NB-C were a departure from this model, in that feedback is provided to the social work units only midway and in the final stages of the program, in a formalized report that is discussed with the parent first (outside of any reporting of imminent risk of harm). It was recognized that this shift is likely to be met with resistance and frustration from the social work units, since this dialogue is at the heart of the social work model. Social workers might also be impacted by perceptions of "their" clients enjoying privileged relationships with facilitators who fed, nurtured, and held the dyads in ways that social workers' roles prevented them from doing. The potential

TABLE 8.3. Implementation Principles

Principle	Aims	Activities	Outcome
Collaboration in program planning, implementation, and review	Ensure program is relevant to commissioning and participants agenda	Focus groups and individual meetings with commissioners and service users before and during program implementation	• Deliver a locally appraised program • Reduce organizational anxiety and increase positive regard for the introduction of a new and different program • Increase participation rates through enhancing relevance and sensitivity to user group
Embeddedness in local services	Infant mental health becomes a locally endorsed and budgeted priority	• Six monthly meetings with statutory social services management • Training of general social work and psychology staff	• Program review and development is an iterative process • Improved referral pathways and risk management
Recognition of the importance of a rolling program of training and supervision to change practice	• Increase knowledge and reflectiveness within the broad professional network regarding infant mental health • Create local specialist resource in the facilitators	• Training of social work and psychology workforce • Training of facilitators	• Up-skilling the local workforce
Culture of reflectiveness and transparency	Offer program participants relational and organizational experiences that increase their trust in professionals	Create and adhere to transparent procedures for reporting back to social workers (who monitor and make decision regarding child welfare)	• Increase participants attendance in the program • Input to considered decisions regarding the future of mother and baby

of bias against the program and/or facilitators made it imperative for program facilitators to prepare the ground with the social work units. Collaboration was achieved with the understanding that the model allowed facilitators more space to build on the clinical hypothesis for each dyad, thereby allowing them to make more considered and robust proposals at the end. However, social worker and facilitator recommendations may conflict, and the possibilities for disagreement and implicit tensions, rare as they may be, need attention.

The parallels between the experiences of the program clients and those of the facilitators in this instance were striking; both were in the position of having to learn to trust the program at a time when there were tensions about how information would be interpreted, shared, and recorded. Both were susceptible to experiencing splitting, which, if not handled sensitively, could undermine the efficacy of the program and diminish outcomes. Supported by the supervisory process, program facilitators subsequently found themselves responsible for the anxieties of both the institution and the dyads.

Over time, the institutional anxieties decreased when positive outcomes for the first NB-C dyads were achieved, thereby increasing confidence in the model and further embedding it in the culture of the social work unit. It has increasingly come to be seen as a provision for families, where concerns about the risks to the baby—and therefore the possibility of separation—are high.

A second challenge pertained to the facilitator–client relations. The delivery model for a situation whereby the very authority that was monitoring child welfare, and therefore seen as bad/persecutory to most of the mothers, was also the agency delivering what they hoped the mothers would experience as a "good" program. Thus, we anticipated that suspicion could initially taint the mothers' trust in the facilitators' intentions and therefore their belief in the authenticity and personal relevance of the program. These expectations were met in a large number of the mothers, who initially challenged the facilitators' trustworthiness ("These people are social workers!!") or withdrew from confiding in the group because of this. However, we also hypothesized that the process of building this trust could indirectly address a central, maladaptive mode of mental functioning in many mothers, typically characterized by splitting between "good" and "bad" objects (people, organizations, baby, etc.). Yet to be tested is whether there is carryover in their relationships with their babies and others over time.

Summary

NB reaches out to the "hardest to reach" families with complex and entrenched sociofamilial difficulties, who are operating under the risk of separation arising from very real child protection needs. These are mothers, therefore, who are in the fright-without-solution predicament (Main & Hesse, 1990) of struggling to forge attachments to their infants in the here and now, while dealing with both past traumatic attachment histories and the prospect of future attachment disruption of the severest kind. The babies, upon commencement of the program, may already show features associated with trauma, such as avoidance, blank face, and freezing (Beebe et al., 2012; Beebe & Lachmann, 2014; Guédeney, Matthey, & Puura, 2013; Lyons-Ruth et al., 2013). NB mobilizes compelling empirical evidence and theoretical insight in a coherent model that can be replicated and applied to support a wide range of families, and is establishing itself with a growing evidence base.

REFERENCES

Abidin, R. R. (1995). *Parenting Stress Index–Short Form: Test manual.* Charlottesville, VA: Pediatric Psychology Press.

Bain, K. (2014). "New Beginnings" in South African shelters for the homeless: Piloting of a group psychotherapy intervention for high-risk mother–infant dyads. *Infant Mental Health Journal, 35*(6), 591–603.

Baradon, T. (2009). *New Beginnings–Facilitators manual.* Unpublished manual, Anna Freud Centre, London.

Baradon, T. (2013). *New Beginnings in the Community (NB-C)–Facilitators manual.* Unpublished manual, Anna Freud Centre, London.

Baradon, T., Fonagy, P., Bland, K., Lénárd, K., & Sleed, M. (2008). New Beginnings—an experience-based programme addressing the attachment relationship between mothers and their babies in prisons. *Journal of Child Psychotherapy, 34*(2), 240–258.

Baradon, T., & Target, T. (2010). New Beginnings—a psychoanalytically informed programme to support primary attachment relationships between mothers and babies in prison. In A. Lemma & M. Patrick (Eds.), *Off the couch: Contemporary psychoanalytic applications* (pp. 11–81). London: Routledge.

Baradon, T., with Biseo, M., Broughton, C., James, J., & Joyce, A. (2016). *The practice of psycho-analytic parent–infant psychotherapy: Claiming the baby* (2nd ed.). London: Routledge.

Beebe, B. (2013). How does microanalysis of mother–infant communication inform maternal sensitivity and infant attachment? *Attachment and Human Development, 15*(5–6), 583–602.

Beebe, B., & Lachmann, F. M. (2014). *The origins of attachment: Infant research and adult treatment.* New York: Routledge.

Beebe, B., Lachmann, F., Markese, S., & Bahrick, L. (2012). On the origins of disorganized attachment and internal working models: Paper I. A dyadic systems approach. *Psychoanalytic Dialogues, 22*(2), 253–272.

Bevington, D., Fuggle, P., Fonagy, P., Target, M., & Asen, E. (2013). Innovations in practice: Adolescent mentalization-based integrative therapy (AMBIT)—a new integrated approach to working with the most hard to reach adolescents with severe complex mental health needs. *Child and Adolescent Mental Health, 18*(1), 46–51.

Bickman, L., Kelley, S. D., Breda, C., de Andrade, A. R., & Riemer, M. (2011). Effects of routine feedback to clinicians on mental health outcomes of youths: Results of a randomized trial. *Psychiatric Services, 62*(12), 1423–1429.

Bollas, C. (1987). *The shadow of the object: Psychoanalysis of the unthought known.* New York: Columbia University Press.

Borelli, J. L., Goshin, L. S., Joestl, S., Clark, J., & Byrne, M. W. (2010). Attachment organization in a sample of incarcerated mothers: Distribution of classifications and associations with substance abuse history, depressive symptoms, perceptions of parenting competency and social support. *Attachment and Human Development, 12*(4), 355–374.

Bronfman, E., Parsons, E., & Lyons-Ruth, K. (1999). *Atypical Maternal Behavior Instrument for Assessment and Classification (AMBIANCE): Manual for coding disrupted affective communication, version 2.* Unpublished manuscript, Harvard Medical School, Cambridge, Massachusetts.

Broughton, C. (2016). The middle phase: Elaboration and consolidation. In T. Baradon, M. Biseo, C. Broughton, J. James, & A. Joyce (Eds.), *The practice of pschoanalytic parent–infant psychotherapy: Claiming the baby* (2nd ed., pp. 87–108). London: Routledge.

Brown, E. R., Khan, L., & Parsonage, M. (2012). *A chance to change: Delivering effective parenting programs to transform lives.* London: Centre for Mental Health.

Csibra, G., & Gergely, G. (2006). Social learning and social cognition: The case for pedagogy. In M. H. Johnson & Y. Munakata (Eds.), *Processes of change in brain and cognitive development: Attention and Performance XXI* (pp. 249–274). Oxford, UK: Oxford University Press.

Csibra, G., & Gergely, G. (2009). Natural pedagogy. *Trends in Cognitive Sciences, 13*(4), 148–153.

Csibra, G., & Gergely, G. (2011). Natural pedagogy as evolutionary adaptation. *Philosophical Transactions of the Royal Society of London B: Biological Sciences, 366*(1567), 1149–1157.

Evans, C., Mellor-Clark, J., Margison, F., Barkham, M., Audin, K., Connell, J., & McGrath, G. (2000). CORE: Clinical Outcomes in Routine Evaluation. *Journal of Mental Health, 9*(3), 247–255.

Feldman, R. (1998). *Coding Interactive Behaviour manual.* Unpublished manuscript, Bar-Ilan University, Ramat Gan, Israel.

Feldman, R. (2007). Parent–infant synchrony: Biological foundations and developmental outcomes. *Current Directions in Psychological Science, 16*, 340–345.

Fonagy, P. (1999, Spring). *The process of change and the change of process: What can change in a good analysis?* Keynote Address presented at the meeting of Division 39 of the American Psychological Association, New York.

Fonagy, P., & Allison, E. (2014). The role of mentalizing and epistemic trust in the therapeutic relationship. *Psychotherapy, 51*(3), 372–380.

Fonagy, P., Gergely, G., Jurist, E., & Target, M. (2002). *Affect regulation, mentalization, and the development of the self.* New York: Other Press.

Fonagy, P., Gergely, G., & Target, M. (2007). The parent–infant dyad and the construction of the subjective self. *Journal of Child Psychology and Psychiatry, 48*(3–4), 288–328.

Fonagy, P., Lorenzini, N., Campbell, C., & Luyten, P. (2014). Why are we interested in attachments? In P. Holmes & S. Farnfield (Eds.), *The Routledge handbook of attachment: Theory* (pp. 38–51). Hove, UK: Routledge.

Fonagy, P., Luyten, P., & Allison, E. (2015). Epistemic petrification and the restoration of epistemic trust: A new conceptualization of borderline personality disorder and its psychosocial treatment. *Journal of Personality Disorders, 29*(5), 575–609.

Fonagy, P., Steele, M., Moran, G., Steele, H., & Higgitt, A. (1993). Measuring the ghost in the nursery: An empirical study of the relation between parents' mental representations of childhood experiences and their infants' security of attachment. *Journal of the American Psychoanalytic Association, 41*(4), 957–989.

Fonagy, P., Steele, M., Steele, H., Moran, G. S., & Higgitt, A. C. (1991). The capacity for understanding mental states: The reflective self in parent and child and its significance for security of attachment. *Infant Mental Health Journal, 12*(3), 201–218.

Fraiberg, S., Adelson, E., & Shapiro, V. (1975). Ghosts in the nursery: A psychoanalytic approach to the problems of impaired infant–mother relationships. *Journal of the American Academy of Child Psychiatry, 14*(3), 387–421.

George, C., & Solomon, J. (2008). The caregiving system: A behavioral systems approach to parenting. In J. Cassidy & P. R. Shaver (Eds.), *Handbook of attachment: Theory, research, and clinical applications* (2nd ed., pp. 833–856). New York: Guilford Press.

Grienenberger, J. F., Kelly, K., & Slade, A. (2005). Maternal reflective functioning, mother–infant affective communication, and infant attachment: Exploring the link between mental states and observed caregiving behavior in the intergenerational transmission of attachment. *Attachment and Human Development, 7*(3), 299–311.

Guédeney, A., Matthey, S., & Puura, K. (2013). Social withdrawal behaviour in infancy: A history of the concept and a review of published studies using the Alarm Distress Baby Scale. *Infant Mental Health Journal, 34*(6), 516–531.

James, J. (2016). Parent–infant psychotherapy in groups. In T. Baradon, M. Biseo, C. Broughton, J. James, & A. Joyce (Eds.), *The practice of pschoanalytic parent–infant psychotherapy: Claiming the baby* (2nd ed., pp. 138–160). London: Routledge.

Kernberg, P. F. (1983). *Reflections in the mirror: Mother–child interaction, self-awareness, and self-recognition.* New York: Basic Books.

Lambert, M. J., Whipple, J. L., Hawkins, E. J., Vermeersch, D. A., Nielsen, S. L., & Smart, D. W. (2006). Is it time for clinicians to routinely track patient outcome?: A meta-analysis. *Clinical Psychology: Science and Practice, 10*(3), 288–301.

Lerner, P. M., & Van-Der Keshet, Y. (1995). A note on the assessment of idealization. *Journal of Personality Assessment, 65*(1), 77–90.

Loewald, H. W. (1979). Reflections on the psychoanalytic process and its therapeutic potential. *Psychoanalytic Study of the Child, 34,* 155–167.

Lyons-Ruth, K. (2002). The two-person construction of defenses: Disorganized attachment strategies, unintegrated mental states, and hostile/helpless relational processes. *Journal of Infant, Child, and Adolescent Psychotherapy, 2*(4), 107–119.

Lyons-Ruth, K., Bureau, J.-F., Easterbrooks, A., Obsuth, I., Hennighausen, K., & Vulliez-Coady, L. (2013). Parsing the construct of maternal insensitivity: Distinct longitudinal pathways associated with early maternal withdrawal. *Attachment and Human Development, 15*(5–6), 562–582.

Main, M., & Hesse, E. (1990). Parents' unresolved traumatic experiences are related to infant disorganized/disoriented attachment status: Is frightened and/or frightening parental behavior the linking mechanism? In M. T. Greenberg, D. Cicchetti, & E. M. Cummings (Eds.), *Attachment in the preschool years: Theory, research, and intervention* (pp. 161–182). Chicago: University of Chicago Press.

Midgley, N., & Vrouva, I. (Eds.). (2013). *Minding the child: Mentalization-based interventions with children, young people and their families.* London, UK: Routledge.

Oates, J. M., & Gervai, J. (2003). *Mothers' Object Relations Scales.* Paper presented at the Poster presented at the 11th European Conference on Developmental Psychology, Milan, Italy.

Prison Reform Trust. (2012). Bromley Briefings Prison Factfile. Retrieved from *www.thebromleytrust.org.uk/Indexhibit/files/bbriefings2012.pdf.*

Radloff, L. S. (1977). The CES-D Scale: A self-report depression scale for use in the general population. *Application of Psychological Measures, 1,* 385–401.

Slade, A., Aber, J. L., Berger, B., Bresgi, I., & Kaplan, M. (2004). *The Parent Development Interview–Revised.* New York: City University of New York.

Slade, A., Bernbach, E., Grienenberger, J., Levy, D., & Locker, A. (2004). *Addendum to Fonagy, Target, Steele, and Steele Reflective Functioning Scoring Manual for use with the Parent Development Interview.* Unpublished manuscript, City College of New York, New York.

Slade, A., Grienenberger, J., Bernbach, E., Levy, D., & Locker, A. (2005). Maternal reflective functioning, attachment, and the transmission gap: A preliminary study. *Attachment and Human Development, 7*(3), 283–298.

Sleed, M., Baradon, T., & Fonagy, P. (2013). New Beginnings for mothers and babies in prison: A cluster randomized controlled trial. *Attachment and Human Development, 15*(4), 349–367.

Stern, D. (2004). *The present moment in psychotherapy and everyday life.* New York: Norton.

Stern, D., Sander, L., Nahum, J., Harrison, A., Lyons-Ruth, K., Morgan, A., . . . Tronick, E. (1998). Non-interpretive mechanisms in psychoanalytic therapy: The "something more" than interpretation. *International Journal of Psycho-Analysis, 79*(5), 903–921.

Stern, D. N., Hofer, L., Haft, W., & Dore, J. (1985). Affect attunement: The sharing of feeling states between mother and infant by means of inter-modal fluency. In T. M. Fields & N. A. Fox (Eds.), *Social perception in infants* (pp. 249–268). Norwood, NJ: Ablex.

Tomas-Merrills, J., & Chakraborty, A. (2010). Babies behind bars: Working with relational trauma with mothers and babies in prison. In T. Baradon (Ed.), *Relational trauma in infancy: Psychoanalytic, attachment and neuropsychological contributions to parent–infant psychotherapy* (pp. 103–115). Hove, UK: Routledge.

Tronick, E. Z., & Weinberg, M. K. (1997. Depressed mothers and infants: Failure to form dyadic consciousness. In L. Murray & P. Cooper (Eds.), *Postpartum depression and child development* (pp. 54–84). New York: Guilford Press.

Waddell, M. (1994). *Owl babies.* London: Walker Books.

ZERO TO THREE/National Center for Clinical Infant Programs. (1994). *Diagnostic classification: 0–3, diagnostic classification of mental health and developmental disorders of infancy and early childhood.* Washington, DC: Author.

ZERO TO THREE/National Center for Clinical Infant Programs. (2005). *Diagnostic classification of mental health and developmental disorders of infancy and early childhood, revised edition (DC:0-3R).* Washington, DC: Author.

Zlotnick, C. (1997). Posttraumatic stress disorder (PTSD), PTSD comorbidity, and childhood abuse among incarcerated women. *Journal of Nervous and Mental Disease, 185*(12), 761–763.

CHAPTER 9

Group Attachment-Based Intervention
A Multifamily Trauma-Informed Intervention

HOWARD STEELE, MIRIAM STEELE, KAREN BONUCK,
PAUL MEISSNER, and ANNE MURPHY

This chapter outlines the main premises of an attachment- and trauma-informed intervention, Group Attachment-Based Intervention (GABI©), specifically developed to target vulnerable families with infants and toddlers. This chapter describes the twin attachment- and trauma-informed nature of the intervention, how this is expressed in the therapeutic stance taken by GABI-trained therapists, and a summary of the findings from the single-group open-enrollment stage of developing the intervention, through to a description of the ongoing pragmatic randomized clinical trial (RCT) comparing GABI to treatment as usual (a parenting training group). The chapter then details the training and supervision processes underpinning GABI. Notably, the development of GABI was informed and developed through clinical work with vulnerable families in a community clinic rather than in an academic setting. And, so the lessons and premises of GABI have much to do with the actual experiences, histories, and dreams of vulnerable parents aiming to keep custody of their birth to 3-year-old child, often against the background of older children who have been placed in foster care, following termination of parental rights. For many families, GABI offers a second chance at the dream of being a good-enough parent whose child succeeds at school, stays out of prison, and finishes school. The GABI model has a vast range of applications for therapeutic work with parents who are living with pronounced feelings of social isolation and stress impeding the parent–child relationship. We therefore conclude the chapter with comments on the potentially wide applications of the GABI model.

Theoretical Basis for GABI

Attachment Theory

There are several sources that inform the underlying theoretical context for GABI, including attachment theory and other psychodynamic models, socioemotional developmental theories, and studies of trauma. We understand vulnerability clinically in terms of attachment theory and contextually with regard to families' histories of adverse childhood experiences. Attachment theory is foremost among the influences that inform GABI, with an emphasis on the centrality of an infant's relationship to a primary caregiver for its immediate and long-term health (Bowlby, 1951). Bowlby (1982) described the attachment figure as someone bigger, stronger, and wiser, who serves as source of security for the child, a base from which the child can explore the external world, knowing that he or she will be welcomed back and protected when he or she is frightened or distressed (Bowlby, 1951, 1982, 1988). Over time, these experiences are consolidated into internal working models comprising expectations about how self and others should behave, which are particularly salient when the attachment system is activated (i.e., in times of emotional distress, when physical hurt, and when distressed at feeling isolated, alone, or ill). Crucial to Bowlby's thinking was the assumption that early attachment experiences not only have a powerful influence on later development, but also that attachment models remain open to, and are further shaped, by favorable and unfavorable influences across the lifespan.

The Adverse Childhood Experiences Literature

GABI is powerfully influenced by the literature that documents the profound long-term effect of health-related experiences that follow from exposure to adverse childhood experiences, consistent with attachment theory. This is the empirical work first reported by Felitti and colleagues (1998), known as the Adverse Childhood Experiences (ACE) study, which surveyed over 17,000 adults and identified 10 categories of adverse childhood experiences, including two categories of neglect, three categories of abuse, and five categories of household dysfunction that tend to co-occur and lead to a range of psychological and physical health problems, including premature death (Chapman et al., 2004; Felitti et al., 1998; Dong, Anda, Dube, Giles, & Felitti, 2003; Dube et al., 2001, 2003; Dube, Anda, Felitti, Edwards, & Croft, 2002). While a dose–response link was observed in this pioneering work, a threshold effect representing increased risk was noted for those adults who had been exposed to four or more categories of childhood adversity, seen in approximately 16% of the original middle-class sample. Among the families that participated in the development of GABI (Murphy et al., 2014) and the ongoing RCT (Murphy et al., 2015), more than 80% of parents have reported four or more ACEs, and this overlapped significantly with unresolved or unclassified responses to the Adult Attachment Interview (Murphy et al., 2014).

From the perspective of the Adult Attachment Interview (AAI; George, Kaplan, & Main, 1985) and the system for rating and classifying AAIs (Main, Hesse, & Goldwyn, 2008), GABI pays close attention to the experiences and psychological mechanisms that help an individual shift a negative trajectory in the direction of attachment security by lessening the impact of adverse experiences (Murphy et al., 2015). In this way, the well-known intergenerational cycles of abuse and trauma may be subverted. Thinking about the GABI model thus emerged from the conjoining of these two bodies of literature: the negative impact of early adversity and its amelioration by interventions that promote secure attachment relationships. As we show below, parents who participated in GABI experienced a large number of ACEs, but their ability to form secure attachments and parent their children with care, protection, and nurturance remains possible and is advanced by participation in GABI.

Promoting Secure Attachment and Preventing Disorganization

The primary goal of GABI is to promote secure parent–child attachment and prevent disorganized attachment relationships in young children with parents whose histories and current adverse contexts place them at risk. *Disorganized attachment* refers to the marked absence of a consistent strategy for organizing a response to the need for comfort and security when under stress (Main & Solomon, 1986, 1990; Lyons-Ruth & Jacobvitz, 2016). A negative trajectory for children who demonstrate this disorganized (fearful) response to the Strange Situation Procedure (Ainsworth, Blehar, Waters, & Wall, 1978), most notably including externalizing disorders, is well documented (e.g., Fearon, Bakermans-Kranenburg, van IJzendoorn, Lapsley, & Roisman, 2010). Disorganized attachment to mother at 1 year has been linked to a wide range of immediate and long-term social and emotional difficulties, including elevated levels of the stress hormone cortisol (Bernard & Dozier, 2010; Spangler & Grossman, 1993), child behavior problems at age 5 (Lyons-Ruth & Jacobvitz, 2016), posttraumatic stress symptoms at age 8 (MacDonald et al., 2008), and externalizing symptoms in preschool and the school-age years (Fearon et al., 2010). This adverse developmental trajectory, for which disorganized attachment is an early marker, interacts with maternal depression and child gender (Munson, McMahon, & Spieker, 2001), and is correlated with dissociation in the adolescent years as reported by self, peers, and teachers (Carlson, 1998). Yet longitudinal research also indicates that maternal sensitivity may moderate the risk that early disorganization will lead to later behavioral and emotional problems. For example, links between disorganized attachment at 1 year and later externalizing behavior at 36–60 months of age may be significantly lessened by maternal sensitivity at 24 months (Wang, Willoughby, Mills-Koonce, & Cox, 2016). Similarly, sociodemographic risk factors (primarily low socioeconomic status [SES]) has been shown to lead to attachment disorganization, but only in the context of maternal insensitivity (Gedaly & Leerkes, 2016).

Taking into consideration the appropriate caution against being unduly alarmist about observations of disorganized/disoriented attachments (Granqvist et al., 2016), it is still the case that disorganized attachment is especially prevalent among children of maltreating parents. These parents often lack positive childhood experiences themselves and experience ongoing sources of stress and trauma that severely challenge their ability to deliver optimal care. Disorganized infant behavior reflects the paradox of "fright without solution," whereby the parent is alternatively comforting and frightening, or frightened, which makes his or her behavior very difficult for the child to understand and predict (Hesse & Main, 2000; van IJzendoorn, Scheungel, & Bakermans-Kranenburg, 1999). Just as the parent's behavior is likely to seem odd, frightening, or anomalous to the child, so the child's behavior with the parent, at times of greatest need, suggests pronounced fear and lacks organization. In other words, what is unthinking and automatic for the distressed child with a secure attachment—seek out the parent and hold on until settled—is unavailable to the child with a disorganized attachment. The antecedents of disorganized attachment are not limited to maltreatment. Behavioral or mental health difficulties often linked to parents' unresolved loss or trauma, depression, and marital discord impact the quality of parental care (Cyr, Euser, Bakermans-Kranenburg, & van IJzendoorn, 2010; Lyons-Ruth & Jacobvitz, 2016; van IJzendoorn et al., 1999).

Preventing disorganization, containing, and understanding fear in toddlers and their parents is the immediate goal of GABI. By focusing on the parent–child relationship while also providing a setting in which parents can engage with clinicians who are sensitive to understanding relational trauma, GABI assists parents in making sense of previous experiences of trauma and loss. GABI works with both parents and children to reduce ACEs and their consequences, and thereby aims to prevent longer-term social, behavioral, and mental health problems that may otherwise transmit across generations (Fraiberg, Adelson, & Shapiro, 1975; Steele, Steele, & Fonagy, 1996).

GABI: An Intergenerational Approach to Trauma-Informed Care

Parenting is a domain that is extremely sensitive to a history of trauma (Elliott, Bjelajac, Fallot, Markoff, & Reed, 2005; Lieberman, 2004). GABI is a trauma-informed practice that acknowledges the social and emotional needs of both the parent and the child, and places the parent–child relationship at the center of the treatment focus. While the primary mission of GABI is to improve the parent–child relationship and support appropriate child development, the program is also sensitive to past and current trauma influencing the parents. To create a trauma-informed practice (Dubowitz, Fiegelman, Lane, & Kim, 2009; Harris & Fallot, 2001) requires an acute understanding of the complex histories and current life stressors of families, as well as the impact of these events on individuals' emotions and actions.

The Frame

Parents with their infants and toddlers (birth to 3 years old) attend GABI up to three times weekly for 2 hours. The schedule's frequency and consistency provides a secure base for families that may have unpredictable schedules. The flexible schedule reflects an understanding of the context in which parents and children live. In general, a trauma-informed approach favors predictability and structure over rigid rules in order to create a culture of understanding, and it avoids inducing shame about minor and ordinary events such as missed sessions. GABI is delivered in a group model, with two lead clinicians and anywhere from two to six graduate students working at once as a team, as well creating the opportunity for individualized attention to each child and parent. Clinicians thus increase their availability to meet the complex, often multisystem needs of families. Maintaining structure and establishing attendance policies not only benefits patients but also aligns with outcomes that matter to the organization (e.g., service utilization, recidivism, cost-effectiveness). GABI expresses responsivity to the needs of clients and makes trauma-informed care attractive to key providers and policymakers, encouraging support both for trauma-specific services and more broadly for the creation of trauma-informed systems. Recommended guidelines include integrating a trauma-informed approach into all aspects of patient care, which involves educating staff members at all levels to create a therapeutic, healing environment for highly stressed families. The GABI frame includes the provision of a safe place for parents and their children ages 0–3 years to experience time together, and time apart from one another. The typical 120-minute session that is offered three times weekly is shown in Table 9.1.

Table 9.1 shows the tripartite structure of every GABI treatment session, with parents and children together at the start of every session, before they separate into two groups: (1) children with therapists; and (2) parents in a parent group, before a final (3) reunion of parents and children before conclusion of the GABI session. In attachment terms, GABI provides repeated practice in separating and reuniting, autonomy and relatedness. During the child-only session, young children are provided a vital learning experience as they have the opportunity to engage with sensitive adults (typically, trainee therapists) in the absence of the parent. The parent group session is often a welcome relief from the burden of 24/7 caregiving. At least once weekly, the parent group is structured around a video-feedback session, in which a 2- to 3-minute video of one parent and child interacting is shown to the target parent in the film, with the other parents as observers. Video feedback as an adjunct to therapeutic change in GABI is the focus of ongoing research efforts (e.g., Steele et al., 2014). There appears no doubt that seeing oneself on video (with one's young child) is a highly evocative and memorable experience that demands reflection, evaluation, and often is accompanied by expressions of a strong wish to change for the betterment of one's child.

TABLE 9.1. The Structure of GABI

2 hours comprised of . . .

  45 minutes of family psychotherapy

  60 minutes of child group sessions and parent group sessions

  15 minutes of parent–child reunion

Typical length of treatment: 26 weeks (the length relied on for the RCT)

GABI sessions are offered three times a week morning and afternoon, creating intensity and flexibility in scheduling. GABI provides 24/7 text availability to clinical team to provide off-hour support.

The Therapeutic Principles Informing GABI, and the Training of GABI Clinicians: REARING

The GABI clinical approach derives much of its heuristic power from its grounding in clinical processes. Clinical evidence of therapeutic action and elaboration of the GABI model as a vehicle to promoting change in parent–child relationships was established through filmed observation of clinical practice. We reviewed over 5 years of video footage collected during the single group open enrollment stage of the study, over 500 hours of film, in order to identify moments of therapeutic action and conceptualize a treatment manual to guide the training and implementation of GABI (Murphy, Steele, & Steele, 2012). The main theoretical components of GABI are operationalized for training purposes in the acronym REARING, which is applied when working with the parent, child, or their relationship. Below we elaborate on this fitting acronym that is also summarized in Table 9.2, indicating how these principles inform the thoughts, emotions, and actions of GABI therapists and in turn, over time, the parents and children participating in GABI.

• *Reflective functioning* (RF) is the ability to think about the thoughts, feelings, and intentions that may cause or result from the behaviors of oneself and others (Fonagy, Target, Steele, & Steele, 1998; Steele & Steele, 2008). RF is the hallmark objective of GABI, the superordinate goal to which all clinical goals and tools are linked.

• *Emotional attunement* is a critical skill in developing secure attachment relationships (Stern, 1995). In GABI, clinicians try to engage parents in a way that facilitates recognition and understanding of their children's emotional states, conveying to the children, and also to parents, a sense of being understood. The GABI clinician monitors in an ongoing way whether an individual parent or child may benefit most from up-regulation (i.e., to have their emotional state clarified/enlivened/awoken) or down-regulation (i.e., to have their emotional state contained/

TABLE 9.2. The REARING Principles Informing the Delivery of GABI

R	Reflective functioning
E	Emotional attunement
A	Affect regulation
R	Reticence
I	Intergenerational patterns
N	Nurture
G	Group

Note. Each GABI session, parents and children, children only or parents only, are sessions in which these themes are held in mind by GABI therapists and may be explicitly enacted or discussed.

calmed/reassured). The GABI therapist is ever-involved in monitoring the emotional temperature in the room, and that in each participant in the room.

• *Affect regulation,* the ability to manage feeling states and maintain emotional homeostasis, has long been recognized as a vital component of individual differences in attachment (Cassidy, 1994), with organized secure attachment being linked to more-or-less accurate acknowledgment and management of diverse emotions, including sadness, fear, and anger. By interacting with GABI clinicians who are trained to respond to the expression of either volatile or flattened affect, parents and children can further develop their own co-regulation and autonomous skills for regulating affect. The clinical task of engaging in affect regulation strategies may be called upon in parent–child, children-only, or parents-only sessions.

• *Reticence* refers to slowing down and observing, and involves giving parents and children the time and space to discover their own feeling states and to enhance self-efficacy. Reticence is often the most difficult skill for the trainee to learn, because it requires the understanding that being quiet, listening, and watching without speaking can be an active therapeutic stance. For the clinician showing reticence, there is no rush to judge, no need to draw conclusions, and no wish to impose an understanding or a solution on the child or the parent (Trevarthen, 1979). Of all GABI principles, reticence is one that most frequently informs the clinician's stance across interactions with parents and children. It is how clinicians observe and attend to what is going on around them (and within them).

• *Intergenerational patterns* refer to understanding how an individual's history of being parented affects how he or she parents (Fraiberg et al., 1975; Main, Kaplan, & Cassidy, 1985; Zeanah & Zeanah, 1989). It is vital for the GABI therapist to keep this transgenerational phenomenon in mind as it promotes an understanding of the complex, deep reasons underlying a parent's behavior. Parents benefit from becoming aware of these links across generations, and this facilitates their wish to make a break and do things differently from what they knew as children. An awareness of intergenerational patterns can help parents to realize their own dreams, and so doing, realize their children's dreams, too.

• *Nurturance* refers to providing sensitive care by being responsive to the needs of the participants, drawing on the rich attachment literature on sensitive responsiveness as articulated by Mary Ainsworth (1979). GABI focuses on nurturing both parents and children, in both emotional and often more tangible terms, to promote the nurturance of children by parents who often feel emotionally depleted. The GABI therapy room is accordingly equipped with healthy snacks and drinks, and other provisions. But the way these are distributed is done in mindful terms, with the aim of privileging the parent or the older sibling, and giving them the pleasure of giving or providing. In other words, GABI therapists aim to be enablers rather than providers.

• *Group context* is the model of delivery. GABI is able to deliver treatment efficiently to multiple families at one time. The group provides important sources of social support to the parents and facilitates peer relationships among the children, combating the social isolation faced by the participants, a well-known toxic influence on parent–child relationships that often combines with the distinct but related toxic influence born of past trauma, that is, poor impulse control. Other members of a group can often be a calming and supportive influence. The supportive influence of peers is seen in children-only sessions just as it is seen in parents-only sessions.

These primary aims of GABI are closely aligned with other approaches articulated in this handbook, and with Layne et al.'s (2011) Core Curriculum on Childhood Trauma, including the core goal of enhancing practitioners' empathic understanding of the nature of traumatic experiences from the child's and the family's perspective, and the ways in which trauma and its aftermath influence their ongoing experiences. Similar to Layne et al.'s Core Curriculum, GABI's REARING principles understand empathy for the families to mean recognizing the uniqueness of each individual's and each family's situation, putting a dual focus on strengths and needs, and respecting the necessity to view them from multiple perspectives.

Additionally, the REARING framework was developed as a model for clinical practice that may also be adapted to a research context. Testing is ongoing to evaluate how effectively GABI training influences clinicians' delivery of the intervention in terms of the REARING components. Beyond their role as therapeutic techniques, then, the REARING principles can be thought of as measureable skills or outcomes that can be identified in therapists, and the parents and the children they aim to help. As such, ongoing research is investigating both clinicians' use of these principles and parents' adoption of, or improvements in, these skills.

Therapeutic Interactions at All Levels

Trauma-informed guidelines recommend policies and procedures to ensure that at every point of contact patients experience a therapeutic approach (Harris & Fallot, 2001). In our center, this begins with developing relationships with referral sources, including pediatric and primary care providers, early intervention providers, and child welfare and family court systems. Not only does outreach to these systems inform clients of the services available, but it also serves as an avenue through which we can educate community partners about the importance of screening for and recognizing the impact of trauma in the populations that they serve.

Particularly in pediatric practices in which families are seen regularly over the first three years of a child's life, coordination of services is helping to establish more integrated pediatric care (e.g., Briggs, Racine, & Chinitz, 2007; Shonkoff & Garner, 2012). Coordinated care allows for direct linkages: Pediatricians refer families to the clinic, ensuring a "warm handover" that increases the likelihood that the referral will result in patient engagement in treatment.

The Setting

The physical space where GABI is held is another avenue through which a sense of safety is established. We aim to create a calm environment with soothing colors and neutral stimuli. In choosing to omit commercial entertainment and traditional holiday decorations, we are mindful of the potential for common, recognizable toys and ornaments to trigger painful reminders of past trauma and deprivations parents may have experienced in childhood. The space, including waiting areas, is also intended to offer nurturance, including basic comforts in terms of seating, toys (carefully selected), snacks (including milk and warm beverages), and diapers. Staff members are instructed to anticipate patients' needs, offering these things in advance rather than assuming that a parent would feel comfortable expressing a need.

The Intake Appointment

The literature on trauma-informed care emphasizes the necessity of assuming and screening for histories of trauma. We recognize that there are often limits on the length of time allowed for intake appointments, and parents may focus solely on immediate concerns. However, asking directly about trauma communicates to parents our understanding that traumatic experiences may contribute to the presenting problems, and establishes the treatment as a place where unconditional respect is available. This is particularly valuable for parents who are struggling with young children. It can be helpful for parents to begin to think about their own histories of abuse and neglect as explanations for current problems, rather than labeling themselves "bad" or incapable parents, a designation they may believe, particularly those who have lost custody of children in the past.

During the GABI intake, a member of the GABI team (social work clinician, psychologist, or graduate-level trainee) uses the Clinical Adverse Childhood Experiences Interview (both parent and child versions; Murphy, Dube, Steele, & Steele, 2007a, 2007b), which was derived from the ACE study and ask about experiences with 10 categories of abuse, neglect, and household dysfunction (Murphy, Steele, Steele, Allman, Kastner, & Dube, 2016). Asking parents first about their own ACEs, then about their children's, sets up a contrast that often illuminates the ways parents have been, and can be, increasingly more effective in protecting their children. This process of reflection helps parents transition from seeing themselves as a child of their parents to seeing themselves as a parent of their child(ren). Even when one's child has been exposed to trauma, going through these questions with a clinician who maintains a nonjudgmental stance signals the understanding that parents strive to be a different kind of parent than the mother or father they recall. The intake process establishes the clinician and parent as partners who will collaborate to help improve the family's relationships. The AAI (George et al., 1985), also administered to parents within their first few weeks of treatment, takes this process further and deeper as parents are asked in detail about childhood memories, experiences of emotional upset, physical hurt, illness, separation, loss and trauma, with a focus (at the end of the interview) on the meaning they attribute to their attachment history (Murphy, Steele, & Steele, 2013). The AAI is a mandatory part of the GABI intake. As Fraiberg et al. (1975) noted, through the act of remembering (in a supportive context), vulnerable parents are saved from the blind repetition of their morbid past. Conducting an AAI at the start of treatment signals that GABI welcomes, at times even encourages and reinforces, this act of memory, articulating connections between past and present experiences, including a focus on evidence that the past is *not* being repeated. This may come into the conversation at any point in the GABI treatment process but most often may be seen when parents are alone (without the children) in the parents-only group component, laying the foundation for change, with the possible release from blind repetition of that morbid past.

The GABI Stance during Treatment

GABI clinicians are trained to be sensitive to potential traumatic triggers that may arise in the context of the therapy, such as group session exchanges or client–clinician interactions that lead to reminders or reexperiencing of trauma. Importantly, when reexperiencing does occur, either within or outside the group, these troubling emotional responses become a central focus of the treatment at that moment. When children are present, clinicians learn how to gently guide parents' attention away from absorption in past trauma to their child(ren) in the present. In this way, parents are helped to become more conscious and better able to manage their reactions in the moment. Clinicians maintain that no trauma is so great that a compassionate listener cannot lessen the burden. Once children are also in the care of a supportive clinician, an opportunity for sharing the trauma is created. For example, when a mother goes into detail about a heated argument that left her overwhelmed, the clinician listens to the mother's retelling of the experience, helping her deescalate, then gently inquires how her young child responded during the event. The clinician redirects the parent's attention to the child, encouraging the parent's capacity for reflective functioning.

Parent, Child, and Dyadic Goals

In GABI, the parent, the child, and the relationship are treated simultaneously. Clinicians work to understand and validate the parents' experiences, with the ultimate goal of helping parents be more attuned to their children's perspectives and experiences. GABI seeks to create a nurturing environment in which the parent may feel less threatened and better able to attend to the child's fear states. In turn, the child may feel safe to relive and repair traumatic experiences through play. Nurturance and containment are established in several important ways. For starters, the hierarchical structure of psychotherapy is minimized as clinicians ally themselves with parents in respectful, collaborative partnerships. Elliott et al. (2005, p. 472) write, "Parents should be empowered as the best sources of information about their children and encouraged to view their own recovery as part of healing the parent–child relationship." Parents do not do this alone however. Autonomy is a goal that parents work toward with supportive clinicians, who make themselves available via 24/7 text messaging for scheduling purposes and brief consultations. Availability builds rapport and signals to patients that they are being held in mind. For many parents, who may have been forced to be prematurely independent early in their lives, connection with a sensitive and responsive clinician can be a transformative relational experience that helps them consolidate their resources and be more attuned parents.

GABI clinicians and staff put great emphasis on the importance of understanding the rationales for the actions of a parent or child rather than quickly labeling a behavior of the parent or child as pathological. We frequently find, for example, that mothers have not received appropriate prenatal care. A trauma-informed approach considers that obstetrical and gynecological examinations and procedures may be perceived as invasive—making a woman with a sexual abuse history feel vulnerable, exposed, or out of control—and may trigger trauma responses or noncompliance with prenatal care. GABI embodies an understanding of how trauma affects individuals' comfort with seeking and obtaining medical care rather than making judgments or applying labels to those who have not done so. In this way, GABI is a strengths-based program in which parents' strengths and abilities are noted, and the barriers they face are understood in the sociopolitical and cultural contexts from which they arise and in which they are embedded. The group format of GABI provides an opportunity for parents to relate with other parents in a mutually supportive way that encourages them to highlight each other's abilities, promote competence and self-worth, and reduce social isolation. Additionally, when clinicians fully appreciate the context of families' lives, they also better realize when and how to link up the parent with other services and agencies (e.g., as concerns housing, medical care, or legal consultation). In this way, continuity of care across diverse but essentially linked services is understood as part of the GABI culture.

We next provide a summary of the evidence base for GABI, and an account of how the evidence base was assembled, culminating in an RCT.

The Evidence Base for GABI

The Single Group Open-Enrollment Phase

The evidence in support of GABI ranges from early studies of the treatment in a single group open-enrollment design (circa 2006–2011) to the ongoing first RCT (2012–2017), and the present effort (2017 and beyond) to further test and disseminate the model. Back in 2006, a partnership took shape between Anne Murphy and Miriam Steele and Howard Steele. Anne was (and remains) the lead GABI clinician, situated in the Rose F. Kennedy Children's Evaluation and Rehabilitations Center, Department of Pediatrics, Montefiore Medical Center/Einstein College of Medicine. This setting serves as the "flagship" treatment program, which includes the training of psychologists, social workers, and pediatricians to meet the needs of vulnerable parents and their young children via the multifamily trauma-informed and attachment-based treatment model that is GABI. Miriam Steele and Howard Steele offered to Anne Murphy the idea of bringing the families Anne was treating in a group context in the Bronx, one at a time, to the Steele's New School attachment laboratory known as the Center for Attachment Research (CAR). CAR is a place where PhD, MA, and undergraduate students work on various attachment projects. Since 2006, a number of cohorts of graduate students have devoted their efforts, and written their MA theses or PhD dissertations on aspects of the collaborative work with Anne Murphy (e.g., Armusewicz, 2016; Bate, 2012, 2016). When Anne Murphy escorted families to CAR, parents were interviewed with the AAI, the parent–child relationship was observed with the Ainsworth Strange Situation, and in a free-play sequence, and parents' completed the Clinical ACEs Parent and Child Questionnaires, as well as the Parenting Stress Index, leading to an initial description of the intervention and clinical findings from the single group open-enrollment phase of research (Steele, Murphy, & Steele, 2010).

Students from the New School filmed the delivery of the treatment at the Kennedy Center at Montefiore/Einstein, and many hundreds of hours of treatment were scrutinized by a team led by Miriam Steele and Anne Murphy, with the aim of identifying the essential ingredients of therapeutic action and preparing a treatment manual. This led, over time, to the articulation of the REARING principles and the assignment of the name GABI to the program of treatment.

Investigation of the treatment in the original single group open-enrollment design yielded a range of clinically significant findings, including lower levels of parenting stress over time in treatment, and improved parent–child relationships (Steele et al., 2010). Steele et al. reported that disorganized infant–mother attachments were significantly less common in families that had experienced 6 months or more of the treatment, compared to entrants.

Another vital early influence on the development of GABI was the collaboration Anne Murphy established with Shanta Dube (one of the original ACE researchers) in order to develop a 25-item Clinical ACE Parent and Child Interviews for clinicians to administer in order to gently but firmly probe for exposure to each of the five forms of abuse/neglect and five forms of household dysfunction (Murphy et al., 2007a, 2007b; 2016). Use of this measure with the parents in the treatment revealed mean levels of exposure to ACEs (on the well-known 0- to 10-point scale) that were between 5 and 6, with more than 80% of parents in the Bronx, receiving GABI, having been exposed to four or more ACEs in the first 18 years of life (Murphy et al., 2014; Steele et al., 2010). In addition, administration of the AAI to the parents revealed levels of unresolved mourning related to past loss or trauma or "can't classify" interviews (indicative of severe disorganization in thinking about attachment) that exceeded 60% of the sample, a phenomenon closely associated with high exposure to ACEs (Murphy et al., 2014).

During the open-enrollment phase of the development and initial testing of GABI, we began integrating video feedback into the parents-only component of GABI treatment sessions (Steele et al., 2014). George Downing, a frequent visitor to New York City from Paris, where his Video Intervention Therapy Institute is based, has been a close adviser on this integration of video feedback into GABI.

The Launch of the RCT

By 2012, GABI was being studied in the context of a federally funded RCT. For that effort, a professor of social work and a clinical trials expert, Karen Bonuck, as well as a public health expert, Paul Meissner, had joined the "core" GABI team, completing the diverse GABI leadership team of five. In the RCT,[1] we have compared 26 weeks of GABI to treatment as usual, a previously validated parent-only group

---

[1] *https://clinicaltrials.gov/ct2/show/nct01641744?term=group+attachment+based+intervention&rank=1*
Birth to Three: A pragmatic clinical trial for preventing child maltreatment (HRSA R40MC23629).

known as Steps Toward Effective Parenting (STEP), and a 12-week parent training program that was the prevailing treatment modality in the same zip code in the Bronx, where the RCT was conducted.

The RCT is set in the Bronx, New York, where the victimization rate (of child abuse) is more than twice the national average (21.4 per 1,000 vs. ≈12). Its catchment area includes the Morrisania section, where the victimization rate climbs to 26.9 (DiNapoli, 2013). These high levels of victimization are linked to poverty, a well-known risk factor for maltreatment. The Bronx is the nation's poorest urban county; its poverty rate among families and children is more than two times the state and national averages. Bronx residents are also young; the Bronx is the youngest county in New York, and one of only five counties in the United States with more than 30% single-family households. The main criterion for inclusion in the RCT was concern about parenting capacity (vs. evidence of symptomatology in the child) due to the parent's own history of maltreatment, social isolation, or having lost custody of a child in the past. Referrals came from pediatricians, Child Welfare, and Court systems throughout the Bronx. Criteria for inclusion were (1) biological parents (2) of a birth to 36-month-old child, (3) with custody of their child. Exclusion criteria were (1) parent's inability to provide informed consent due to mental illness or cognitive impairment, (2) parent's lack of fluency in English, or (3) child has a diagnosis of an autistic spectrum disorder or severe cognitive delay.

Implementation of the RCT Comparing GABI to STEP

Our central question informing the ongoing RCT concerns the expectation that participation in GABI will lead to changes in the child–mother attachment relationship. To explore this question, we are administering the Ainsworth Strange Situation Procedure at baseline, prior to random assignment to group, and again at the end of treatment, as well as at 6-month follow-up. In addition, we are filming 10 minutes of free play between parent and child at each of these three time points. The first 5 minutes of filmed interaction are being scored with the Coding Interactive Behavior (CIB) guidelines (Feldman, 1998), a system for observing parent–child interactions that has been extensively validated (Feldman, 2007). Five-point rating scales are applied, resulting in separate sets of scores for maternal behavior, child behavior, and interactive behavior. Thus, we have a picture of how the child responds to the stress of two separations in the Strange Situation Procedure, and also how the child and mother behavior in the nonstressful circumstance of free play. Two distinct teams of graduate students rate the Strange Situation observations and CIB observations; each group is blind to whether the observation it is viewing comes from baseline, end of treatment, or 6-month follow-up, and to which arm of the RCT the family is participating in. The study will end when 35 families in each arm of the study has been observed at each of the three time points. The RCT is taking almost twice as long as planned, because attrition is twice more than expected. Attrition in intervention work with low-risk samples is typically 15%. We estimated that attrition would be 30%, and we have found that attrition is 60%. Reasons for this attrition have mainly to do with mothers who are in full-time paid work or full-time training/study and are not free to attend GABI, in addition to more stressful situations such as out-of-borough housing placements for homeless families.

With respect to the ongoing trio of assessments from baseline, end of treatment, and 6-month follow-up, we are also taking measurements with widely used and previously validated tools of maternal mental health, social support, parenting stress, hair cortisol samples, and body mass index. With respect to the children's development, we are assessing their cognitive development with the Bayley Scales.

While we expect participants in the GABI arm of treatment to show significant improvements in the quality of the child–mother attachment and in free play, we do not necessarily expect group differences in reported levels of social support, stress, or mental health, as the STEP control group is known to positively impact self-report in these domains. We are curious about the extent to which self-reported conscious reports of stress will be correlated with the "under-the-skin" hair cortisol measures being collected.

Training in the GABI Model

Within the GABI Research Program

Since the first clinical evidence of the model appeared (Steele et al., 2010), there has been an ongoing effort to identify therapeutic action and train new GABI therapists in the core principles (REARING) of the treatment, as well as to assess the effectiveness of the training processes and the eventual competence of GABI therapists. Though manual-based teaching of structured treatments and prescriptive techniques has been the status quo for decades and we developed a GABI manual (Murphy et al., 2012), criticisms of these approaches emphasize the need for integration across orientations, as well as between research and practice, and the implementation of principles-based trainings that can be flexibly employed and monitored (Skovholdt & Starkey, 2010; Chorpita & Daleiden, 2009). Abramowitz (2006) theorized, "One does not need to be totally bound to a treatment manual to be an effective clinician, especially if he or she understands how to apply the experimentally established principles of behavior . . . to clinical problems" (p. 164). Regarding GABI, we found the REARING principles to be key to training GABI therapists who are capable of helping families considered to be at risk of child abuse and neglect, and that present with myriad needs and challenges, including trauma, poverty, social isolation, and discrimination. The REARING principles, broad in their focus and drawing on diverse bodies of evidence, appear to meet the ideal of Chorpita and Daleiden (2009), who suggested that broad principles of treatment can serve as a foundation and be flexibly applied as needed, rather than emphasizing specific protocols, and this strategy is most appropriate when treating such complex problems, including intergenerational trauma.

In line with these recommendations, the training program in GABI is designed to deepen clinicians' understandings of the seven REARING principles and how they relate to clinical practice, from the perspectives of attachment theory, developmental research, and trauma research. While descriptions of specific techniques are included to provide clinical trainees with a sense of how an attachment-based approach looks in practice, often in the form of video examples and vignettes, the training is designed to allow for flexibility and creativity within each of these general overarching REARING principles.

Our Web-Based Curriculum Supporting Training

The GABI curriculum begins with trainees begin given access to a password pro-tected website that includes 8 hours of videos on attachment theory and research, trauma-informed clinical work, and illustrations of GABI being delivered. Trainees are expected to have viewed the online curriculum once through, and to have read the GABI print manual prior to joining a two-day in-person GABI workshop. The in-person workshop is a chance for trainees to meet seasoned GABI therapists as they elaborate, with case examples, on the core (REARING) concepts of GABI and establish a nonjudgmental approach to assessment, risk, and child protection issues. The details of how to set up a GABI therapy room and how to begin, man-age, and end a GABI session are provided. These 2-day trainings are organized to create a foundation for trainees to maximally benefit from the ongoing GABI expe-riences of working in parent–child groups, children-only groups, and parents-only groups, including video-feedback for a target parent within the group, and partici-pating in reflective supervision groups following GABI sessions. Ongoing training is provided through phone consultations and reviews of videotaped clinical work to ensure fidelity to the GABI model.

Reflective Supervision

In *reflective supervision,* the model we use in GABI, the lead clinician practices and encourages paying attention to (1) one's own inner experience, (2) the experience of the infant or child, and (3) the experience of the parent (Eggbeer, Shahmoon-Shanok, & Clark, 2010; Murphy, Steele, & Steele, 2013). Supervision is provided after every GABI session, permitting review of reactions and concerns, and the planning of targeted, relationship-specific interventions to pursue at the next GABI session.

Assessment of Training Outcomes

We have developed a set of assessments to assess three training outcomes across the training process: knowledge, adherence, and competence. Multicomponent training programs, like the one employed in GABI, which include a manual, work-shop, and supervision, have generally been found to be most consistent in produc-ing changes in therapist skills across orientations (Herschell, Kolko, Baumann, & Davis, 2010).

Active observation is a critical part of clinical work and a foundation for the implementation of interventions (Sternberg, 2005; Harris & Bick, 1976). This is particularly true for parent–child psychotherapies that require the therapist to hold both parent and child, past and present, in mind. Honing observational skills that guide clinical thinking, conceptualization about the patient, and ultimately deci-sions about how to intervene is a central part of GABI training that has deep child psychoanalytic roots (Freud, 1966). Additionally, the content of clinicians' obser-vations, in theory, provides information about how they apply the knowledge of their framework for intervention. As Anna Freud (1951, p. 20) said, "The material which presents itself is seen and assessed not by an instrument, nor by a blank and therefore unprejudiced mind but on the basis of pre-existent knowledge, preformed ideas and personal attitudes (though these should be conscious in the case of the analyzed observer)."

Because clinical observations contain important information about a clinician's assumptions, orientation, and treatment approach, we chose to use trainees' observations of clinical situations as the way to assess their understanding of the clinical applications of attachment theory generally, and their internalization of the GABI approach specifically. Myles and Milne (2004) have used a video assessment task to study the effectiveness of training in cognitive-behavioral therapy (CBT) for adult patients, and found that as a result of training, clinicians improved significantly in their knowledge of and abilities to identify symptoms and name appropriate CBT strategies. Building on their methodology, and looking at clinicians' observations, as distinct from their treatment delivery (which we also measure), we capture some of the more nuanced changes in clinical approach and skills that happen early on in training, as well as the further development of their observational skills after months of practice, with our Application of Clinical Training Assessment (ACTA), developed by Jordan Bate (2016) in conjunction with the GABI leadership team.

The ACTA paradigm uses trainees' observations of real-life clinical situations captured on videotape to evaluate their understanding and application of the GABI treatment model. The task utilizes 3-minute-long video clips edited from footage of GABI from real-life parent–child sessions of GABI in the Bronx setting. This use of videotape allows for standardization, and using clips from the intervention as it is actually delivered in practice with patients maintains ecological validity and reflects the complexity of this clinical work (Muse & McManus, 2013). After viewing each clip, trainees are asked to respond in writing to three open-ended questions about their observations:

1. What do you see happening in this video? What struck you about this situation?
2. Imagine that you are the clinician in this situation, and bringing it to supervision for discussion. What would you talk about?
3. Did you see any therapeutic interventions being used? Please describe.

Videos were chosen based on their coverage of the full range of GABI REARING concepts as they appear in parent–child and children-only sessions, where new GABI trainees are first deployed. Responses are rated on 5-point scales assessing extent of understanding of the REARING principles underlying delivery of GABI.

Pilot Results with ACTA

We are currently using the ACTA to evaluate training of clinicians at our Bronx site, who have completed a 2-day, face-to-face GABI training, have access to training materials, work in the GABI groups, and participate in reflective supervision. These trainees complete the ACTA task at three time points: (1) before beginning training, (2) after the workshop and review of the manual, and (3) following 6–8 months of clinical work in GABI and supervision. Results from 75 trainees show that the current 2-day workshop format plus access to the written manual resulted in statistically significant improvements in trainees' abilities to recognize and apply all of the REARING principles to clinical observations, as well as statistically significant improvements in the overall quality of trainees' observations (Bate, 2016). Efforts are well under way to show that training in the GABI REARING model leads to competence in GABI parent–child sessions months later.

Wider Applications of GABI

GABI brings together parents who lack family support, and who, when growing up, very often never knew the experience of being regarded as special, worthy of protection, and loved. So GABI provides these essential experiences, through GABI sessions up to three times a week, and by 24/7 text access to the GABI clinical team. In turn, vulnerable parents are learning through GABI to provide nurturance and support to their young children, creating fresh opportunities for their children (and themselves) to function successfully in social relationships and school–work. GABI brings together socially isolated parents and their children from birth to age 3, where they work together to achieve the often stated goal of "becoming a different kind of parent" (Murphy, Ponterotto, Cancelli, & Chinitz, 2010). The intensity and frequency of GABI, coupled with the flexibility the group context affords increases its capacity to reach many families. In addition, the GABI model provides social work and psychology trainees a unique opportunity to train alongside experienced clinicians in an apprentice model.

Among the range of attachment-based interventions aimed at families with children under age 3, many of which are detailed in this handbook, GABI is likely to be most relevant in crowded urban centers in which parents are living with poverty, as well as with past and current exposure to trauma, and are at risk of losing their children to Child Protective Services. For such parents, GABI provides a meeting place for supportive peer relationships to develop, for parents to redirect their lives and not only maintain custody of their children but also come to be seen by their children (and by themselves) as a safe haven when feeling fearful or anxious, and a secure base from which to explore, leading, as we know from a half-century of longitudinal attachment research, to substantial gains in social and emotional well-being, school readiness, and job-related skills. The path is not linear; one may expect, many moments of being stuck, and moving sideways or backwards. But the REARING principles of GABI are likely to promote hope, resilience, and recovery.

ACKNOWLEDGMENTS

During the preparation of this chapter, we have been grateful to the New York Health Foundation for a grant (No. 20140216) that enabled us to establish the GABI Learning Collaborative, which involved us in refining our training materials and curriculum to better communicate what is required to be a competent GABI therapist. We have also received support from an R40 MC 23629-01-00 grant from the Maternal and Child Health Research Program, Maternal and Child Health Bureau (Title V, Social Security Act), Health Resources and Services Administration, Department of Health and Human Services.

REFERENCES

Abramowitz, J. S. (2006). Toward a functional analytic approach to psychologically complex patients: A comment on Ruscio and Holohan (2006). *Clinical Psychology: Science and Practice, 13,* 163–166.

Ainsworth, M. D. (1979). Infant–mother attachment. *American Psychologist, 34,* 932–937.

Ainsworth, M. D. S., Blehar, M. C., Waters, E., & Wall, S. (1978). *Patterns of attachment: A psychological study of the Strange Situation.* Hillsdale, NJ: Erlbaum.

Armusewicz, K. (2016). *Towards validation of a competence coding system using the REARING model of therapeutic action for GABI clinicians.* Unpublished master's thesis, Center for Attachment Research, The New School for Social Research, New York, NY.

Armusewicz, K., Bate, J., Steele, H., Steele, M., & Murphy, A. (2015). *Validation of a competence coding system using the REARING model of therapeutic action for GABI clinicians.* Poster presentation at the 7th International Attachment Conference, New York, NY.

Bate, J. (2012). *Evaluating the efficacy of clinical training in group attachment-based intervention for vulnerable families.* Unpublished master's thesis, Center for Attachment Research, The New School for Social Research, New York, NY.

Bate, J. (2016). *Evaluating the effectiveness of clinical training in an attachment-based parent–child intervention.* Unpublished doctoral dissertation, The New School for Social Research, New York, NY.

Bernard, K., & Dozier, M. (2010). Examining infants' cortisol responses to laboratory tasks among children varying in attachment disorganization: Stress reactivity or return to baseline? *Developmental Psychology, 46*(6), 1771–1778.

Bowlby, J. (1951). Maternal care and mental health. *Bulletin of the World Health Organization, 51*(3), 355–534.

Bowlby, J. (1980). *Attachment and loss: Vol. 3. Loss: Sadness and depression.* New York: Basic Books.

Bowlby, J. (1982). *Attachment and loss: Vol. 1. Attachment.* New York: Basic Books. (Original work published 1969)

Bowlby, J. (1988). *A secure base: Parent–child attachment and healthy human development.* New York: Basic Books.

Briggs, R. D., Racine, A. D., & Chinitz, S. (2007). Preventive pediatric mental health care: A co-location model. *Infant Mental Health Journal, 28*(5), 481–495.

Carlson, E. A. (1998). A prospective longitudinal study of attachment disorganization/disorientation. *Child Development, 69*(4), 1107–1128.

Cassidy, J. (1994). Emotion regulation: Influences of attachment relationships. *Monographs of the Society for Research in Child Development, 59*(2–3), 228–249.

Chapman, D. P., Whitfield, C. L., Felitti, V. J., Dube, S. R., Edwards, V. J., & Anda, R. F. (2004). Adverse childhood experiences and the risk of depressive disorders in adulthood. *Journal of Affective Disorders, 82*(2), 217–225.

Chorpita, B. F., & Daleiden, E. L. (2009). Mapping evidence-based treatments for children and adolescents: Application of the distillation and matching model to 615 treatments from 322 randomized trials. *Journal of Consulting and Clinical Psychology, 77,* 566–579.

Cyr, C., Euser, E. M., Bakermans-Kranenburg, M. J., & van IJzendoorn, M. H. (2010). Attachment security and disorganization in maltreating and high-risk families: A series of meta-analyses. *Development and Psychopathology, 22,* 87–108.

DiNapoli, T. P. (2013). *An economic snapshot of the Bronx* (Report No. 4-2014). New York: Office of the New York State Comptroller.

Dong, M., Anda, R. F., Dube, S. R., Giles, W. H., & Felitti, V. J. (2003). The relationship of exposure to childhood sexual abuse to other forms of abuse, neglect and household dysfunction during childhood. *Child Abuse and Neglect, 27,* 625–639.

Dube, S. R., Anda, R. F., Felitti, V. J., Chapman, D. P., Williamson, D. F., & Giles, W. H. (2001). Childhood abuse, household dysfunction, and the risk of attempted suicide throughout the life span: Findings from the Adverse Childhood Experiences Study. *Journal of the American Medical Association, 286*(24), 3089–3096.

Dube, S. R., Anda, R. F., Felitti, V. J., Edwards, V. J., & Croft, J. B. (2002). Adverse childhood experiences and personal alcohol abuse as an adult. *Addictive Behaviors, 27,* 713–725.

Dube, S. R., Felitti, V. J., Dong, M., Chapman, D. P., Giles, W. H., & Anda, R. F. (2003). Childhood abuse, neglect, and household dysfunction and the risk of illicit drug use: The adverse childhood experiences study. *Pediatrics, 111*(3), 564–572.

Dubowitz, H., Feigelman, S., Lane, W., & Kim, J. (2009). Pediatric primary care to help prevent child maltreatment: The Safe Environment for Every Kid (SEEK) model. *Pediatrics, 123,* 858–864.

Eggbeer, L., Shahmoon-Shanok, R., & Clark, R. (2010). Reaching toward an evidence base for reflective supervision. *ZERO TO THREE, 31*(2), 39–45.

Elliott, D. E., Bjelajac, P., Fallot, R. D., Markoff, L. S., & Reed, B. G. (2005). Trauma-informed or trauma-denied: Principles and implementation of trauma-informed services for women. *Journal of Community Psychology, 33,* 461–477.

Fearon, R. P., Bakermans-Kranenburg, M. J., van IJzendoorn, M. H., Lapsley, A. M., & Roisman, G. I. (2010). The significance of insecure attachment and disorganization in the development of children's externalizing behavior: A meta-analytic study. *Child Development, 81*(2), 435–456.

Feldman, R. (1998). *Coding interactive behavior manual.* Unpublished manual, Bar-Ilan University, Ramat Gan, Israel.

Feldman, R. (2007). Maternal versus child risk and the development of parent–child and family relationships in five high-risk populations. *Development and Psychopathology, 19,* 293–312.

Felitti, V. J., Anda, R. F., Nordenberg, D., Williamson, D. F., Spitz, A. M., Edwards, V., . . . Marks, J. S. (1998). Relationship of childhood abuse and household dysfunction to many of the leading causes of death in adults: The Adverse Childhood Experiences (ACE) Study. *American Journal of Preventive Medicine, 14*(4), 245–258.

Fonagy, P., Target, M., Steele, H., & Steele, M. (1998). *Reflective-functioning manual, version 5.0, for application to Adult Attachment Interviews.* London: University College London.

Fraiberg, S., Adelson, E., & Shapiro, V. (1975). Ghosts in the nursery: A psychoanalytic approach to the problems of impaired infant–mother relationships. *Journal of the American Academy of Child Psychiatry, 14*(3), 387–421.

Freud, A. (1951). Observations on child development. *Psychoanalytic Study of the Child, 6,* 18–30.

Freud, A. (1966). *Normality and pathology in childhood.* London: Hogarth Press.

Gedaly, L. R., & Leerkes, E. M. (2016). The role of sociodemographic risk and maternal behavior in the prediction of infant attachment disorganization. *Attachment and Human Development, 18,* 554–569.

George, C., Kaplan, N., & Main, M. (1985). *The Berkeley Adult Attachment Interview.* Unpublished protocol, Department of Psychology, University of California, Berkeley, Berkeley, CA.

Granqvist, P., Hesse, E., Fransson, M., Main, M., Hagekull, B., & Bohlin, G. (2016). Prior participation in the Strange Situation and overstress jointly facilitate disorganized behaviors: Implications for theory, research and practice. *Attachment and Human Development, 18,* 235–249.

Harris, M., & Bick, E. (1976). The contribution of observation of mother–infant interaction and development to the equipment of a psychoanalyst or psychoanalytic psychotherapist. In M. H. Williams (Ed.), *Collected Papers of Martha Harris and Esther Bick* (pp. 225–239). Pertshire, Scotland: Clunie Press.

Harris, M. E., & Fallot, R. D. (2001). *Using trauma theory to design service systems.* San Francisco: Jossey-Bass.

Herschell, A. D., Kolko, D. J., Baumann, B. L., & Davis, A. C. (2010). The role of therapist training in the implementation of psychosocial treatments: A review and critique with recommendations. *Clinical Psychology Review, 30,* 448–466.

Hesse, E., & Main, M. (2000). Disorganized infant, child, and adult attachment: Collapse in behavioral and attentional strategies. *Journal of the American Psychoanalytic Association, 48,* 1097–1127.

Layne, C. M., Ippen, C. G., Strand, V., Stuber, M., Abramovitz, R., Reyes, G., . . . Pynoos, R. (2011). The core curriculum on childhood trauma: A tool for training a trauma-informed workforce. *Psychological Trauma: Theory, Research, Practice, and Policy, 3*(3), 243–252.

Lieberman, A. F. (2004). Traumatic stress and quality of attachment: Reality and internalization in disorders of infant mental health. *Infant Mental Health Journal, 25*(4), 336–351.

Lyons-Ruth, K., & Jacobvitz, D. (2016). Attachment disorganization from infancy to adulthood: Neurobiological correlates, parenting context, and pathways to disorder. In J. Cassidy & P. Shaver (Eds.), *Handbook of attachment: Theory, research, and clinical applications* (3rd ed., pp. 667–695). New York: Guilford Press.

MacDonald, H. Z., Beeghly, M., Grant-Knight, W., Augustyn, M., Woods, R. W., Cabral, H., . . . Frank, D. A. (2008). Longitudinal association between infant disorganized attachment and childhood posttraumatic stress symptoms. *Development and Psychopathology, 20,* 493–508.

Main, M., Hesse, E., & Goldwyn, R. (2008). Studying differences in language usage in recounting attachment history: An introduction to the AAI. In H. Steele & M. Steele (Eds.), *Clinical applications of the Adult Attachment Interview* (pp. 31–68). New York: Guilford Press.

Main, M., Kaplan, N., & Cassidy, J. (1985). Security in infancy, childhood, and adulthood: A move to the level of representation. *Monographs of the Society for Research in Child Development, 50*(1/2), 66–104.

Main, M., & Solomon, J. (1986). Discovery of an insecure-disorganized/disoriented attachment pattern. In T. B. Brazelton & M. W. Yogman (Eds.), *Affective development in infancy* (pp. 95–124). Westport, CT: Ablex.

Main, M., & Solomon, J. (1990). Procedures for identifying infants as disorganized/disoriented during the Ainsworth Strange Situation. In M. T. Greenberg, D. Cicchetti, & E. M. Cummings (Eds.), *Attachment in the preschool years: Theory, research, and intervention* (pp. 121–160). Chicago: University of Chicago Press.

Munson, J. A., McMahon, R. J., & Spieker, S. J. (2001). Structure and variability in the developmental trajectory of children's externalizing problems: Impact of infant attachment, maternal depressive symptomatology, and child sex. *Development and Psychopathology, 13,* 277–296.

Murphy, A., Dube, S. R., Steele, H., & Steele, M. (2007a). *Clinical Adverse Childhood Experiences Questionnaire.* Unpublished document, Department of Clinical Pediatrics, Albert Einstein College of Medicine, New York, NY.

Murphy, A., Dube, S. R., Steele, H., & Steele, M. (2007b). *Child Clinical Adverse Childhood Experiences Questionnaire.* Unpublished document, Department of Clinical Pediatrics, Albert Einstein College of Medicine, New York, NY.

Murphy, A., Ponterotto, J., Cancelli, A., & Chinitz, S. (2010) Daughters' perspectives on maternal substance abuse: Pledge to be a different kind of mother. *Qualitative Report, 15,* 1328–1364.

Murphy, A., Steele, H., Bate, J., Nikitiades, A., Allman, B., Bonuck, K., . . . & Steele, M. (2015). Group attachment-based intervention: Trauma-informed care for families with adverse childhood experiences. *Journal of Family and Community Health, 38,* 268–279.

Murphy, A., Steele, H., Steele, M., Allman, B., Kastner, T., & Dube, S. R. (2016). The Clinical Adverse Childhood Experiences (ACEs) Questionnaire: Implications for trauma-informed behavioral health care. In R. D. Briggs (Ed.), *Integrated early childhood behavioral health in primary care* (pp. 7–16). New York: Springer International.

Murphy, A., Steele, M., Dube, S. R., Bate, J., Bonuck, K., Meissner, P., . . . Steele, H. (2014). Adverse Childhood Experiences (ACEs) questionnaire and Adult Attachment Interview (AAI): Implications for parent child relationships. *Child Abuse and Neglect, 38*(2), 224–233.

Murphy, A., Steele, M., & Steele, H. (2012). *Group attachment-based intervention: Clinical training manual.* Unpublished document, Center for Attachment Research, Psychology Department, The New School for Social Research, New York, NY.

Murphy, A., Steele, M., & Steele, H. (2013). From out of sight, out of mind to in sight and in mind: Enhancing reflective capacities in a group attachment-based intervention. In J. E. Bettmann & D. D. Friedman (Eds.), *Attachment-based clinical work with children and adolescents* (pp. 237–258). New York: Springer.

Muse, K., & McManus, F. (2013). A systematic review of methods for assessing competence in cognitive-behavioral therapy. *Clinical Psychology Review, 33,* 484–499.

Myles, P. J., & Milne, D. L. (2004). Outcome evaluation of a brief shared learning programme in cognitive behavioural therapy. *Behavioural and Cognitive Psychotherapy, 32,* 177–188.

Shonkoff, J. P., & Garner, A. S. (2012). The lifelong effects of early childhood adversity and toxic stress. *Pediatrics, 129,* 232–246.

Skovholt, T. M., & Starkey, M. T. (2010). The three legs of the practitioner's learning stool: Practice, research/theory, and personal life. *Journal of Contemporary Psychotherapy, 40,* 125–130.

Spangler, G., & Grossmann, K. E. (1993). Biobehavioral organization in securely and insecurely attached infants. *Child Development, 64*(5), 1439–1450.

Steele, H., & Steele, M. (2008). On the origins of reflective functioning. In F. Busch (Ed.), *Mentalization: Theoretical considerations, research findings, and clinical implications* (pp. 133–158). New York: Analytic Press.

Steele, H., Steele, M., & Fonagy, P. (1996). Associations among attachment classifications of mothers, fathers, and their infants. *Child Development, 67*(2), 541–555.

Steele, M., Murphy, A., & Steele, H. (2010). Identifying therapeutic action in an attachment-based intervention with high-risk families. *Clinical Social Work Journal, 38,* 61–72.

Steele, M., Steele, H., Bate, J., Knafo, H., Kinsey, M., Bonuck, K., . . . Murphy, A. (2014). Looking from the outside in: The use of video in attachment-based interventions. *Attachment and Human Development, 16,* 402–415.

Stern, D. N. (1995). *The motherhood constellation: A unified view of parent–infant psychotherapy.* London: Karnac Books.

Sternberg, J. (2005). *Infant observation at the heart of training.* London: Karnac Books.

Trevarthen, C. (1979). Communication and cooperation in early infancy: A description of primary intersubjectivity. In M. Bullowa (Ed.), *Before speech: The beginning of interpersonal communication* (pp. 321–347). London: Cambridge University Press.

van IJzendoorn, M. H., Schuengel, C., & Bakermans-Kranenburg, M. J. (1999). Disorganized attachment in early childhood: Meta-analysis of precursors, concomitants, and sequelae. *Development and Psychopathology, 11,* 225–250.

Wang, F., Willoghby, M., Mills-Koonce, R., & Cox, M. (2016). Infant attachment disorganization and moderation pathways to level and change in externalizing behavior during preschool ages. *Attachment and Human Development, 18,* 534–553.

Zeanah, C. H., & Zeanah, P. D. (1989). Intergenerational transmission of maltreatment: Insights from attachment theory and research. *Psychiatry, 52*(2), 177–196.

CHAPTER 10

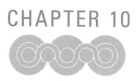

CAPEDP Attachment
An Early Home-Based Intervention Targeting Multirisk Families

SUSANA TERENO, NICOLE GUÉDENEY,
TIM GREACEN, ANTOINE GUÉDENEY,
and THE CAPEDP STUDY GROUP

We begin this chapter with a summary of the background and contextual factors that informed the development of the CAPEDP (*Compétences Parentales et Attachement dans la Petite Enfance: Diminution des risques lies aux troubles de santé mentale et Promotion de la resilience*—i.e., Parental Skills and Attachment in Early Childhood: Reduction of Risks Linked to Mental Health Problems and Promotion of Resilience) intervention, an account of infant attachment quality, maternal disruptive behavior, and related risk factors. We then describe methods, including a detailed presentation of the project intervention protocol, and present results on infants' attachment security and maternal disruptive behavior, which subsequently give way to the final global section in which we discuss these results, as well as attrition issues and future research proposals.

Developmental theories recognize that the social and family environment has long-term effects on the individuals' psychological functioning (Bowlby, 1988). Early secure attachment relationships allow infants to explore their environment safely and contribute to the establishment of a broad range of social skills. Moreover, infants are particularly sensitive to contexts that generate stress within the family. Their parents' psychological problems and the vulnerable social contexts into which they are born can have a deleterious effect on their later development. Mental health disorders in childhood have long-term consequences throughout the lives of the individuals in question, their families, and the social environment as a whole (World Health Organization, 2003). Infant mental health is therefore a public health priority both internationally (World Health Organization, 2010) and in France (Cléry-Melin, Kovess, & Pascal, 2003).

The prevalence of psychiatric disorders in infants is related to a variety of psychosocial vulnerability factors. More emotional and behavioral disorders are seen in children of young, first-time mothers (Olds et al., 1997; Nagin & Tremblay, 2001); in children of mothers with postnatal depression (Murray & Cooper, 1999; Hay, Pawlby, Angold, Harold, & Sharp, 2003); in children whose mothers lack parenting skills (Coleman & Denisson, 1998) or whose parents have deficits in insightfulness (Oppenheim, Goldsmith, & Koren-Karie, 2004); in children whose parents are in situations of psychosocial stress (Hungerford & Cox, 2006) or have less perceived social support (Warren, 2005); in children of mothers showing attachment disorganization (Fearon, Bakermans-Kranenburg, van IJzendoorn, Lapsley, & Roisman, 2010); in preschoolers whose parents do not live together (Wichstrøm et al., 2011); and in children of families with low socioeconomic status and educational level (Wichstrøm et al., 2011). Furthermore, individual vulnerability appears to be linked to the accumulation of vulnerability factors rather than being a direct result of one particular factor (Dyrbye, Thomas, & Shanafelt, 2006).

Infant Attachment Quality and Risk Factors

Attachment is considered a vital component of social and emotional development in the early years. The quality of attachment is an important early indicator of infant mental health (Bowlby, 1988), among other reasons, because it influences the child's ability to manage stressful situations. Whereas attachment security is largely determined by caregiver sensitivity, disorganization is associated with disruptive interactions that frighten the infant. Disruptive caregiving behavior and difficult psychosocial contexts have been shown to be significantly associated with the development of attachment disorganization. If the mother is unable to adapt her caregiving responses despite repeated signs from her child, and manifests disorganizing or disruptive behavior, this can lead to attachment disorganization in the child (Lyons-Ruth, Bronfman, & Parsons, 1999).

A number of researchers have found that cumulative risk portends a variety of negative outcomes (Deater-Deckard, Dodge, Bates, & Pettit, 1998; Greenberg, Speltz, DeKlyen, & Jones, 2001; Jones, Forehand, Brody, & Armistead, 2002; Rutter, 1979). The cumulative risk hypothesis asserts that the accumulation of such factors, independent of the presence or absence of particular ones, impacts developmental outcomes: The greater the number of risk factors, the greater the prevalence of clinical problems (Rutter, 1979; Sameroff, 2000).

The link between child maltreatment and attachment disorganization has been the object of numerous studies (Cyr, Euser, Bakermans-Kranenburg, & van IJzendoorn, 2010). Strangely, the association between socioeconomic risk and disorganization has received less attention. Socioeconomic risks are pervasive, often prolonged, and have the propensity to co-occur and cluster in the same families and individuals (Belsky & Stratton, 2002). Empirical studies have shown that the cumulative and enduring effect of multiple risks creates precarious situations in which children are more prone to distress and less securely attached. In a high-risk sample, Shaw and Vondra (1993) found that, with families with at least three or more stressors, the greater the number of risk factors, the greater the likelihood that the children in question would develop an insecure attachment. With low-risk subjects, research conducted by Belsky and colleagues (Belsky, 1996; Belsky & Isabella, 1988; Belsky, Rosenberger, & Crnic, 2000) also supports the cumulative risk hypothesis. The meta-analysis of Cyr and colleagues (2010) reveals that the accumulation of socioeconomic risks appears to have a similar impact to maltreatment with regard to attachment disorganization.

Maternal Disruptive Behavior and Risk Factors

Cyr and colleagues (2010) suggest multiple possible pathways leading to attachment disorganization, involving either child maltreatment by abusive parents or parental neglect. Although these disruptive parental behaviors are not limited to multiple-risk family environments, the accumulation of risk factors makes parents less psychologically accessible, lowers their tolerance to stress, and is associated with parents losing their self-control more frequently.

Disruptive maternal behavior can manifest itself in several ways. *Frightening/ frightened* parental behaviors, first identified by Main and Hesse (1990) and Solomon and George (1999), are directly related to parent–infant interaction. *Parental Unresolved Trauma and Loss* is frequently identified as being at the origin of this kind of behavior (Main & Hesse, 1990). Multiple-risk environments are associated with parents experiencing more losses and other traumatic events that may remain unresolved and trigger further frightening/frightened parenting behavior (Lynch & Cicchetti, 1998; Schuengel, Bakermans-Kranenburg, & van IJzendoorn, 1999; Guédeney & Tereno, 2012). Child maltreatment, such as physical or sexual abuse by parents, induces "fright without solution" for the child, who is unable to handle the paradox of a potentially protective but, at the same time, abusive attachment figure, resulting in attachment disorganization in the child (Madigan et al., 2006). Cicchetti and Lynch (1993) and Zeanah and colleagues (1999) argue that *marital discord* and *domestic violence* may also lead to elevated levels of disorganization if the child witnesses an attachment figure unable to protect him- or herself in a struggle with his or her partner (Guédeney, Guédeney, & Rabouam, 2013).

Other types of disruptive maternal behavior impact infant attachment more indirectly. Parents who withdraw from interacting with their children due to urgent problems or difficulties in other areas of functioning, such as securing an income, losing a job, having housing problems or being victims of discrimination, can create chronic hyperaroused attachment systems in children who do not know who to turn to for consolation in times of stress (Cyr et al., 2010; Lyons-Ruth et al., 1999). Although these microcontextual variables are not specific to multiple-risk families, in a wider ecological perspective, the more chaotic, multiple-risk environments increase neglectful behavior with regard to infant attachment needs, because the accumulation of stress factors seems to decrease parental sensitivity and responsivity to children's needs (Lyons-Ruth et al., 2013).

Intervention Programs

Intervention programs targeting psychosocially high-risk populations have been developed in North America and in other contexts from as early as the 1960s. Since Olds's (1998) initial work in Elmira, other studies have confirmed the efficacy of home-based preventive interventions. With high-risk mothers, several studies have shown that home-based interventions conducted jointly by nurses and infant mental health workers yield significant results, particularly with regard to reducing externalizing behavior problems (Guédeney et al., 2011). Lyons-Ruth and Melnick (2004) showed that targeting early prevention can help prevent later externalizing behavior, with a clear dose–response effect; furthermore, the intervention model created by Boris and colleagues, with joint intervention by nurses and infant mental health practitioners (Boris, Larrieu, Zeanah, Nagle, & Steier, 2006; Zeanah, Larrieu, Boris, & Nagle, 2006), confirmed this effect with vulnerable populations. Moss, Karine, Cyr, Tarabulsy, and Bernier (2011) underline the fact that extensive training of those providing the intervention, backed up by frequent supervision, are essential ingredients for the success of this kind of program. A meta-analysis on the impact of attachment-focused interventions by Bakermans-Kranenburg, van IJzendoorn, and Juffer (2003) demonstrated that these interventions can indeed increase attachment security by enhancing maternal sensitivity, although generally with a small effect size. According to these authors, short interventions with precise goals seem to be more effective than lengthy, multifocal interventions.

In France, a national mother–child support and prevention network, the *Protection Maternelle et Infantile* (PMI), was implemented after World War II, parallel to the creation of free public mental health services for both adults and children across the country. Mothers can consult PMI centers free of charge at any point during pregnancy and the first 3 years postpartum. Certain checkups and vaccinations are compulsory if the mother wishes to access local government family support funds. Widely used, even by middle-class families, this system has never really been evaluated with regard to cost-efficiency (Ikounga N'Goma, & Brodin, 2001). In Paris, PMI home visits to vulnerable families are frequently limited to a single visit (60% of cases); few families receive more than three home visits. Furthermore, PMI nurses do not receive specific training in mental health issues for mothers and children, and receive little organized psychological supervision (DASES 75, 2003). However, they can and do refer families directly to their local community child and adolescent mental health services. As with PMI services, the functioning, outcomes and cost-efficiency of these mental health services have undergone little systematic evaluation.

The CAPEDP Study

The CAPEDP study is the first randomized, controlled trial, assessing an evidence-based, home-visiting program to take place in France. Toward the end of the 1990s, despite the existence in every neighborhood of the above-mentioned government-run PMI services, as well as community mental health services for both children and adults with no out-of-pocket payment, mental health professionals were becoming increasingly concerned by the number of children living in vulnerable social situations being referred for care, typically for behavioral problems. An international conference (Haddad, Guédeney, & Greacen, 2004) confronting evidence-based preventive programs from different national contexts provided the impetus for developing the first French home-visiting program that specifically targeted infant mental health, in line with international best practices criteria (Daro, McCurdy, Falconnier, & Stojanovic, 2003; Kahn, Moore, & Haven, 2004; Gomby, 2005; Durlak & DuPre, 2008) and adapted to the particularities of the French context. The resulting CAPEDP project involved designing, implementing, and evaluating an early long-term, supervised, home-based intervention targeting the determinants of infant mental health in families presenting multiple psychosocial vulnerability factors (Tubach et al., 2012).

The CAPEDP program has two major specificities with regard to most other home-visiting programs targeting mental health promotion. The first specificity was to address child mental health promotion in families that already have, at least theoretically, free access to one of the most extensive, comprehensive, and long-standing social and health care systems in the Western world. The second major specificity was that qualified psychologists conducted the entire home-visiting program. It was hypothesized that professionals who were more highly trained in psychology would be more competent in recognizing the elements in play with regard to the determinants of infant mental health and more skilled in acting on these determinants.

An Ancillary Project: The CAPEDP Attachment Study

Assessment of attachment security and caregiver behavior, which is particularly complex from a procedural point of view, was the focus of an ancillary study involving a subsample of the CAPEDP population designed to investigate these attachment-relevant points: the CAPEDP Attachment (CAPEDP-A) study. The objectives of this ancillary study were to assess the impact of the CAPEDP intervention in terms of increasing infant attachment security and maternal reflective functioning, and reducing infant attachment disorganization and maternal disorganizing behavior when the child was 12 to 17 months old. In a second phase of the attachment study, currently under way, children are being followed up and assessed at their fourth birthday. The aim of this second study is to verify the stability of observed effects and detect any other sleeper effects of the intervention program on infants' and mothers' attachment quality. To our knowledge, CAPEDP-A is the first study to describe the distribution of infant attachment in a French multirisk population and CAPEDP-A Phase II, the first French longitudinal study on infant–mother attachment (see Table 10.1).

Methods

Recruitment Procedures

The first subject was recruited in December 2006, and the final visit of the last participant in the main CAPEDP study took place in July 2011. Participants were recruited by the research team at 10 maternity hospitals in Paris and the surrounding

TABLE 10.1. CAPEDP-A Measures and Training Procedures

Infant age	Measure	Trainees	Trainers	Institution
CAPEDP general				
6–9 and 12–15 months	Video intervention therapy	All teams: 3-day workshop; ST, AG, and NG: 9-day workshop	George Downing	International Institute of Video Intervention Therapy
18 months	Alarme Détresse BéBé Scale (Alarm Distress Baby Scale [ADBB]; Guédeney & Fermanian, 2001)	Assessment team: 5-day workshop	Antoine Guédeney	University Paris Diderot, Sorbonne Paris Cité, France
18 months	Attachment Q-Sort (Waters & Deane, 1985)	All teams: 3-day workshop	Manuela Verissimo	Applied Psychology of Lisbon, Portugal
CAPEDP-A Phase I				
12–17 months	Strange Situation Procedure (A/B/C) (Ainsworth et al., 1978)	ST, AG, and NG: 5-day workshop	Karin Grossmann; Fabienne Becker-Stoll	University of Regensburg, Germany
12–17 months	Strange Situation Procedure (D) (Main & Solomon, 1990)	ST: 5-day workshop	Alan Sroufe and Elizabeth Carlson	University of Minnesota, Minneapolis, USA
12–17 months	Insightfulness Assessment (Oppenheim, & Koren-Karie, 2002)	NG and ST: 5-day workshop	David Oppenheim and Nina Karin-Koren	Haifa University, Israel
12–17 months	AMBIANCE (Bronfman, Parsons, & Lyons-Ruth, 2004)	ST, AG, NG, RD, and JW: 3-day workshop	Karlen Lyons-Ruth and Elisa Bronfman	Harvard University, Boston, MA, USA
CAPEDP-A Phase II				
48 months	Strange Situation paradigm for preschoolers (Cassidy, Marvin, & MacArthur Working Group on Attachment, 1992)	NG, AG, ST, JW, and RD: 5-day workshop	Robert Marvin	University of Virginia Medical Center, Charlottesville, VA, USA
48 months	Attachment Story Completion Workshop (Bretherton, Ridgeway, & Cassidy, 1990)	ST, AG and assessment team; 2-day training	Manuela Verissimo	Institute of Applied Psychology of Lisbon, Portugal
48 months	Puppet Interview, Self (Cassidy, 1988; Ackerman, & Dozier, 2005)	ST, AG, and assessment team: 1-day workshop	Manuela Verissimo	Institute of Applied Psychology of Lisbon, Portugal
48 months	Adult Attachment Narratives (Waters & Deane, 1985)	ST, AG, and assessment team: 3-day workshop	Manuela Verissimo	Institute of Applied Psychology of Lisbon, Portugal

Note. ST, Susana Tereno; AG, Antoine Guédeney; NG, Nicole Guédeney; RD, Romain Dugravier; JW, Jaqueline Wendland.

suburbs. Participation in the study was proposed to eligible women in the waiting room of the maternity hospital or prior to a checkup appointment. During this meeting, or later, if the woman requested time to make up her mind, she signed the informed consent form and was included in the study.

Eligibility criteria limited participation to women in situations of medium to high vulnerability with regard to their future child's mental health. All consecutive women consulting in the second trimester of pregnancy in 10 public maternity wards in Paris and its surrounding suburbs were assessed for eligibility. Women were eligible if they presented the following characteristics: living in the intervention area (Paris and its inner suburbs); fluent enough in French to give valid informed consent; able to participate in assessment sessions; less than 27 weeks after their last menstrual period at their first assessment interview; and, as required by French law relative to clinical research, registered with the national health insurance scheme or its equivalent for non-French participants. In terms of risk factors for their future children's mental health, they also had to be first-time mothers; less than 26 years old; and meet at least one of the following three criteria: (1) have less than 12 years of education, (2) plan to bring up their child without the child's father, or (3) have a low income, defined as being eligible for French national social welfare health insurance (*Couverture Maladie Universelle Complémentaire*) or, for undocumented migrants, Government Medical Aid (*Aide Médicale d'Etat*). The benchmark used in the CAPEDP study was that of vulnerability as a result of an accumulation of risk factors and not as a direct result of one factor in particular (Tubach et al., 2012).

Exclusion criteria pertained to women who would be impossible to follow-up (e.g., women who were planning to move away from the greater Paris area after their child was born), women receiving social or medical care for reasons other than those listed in the inclusion criteria (e.g., substance abuse, serious mental illness, or other chronic diseases requiring close follow-up), and women who did not consent to participate.

Randomization and Masking Procedures

Randomization took place after this inclusion phase. After completing baseline screening and informed consent procedures, participants were randomly assigned in a 1:1 ratio to either the CAPEDP intervention or the usual care group, using a computer-generated randomization sequence, stratified by recruitment center, with random block sizes of two, four, or six participants. The Clinical Research Unit of Bichat Hospital, Paris, France, centrally generated this sequence. Assignment of participants was concealed using centralized randomization through fax in the Clinical Research Unit. Investigators therefore had no knowledge of the next assignment in the sequence in this open-label trial. All investigators, all psychologists performing the CAPEDP intervention, and all participants were blinded to assignment before, but not after, randomization. However, in accordance with multicenter randomized controlled parallel trial (PROBE) methodology, all outcome assessors were blinded to assignment, and no investigators, intervention psychologists, or participants had any knowledge of aggregate outcomes at any point during the course of the study. The families were therefore divided at random between the two arms of the trial: The control group received usual care and seven assessment visits across the trial period. The intervention group, in addition to usual care, received the CAPEDP intervention (Tubach et al., 2012).

When their child reached 12 months of age, all families participating in the main CAPEDP trial were consecutively invited to participate in the CAPEDP-A study. The mothers were informed about this ancillary study, and if they agreed to participate with their child, they signed an informed consent form, and an appointment was made for a 2-hour assessment within the following 2 weeks. Inclusion was terminated when the required 120 mother–infant dyads had accepted to participate. Mothers received a gift check of 50 euros for participating in CAPEDP-A.

At the children's fourth birthday, 2 years after the end of the main CAPEDP study, we then tried to contact all 440 mothers by letter or by telephone to invite them to participate in a follow-up study concerning attachment issues (CAPEDP-A Phase II). Only 114 families could be contacted. They were informed about this second phase of the study and, if they agreed to participate with their child, they signed a new informed consent form and an appointment was made for a 2-hour assessment meeting in next 2 weeks. Of the 114 contactable mothers, 13 refused or were not available to participate. The resulting 101 mothers received 70 euros gratification for their participation. Results from the follow-up study are currently being analyzed.

The General CAPEDP Intervention[1]

The general intervention sought to act on the major modifiable determinants of infant mental health from the third trimester of pregnancy to the child's second birthday. Psychologists visited families on average six times during the prenatal period (starting from the 27th week of pregnancy), eight times in the first 3 months of the child's life, 15 times when the child was between 4 and 12 months of age, and another 15 times during the child's second year, resulting in a total of 44 home visits during the entire intervention. Each session was approximately 60 minutes in duration. Additional details regarding the content of the manualized CAPEDP intervention can be found elsewhere (Saïas et al., 2013).

The CAPEDP home-visiting program used an intervention manual based on Services Intégrés Pour la Périnatalité et la Petite Enfance (Integrated Services for Perinatal Health and Early Childhood), a Canadian adaptation of the Nurse–Family Partnership intervention program. The manual proposes that 39 different intervention brochures be used during home visits. Each brochure addresses a specific health or mental health topic, based on a common theme of promoting quality mother–child relationships. The intervention manual also drew from Weatherston's (2000) guidelines concerning the most practical aspects of home visiting, as well as best practice recommendations for home visiting from the 2007 State University Prevention and Early Intervention Policy (2009). The manual proposed a series of reference points for addressing different topics at different periods during the intervention (prenatal, 0–6 months, 6–15 months, and 15–24 months). Each intervention was based around four themes: the family and its social and cultural

---

[1] Saïas et al. (2013); Tubach et al. (2012).

network; the mother's needs and health; creating a safe and stimulating environment for the baby; and the baby's development. The psychologists were instructed both to adapt their interventions to the needs of each family being visited and to encourage the family to make the most of available PMI centers, social services, and community resources in general.

Home-visiting psychologists were also provided a set of items they could discuss with the families being visited: (1) family information brochures, each addressing a specific topic and designed to facilitate discussion and to be left with the family; (2) a series of six DVDs, including short films on pregnancy, child care, and child development, which were used by the home-visiting psychologists to facilitate forming a working alliance with each family, particularly in the antenatal period; and (3) a comprehensive document, collated by the research team, on promoting infant emotional development and mother–child attachment quality. Furthermore, the home-visiting team systematically proposed, with the mothers' approval, to film short sequences of everyday interactions between the mothers and their children: bathtime, mealtime, play, changing nappies, and so forth. During subsequent visits, mothers would watch the video and discuss what they saw with the home-visiting psychologist.

The CAPEDP-A Intervention[2]

With regard to promoting quality attachment, the intervention drew largely from three international programs, with adaptations concerning local cultural specificities: the Olds (1998) model, which shaped the program as a continuum; the STEEP™ (Steps Toward an Effective, Enjoyable Parenting model; Egeland & Erickson, 1999); and the Mind the Baby (Slade, Grienenberger, Bernbach, Levy, & Locker, 2005) models, during the period after birth. In parallel, video feedback was used base on the Video-Feedback Intervention Program to Promote Positive Parenting (VIPP; Juffer, Bakermans-Kranenburg, & van IJzendoorn, 2007) approach, to promote maternal sensitivity and prevent/repair atypical maternal behavior. In general, with regard to attachment, the intervention aimed to help mothers answer their babies' attachment and exploration needs in a more sensitive way, without manifesting atypical/disorganizing behavior.

Three intervention themes structured psychologists' home visits with regard to promoting attachment quality:

1. Caring for the caregiver: Providing mothers with a solid working alliance and a secure base to enable them to take care of their infants (Kobak & Mandelbaum, 2003).

2. Infant attachment security: Promoting maternal sensitive interactions.
   a. Learning how to detect, interpret, and rapidly respond to infants' signs in an adequate way.
   b. Promoting maternal mentalizing skills (Lyons-Ruth & Melnick, 2004; Marvin, Cooper, Hoffman, & Powell, 2002; Slade et al., 2005).

---

[2]Tereno et al. (2013).

3. Maternal self-efficacy: Promoting mothers' self-efficacy with regard to their own behavior (Bandura, 1977).

   a. Parental guidance on babies' attachment and development ("Infants' Emotional Development" pamphlet).

   b. Providing mothers with strategic and operational support in order to help them find solutions for their practical needs.

Other themes were addressed when necessary:

1. Maternal representations, at the caregiving and transgenerational levels, were addressed in a systematic way, with maternal attachment traumatic representations being worked on only if mothers spontaneously evoked these issues or if disruptive maternal behavior was detected.

2. Maternal disruptive behaviors and infant disorganized attachment.

   a. Detection, prevention, and reparation of maternal disruptive behavior. If relevant, associated traumatic representations were addressed.

   b. Detection and regulation of infants' disorganized attachment behavior.

   c. Handling infants' oppositional behavior, associated with increased parental stress and greater risk of disruptive behavior.

Home-visiting psychologists were encouraged to refer participants to mental health services if more intense psychotherapeutic help was deemed necessary. Specific tools were developed to support the intervention team with regard to attachment issues.

• Home-visiting psychologists were provided with two manuals aiming at structuring their interventions: The first manual, for the period when the child was between 6 and 12 months of age, focused on attachment issues, and the second, for the period between 12 and 15 months, on oppositional behavior.

• A *pamphlet* drafted by the research team and focusing on the emotional development of young children was distributed to the families when the children were 3 months old, with the aim of making families aware of the importance of early attachment bonds. This document, developed from a literature review conducted by the first author (S. T.; Tereno, Soares, Martins, Sampaio, & Carlson, 2007), introduces, in everyday language, the concept of attachment and the four *Bowlbian* phases of attachment development. Guidelines for promoting maternal sensitivity are proposed in several domains: crying, sleeping, feeding, separation, and play. It concludes with signs to help mothers detect when they should ask for professional help. Use of the pamphlet was particularly recommended when the babies were 3 months old, a sensitive period for attachment bonds. Using it before 3 months was considered too soon: In the first trimester, mothers with their first child are still adapting to their infants' physiological needs, leaving little time for emotional and psychological issues. Using it too late would also be problematic: Maternal sensitivity, assessed at infant age 4 months, is already associated with later attachment quality (Grossmann, Grossmann, Spangler, Suess, & Unzner, 1985).

- *Video feedback* was used at two time points to encourage parents to reflect on their parenting practices and experiences: when the child was between 6 and 9 months old (two videos focusing on attachment), then between 12 and 15 months (two videos focusing on oppositional behavior). For each of these four video-feedback sessions, the intervention psychologist would propose to film a short sequence of mother–child interactions during a home visit, for example at bathtime, mealtime, free play, or nappy change. At the following home visit, the mother and the home-visiting psychologist would watch and discuss the video together.

Video intervention, relatively recent in this kind of program, was felt to be particularly effective, allowing mothers and home visitors to (1) focus on the baby's signals and expressions; (2) focus on the infant's perspective; (3) stimulate the mother's observation skills and her empathy with the child; (4) enable positive reinforcement moments of sensitive behavior evidenced on the video; (5) stimulate maternal narcissism, allowing mothers to be aware of their own strengths and weakness; and (6) see the difference between maternal intentions and manifested behavior (especially in moderate to highly stressful situations).

The video strategy is all the more successful as it occurs within a supportive relationship that continually recognizes the individual's and the family's strengths and acknowledges the broader context to which they belong.

The CAPEDP Assessment Procedures

Assessments were conducted during specific home visits by a team of four trained psychologists, working independently from the psychologists performing the CAPEDP intervention, and with no knowledge of whether the women being evaluated were in the intervention group or the control group. Assessment took place at baseline for demographic and health characteristics and then at 3, 6, 12, 18, and 24 months after the child's birth for both groups. The assessment team received specific training on each of the assessment instruments. Individual and group supervision was provided for all members of the assessment team, to support them in handling difficult situations during evaluation, for example, in situations of abuse or neglect, developmental delay, suicidal ideation in the mother, or serious social problems. Whenever necessary, families were addressed to social or medical services (Dugravier et al., 2013).

In the CAPEDP-A study, a specific and parallel attachment assessment team received training, and systematic supervision by the first author (S. T.), on the procedures and instruments that were used. Parallel coding teams for each instrument were put into place in order to ensure a blinded coding system, in which coders were aware of neither the subject's group nor other assessment results.

Assessment measures targeting attachment issues are listed in Table 10.1 (for a full list of CAPEDP general project measures, see Tubach et al., 2012).

Statistical Analysis Procedures

To account for possible attrition and have sufficient power to answer all three primary objectives, the CAPEDP project needed to recruit 440 families. Including all families into the CAPEDP-A ancillary study was not possible due to the demanding assessment and coding procedures. In the CAPEDP-A study, the first 120 mothers of the general sample who agreed to participate were recruited. Only the data on infant attachment distribution and maternal disruptive behavior are presented here. Infant attachment quality categorical variables were compared using Pearson's chi-square test, and risk factors for maternal disruptive behavior were explored using logistic regression. Other continuous variables are expressed as means and standard deviation and categorical variables as percentages and frequencies. All statistical analyses were deemed significant at a 5% confidence level using two-sided tests. Statistical analyses were performed using Statistical Analysis System (SAS) software version 9.2 (SAS Institute Inc., Cary, North Carolina).

Results

Sample Description

At baseline and, when appropriate, at follow-up visits, the following data were collected for all participants (N = 440): Demographic data included age, sex, marital status, ethnicity, family characteristics, household composition, characteristics of the partner, and, if different, the father of the coming child, whether the pregnancy was planned or not, educational level attained, employment status, and income; health variables included maternal postnatal depression assessed using the Edinburgh Postnatal Depression Scale (EPDS; Cox, Holden, & Sagovsky, 1987; Guédeney & Fermanian, 1998) and maternal psychiatric symptoms using the Symptom Checklist (SCL-90; Derogatis, 1994), self-perceived state of health, and use of tobacco, alcohol, or drugs.

Of the 120 mother–infant dyads recruited into the CAPEDP-A protocol, 117 had their Strange Situation videos coded with the Strange Situation Procedure (SSP) and the Atypical Maternal Behavior Instrument for Assessment and Classification (AMBIANCE) system. Three dyads could not be coded because of technical problems with the video recordings. A total of 65 of these dyads belonged to the intervention group and 52, to the control group (usual care).

The sociodemographic analyses indicated that, at inclusion in the main CAPEDP study during the 27th week of pregnancy, the mothers presented the following characteristics:

1. Almost half (n = 57; 47.9%) were first-generation immigrants.
2. Of the mothers, 15.1% (n = 18) had less than 9 years of education, but a large majority (n = 100; 83%) had less than 12 years of education.
3. Of the households, 39.5% (n = 45) had a monthly income of less than 840 euros.
4. Of the mothers, 40.3% (n = 48) declared they were not living in a couple, and 59.7% (n = 71) were married to or living with the father of the child.

5. Of the mothers, 24.2% (n = 29) declared themselves to be isolated, intending to raise their child without the father.

6. Of the mothers, 42.9% (n = 51) were sufficiently poor to be eligible for free state-funded health care.

The average age of the infants when assessment took place was 14.2 (SD = 2.8) months. The mothers' average age at assessment was 22.3 (SD = 2.5; median age = 23.0 [20.0–24.5]).

No significant differences were observed between intervention and control groups on any sociodemographic variable, with the exception of the following:

1. There were more women less than age 20 years in the intervention group (n = 20; 37.7%) than in the control group (n = 14; 20.9%); $\chi^2(1)$ = 6.52; p = .01).

2. Women in the intervention group declared more tobacco and/or alcohol use during pregnancy (n = 24; 35.8%) than those in the control group (n = 9; 17.3%; $\chi^2(1)$ = 5.01; p = .03).

With regard to risk factor accumulation, 75.6% (n = 90) of women presented at least three risk factors at inclusion and 37.8% (n = 45), at least five, with no differences between groups.

Infant Attachment Distributions[3]

The SSP was used to describe the infants' attachment distribution in four categories (Ainsworth, Blehar, Waters, & Wall, 1978). The SSP is a laboratory paradigm with a series of eight 3-minute, increasingly stressful episodes for 12- to 18-month-olds. The SSP is videotaped, and infant behavior is coded using four 7-point anchored scales for proximity seeking, maintaining contact, avoidance, and resistance, and one 9-point scale for disorganization (Main & Solomon, 1990). For the secure, avoidant, and ambivalent-resistant SSP scores, two coders were trained by Karin Grossman and Fabienne Becker-Stoll, obtaining reliability greater than .85. Fifty percent of the SSPs were coded by a second independent rater, and intercoders reliability for the three-way classification was 85%. An expert coder, who was blind to intervention group status, coded all SSPs for disorganization. The concordance for the disorganized versus not-disorganized classification (N = 18) between the primary coder and a second trained and reliable coder was 86.3%.

Table 10.2 compares the intervention and control groups for infants' attachment quality. In the control group (care as usual; n = 52), 48.1% (n = 25) were classified as secure, 25% (n = 13) as insecure-avoidant, 7.7% (n = 11) as insecure-ambivalent/resistant, and 19.2% (n = 10) as disorganized/disoriented. In the intervention group (n = 65), 58.5% (n = 38) were classified as secure, 13.8% (n = 9) as insecure-avoidant, 20% (n = 13) as insecure-ambivalent/resistant, and 7.7% (n = 5) as disorganized/disoriented. There were no significant difference between the

[3]Tereno et al. (2016, 2017).

TABLE 10.2. Strange Situation Classification by Treatment Group

	Intervention group (*N* = 65) *n* (%)	Care as usual group (*N* = 52) *n* (%)
Secure	38 (58.5)	25 (48.1)
Ambivalent/Resistant	13 (20.0)	4 (7.7)
Avoidant	9 (13.8)	13 (25.0)
Disorganized/Disoriented	5 (7.7)	10 (19.2)

intervention group and the control group for infant attachment security, $\chi^2(2)$ = 2.40, p > .05. However, there were significant differences between the intervention and the control groups on classifications of disorganized attachment, $\chi^2(1)$ = 4.44, p < .05.

Predictive Risk Factors for Maternal Disruptive Behavior[4]

The AMBIANCE scale codes disruptive caregiver behavior during videotaped caregiver–infant interactions, in this case using the SSP videos. After producing a written register of all instances of mothers' disruptive behavior, a frequency score was derived for each of the five dimensions of the AMBIANCE scale: Affective Communication Errors, Role/Boundary Confusion, Fearful/Disorientation, Intrusive/Negative, and Withdrawing Behavior. The AMBIANCE coding system also involves using a continuous 7-point scale to assess the global level of disruptive communication, where 1 corresponds to "high normal behavior," 3 to "low normal behavior," 5 to "clear evidence of disruption in affective communication," and 7 to "disruptive communication with few or no ameliorating behaviors." The global disruptive communication score is based on the frequency and intensity of disruptive behaviors displayed by the caregiver. A binary classification is then attributed in which scores of 5 or above are classified as "disruptive" and scores of less than 5 as "nondisruptive" (Bronfman, Parsons, & Lyons-Ruth, 2004).

In order to identify risk levels at inclusion, four kind of variables were identified according to risk type:

1. *Socioeconomic risk* (4 items: educational level less than 9 years of schooling; low income, defined as being sufficiently poor to be eligible for free health care; first-generation immigrant; feeling isolated (defined as intending to bring up the child without the presence of the child's father).

2. *Psychological risk* (2 items: EPDS > 11; SCL-90 global score; tobacco and/or alcohol use during pregnancy).

---

[4]Tereno et al. (submitted, 2017).

3. *Parenting risk* (4 items: perinatal complications; unplanned/unwanted pregnancy; early loss of attachment figure (when less than 11 years old); less than 20 years old).

4. *Infant risk* (2 items: premature baby; tobacco and/or alcohol use during pregnancy).

Logistic regression shows that mothers with disruptive communication, assessed when the child was 12 months old, when they were included in the study toward the end of their pregnancy, were more likely:

1. To have sufficiently low income to have the right to free health care with no out-of-pocket payment, $\chi^2(1) = 4.21$; $p = .04$; disruptive mothers: n (%) = 26 (54.2%) versus nondisruptive mothers: n (%) = 22 (33.8%).

2. To have given birth prematurely, $\chi^2(1) = 4.24$; $p = .04$; disruptive mothers: n (%) = 6 (13.0) versus nondisruptive mothers: n (%) = 2 (3.2%).

From a cumulative perspective, mothers with disruptive communication were more likely to have had:

3. A superior number of risk factors, $F(1) = 6.74$; $p = .01$; disruptive mothers: mean (SD) = 4.4 (2.1) versus nondisruptive mothers: mean (SD) = 3.4 (2.0%).

4. At least five risk factors, $\chi^2(1) = 5.61$; $p = .02$; disruptive mothers: n (%)= 24 (50.0) versus nondisruptive mothers: n (%) = 20 (30.3%).

No association with the number of intervention visits was observed, $\chi^2(1) = 0.10$; $p = .75$; disruptive mothers: n (%) = 18.5 (7.05%) versus nondisruptive mothers: n (%) = 19 (7.7%).

Discussion

Infants' Attachment Distributions

Results concerning attachment distributions are consistent with those described elsewhere in moderate to high-risk populations. Attachment security is underrepresented compared to the general population, where it is generally between 60 and 70% (van IJzendoorn, Schuengel, & Bakermans-Kranenburg, 1999). Although the intervention group's security distribution (58.5%) is closer to that of the general population than that of the control group (48.1%), the CAPEDP intervention had no significant statistical impact on infant attachment security (Tereno et al., 2016), no doubt linked to the fact that in France the control group cannot be considered to have received no intervention given that "care as usual" is particularly generous in the French health and social care system. The overrepresentation of insecure-ambivalent/resistant (20%) infants compared to the insecure-avoidant (13.8%), in the intervention group, may be seen, however, as a transitory intervention effect. Interestingly, when assessing infants' withdrawal, with the Alarm

Distress Baby Scale (ADBB) at 18 months of age, the total score was significantly lower in the intervention group (p = .03) than in the group in the CAPEDP-A sub-sample (Guédeney et al., 2013). Indeed, transition from disorganized attachment to a more secure relationship may pass through an insecure-ambivalent/resistant phase before reaching attachment security. Given that infant attachment quality in this study was assessed around the children's first birthdays, with one-third of the home visits still to come, it can be hypothesized that these less secure infants may become secure later on. This hypothesis is being explored in the second phase of the attachment project (CAPEDP-A Phase II follow-up study), with attachment assessments at the children's fourth birthday.

The results of this study also demonstrated that there are significant differences between the intervention and the control groups in terms of infant disorganization (Tereno et al., 2017). In the intervention group, the percentage of disorganized attachment was 7.7%, whereas, in the control group, it was 19.2%. Again, the proportion of disorganized attachment in the control group was comparable to other high-risk samples (25%; van IJzendoorn et al., 1999). The cumulative effect of multiple vulnerability factors should be taken into account when analyzing these results: Three out of four women (75.6%) presented with at least three risk factors at inclusion during pregnancy, and 37.8% with at least five. Most were young, first-time mothers, first- or second-generation immigrants, with low educational levels and relatively little income. Without intervening services, the cumulative effect of multifaceted familial and ecological risks may have created repercussions for the development of the parent–child attachment relationship (Cyr et al., 2010).

Predictive Risk Factors of Maternal Disruptive Behavior

Although Cyr and colleagues (2010) have described the impact of *independent* versus *cumulative* socioeconomic factors on infant attachment disorganization, to our knowledge, the impact on parental disruptive behavior has yet to be explored. This study shows that *high levels of poverty* and *giving birth prematurely* were predictive of later maternal disruptive behavior. It may therefore be hypothesized that social stress associated with prematurity has a direct effect on the parental behavior with a more disruptive communication. These results underscore the importance of seeing socioeconomic vulnerability as a risk factor for maternal disruptive behavior, with poverty directly influencing parental behavior. This is in line with others studies, in which we see that low income, as well as ethnic-minority status, may increase the number and intensity of daily stresses that parents experience, which in turn may decrease sensitive parenting behavior (Bakermans-Kranenburg, van IJzendoorn, & Kroonenberg, 2004), increase disruptive behavior, and therefore negatively impact the child's attachment security.

Although only two prenatal risk factors (poverty, prematurity) were significantly associated with later disorganized maternal behavior, the accumulation of many factors (i.e., socioeconomic, psychopathological, infant, parenting), at least five in the present study, proved also to be significant. Handling a multitude of problems in everyday life is clearly a major issue for young first-time mothers, with a significant impact on the quality of their relationship with their child and later child mental health.

Additional Commentary on Program Attrition Issues

In the CAPEDP trial, 50% of eligible future mothers declined when participation was proposed to them. Of the remaining 50%, 55.2% (27.6% of the overall sample of eligible women) dropped out of the intervention at some point (Foulon et al., 2015). The attrition rate from assessment in the CAPEDP trial at the time the children were 3 months old (i.e., early attrition—6 months after the beginning of the trial) is similar to that observed in other randomized trials evaluating home-visiting programs (Katz et al., 2001; St Pierre & Layzer, 1999; Koniak-Griffin et al., 2003). Predictors of early attrition included having had an abortion and having higher attachment insecurity, as measured by the Vulnerable Attachment Style Questionnaire (VASQ; Bifulco, Mahon, Kwon, Moran, & Jacobs, 2003). The only predictor of later attrition was early parental loss (death or separation of the woman's own parents before she was 11 years old). Being employed or currently studying or doing training, tobacco consumption during pregnancy, and presence of psychiatric symptoms were positively associated with early retention. So signs of (1) organization and planning and (2) addiction and vulnerability were linked to retention.

The higher VASQ insecurity scores in subjects who prematurely abandoned the study, as well as the association between later attrition and parental loss, can be understood in the light of attachment theory. Attachment insecurity is associated with having an idea of oneself as not being worthy of other people's interest, of not being able to count on other people, and of being felt to be unreliable or even ill-meaning. Insecure subjects undervalue the impact they might have on other people or on a given situation, particularly when under stress. Early parental loss has been associated with unresolved attachment and consequent relational difficulties, namely, via maternal depression (Brown, Craig, & Harris, 2008). Both insecure and unresolved persons may therefore be more prone to dropping out, because they have a negative perception of the assessment team or see themselves and their participation as being unimportant, as having no possible effect on the research process. They cannot believe that it would make any difference to anyone if they left the study: No one would care. The insecure subject also finds it hard to believe that the support the program claims that it is going to provide will be of any real help. Paton, Grant and Tsourtos (2013) have proposed that program engagement depends on managing participants' apprehension, trust, respect, social support, and challenges. Mutual trust and acceptance impact on the quality of the intervention and are influenced by the personal characteristics and perceived relationship styles of both parties (Brookes, Summers, Thornburg, Ispa, & Lane, 2006).

The fact that having a higher initial attachment insecurity score is not associated with later attrition can be understood in light of research on therapeutic alliances: In relationships with professionals that have been maintained over a certain time, the quality of the relationship itself becomes a determining retention factor, counteracting the negative impact of the individual's insecure attachment profile. Another highly interesting result is the finding that women with higher psychiatric symptom scores (SCL-90) were more likely to remain in this trial. This phenomenon is probably related to one of the major specificities of the CAPEDP study: All members of both the home-visiting and the assessment teams were qualified clinical psychologists. Seemingly, providing professional skills corresponding to the needs of participants in this French perinatal health promotion programs increased the likelihood that they would remain in the program (Foulon et al., 2015).

In the literature, authors such as Clarke, King, and Prost (2013) defend the point of view that psychological interventions delivered by nonspecialists are beneficial in perinatal mental health promotion programs, because they extend access to these interventions to low resource settings. However, Moss and colleagues (2011), who, as in the present study, used trained psychologists to do the home visits, consider that extensive training of those providing the intervention, backed up by frequent supervision, are essential ingredients if programs of this sort are to be successful. Our study supports the perspective of Moss and colleagues (Chapter 14, this volume). In order to correct very dysfunctional caregiver–infant interactions (e.g., parental disruptive behavior and infants' disorganized attachment), very well trained (on attachment issues and dysfunctional interactions) and supervised psychologists seem to be essential components of the study design (Guédeney et al., 2017).

Study Limitations, Strengths and Future Research Directions

This study has several limitations. First, the control group cannot be considered to have received no intervention given that "usual care" is particularly generous in the French health and social care system. In future studies, including a comparison group recruited from the general population would clearly help in identifying optimal target population characteristics for home-visiting approaches. Second, it must be remembered that women who were not fluent enough in French to give informed consent were not eligible for inclusion in the present study. Future works should take into account that socially at-risk families often belong to immigrant population groups. Finally, it has been suggested that observing disruptive parental behavior using the SSP raises the possibility of common method variance. This could lead to contamination with the observation of infant attachment behavior during the same procedure. In our study, this possible contamination was controlled by using AMBIANCE coders, with no specific training with regard to infant attachment behavior, but future work should consider the use of two distinct coding supports.

Despite these limitations, the CAPEDP study has a number of major strengths: (1) the use of a large number of validated psychological scales to explore different aspects of the mothers' psychological situations and their eventual interactions with their child; (2) a homogeneous collection of potential predictors with little missing data; and (3) a dynamic approach identifying predictors of later attrition in women who had initially adhered to the study, thus allowing us to describe vulnerability factors in the postpartum period that may have differed from those observed during pregnancy (e.g., maternal employment, presence of psychiatric symptoms) or that were not available during pregnancy (e.g., parenting scales). Particularly, in the CAPEDP-A study (see Table 10.1), attachment was assessed (4) on a basis of multiple measures (infants: Strange Situation Procedure Preschoolers [SSP], Attachment Q-Sort [AQS]; mothers: VASQ, Relationship Style Questionnaire [RSQ], Adult Attachment Narratives [AAN]) and a multijudge method with parallel coding teams; and (5) in a longitudinal perspective (infants 12, 18, and 48 months of age; mothers of infants 12 and 48 months of age).

Conclusion

A primary pathway to enhancing children's well-being is through interventions designed to increase the quality of their parents' parenting skills. CAPEDP-A was the first study to present infant attachment distributions and the impact of a preventive program on infant attachment quality in a French multirisk sample. To our knowledge, it was also the first to address the link between socioeconomic vulnerability and parental disruptive behavior. Our results confirm that this exploration is essential to understand the link between the latter and the development of infants' attachment disorganization. Intervention programs targeting infants' attachment quality should privilege a twofold approach: here disruptive maternal behavior is addressed, in an integrated way, with a risk factors' accumulation perspective. Taking into account predictors of early and later attrition is another key point. It allows project managers to adapt retention procedures, according to each participant's personal psychosocial characteristics, which may well vary across the study.

ACKNOWLEDGMENTS

We would like to thank the CAPEDP Study Group (Elie Azria, Emmanuel Barranger, Jean-Louis Benifla, Bruno Carbonne, Marc Dommergues, Romain Dugravier, Bruno Falissard, Tim Greacen, Antoine Guédeney, Nicole Guédeney, Alain Haddad, Dominique Luton, Dominique Mahieu-Caputo, Laurent Mandelbrot, Jean-François Oury, Dominique Pathier, Diane Purper-Ouakil, Thomas Saïas, Susana Tereno, Richard E. Tremblay, Florence Tubach, Serge Uzan, and Bertrand Welniarz), the 440 families who participated in the study, the assessment and coding teams, the members of the home-visiting team, and the research assistants, without whom this project would not have been possible. Our special thanks to the CAPEDP steering committee: Romain Dugravier, Thomas Saïas, and Florence Tübach.

CAPEDP-A was supported by research grants from the French Ministry of Health (Hospital Clinical Research Programme: PHRC AOM05036), the French National Institute for Promotion and Health Education (INPES), the French National Institute of Health and Medical Research (INSERM), and the French Public Health Research Institute (IReSP, PREV0702). The Foundation Pfizer funded CAPEDP-A Phase II. The CAPEDP general project was financed with a grant from the National Ministry of Health Hospital Clinical Research Program (PHRC AOM 05056) and the French Institute for Health Promotion and Health Education. The sponsor was the Clinical Research and Development Department of the APHP. The funders had no role in study design, data collection and analysis, the decision to publish, or the preparation of the chapter.

CAPEDP-A received ethical approval from the *Comité de Protection des Personnes Ile de France IV,* Institutional Review Board and from the Commission Nationale de l'Informatique et des Libertés (CNIL, 907255), with Clinical Trial Registration Number: NCT00392847.

REFERENCES

Ackerman, J., & Dozier, M. (2005). The influence of foster parent investment on children's representations of self and attachment figures. *Applied Developmental Psychology, 26,* 507–520.

Ainsworth, M. D. S., Blehar, M., Waters, E., & Wall, S. (1978). *Patterns of attachment: A psychological study of the Strange Situation.* Hillsdale, NJ: Erlbaum.

Bakermans-Kranenburg, M. J., van IJzendoorn, M., & Juffer, F. (2003). Less is more: Meta-analyses of sensitivity and attachment interventions in early childhood. *Psychological Bulletin, 129*(2), 195–215.

Bakermans-Kranenburg, M. J., van IJzendoorn, M. H., & Kroonenberg, P. M. (2004). Differences in attachment security between African-American and white children: Ethnicity or socio-economic status? *Infant Behavior and Development, 27*(3), 417–433.

Bandura, A. (1977). Self-efficacy: Toward a unifying theory of behavioral change. *Psychological Review, 84*, 191–215.

Belsky, J. (1996). Parent, infant, and social-contextual antecedents of attachment security. *Developmental Psychology, 32*, 905–913.

Belsky, J., & Isabella, R. (1988). Maternal, infant, and social-contextual determinants of attachment security. In J. Belsky & T. Nezworski (Eds.), *Clinical implications of attachment* (pp. 41–94). Hillsdale, NJ: Erlbaum.

Belsky, J. B., Rosenberger, K., & Crnic, K. (2000). The origins of attachment security: "Classical" and contextual determinants. In S. Goldberg, R. Muir, & J. Kerr (Eds.), *Attachment theory: Social, developmental, and clinical perspectives* (pp. 153–184). New York: Analytic Press.

Belsky, J., & Stratton, P. (2002). An ecological analysis of the etiology of child maltreatment. In K. Browne, H. Hanks, P. Stratton, & C. Hamilton (Eds.), *Early prediction and prevention of child abuse: A handbook* (pp. 95–110). Chichester, UK: Wiley.

Bifulco, A., Mahon, J., Kwon, J. H., Moran, P. M., & Jacobs, C. (2003). The Vulnerable Attachment Style Questionnaire (VASQ): An interview-based measure of attachment styles that predict depressive disorder. *Psychological Medicine, 33*, 1099–1110.

Boris, N., Larrieu, J. A., Zeanah, P. D., Nagle, G. A., & Steier, A. (2006). The process and promise of mental health augmentation of nurse home-visiting programs: Data from the Louisiana nurse–family partnership. *Infant Mental Health Journal, 27*(1), 26–40.

Bowlby, J. (1988). Developmental psychiatry comes of ages. *American Journal of Psychiatry, 145*(1), 1–10.

Bretherton I., Ridgeway, D., & Cassidy, J. (1990). Assessing the internal working models of the attachment relationship: An attachment story completion task for 3-year-olds. In M. T. Geenberg, D. Ciccetti, & E. M. Cummings (Eds.), *Attachment in the preschool years: Theory, research and intervention* (pp. 273–308). Chicago: University of Chicago Press.

Bronfman, E., Parsons, E., & Lyons-Ruth, K. (2004). *Atypical Maternal Behavior Instrument for Assessment and Classification (AMBIANCE): Manual for coding disrupted affective communication* (2nd ed.). Unpublished manual, Harvard University Medical School, Cambridge, MA.

Brookes, S. J., Summers, J. A., Thornburg, K. R., Ispa, J. M., & Lane, V. J. (2006). Building successful home visitor–mother relationships and reaching program goals in two Early Head Start programs: A qualitative look at contributing factors. *Early Childhood Research Quarterly, 21*, 25–45.

Brown, G. W., Craig, T. K., & Harris, T. O. (2008). Research report: Parental maltreatment and proximal risk factors using the Childhood Experience of Care and Abuse (CECA) instrument: A life-course study of adult chronic depression—5. *Journal of Affective Disorders, 110*, 222–233.

Cassidy, J. (1988). Child–mother attachment and the self in six-year-olds. *Child Development, 59*, 121–134.

Cassidy, J., Marvin, R. S., & the MacArthur Working Group on Attachment. (1992). *Attachment organization in preschool children: Procedures and coding manual*. Unpublished manual, University of Pennsylvania, Philadelphia.

Center for Early Education and Development. (2009). *Steps Toward Effective, Enjoyable Parenting* (STEEP™) manual. Minneapolis: University of Minnesota.

Cicchetti, D., & Lynch, M. (1993). Toward an ecological/transactional model of community violence and child maltreatment: Consequences for children's development. *Psychiatry, 56*, 96–118.

Clarke, K., King, M., & Prost, A. (2013). psychosocial interventions for perinatal common mental disorders delivered by providers who are not mental health specialists in low- and middle-income countries: A systematic review and meta-analysis. *PLOS Medicine, 10*(10), 1001541.

Cléry-Melin, P., Kovess, V., & Pascal, J.-C. (2003). Plan d'actions pour le développement de la psychiatrie et la promotion de la santé mentale [Action plan for the development of psychiatry and the promotion of mental health]. *French Social Affairs Review, 1*, 215–220.

Coleman, J., & Dennison, C. (1998). Teenage parenthood. *Children and Society, 12*(4), 306–314.

Cox, J. L., Holden, J. M., & Sagovsky, R. (1987). Detection of postnatal depression. Development of the 10-item Edinburgh Postnatal Depression Scale. *British Journal of Psychiatry, 150*, 782–786.

Cyr, C., Euser, E., Bakermans-Kranenburg, M., & van IJzendoorn, M. (2010). Attachment security and disorganization in maltreating and high-risk families: A series of meta-analyses. *Development and Psychopathology, 22*, 87–108.

Daro, D., McCurdy, K., Falconnier, L., & Stojanovic, D. (2003). Sustaining new parents in home visitation services: Key participant and program factors. *Child Abuse and Neglect, 27*, 1101–1125.

DASES 75. (2003). *La santé de la mère et de l'enfant à Paris: Evolution 1980–2002* [Infants' and mothers' health in Paris]. Paris: Département de Paris, DASES-PMI.

Deater-Deckard, K., Dodge, K. A., Bates, J. E., & Pettit, G. S. (1998). Multiple risk factors in the development of externalizing behavior problems: Group and individual differences. *Development and Psychopathology, 10*(3), 469–493.

Derogatis, L. R. (1994). *SCL-90 Administration, scoring, and procedures manual* (3rd ed.). Minneapolis: National Computer Systems.

Dugravier, R., Tubach, F., Saias, T., Guédeney, N., Pasquet, B., Purper-Ouakil, D., . . . Greacen, T. (2013). Impact of a manualized multifocal perinatal home-visiting program using psychologists on postnatal depression: The CAPEDP randomized controlled trial. *PLOS ONE, 8*(8), e72216.

Durlak, J. A., & DuPre, E. P. (2008). Implementation matters: A review of research on the influence of implementation on program outcomes and the factors affecting implementation. *American Journal of Community Psychology, 41*, 327–350.

Dyrbye, L. N., Thomas, M. R., & Shanafelt, T. D. (2006). Systematic review of depression, anxiety, and other indicators of psychological distress among U.S. and Canadian medical students. *Academic Medicine: Journal of the Association of American Medical Colleges, 81*, 354–373.

Egeland, B., & Erickson, M. F. (1999). Findings from the Parent–Child Project and implications for early intervention. *ZERO TO THREE, 20*, 3–10.

Fearon, R. P., Bakermans-Kranenburg, M. J., van IJzendoorn, M. H., Lapsley, A.-M., & Roisman, G. I. (2010). The significance of insecure attachment and disorganization in the development of children's externalizing behavior: A meta-analytic study. *Child Development, 81*, 435–456.

Florida State University Center for Prevention and Early Intervention Policy. (2007). *Partners for a Healthy Baby Home Visiting curriculum.* Tallahassee: Florida State University

Foulon, S., Greacen, T., Pasquet, B., Dugravier, R., Saïas, T., Guédeney, N., . . . CADEDP Study Group (2015). Predictors of study attrition in a randomized controlled trial evaluating a perinatal home-visiting program with mothers with psychosocial vulnerabilities. *PLoS ONE, 10*(11), e0142495.

Gomby, D. S. (2005). *Home visitation in 2005: Outcomes for children and parents* (Working Paper No. 7). Washington, DC: Invest in Kids Working Group.

Greenberg, M. T., Speltz, M. L., DeKlyen, M., & Jones, K. (2001). Correlates of clinic referral for early conduct problems: Variable- and person-oriented approaches. *Development and Psychopathology, 13*, 255–276.

Grossmann, K., Grossmann, K. E., Spangler, G., Suess, G., & Unzner, L. (1985). Maternal sensitivity and newborns' orientation responses as related to quality of attachment in Northern Germany. *Monographs of the Society for Research in Child Development, 50*(1/2), 233–256.

Guédeney, A., & Fermanian, J. (2001). A validity and reliability study of assessment and screening for sustained withdrawal reaction in infancy: The Alarm Distress Baby Scale. *Infant Mental Health Journal, 22*, 559–575.

Guédeney, A., Guédeney, N., Tereno, S., Dugravier, R., Greacen, T., Welniarz, B., . . . Tubach, F. (2011). Infant rhythms versus parental time: Promoting parent–infant synchrony. *Journal of Physiology–Paris, 105*(4–6), 195–200.

Guédeney, A., & Tereno, S. (2012). La vidéo dans l'observation d'évaluation et d'intervention en santé mentale du jeune enfant: Un outil pour la transmission [Video in early childhood mental health assessment and intervention: A tool for transmission]. *Neuropsychiatrie de l'Enfance et de l'Adolescence, 60*(4), 261–266.

Guédeney, A., Welniarz, B., Weatherston, D., Purper-Ouakil, D., Wendland, J., Tereno, S., Saïas, T., . . . Greacen, T. (2017). Best practice in individual supervision of psychologists working in the French CAPEDP Preventive Perinatal Home-Visiting Program: Results of a Delphi consensus process. *Infant Mental Health Journal, 38*(2), 267–275.

Guédeney, A., Wendland, J., Dugravier, R., Saïas, T., Tubach, F., Welniarz, B., . . . Pasquet, B. (2013). Impact of a randomized home-visiting trial on infant social withdrawal in the CAPEDP prevention study. *Infant Mental Health Journal, 34*(6), 594–601.

Guédeney, N., & Fermanian, J. (1998). Validation study of the French version of the Edinburgh Postnatal Depression Scale (EPDS): New results about use and psychometric properties. *European Psychiatry, 13*, 83–89.

Guédeney, N., Guédeney, A., & Rabouam, C. (2013). Violences conjugales et attachement des jeunes enfants: Une revue de la littérature [Spousal violence and attachment of young children: A review of the literature]. *Perspectives Psychiatriques, 52*, 222–230.

Haddad, A., Guédeney, A., & Greacen, T. (2004). *Santé Mentale du jeune enfant: Prévenir et intervenir* [Early childhood mental health: Prevention and intervention]. Ramonville Saint-Agne, France: Erès.

Hay, D. F., Pawlby, S., Angold, A., Harold, G. T., & Sharp, D. (2003). Pathways to violence in the children of mothers who were depressed postpartum. *Developmental Psychology, 39*, 1083–1094.

Hungerford, A., & Cox, M. J. (2006). Family factors in child care research. *Evaluation Review, 30*, 631–655.

Ikounga N'Goma, G., & Brodin, M. (2001). Les certificats de santé: Intérêt et limites [Health certificates: Interests and limits]. *Médecine et Enfance, 21*(9), 478–482.

Jones, D. J., Forehand, R., Brody, G., & Armistead, L. (2002). Psychosocial adjustment of African American children in single-mother families: A test of three risk models. *Journal of Marriage and the Family, 64*, 105–115.

Juffer, F., Bakermans-Kranenburg, M., & van IJzendoorn, M. (2007). *Promoting positive parenting: An attachment-based intervention.* New York: Erlbaum.

Kahn, J., Moore, K. A., & Haven, N. (2010). What works for home visiting programs: Lessons from experimental evaluations of programs and interventions. *Child Trends Fact Sheet, 20008*, 1–33.

Katz, K. S., El-Mohandes, P. A., Johnson, D. M., Jarrett, P. M., Rose, A., & Cober, M. (2001). Retention of low income mothers in a parenting intervention study. *Journal of Community Health, 26*, 203–218.

Kobak, R., & Mandelbaum, T. (2003). Caring for the caregiver: An attachment approach to assessment and treatment of child problems. In M. Johnson & V. E. Whiffen (Eds.), *Attachment processes in couple and family therapy* (pp. 144–164). New York: Guilford Press.

Koniak-Griffin, D., Verzemnieks, I. L., Anderson, N. L. R., Brecht, M.-L., Lesser, J., Kim, S., & Turner-Pluta, C. (2003). Nurse visitation for adolescent mothers: Two-year infant health and maternal outcomes. *Nursing Research, 52*, 127–136.

Lynch, M., & Cicchetti, D. (1998). An ecological–transactional analysis of children and contexts: The longitudinal interplay among child maltreatment, community violence, and children's symptomatology. *Development and Psychopathology, 10*, 235–257.

Lyons-Ruth, K., Bronfman, E., & Parsons, E. (1999). Atypical maternal behaviour and disorganized infant attachment strategies: Frightened, frightening, and atypical maternal behaviour and disorganized infant attachment strategies. *Monographs of the Society for Research in Child Development, 258*, 67–96.

Lyons-Ruth, K., Bureau, J.-F., Easterbrooks, M. A., Obsuth, I., Hennighausen, K., & Vulliez-Coady, L. (2013). Parsing the construct of maternal insensitivity: Distinct longitudinal pathways associated with early maternal withdrawal. *Attachment and Human Development, 15*(5–6), 562–582.

Lyons-Ruth, K., & Melnick, S. (2004). Dose–response effect of mother–infant clinical home visiting on aggressive behaviour problems in kindergarten. *Journal of the American Academy of Child and Adolescent Psychiatry, 43*, 699–707.

Madigan, S., Bakermans-Kranenburg, M., van IJzendoorn, M., Moran, G., Pederson, D., & Benoit, D. (2006). Unresolved states of mind, anomalous parental behavior, and disorganized attachment: A review and meta-analysis of a transmission gap. *Attachment and Human Development, 8*(2), 89–111.

Main, M., & Hesse, E. (1990). Parents' unresolved traumatic experiences are related to infant disorganized attachment status: Is frightened and/or frightening parental behavior the linking mechanism? In M. T. Greenberg, D. Cicchetti, & E. M. Cummings (Eds.), *Attachment in the preschool years: Theory, research, and intervention* (pp. 161–182). Chicago: University of Chicago Press.

Main, M., & Solomon, J. (1990). Procedures for identifying infants as disorganized/disoriented during the Ainsworth Strange Situation. In M. T. Greenberg, D. Cicchetti, & E. M. Cummings (Eds.), *Attachment in the preschool years: Theory, research, and intervention* (pp. 121–160). Chicago: University of Chicago Press.

Marvin, R. S., Cooper, G., Hoffman, K., & Powell, B. (2002). The Circle of Security project: Attachment-based intervention with caregiver–preschool child dyads. *Attachment and Human Development, 4*, 107–124.

Moss, E., Karine, D.-C., Cyr, C., Tarabulsy, S.-L., & Bernier, A. (2011). Efficacy of a home-visiting intervention aimed at improving maternal sensitivity, child attachment, and behavioral outcomes for maltreated children: A randomized control trial. *Development and Psychopathology, 23*, 195–210.

Murray, L., & Cooper, P. J. (1997). *Postpartum depression and child development.* New York: Guilford Press.

Nagin, D. S., & Tremblay, R. E. (2001). Parental and early childhood predictors of persistent physical aggression in boys from kindergarten to high school. *Archives of General Psychiatry, 58*, 389–394.

Olds, D. (1998). Prenatal and infancy home visitation by nurses: A program of research. In

C. Rovee-Collier, L. Lipsitt, & H. Hayne (Eds.), *Advances in infancy research* (pp. 79–130). Stanford, CA: Ablex.

Olds, D. L., Eckenrode, J., Henderson, C. R., Kitzman, H., Powers, J., Cole, R., . . . Luckey, D. (1997). Long-term effects of home visitation on maternal life course and child abuse and neglect: Fifteen-year follow-up of a randomized trial. *Journal of the American Medical Association, 278*, 637–643.

Oppenheim, D., Goldsmith, D., & Koren-Karie, N. (2004). Maternal insightfulness and preschoolers' emotion and behavior problems: Reciprocal influences in a therapeutic preschool program. *Infant Mental Health Journal, 25*, 352–367.

Oppenheim, D., & Koren-Karie, N. (2002). Mothers' insightfulness regarding their children's internal worlds: The capacity underlying secure child–mother relationships. *Infant Mental Health Journal, 23*, 593–605.

Paton, L., Grant, J., & Tsourtos, G. (2013). Exploring mothers' perspectives of an intensive home visiting program in Australia: A qualitative study. *Contemporary Nurse, 43*, 191–200.

Rutter, M. (1979). Protective factors in children's responses to stress and disadvantage. In M. W. Kent & J. E. Rolf (Eds.), *Primary prevention in psychopathology: Vol. 3. Social competence in children* (pp. 324–338). Hanover, NH: University Press of New England.

Saïas, T., Greacen, T., Tubach, F., Dugravier, R., Marcault, E., Tereno, S., . . . CAPEDP Study Group. (2013). Supporting families in challenging contexts: The CAPEDP project. *Global Health Promotion, 20*(Suppl. 2), 66–70.

Sameroff, A. J. (2000). Developmental systems and psychopathology. *Development and Psychopathology, 12*, 297–312.

Schuengel, C., Bakermans-Kranenburg, M. J., & van IJzendoorn, M. H. (1999). Frightening maternal behavior linking unresolved loss and disorganized attachment. *Journal of Consulting and Clinical Psychology, 67*, 54–63.

Shaw, D. S., & Vondra, J. (1993). Chronic family adversity and infant attachment security. *Journal of Child Psychology and Psychiatry, 34*, 1205–1215.

Slade, A., Grienenberger, J., Bernbach, E., Levy, D., & Locker, A. (2005). Maternal reflective functioning, attachment, and the transmission gap: A preliminary study. *Attachment and Human Development, 7*, 283–298.

Solomon, J., & George, C. (1999). The place of disorganization in attachment theory: Linking classic observations with contemporary findings. In J. Solomon & C. George (Eds.), *Attachment disorganization* (pp. 3–32). New York: Guilford Press.

St Pierre, R. G., & Layzer, J. I. (1999). Using home visits for multiple purposes: The Comprehensive Child Development Program. *The Future of Children, 9*, 134–151.

Tereno, S., Guedeney, N., Dugravier, R., Greacen, T., Saïas, T., Tubach, F., & Guédeney, A. (2013). Early home-based intervention on infant attachment organisation: The CAPEDP Attachment Study in France. *Global Health Promotion, 20*, 71–75.

Tereno, S., Guédeney, N., Dugravier, R., Greacen, T., Saïas, T., Tubach, F., . . . Guédeney, A. (2016). Sécurité de l'attachement des jeunes enfants dans une population Française vulnérable [Infants' attachment security in a vulnerable French sample]. *Encéphale, 43*(2), 99–103.

Tereno, S., Guédeney, N., Wendland, J., Tubach, F., Lamas, C., Vulliez-Coady, L., . . . CAPEDP Group. (submitted). Predictive and associated risk factors of maternal disruptive behavior. *Attachment and Human Development*.

Tereno, S., Madigan, S., Lyons-Ruth, K., Plamondon, A., Atkinson, L., Guédeney, N., . . . Guédeney, A. (2017). Assessing mechanisms of effect in a randomized home-visiting trial: Reduced disrupted maternal communication decreases infant disorganization. *Development and Psychopathology, 29*(2), 637–649.

Tereno, S., Soares, I., Martins, E., Sampaio, D., & Carlson, E. (2007). La théorie de l'attachement: Son importance dans un contexte pédiatrique [The theory of attachment: Its importance in a pediatric context]. *Devenir, 19*(2), 151–188.

Tubach, F., Greacen, T., Saïas, T., Dugravier, R., Guédeney, N., Ravaud, P., . . . Guédeney, A. (2012). A home-visiting intervention targeting determinants of infant mental health: The study protocol for the CAPEDP randomized controlled trial in France. *BMC Public Health, 12*(1), 648.

van IJzendoorn, M. H., Schuengel, C., & Bakermans-Kranenburg, M. J. (1999). Disorganized attachment in early childhood: Meta-analysis of precursors, concomitants, and sequelae. *Development and Psychopathology, 11*, 225–249.

Warren, P. L. (2005). First-time mothers: Social support and confidence in infant care. *Journal of Advanced Nursing, 50*, 479–488.

Waters, E., & Deane, K. (1985). Defining and assessing individual differences in attachment relationships: Q-methodology and the organization of behaviour in infancy and early childhood. *Monographs of the Society for Research in Child Development, 50*(Serial No. 209), 41–65.

Weatherston, D. (2000). The infant mental health specialist. *ZERO TO THREE, 21*, 3–10.

Wichstrøm, L., Berg-Nielsen, T. S., Angold, A., Egger, H. L., Solheim, E., & Sveen, T. H. (2011). Prevalence of psychiatric disorders in preschoolers. *Journal of Child Psychology and Psychiatry and Allied Disciplines, 53*, 695–705.

World Health Organization. (2003). *Caring for children and adolescents with mental disorders: Setting WHO directions.* Geneva: Author.

World Health Organization. (2010). *Mental health: Strengthening our response.* Geneva: Author.

Zeanah, C. H., Danis, B., Hirschberg, L., Benoit, D., Miller, D., & Heller, S. (1999). Disorganized attachment associated with partner violence: A research note. *Infant Mental Health Journal, 20*, 77–86.

Zeanah, P. D., Larrieu, J., Boris, N. W., & Nagle, J. A. (2006). Nurse home visiting: Perspectives from nurses. *Infant Mental Health Journal, 27*(1), 41–54.

CHAPTER 11

Mom2Mom
An Attachment-Based Home-Visiting Program
for Mothers of Young Infants

MARSHA KAITZ

in collaboration with MIRIAM CHRIKI, NAOMI TESSLER,
JUDITH LEVY, and SARA BURSTIN

Mom2Mom (M2M) was born in 2000 as an innovative home-visiting project in Israel, aimed at providing emotional support to mothers in the year that follows childbirth. Home visitors are volunteers, trained and supervised by project coordinators who are professionals in the field of child development and social work. Basic tenets of the project are in keeping with attachment theory and with a broad literature that shows that mothers who are well supported by family, friends, and their community enjoy parenting more, feel better about themselves, are less likely to be anxious and depressed, and are more sensitive to their infants' needs. Furthermore, there is strong evidence that infants of these mothers develop more optimally, according to many outcome measures, including felt-security and resilience to stress. In this chapter, we describe the development and implementation of M2M. We outline its basic tenets, describe the processes that underlie the project (e.g., training, supervision, and evaluations), as well as our challenges, and our plans and dreams for the future. Our hope is that a description of the development of M2M will acquaint readers with the project. More generally, we hope that our account offers a general plan and tips for other professionals who are thinking about founding or those planning or already working on the same or similar projects. We consider the information worthy of sharing because, quite simply, the development plan has worked for us, for our home visitors, and for most of the families we have served.

The Past, Present, and Future of M2M

The M2M project is modeled after the Visiting Moms (Boston, Massachusetts) program (see Paris & Dubus, 2005; Paris, Gemborys, Kaufman, & Whitehill, 2007)—grounded in both attachment theory and a broad literature showing that emotional support during the months after childbirth can reduce mothers' stress level, counter loneliness and feelings of isolation, and encourage feelings of self-efficacy and self-esteem (Cutrona & Troutman, 1986; for meta-analysis, see Andresen & Telleen, 1992; for reviews, see Cobb, 1976; Hoffman, & Hatch, 1996). Importantly, the literature indicates that support, well-timed and well-tuned to mother and family, predicts more sensitive maternal behavior (Andresen & Telleen, 1992; Crockenberg, 1981) and mothers' greater resilience in the face of the challenges that may arise during the course of this period of profound transition (Dunkel Schetter, 2011). Consequently, efforts to support mothers during this time can benefit their children and family as a whole and therefore contribute to the future health and wealth of a culture and society (Harris, Lieberman, & Marans, 2007; Odgers, Caspi, Russell, Sampson, Arsenault, & Moffitt, 2012). In this regard, maternal emotional support may be especially important because stress, dangers, and uncertainty are often part of daily life, for example, as in many countries (like Israel) where war is a recent memory and peace is elusive, or in families anywhere that contend with serious internal dysfunction or a significant lack of personal or familial resources. M2M offers support to women during one of the most important periods in their lives and in the lives of their children. Moreover, M2M helps the helper to realize her own strengths, and harness them in an effort to provide support to a woman who just had a new baby.

M2M in Israel began in the year 2000 and as of 2015,[1] has 25 branches (throughout the country), serving hundreds of families every year. We advertise in hospitals and well-baby clinics, and receive referrals from professionals (e.g., psychiatrists, family doctors) and concerned relatives and neighbors. About half of the women who join the project are self-referred. We work together with offices within municipalities, ministries (e.g., social services, health ministry) and special offices (immigration). We lobby in the Parliament; we put mothers in contact with needed resources that range from free baby equipment to a volunteer doula. We support mothers through difficult judicial proceedings (divorce, custody), help them reach out to social services, and connect them with psychological services, if needed. We have trained more than 250 volunteers (in Jerusalem alone) and paired them with more than 500 mothers for a year of home visiting. We run a weekly play group for mothers and infants up to age 1 year. The project is called *eml'em* in Hebrew (Mom2Mom, in English; website: *www.emlem.co.il*), and today is a well-known and well-used fixture in the Jerusalem landscape of resources for families.

What follows is select parts of our story, particularly those that may further understanding of our goals, steps toward implementation, and some of the underlying processes that have made M2M the success story that it is. We share the M2M history by drawing on a lifespan metaphor for becoming parents, starting with the "joining of hands" and continuing through "pregnancy/gestation" and the birth of

---

[1]As of 2017, there are 41 branches of M2M in Israel and 3 branches outside of the country. In 2016, the National Network of Mom2Mom Coordinators and Directors was founded.

the "infant." We discuss the development of M2M during the project's early years and compare that with its present status, which involves diverse, interlocking tiers providing support to one another. Accordingly, our logo, representing our project, is drawn as concentric circles reflecting interlacing connections between coordinators and home visitors, between home visitors, between home visitors and "our moms" (the clients); and, at the center of it all, are the mothers and their babies. At the end of this chapter, we share our challenges and dreams.

A Historical Perspective: From Conception Onward

Joining Hands

Relationships are at the heart of the M2M model. At the inception of the project, two relationships were of crucial importance, and they have continued to be among the most important relationships that "we" have. One was between Marsha Kaitz and a former student Miriam Chriki, who practices as a developmental clinician in the field. Miriam has been a founding partner of M2M, and together with Kaitz, put the first "bricks" of the project into place. This relationship has been so important that we now suggest strongly that all persons considering the founding of M2M in their community find a partner (a passionate and committed confidante) as a first step on their "to-do list." The second relationship that is a solid cornerstone for the M2M project is with the Irving Harris Foundation based in Chicago, and with the Harris-funded Professional Development Network (PDN). The former has supported us financially and the latter, emotionally and academically from the start of the project.

Pregnancy: Defining Basic Tenets

At the outset (1999–2000), we were privileged to have time to plan the project, without pressure to "open our doors" right away. This period of gestation gave us the luxury of time to attend mindfully to the project's "needs," including careful consideration of focal aims, basic tenets, and core processes such as training, supervision, and evaluation—down to the fine details, including the project's name, logo, and color of the stationery.

Some of the important issues and decisions made at this stage are listed and described below.

Attachment Theory as Our Guide

Following Visiting Moms, we grounded our support project in attachment theory (Bowlby, 1969/1982), which means that our primary tenet is that secure relationships are essential for individuals' good health and development, especially in times of distress or transition. With attachment figures by their side (and secure representations "in their head"), individuals perceive themselves and others in a more positive light (Mikulincer & Shaver, 2016), are better able to regulate their emotions and behavior (Mikulincer, Shaver, & Pereg, 2003), and develop more optimally than persons who are not privy to attachment security (Raby, Lawler, Shlafer, Hesemeyer, Collins, & Sroufe, 2015).

For parents, a history of secure relationships makes it easier for them to open their hearts freely to their children, without fear, and respond consistently to their needs in a manner that balances sensitivity and appropriate demands (Karavasilis, Doyle, & Markiewicz, 2003). These parents also tend to perceive their children's motives and needs with reasonable accuracy (Haft & Slade, 1989), adjust their expectations and attention to fit their children's developmental level (Karavasilis et al., 2003), and are more likely to cope effectively with the significant challenges that often accompany the postpartum period (Mikulincer & Florian, 1998). Research indicates that parents with secure attachment enjoy parenting more (Slade, Belsky, Aber, & Phelps, 1999), seem to get along with their spouses better (Feeney, 2002; Hazan & Shaver, 1987), and have lower incidence rates of anxiety and depression before and after childbirth (Bifulco et al., 2004; McMahon, Trapolini, & Barnett, 2008). Importantly, children of parents who are securely attached, according to attachment assessment tools, are more sensitive and more positive with their children (Ainsworth, 1979; Slade et al., 1999; Wolff & van IJzendoorn, 1997), and are more likely to have children who are secure and well adjusted than parents who have an insecure (dismissing, preoccupied or unresolved regard to loss and/or trauma) pattern of attachment (Cowan, Cohn, Cowan, & Pearson, 1996; Fonagy, Steele, & Steele, 1991).

On these bases, M2M offers emotional support—a partner in the form of a volunteer home visitor from the community, who is also a mother—to share the lows and highs and uncertainties that are often part and parcel of the important first year after childbirth (Kaitz & Katzir, 2004). Attachment theory contends that partnering in this way can promote a secure emotional bond between individuals (Ainsworth, 1989). It is our hope that such a bond forms between mothers and volunteers, and that it helps mothers achieve their goal of being the best caregiver they can be and to cope with barriers that interfere with that aspiration. Furthermore, closely aligned theories, particularly relational regulation theory (RRT; Lakey & Orehek, 2011), stress the contribution of relationships and shared activities for regulation of the "recipient," which is exactly the nature of the supportive intervention offered by M2M (also see Heinicke, Ruth, Recchia, Guthrie, Rodning, & Fineman, 1999; Paris & Dubus, 2005; Paris et al., 2007; Stern, 1995; Slade, 2002).

Our anchor in attachment theory also prompts our continual efforts to nurture secure connections between home visitors and staff members. For this, we try to be available to home-visitors 24/7 by phone or e-mail, and to foster and reinforce a sense of belonging to the project as a whole. In these ways, we try to make the "job" of home visitor enjoyable, secure, and enriching, despite the difficult circumstances that some of our volunteers confront during their home visits. We also hope that through our efforts, volunteers feel secure enough to freely share their home-visiting experiences with coordinators and other volunteers during monthly group supervision sessions. In this way, group facilitators can help guide home visitors through dilemmas, contain their distress and uncertainties, help them to digest their experiences, and offer insights that may be helpful in the quest to forge a close relationship with "their mom." With trust in hand, volunteers can more effectively regulate themselves during home visits and successfully balance the need to "be present" and emotionally available to their mom, while maintaining personal space considerations and boundaries that are comfortable and appropriate for the individual, place, and time (Cole, 2014; Hauer, ten Cate, Boscardin, Irby, Iobst, & O'Sullivan, 2014; Kaitz, Bar-Haim, Lehrer, & Grossman, 2004).

The focus on relationships extends to the circle of home visitors themselves. This is important, because volunteers' support of one another, through the sharing of feelings, experiences, and ideas, can be mutually regulating and lead to creative strategies for dealing with issues that arise during training and supervision. In one recent supervision session, a volunteer was down-hearted because her "mom" moved away without saying good-bye, leaving her feeling despondent and unable to "let go" of the case without closure. In supervision, the volunteer was able to find closure through open discussion of the challenges of separations and what she, personally, had gained, and what her "mom" had gained during their time together. Mutual support and working on shared goals also enhance feelings of closeness between the volunteers and remind them that they are part of a larger group and not alone in the field.

Finally, secure relationships between us, the coordinators, are paramount to the health of the project. Our mutual closeness and trust makes it possible for us at the helm to continue to work in the field with confidence, knowing that should we falter or fall, there is trusted help readily available. This prevents burnout, protects our mental and physical health, and endows the project with viability and strength that it might not otherwise have.

Free Services

The widely quoted line "It takes a village to raise a child" (Clinton, 1996) reflects the difficulty of going it alone as a family with young children and the universal need for support when rearing them. For some families, support is "built in" and members of the family gather round to provide the practical, informational, and emotional support needed in times of stress and transition, including the early months after childbirth. For other families, support is less or not accessible because of logistics, practicalities, interpersonal relations, history, and/or family culture. With this, we believe that regardless of where a family is positioned on the continuum of "support accessibility," mothers can benefit from a home visitor who is "there" for the sole purpose of supporting their efforts to be a good mother (Lakey & Orehek, 2011). Certainly, in families contending with significant difficulties and risk, weekly home visits that afford mothers the opportunity to "download" their feelings, sort them out, prioritize issues, and strategize can go far in helping them to feel better about themselves and move forward with confidence (Cohen & Wills, 1985).

On these bases, we hold close the tenet that all services related to M2M are provided free of charge. In addition, we train and supervise professionals and share our project-related materials (e.g., posters, flyers, and training tools) free of charge with those who want to start M2M in their community. Our only stipulations are that all services based on our material are provided to clients free of charge and that the staff members of the new project attend our training course. The rule of free services is important to us, because we do not want M2M to be a business, but rather a community-based project developed out of need and dependent on the good will of dedicated volunteers who want to help mothers, infants, and families.

Most importantly, our provision of free services assures us that, within the M2M network, money will not come between a family's need and the support we offer.

Home Visitors from the Community

These tenets are shared with the Boston-based project Visiting Moms (also see Donovan, 2011), but set us apart from most home-visiting projects for mothers of young infants, which typically use salaried professionals as home visitors (e.g., Goldblatt, Yahav, & Ricon, 2014; see meta-analyses in Drummond, Weir, & Kysela, 2002; Olds, Sadler, & Kitzman, 2007; Sweet & Appelbaum, 2004; see reviews in Segal, Opie, & Dalziel, 2012). To our way of thinking, the idea of neighborhood women visiting other women in their community after childbirth for up to a year is appropriate given that our primary goal is to support mothers emotionally, and to accomplish that, the women need quality time together to build a relationship (also see Landy, Jack, Wahoush, Sheehan, & MacMillan, 2012). Our basic assumption is that the close relationship forged between home visitor and mother is the mediator—the underlying foundation—of successful home visits (Landy et al., 2012; Watkins & Riggs, 2012), defined in our evaluations by mothers' ratings of satisfaction with the project, and what and how much they gained from it.

Focus on Mothers of Young Infants (0–1 Year of Age)

The decision to focus on families with infants under age 1 was based on several considerations. First, the first year after childbirth is considered a particularly important period in children's development because of the substantial neural/brain growth and pruning that occur during this time and the strong impact that infants' early experiences have on their "present" and future development (Bell & Fox, 1994; Fox, Levitt, & Nelson, 2010). Second, we know that the first year of life is the time when mothers and infants get to know each other and, through their mutual, dynamic social interactions, come to forge an attachment relationship (Ainsworth, Blehar, Waters, & Wall, 1978/2014). According to attachment theory, mothers' early responses to their infants' distress signals play a significant role in determining whether infants develop a secure bond with their caregiver as a result of consistent and sensitive caregiving or an insecure bond due to maternal behavior that is ill tuned, inconsistent, and/or frightening to the child (Ainsworth, 1979; Bowlby, 1969/1982; Isabella, 1993). Third, the first postpartum year is one of transition and challenge for parents, so that extra support can be particularly beneficial at this time (Cowan & Cowan, 1995).

Nesting: Getting Ready

Defining our identity entailed setting criteria for accepting women into the program as volunteers and clients, though we have kept such rules to a minimum in order to welcome a broad spectrum of participants. To be a volunteer, the only criterion is to be a mother with free time for home visiting (2 hours a week) and supervision (2 hours a month). The criterion of being a mother seemed important for sharing experiences during training and supervision, but mostly because we reasoned that mothers seeking support after childbirth are likely to see a woman who is herself a mother as a viable "partner," mentor, or friend. As for the clients, almost all are accepted, with the exception of extreme cases in which there is violence or abuse of hard drugs in the immediate family. This rule was put into place in order to protect the volunteers from circumstances that are potentially dangerous and beyond what they can handle. Finally, we decided to prioritize cases on a first come, first serve basis, with some flexibility to accommodate cases that are in need of immediate help. This decision was based on our wish to avoid ranking the (espoused) needs of mothers who have asked us to help them.

Toward our opening, we readied core processes, including training, supervision, and evaluation. We also prepared the organizational material we would need in the course of running the project, so that we would be ready to start training, matching, pairing, and supervising as soon as we opened our doors. This material included succinct and catchy abstracts to distribute to professionals and laypersons, a manual to accompany the training sessions, advertising material (e.g., posters and flyers, business cards, budget spreadsheets) and questionnaires used to obtain participants' evaluations of the project. Of especial importance was the creation of the spreadsheet endearingly called "the demo," which essentially tracks each mom and volunteer and also lists their contact information for easy access. Also essential was the creation of a Statistical Package for the Social Sciences (SPSS) file into which we enter data related to participants' demographics, dates of beginning and end of visits, feedback gleaned from evaluation forms, presenting problems, family and personal risk factors (e.g., mothers' health issues), and availability of other sources of support, among other information. This file and "the demo" are updated at least weekly and are the basis of analyses reported here.

As a final step in our planning stage, we organized a brunch for the heads of family-centered projects in the city. This was our way of thanking those who had helped us in our planning stage, of introducing ourselves to professionals in the community whom we had not yet met, and for transmitting our desire to network and work together toward a common goal of helping families. The connections made in that forum were important ones, and they have remained strong over time despite changes in personnel. The brunch also was a good way to celebrate the end of our planning stage and begin the next stage of implementation.

The Birth

Encouraged and ready, we opened our doors to a sliver and enlisted good friends, whom we asked to be our first home visitors. The locale of training was the home of the first author (M. K.), and we trained around the kitchen table. Then, with processes in place and our first volunteers trained and waiting, we began to advertise the project in community papers, well-baby clinics, and hospitals in the area. Referrals began to roll in; mothers called, and we were officially off and running. M. K. took the first mother and M. C. took the second, then subsequent referrals were matched with the other volunteers. In short order, we hired a student to man the phone lines and enter data into "the demo" and SPSS file. We began to train on a regular basis, provide supervision, and reach out to a wider circle of resources. We gained recognition by giving interviews to the media that had regarded our project, since its inception, as a *nice* one that can temper turmoil that often marks news of daily life in Israel.

At this point in time, we also found another "home" in which to train and run supervision groups. For this, we connected with the municipality that offered us rooms, free of charge, in a community center in the middle of town. The office and phone lines of M2M were and still are located in M. K.'s lab in Hebrew University, so that research assistants and M2M staff share facilities, thus affording the two teams opportunities to learn from each other. The sharing of space has enabled cross talk between students and staff working on varied projects, and this has enriched the experience for all. Notably, Hebrew University administers the financial end of M2M, for the price of "overhead," and this allows the project to be a tax writeoff for donors.

"Postpartum"

As our reputation as a quality project has spread, requests from professionals to disseminate the project to areas outside Jerusalem have burgeoned. In response, we have written up a "to-do" manual that describes the initial steps to set up a branch of M2M and designed a training and supervision protocol to help new directors get the project off of the ground. We now have branches of M2M and offshoots (e.g., mothers' support groups, play groups) in cities and communities throughout Israel. Some of the branches are integral parts of municipal services; others are located in community centers or universities. What they have in common is that the head of the project and/or the staff members were trained by us, or by professionals trained by us; the projects aim to support mothers with young infants; and their services are provided free of charge.

The expansion of M2M sites allows directors and staff members of the different projects to work as a network—passing on volunteers and moms to the most fitting locale, and sharing knowledge and skills. We also share our experience and expertise with directors and personnel of other family-centered projects and institutions. Shared activities include giving lectures and seminars on the project and its development. In addition, students from the Hebrew University, the Open University, David Yellin College, and Bar Ilan University have received academic credit for their participation in the project or for their use of M2M data for seminar papers or theses.

Processes and Implementation

Intakes

Intakes constitute the first face-to-face meeting that coordinators have with volunteers and mothers who have requested support from the project. The meetings are usually one-on-one and take place in the mother's or volunteer's home. Intakes provide coordinators with the opportunity to explain the project to potential participants and to begin to get to know them and for them to get to know us. Intakes of mothers are aimed at explaining the goals of M2M and the "mandate" of volunteers.

The coordinators also can use the time to assess the safety of the home venue for the volunteer and home visiting. During intakes, mothers are asked pointed questions about their needs, what they would like to gain from the project, and their preferences for a volunteer. Those women who are interested in joining the project provide demographic information as well the name and number of professionals (social workers, psychiatrists), who are in contact with them "at present." In most cases, we contact the professionals to say that we are "in the picture," but mostly we keep the information on file in case of a crisis that is beyond the capability of M2M to deal with (e.g., sudden homelessness, psychotic breakdown, threat of or actual violence in the home). For volunteers, the intake is done before training, and is the start of what we hope will be a long lasting relationship with M2M. The intake provides the volunteers with an opportunity to talk freely about themselves and to tell us why they want to volunteer in M2M. For both mothers and volunteers, intakes are the gateway to the project, and we use them to reduce participants' anxieties by answering questions candidly so that training (for volunteers) and home visiting (for mothers and volunteers) can start out on the right foot.

Training

The primary aims of training are to become familiar with M2M, to bond with the project, to develop a relationship with staff members and other volunteers, to reflect on processes that make relationships happen, and to practice home-visiting skills. For these purposes, the course is highly interactive and, practically speaking, it is 8 hours long, scheduled 2 hours per session, for 4 consecutive weeks, with the participation of four to eight volunteers in each group. Days and times of the course are scheduled according to preferences of the participants, with most scheduled during evening hours (20:00–22:00) to accommodate volunteers who work full time and those who have young children. A training booklet accompanies the course and is used as a reference during training and home visiting.

The course introduces the program and personnel to the volunteers and takes them through first contacts with a mother seeking support, solving problems *with* the mother and not *for* the mother, and finally teaches some observational skills. Specifically, the first session introduces coordinators to the new volunteers and the volunteers to each other, to the coordinators, and to the project as a whole. To facilitate this, we ask volunteers to share an experience that they had in the months that followed the birth of one of their children, and then we talk about sources of support that were particularly helpful to them at that time. This exercise is a good start to getting acquainted, prompts a discussion of the meaning of support, and raises questions as to what makes for effective support and why it is so important for our well-being. It also "ups" the intimacy level between volunteers. In the first session, we also facilitate an exercise that demands active listening (without speaking), which affords participants a chance to practice *really* listening to another person, which is central to their home-visiting job. This listening task involves pairing up volunteers and giving each member of the pair 2 minutes to speak, without the other speaking at all, though the other can express emotions through nonverbal cues. Then they switch roles. Volunteers are surprised that refraining from speaking promotes real listening. Some are quite challenged during their "quiet time," and this can be a powerful experience for them. The second training session focuses on the volunteer's first phone call to the mom in which she introduces herself and negotiates a time and day for their first meeting. Volunteers also role-play a first visit with a mom, so that they can practice and acclimate to their role. We spend time on these introductory meetings, because first impressions can be lasting ones (Bar, 2007; Bar, Neta, & Linz, 2006), and it is important for the "pair" to get off on the right foot, so to speak. In the third session, we talk about stress and present a model for solving problems *with* someone instead of *for* the person. The volunteers then practice using the method in interactive exercises with structured scenarios that might arise in real life. Using these exercises, among others, volunteers can practice their role as a home visitor, reflect on their feelings, and receive feedback from their trainer and other volunteers. The fourth and final session focuses on social cues that help us get to know another person. For this, we watch video clips of mother–child play interactions in an effort to hone observational skills and learn about features of interactions, such as the synchrony and shared affect that predict secure attachment and healthy development. Finally, we discuss "barriers to home visiting" such as the ones listed in Table 11.1.

As in the Boston-based project, our training sessions are facilitated by the project coordinators. We all attend the first session; the other sessions are split among us. This roster is important, because it affords each coordinator ample opportunity to get to know the new volunteers, which is imperative for being able to effectively match them with a client after training. Likewise, the roster offers the volunteers opportunities to get acquainted with the staff members, which is an essential first step for bonding with us and with the project. To nurture these connections, we take special care to transmit our thankfulness to the volunteers for their participation

TABLE 11.1. Barriers to Home Visiting and a Sample of Issues Discussed in Supervision

Barriers between volunteers and moms

1. Difficulties in maintaining comfortable and appropriate personal borders
2. Bad match
3. Clash of values between volunteer and client
4. Personal issues interfere with the home-visiting schedule and emotional availability
5. Interpersonal style

Barriers from moms

6. Client's lack of commitment
7. Problem trusting others
8. Difficulties in focusing on relevant Mom2Mom issues

Barriers from volunteers

9. Espousing solutions
10. Frustration at no or slow progress
11. Unclear why mother needs Mom2Mom support

both in our words and actions. We encourage interactions between volunteers, so that they will get to know each other and form a relationship between themselves. In the end, we hope that the group meetings are demonstrations that no special skills are necessary to forge ties with another. Availability, sensitivity, consistency, and mindfulness are the keys.

Supervision

Supervision in M2M is "reflective," which means that the sessions provide a secure base in which volunteers can step back from their field experiences and take time to process them (Gilkerson, 2004). Through reflection, volunteers can assess their own performance and become aware of their strengths, limits, and vulnerabilities, which in turn promotes realistic and effective strategic decisions regarding the directions that they should take to help the mother they visit (Ruch, 2005). Reflection also prompts volunteers to consider the mother's perspective of her own life and the reason that she turned to M2M. In this way, the volunteer can speak to her mom on the mother's own terms, from her own belief system and principles, without judgment; and this fosters sensitive responsiveness on the part of the volunteer and trust on the part of the mother who is seeking support.

We consider a well-functioning supervision group to be one whose members work as a team to support each participant's feelings about the work and the issues that arise. As a team, the participants work to identify appropriate next steps, empathize with difficulties, and rejoice in each other's successes. The role of the supervisor in this process is to help the supervisees answer their own questions and to provide the support and knowledge necessary to guide healthy decision making. The issues listed in Table 11.1 are among the important themes that are discussed thoroughly and frequently revisited in supervision sessions. During these discussions, the supervisor serves as an empathetic and nonjudgmental sounding board for the supervisees, in the hope that they will provide the same to each other. Working through complex emotions in a "safe place" allows the supervisees to freely explore their feelings, and the security derived from the relationship with the supervisor and the group as a whole can reduce stress in the field (Bennett & Saks, 2006; Pistole & Watkins, 1995; Watkins, 1995; see review in Watkins & Riggs, 2012). It also allows the supervisees to experience the same sort of relationship that we hope they will nurture with the mothers they visit (also see Jarrett & Barlow, 2014). Supervisors also support home visitors by using supervisory meetings as opportunities to acquire new knowledge. One way of doing this is to encourage supervisees to analyze their own work and its implications. Another way is to discuss topics associated with home visiting that can enrich the volunteers' knowledge base and experiences (e.g., new applications of attachment theory to clinical endeavors, new therapeutic advances, and relevant research findings about children and development). Practically speaking, monthly group supervision is required of all home visitors in our project, and to encourage attendance, we offer supervision on several days, at several times, and in a locale that is easy to reach by public transportation. If, despite this, a volunteer cannot make a session, supervision may take the form of a phone or private meeting, so that, at the very least, the coordinators receive an update, and volunteers can download their feelings.

Staff Meetings

For many years, M2M staff meetings have been held once a week, at the same time and in the same place (a university office). The primary goal of the meetings is to assign mothers who have called or were referred in the past week to the coordinators; match mothers with volunteers, and split between us whatever other tasks are on the agenda. Such tasks might include meeting with professionals who are interested in starting a project in their place of work or in their community, advising a student who seeks consultation about a study or thesis, or the planning of peripheral activities such as our coming roundtable meeting that is aimed at gathering together heads of family-centered projects in Jerusalem for networking and strategic planning. Once or twice a year, the coordinators plan a special staff meeting to consider new processes or revisit old ones that need to be revised.

Staff meetings, like supervision and training, are reflective. We reflect on ourselves and our feelings regarding any aspects of the project or our lives that seem relevant or worthy of mention. At least 15 minutes are devoted to talking about our personal lives, which draws us close and keeps us informed.

Matching

The coordinators agree that the most fun part of our work is matching moms with volunteers. Likely, this is because the addition of a new pair to our "active list" marks the end of a long process that began with the mother's call, followed by an intake in the mom's home, the search for and negotiations with a volunteer, and the OK from both mother and volunteer to give it a try. Hope is inherent in the process: hope that the pair will work, hope that it is a new beginning of a close relationship, and hope that volunteer and mother will gain from participation in the project and their time together.

Matching is not a simple process, because it takes into account many complex factors, some related to logistics and others that have to do with the individuals themselves and their life stories. Logistics are the easy part, and the general rule is to try to pair women who live close to each other, so that the volunteers do not waste time on the road. This is not only important for our volunteers who depend on public transportation, but it also is true for those with cars, since time is precious and we do not pay for gas or auto upkeep. With this, some clients may voice concerns about working with a volunteer from their neighborhood, because they may have common friends and would feel uncomfortable running into each other outside of the home-visiting context. Other requests may include a preference for a volunteer with a similar belief system (religiosity), because it relates to so many important and basic issues inside and outside the home, including dietary restrictions and the style of clothes deemed appropriate for wearing in public. Women also may have a certain age range in mind for their volunteer, particularly if they are seeking a mother figure or a friend who is a young mother herself. Language also is an issue, since some of the mothers in the program are new immigrants who want a home visitor who speaks their mother tongue. In all cases, we try to match women who we think will "dance" well together—either because their speed, tempo, and rhythm are the same or complementary or, in keeping with the analogy, because they know or like the same "music."

It should be noted here that sometimes we intuitively feel that a match is a good one, and sometimes we are less than sure, even though it is the best option that we have available. In the latter circumstance, we make the match with some trepidation but hold firm to the belief that a bond will form between volunteer and mother if visiting conditions are right (consistency, openness to the relationship, sensitivity, mindfulness), and if they both want it to happen. By the same token, a seemingly excellent match can go wayward, if conditions do not foster a close relationship between visitor and mom. This can happen for many reasons, most frequently because the mother is not emotionally ready or able to work on nurturing *another* new relationship (besides the one with her infant) or she cannot commit to weekly visits because of her busy schedule, or because commitment is generally difficult for her or she feels that she cannot focus on her emotional needs because the challenges she is facing are too overwhelming. Sometimes, these mothers reconsider; other times they do not. Sometimes they miss the opportunity with their first child but join after the birth of their second.

Evaluations

Evaluations of our project take three forms. The first comprises case reports of mothers who joined the project. These case reports illustrate the processes by which gains are made within the framework of M2M and help identify factors that may interfere with the development of a relationship between mom and volunteer. The second means of evaluation is based on empirical data reflecting our progress, including a tally of total intakes, matches, and volunteers trained each year. The third method of evaluation is based on data derived from feedback of mothers and volunteers on the questionnaire that we administer at the end of the visiting period. The questionnaire has three parts. One part assesses mothers' global satisfaction with the project and is calculated as the mean of ratings on two scales (rating 1 for low to 5 for high): (1) Are you glad that you joined the project? and (2) Would you recommend the project to someone else? The second part of the questionnaire taps mothers' perception of the closeness of the relationship between volunteer and mother, and it is derived by averaging mothers' ratings (1 for none to 5 for a great deal) on four items: (1) intimacy of the relationship with the volunteer, (2) fit of match with volunteer, (3) difficulty in separating from the volunteer, and (4) "closeness" between volunteer and mom. The third and final part of the questionnaire comprises 14 rating scales (1 for none to 5 for a great deal) referring to potential gains (e.g., increased self-confidence) resulting from the home-visiting experience. From these scales, a measure of Overall Gains is derived, and for more detail, measures of Gains on two internally consistent factors: Personal Gains (e.g., mood, confidence) and Gains in Child Care and Child Understanding (e.g., valuing the infant more). All three measures of Gains are derived by calculating the average score across relevant items. All Gain items are listed in Table 11.2. For presentation, we have collapsed the 5-point Gain scales into 3-point scales (rating 1–2, 3, 4–5) because of the low counts in some of the cells. In all, the aim of these three modes of evaluation is to derive empirical data on (1) what mothers gain from the project, (2) whether the mothers are generally satisfied with the project, and (3) whether mothers' feelings of closeness with their volunteer predict mothers' satisfaction and their gains.

Analyses of the data ($N = 226$; 40% of the total) suggest that, overall, mothers are very satisfied with the project (mean rating = 4.61, $SD = .92$) and develop a close relationship with their home visitor (mean rating = 3.95, $SD = .75$) Furthermore, the women who filled out the questionnaire reported moderate to strong "gains" across 14 domains (see Table 11.2). According to mean ratings, the most notable gains are in terms of feeling less isolated and more positive. Interestingly, items having to do with self (bold, in Table 11.2) were rated higher than the ratings of gains on items related to their infant: mean, SD: 3.67, 1.11 vs. 3.11, 1.31, respectively; repeated measures general linear model, $F(1, 225) = 63.22$, $p = .001$. This latter finding may be related to the fact that a substantial proportion (39.7%) of participants were multiparae and therefore, already highly experienced in caregiving before they joined the project.

TABLE 11.2. Gain Items Listed on Evaluation Forms, Mean Ratings of Each One, and Percent of the Sample That Rated Each Item as Low (Rating 1–2), Moderate (Rating 3), or High (Rating 4–5)

Gains from M2M	Mean	Percent mothers ($N = 226$)		
		Low	Moderate	High
Feel less isolated	**3.99 (1.23)**	5.3	25.3	73.7
Be more positive	**3.98 (1.24)**	6.6	19.8	73.2
Comfort with feelings	**3.85 (1.30)**	8.6	21.6	69.8
Self-worth	**3.73 (1.37)**	11.7	24.7	63.6
Self-confidence	**3.68 (1.45)**	14.5	20.6	64.8
Get out of the house	**3.44 (1.53)**	17.4	26.8	55.7
Reduce anxiety	**3.41 (1.42)**	15.7	28.3	57.1
Solve problems	**3.43 (1.33)**	11.9	31.0	56.4
Trust others	**3.12 (1.43)**	21.0	31.1	47.9
Meet infant's needs	3.09 (1.51)	24.6	28.3	47.1
Value infant	3.06 (1.58)	27.3	27.3	45.5
Reach resources	**3.04 (1.69)**	32.8	20.1	47.0
Learn caregiving	3.03 (1.43)	22.0	37.1	40.9
Sensitivity to baby	2.94 (1.55)	30.9	25.9	43.2

Note. **Bold type** identifies items related to Self; regular type identifies items related to Infant.

As predicted, the relations between (scores reflecting) the closeness of the mother–volunteer relationship and mothers' satisfaction and gains were highly significant: Spearman r's = .49, p = .0001; .58, p = .0001, respectively. These findings are important for us, because they examined a basic tenet of the project, which states that the benefits that mothers derive from the project are related to the support garnered from the relationship with their volunteer.

Together, our evaluative data suggest that mothers benefit from M2M, mostly in the extent to which they see themselves in a positive light. The data also are consistent with the contention that M2M is attachment-based and, accordingly, that the benefits procured by mothers are related to forging a close and secure relationship with their volunteer.

From the beginning of the project, we accumulated evaluative data, because it was important for us to receive immediate feedback about the project. We chose the format, reasoning that questions that directly probed women's satisfaction with and benefits derived from the project were the most efficient route to take at that time. Though a more sophisticated approach using a randomized control design (Concato, Shah, & Horwitz, 2000) and a broader spectrum of outcome measures, including symptoms of depression, maternal behavioral sensitivity, and stress, would be very informative, the questionnaire that that we have relied on until now has content validity and offers insight into our efficacy in running the project and the benefits that women derive from it (Sackett, Rosenberg, Gray, Haynes, & Richardson, 1996). It also is within our budget.

Annual Data, Diversity, and Dissemination

According to our annual data, there has been a steady accumulation of referrals and training groups over the years. These data are presented visually in Figure 11.1 (A and B), and they reflect a "caseload" of 30–40 pairs in the field at any given time, with another 5–15 in various stages of the matching and pairing process. At present, this load represents the maximum that the project can handle given its staff and resources, and still provide quality supervision and backup for volunteers in the field.

Table 11.3, showing the demographics of a sample of mothers (N = 567) and volunteers (N = 235) who have participated in the project since 2000, indicates that it is used by a broad spectrum of women. In this regard, 11.7% of the mothers and 11.0% of the volunteers described themselves as ultraorthodox. This is impressive because members of that sector tend to isolate themselves from the general population and, if they volunteer, tend to do so within their own community. We also point out the high proportion (12.0%) of young volunteers (ages 20–29 years), most with young children, and the significant proportion (25.3%) of volunteers who work full time. More than half of mothers and volunteers were born in Israel; the others were immigrants from all over the world (North America, South America, West Europe, East Europe, Russia and the USSR, Australia and New Zealand, Eastern Asia, West Africa, South Africa). Sixty-one percent of the women who have used us for support were first-time mothers, and, across the sample, parity ranged from 1 to 14.

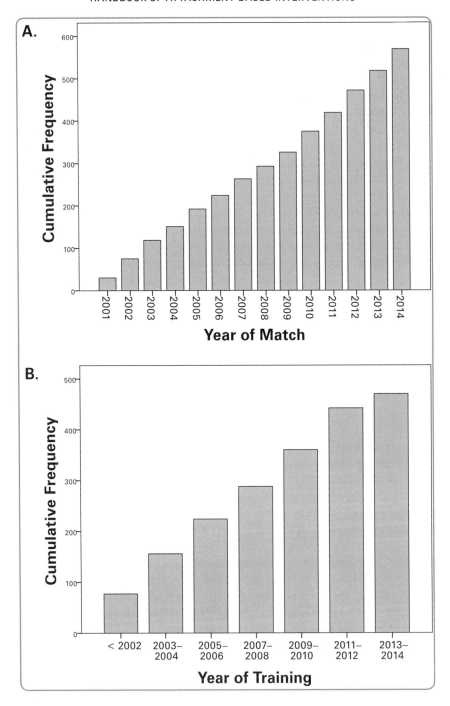

FIGURE 11.1. (A) Cumulative frequency of pairs in the field. (B) Cumulative frequency of training groups.

TABLE 11.3. Select Demographics of Volunteers (*N* = 225) and Mothers (*N* = 567) in the Program

	Volunteers	Mothers		Volunteers	Mothers
Age			**Religiosity**		
Mean	44.38	32.86	Secular (Jewish, non-Jew)	34.9	32.7
Range	21–78	18–56	Religious/traditional	54.1	55.6
< 20	0	1.2	Ultra-Orthodox	11.0	11.7
20–29	12.0	34.3	**Occupation**		
30–39	31.3	47.3	Housewife	3.3	3.6
40–59	17.2	17.1	Health related	21.1	10.3
60+	39.5	0.0	Clerk, secretary	17.4	27.7
Education			Teacher	25.4	24.1
< High school	0	1.7	Academic, lawyer	9.4	13.9
High school	8.0	14.9	Independent, student	10.8	13.3
Professional training	17.3	17.5	Police, army	0.9	1.0
BA	47.3	27.1	Social services	11.3	5.1
Graduate	27.4	17.1	Manual labor	0.5	1.0
No. of children			**Work status**[a]		
Mean	3.12	1.63	Unsalaried/retired/mat	39.3	40.0
Range	1–14	1–14	**Work time**		
1	14.9	61.3	Part time	35.4	16.5
2–4	57.4	33.7	Full time	25.3	43.5
4–6	22.1	3.7	**Immigrants**		
6 +	5.5	1.4	Non-natives	45.7	39.4
Family status					
Married/cohabitating	86.4	76.5			
Single/divorced/widowed	13.6	23.5			

[a]Work status at the time of intake, includes maternity leave (mat).

Diversity also is seen in the presenting issues of the mothers who join the project. As noted in Table 11.4, nearly one-fourth of mothers were single at the time of enrollment, and nearly one-third had mental health problems, according to the mothers themselves or the professional who referred them. Approximately one-third (35.2%) were listed as recipients of social services from the Department of Social Welfare. Also notable is the high prevalence of pregnancies induced after fertility treatments (7.3%) and the percentage of women with twins, triplets, or quadruplets (9.0%).

We also mention that most (64.1%) of our volunteers take on one mom after another, which, we believe, speaks to the meaningfulness of their home-visiting experience. In fact, 22.2% of volunteers have taken on two mothers in succession; 11.6% have taken on three; and 21.3% have taken on four to nine.

Figure 11.2 shows the number of branches founded in the country until now, including four branches located in and around Jerusalem (Modiin, Maale Adumim, Mate Binyamin, and the central headquarters in the center of the city). Besides these, there are 10 branches in the center of the country, five in the south, and eight in the north. Notably, some of the branches are considered "cousins" rather than offspring, as they were direct products of a training course for coordinators, offered in Oranim College, under the supervision of Daphna Noyman, MSW. At present, four new branches of M2M are in various stages of development and not yet marked on the map (Figure 11.2).

Challenges

There are many challenges in our work. Some of them are related to inherent features of the project, for instance, issues related to the fact that our home visitors are community-based volunteer mothers (also see Hiatt, Sampson, & Baird, 1997). Others are acute problems, for example, having to do with a particularly difficult case or a problematic mother–volunteer pair. A third category of challenges has to do with the administration and management of the project. We discuss here a few of the leading challenges.

TABLE 11.4. Issues Raised during Intakes of Mothers and Their Prevalence in the Sample ($N = 567$)

1. Isolation/loneliness	66.5%
2. Poverty	50.9%
3. Pregnancy complications[a]	35.8%
4. Mothers' mental health	31.7%
6. Infants' health (postpartum)	18.1%
7. Mothers' physical health	10.0%

Note. More than one issue could be listed for each mother.
[a]Includes *in vitro* fertilization, multiple fetuses.

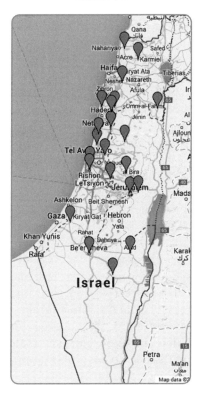

FIGURE 11.2. Branches of Mom2Mom as of January 2015. From Google.

Volunteer Home Visitors

Using volunteer home visitors means that we cannot demand work-hours, but rather depend on the volunteers to understand the necessity of meeting frequently and regularly with their moms in order to develop their relationship. Volunteers take vacations, have family obligations, and change work schedules; and these or other time-limiting factors can interfere with the home-visiting schedule, which can degrade the volunteer–mother relationship and sometimes stymie it altogether. Volunteers may take incidents personally, become dysregulated by their moms' distress, become frustrated by a lack of progress, and may find themselves at a loss as what to do and how to do it in order to help the mothers they visit (see Table 11.1). For all this, the staff members need to be available to the volunteers, supervise them, and monitor the progress of visits carefully. For their part, the volunteers need to trust that the staff members are there for them and use them as a source of support and backup as needed.

Related to these issues are problems that arise because some volunteers are more difficult to train than others. This is sometimes because of volunteers' tendency to act first and reflect later, or because their interpersonal style is more authoritarian than the style that we encourage (Hiatt et al., 1997). Difficulties also may be related to the volunteers' own insecure attachment style, as noted by others (Pistole & Watkins, 1995). Though role playing, feedback, supervision, and exercises in reflection go far in demonstrating "another way," old habits are often difficult to break, and coordinators can find themselves repeatedly trying to nurture a more relationship-based stance in some volunteers, with varying degrees of success.

Similarly, we find that some volunteers are easier to match to a mom than others (also see Lutz & Lakey, 2001). Again, this could be due to their interpersonal style (Hiatt et al., 1997) or because of logistical issues, such as the volunteer's limited free time. In addition, we are very careful not to pair volunteers with particularly difficult cases if they themselves are dealing with considerable challenges in their own lives. By the same token, some volunteers specifically request mothers with complex histories and circumstances, because they want to be absolutely certain why they are "there." For these reasons and others, it can take weeks to find a good match for a particular volunteer, and during that time, she may become disappointed, angry, or sad that she has not been matched as quickly as she thought she would be. In this context, we also mention special challenges in training and supervising volunteers who are themselves professionals who work with families in their day jobs (e.g., doctors, social workers, psychologists), because their habits of dealing with "cases" may be more directive then the kind of support that we offer in M2M. Helping these volunteers to make a shift in their heads and behavior toward a more relationship-based and reflective style during home visits is not always easy. Nonetheless, it is our hope that the experiences these professionals gain in M2M will enhance their professionalism both within and outside the home-visiting project, and the feedback that we receive from these professionals suggests that it does.

Mothers/Clients

Another set of challenges centers on the moms (i.e., the clients), who, by definition, have an infant under the age of 1. Given the exhaustion and workload associated with caregiving for a young infant, it can be difficult for our mothers to focus on feelings or to consider their own emotional needs, especially if they are dealing with entrenched and multiple problems in their lives. Not a few mothers in the project have had trouble committing to the home-visiting relationship because they have issues with trust. We also know well that mental health issues, and sometimes the side effects of medication, may challenge mothers' ability to commit to home visits and to participate in building a relationship with their home visitor. Mothers may overstep bounds and ask their volunteer to do chores or share in other activities that are outside of the home-visiting mandate, and this can put volunteers in a difficult position; furthermore, a negative response by the volunteer to the mothers' request can undermine and derail their relationship, especially if it is a new pair at the start of their "journey" together.

Administration and Management

Other challenges have to do with administration and management of the project. The two biggest challenges in these domains are budgetary restrictions and the constant attempt to balance quality and quantity. In this context, *quality* is defined as the degree to which M2M serves as a reliable source of support for mothers with young infants and succeeds in helping mothers to feel better about themselves, bond with their infant, and be better able to cope with the issues that they are facing. *Quantity* is defined as the number of training groups that we are running, the number of active pairs in the field, and the breadth of related activities in which we are involved. As caregivers of the project, we are cognizant of the fact that an imbalance (quantity > quality) can mean that we are spread too thin, which makes quality supervision difficult and may cause time delays in our responses to questions or problems that may arise in the field. With all that, it is very difficult to limit the size of the project, because that entails refusing women who call us for help.

Future Plans and Dreams

Networking and expansion are the focus of our future plans. In this section, we describe some of these plans and also our dreams, roughly ordered from the ones that are in process and require relatively small modifications in the structure or content of M2M to those that we dream of and that entail more substantial change.

Plans that are in progress include expanding the window of home visiting, so that it extends to the antenatal period. This modification is being implemented because the antenatal period can be an anxious time for women (Kaitz & Katzir, 2004), and beginning home visiting then would offer them a time for mindful contemplation, guided and supported by their volunteer. Furthermore, a volunteer's presence and help from the start of the transition period, including childbirth, is a wonderful way to begin the mom–volunteer relationship, as we have seen in a number of pairs that began prior to delivery. This change in the time frame for home visits requires expanding outreach to professionals who care for women during pregnancy and to places that women frequent during pregnancy (e.g., antenatal ultrasound clinics). The expansion also requires some modification in the supervision and training of volunteers, due to differences in the content and structure of the home visits before and after the infant is born, although the fundamental aims, themes, and strategies of the project would remain the same.

At this time, we also are expanding services offered to clients in M2M by incorporating new and evidence-based intervention models for parents with specific challenges. For this, three coordinators (J. T., J. L., and M. K.) are being trained in Fussy Baby©, created by Professor Linda Gilkerson from Erikson Institute in Chicago, which is geared to parents with colicky and otherwise difficult babies (Gilkerson et al., 2012). One coordinator (M. C.) has been trained in child–parent psychotherapy (CPP), created by Selma Fraiberg in the 1970s and adapted by Professors Alicia Lieberman and Patricia Van Horn from University of California San Francisco, for treatment of persons with a history of trauma (Lieberman & Van Horn, 2005, 2008; see Toth, Michl-Petzing, Guild, & Lieberman, Chapter 13, this volume). A central goal of both models is to support and strengthen caregiver–child relationships and protect or restore mothers' and children's mental health. Also, both models center on processes of mindful reflection, so that their approaches are very much aligned with those of M2M. With the aid of our expanded repertoire of tools, we already are providing some clients in M2M with specialized short-term interventions, in addition to those offered by regular home visiting. For mothers with a history of trauma, we hope that a brief exposure to CPP within M2M will motivate them to seek long-term therapy outside of the project, and we do what we can to see that this happens.

We also mention plans to improve and expand on our strategy for evaluation. Most important for this will be our careful consideration of the outcomes to assess and the methods by which to assess them. At present, our nominations for outcomes fall within two time windows: just after home visiting and a year later, to assess the stability of skills and state (well-being) of mother and child. At the first time point, we would continue to assess gains of mothers by subjective reports but would add objective indices, such as the degree of order in the household, as assessed by the Home Observation for Measurement of the Environment (HOME) questionnaire (Caldwell & Bradley, 1979), and maternal sensitivity, as observed during caregiving or structured or free-play mother–infant interactions, using one of the available Maternal Sensitivity Scales (e.g., Feldman, 1998).

For longer term outcomes, we would ask again about gains to determine whether they were sustained over time. We also would add indices that speak directly to infants' developmental outcomes, such as infants' self-regulation and physical health (e.g., Bayley, 2006). For all measures, we would utilize reliable and valid tools to assess them. In addition to these efforts, we need to find ways to up the percent return of the questionnaires so that our data reflect answers from a larger, representative sample. According to our analyses, women who filled out evaluations were more educated than those who did not, but they did not differ in age, marital status, or indices of risk (e.g., low socioeconomic status [SES], use of social services).

Closely aligned are plans to analyze in more detail the data collected so far. Such analyses could impart information on factors that contribute to the variation in Gains and Satisfaction of the mothers in the project and the conditions that make M2M most and least effective (see Weiss, Bloom, & Brock, 2014). They also could address more complex questions, such as whether mothers from high-risk families benefit more from the project if their home visitor is experienced and professional (i.e., works with families in her day job). On the one hand, high-risk families may find it difficult to trust a professional, if they have had uncomfortable dealings with social services in the past; on the other hand, a professional with experience may be more helpful to a family facing complex and difficult problems (Hiatt et al., 1997). These data would be informative to others who are involved in home-visiting projects, and publication of the findings would be a good means of disseminating information about M2M.

Also important at this time are plans for knitting our own M2M branches more closely together for mutual support and education. In this regard, we dream of adding a professional to the staff whose job would be to travel between branches, testing their efficacy and fidelity to the M2M model, networking, and providing backup and support to directors, as needed. Toward the same goals, we would like to bring the directors together for informative seminars and conferences as well as "play days," so that we can support each other, as the volunteers do for their moms, and as coordinators do for the volunteers. In effect, we would be adding a new dimension to our logo of concentric circles that represents the combined metasupport fostered by all the branches, mutually supporting each other.

We also are continuing to push ahead with plans to integrate M2M into larger, existing systems, so that M2M is more accessible to those who may benefit from its services (see Shonkoff, 2010). In this context, integration means that M2M would be formally included on the "map" of resources in the city and country, so that all women who could benefit from more support and are willing to hear about the project would be automatically referred to it before or after the birth of their children. From there, coordinators would call the mother and offer explanations and schedule an intake, if the mother is interested. In fact, we dream of making our intakes the gateway for many possible interventions for families, as in large-scale programs being implemented in the United States as part of the national effort to strengthen families (e.g., Maternal, Infant, and Early Childhood Home Visiting (MIECHV; *mchb.hrsa.gov/programs/home visiting*). In this way, Jerusalem-based professionals who are working with children and families could operate collaboratively. This, in turn, would facilitate referrals, enhance the effectiveness of individual outreach efforts, and ensure that families get what they need when they need it.

On our dream list is the founding of playgroups for fathers (e.g., see Guterman, 2012) that would offer dads company, support, and a safe place outside their homes to "hang out" with their infants. This project has not been funded yet, and we are still looking for a father who is willing to come on board as a group leader. Though one solution to the budgetary problem would be to integrate fathers into the already established (women-only) play groups, women in the groups have objected to the inclusion of men, because they say that they would not be comfortable talking about intimate topics in front of men they do not know; among some religious women, it is also forbidden. Furthermore, nursing would become impossible for many women in an integrated group. For these reasons, we need to either establish men-only groups or even better (in our opinion), find some way for mothers in our play groups to perceive fathers who want to join the groups as parents first, and men second.

Finally, we dream of bringing M2M to communities in which there is a large proportion of Arab Israelis and to Arab communities beyond the Green line (the demarcation lines that effectively divide Israel proper from areas disputed with Arab neighbors). This expansion would require considerable thought in regard to logistics, content, and security. However, with funding, we would be willing to try despite the challenges, because we would love to see M2M as a vehicle of peace, "driven" by a cohort of mothers caring for other mothers, who need their help.

Summary

We offer the services of M2M to mothers of young infants who need more support than they have available to them. The aim of the project is to strengthen mothers and their families by pairing them with a volunteer home visitor for up to a year after childbirth. According to attachment theory, the "hug" afforded by such a partnership, bound in trust and understanding, empowers, validates, and provides an excellent venue for mindfully sorting out the complexities that may arise after a new baby is born into the family. Evidence from data collected from participants thus far attests to mothers' gains in the project and their satisfaction with it. Challenges, plans, and dreams abound, including expansion of the project to the antenatal period and to dads. In the future, we hope to see M2M used as a hub for referrals and for training and supervision of professionals working with families. In this way, M2M could work most effectively toward the best interests of society, which should prioritize the health and well-being of mothers, fathers, infants, and families (see Harris et al., 2007).

ACKNOWLEDGMENTS

M2M is supported by a grant from the Irving Harris Foundation, Chicago, Illinois; the C & L Foundation; and The Elia & Fannie Karas Foundation.

We thank our supporters and the Jerusalem-based board of the Harris Foundation for their support from the inception of the project and professionals from all over the city and country for their trust in us. We also thank the mothers who join the project. We are indebted to the volunteers, who give freely of their time and themselves, and without whom there would be no M2M. M2M is greatly indebted to the Irving Harris Professional Development Network of passionate, caring, world-class professionals who have designed and directed intervention or prevention programs aimed at reducing risk and fostering resilience of infants and families throughout America and in several sites in Israel. These colleagues have shared their knowledge and have encouraged our efforts every step of our way. The Harris Board in Jerusalem, founded by Professor Charles Greenbaum and Professor Arthur Eidelman, has supported our efforts from the time that M2M was conceived through the present. Many thanks to Professor Julie Cwikel, head of M2M in Beersheba and of the Women's Health Center in Ben Gurion University of the Negev, for her support and friendship. We also acknowledge the annual donations of several Boston-based foundations that have remained solid supporters of M2M through the years.

Staff members (coordinators) of the M2M program are crucial to its ongoing success. Miriam Chriki, a founder of M2M, is a developmental psychologist. Naomi Tessler, a social worker and breast-feeding counselor, joined M2M as a home visitor in 2001 and was hired as a coordinator in 2003. In 2009, Naomi founded and continues to facilitate the weekly M2M play group, located in a community with many young, low SES families. Our newest coordinator, Judith Levy, came to M2M as a volunteer to earn credit toward her BA degree at Hebrew University, then was hired as a staff member in 2014. In addition to working as a project coordinator, Judith is working toward her MA in Early Child Development at Hebrew University. The coordinators are salaried; Marsha Kaitz is not. The four of us make up the Jerusalem-based branch of M2M and wake up each morning with a firm sense of love for the work.

REFERENCES

Ainsworth, M. D. S. (1979). Attachment as related to mother–infant interaction. In J. Rosenblatt, R. Hinde, C. Beer, & M. Bushel (Eds.), *Advances in the study of mother–infant interaction* (Vol. 9, pp. 1–51). New York: Academic Press.

Ainsworth, M. D. S. (1989). Attachments beyond infancy. *American Psychologist, 44,* 709–716.

Ainsworth, M. D. S., Blehar, M. C., Waters, E., & Wall, S. (2014). *Patterns of attachment: A psychological study of the strange situation.* New York: Psychology Press. (Original work published 1978)

Andresen, P. A., & Telleen, S. L. (1992). The relationship between social support and maternal behaviors and attitudes: A meta-analytic review. *American Journal of Community Psychology, 20*, 753–774.

Bar, M. (2007). The proactive brain: Using analogies and associations to generate predictions. *Trends in Cognitive Sciences, 11*, 280–289.

Bar, M., Neta, M., & Linz, H. (2006). Very first impressions. *Emotion, 6*, 269–278.

Bayley, N. (2006). *Bayley Scales of Infant and Toddler Development.* San Antonio, TX: Harcourt Assessment.

Bell, M. A., & Fox, N. A. (1994). Brain development over the first year of life In C. D. Lawson & K. W. Fischer (Eds.), *Human behavior and the developing brain* (pp. 314–345). New York: Guilford Press.

Bennett, S., & Saks, L. V. (2006). Field notes: A conceptual application of attachment theory and research to the social work student–field instructor supervisory relationship. *Journal of Social Work Education, 42*, 669–682.

Bifulco, A., Figueiredo, B., Guedeney, N., Gorman, L. L., Hayes, S., Muzik, M., . . . Henshaw, C. A. (2004). Maternal attachment style and depression associated with childbirth: Preliminary results from a European and US cross-cultural study. *British Journal of Psychiatry, 184*, s31–s37.

Bowlby, J. (1982). *Attachment and loss: Vol. 1. Attachment* (2nd ed.). New York: Basic Books. (Original work published 1969)

Caldwell, B. M., & Bradley, R. H. (1979). *Home observation for measurement of the environment.* Little Rock: University of Arkansas Press.

Clinton, H. (1996). *It takes a village to raise a child.* New York: Touchstone Books.

Cobb, S. (1976). Social support as a moderator of life stress. *Psychosomatic Medicine, 38*, 300–314.

Cohen, S., & Wills, T. A. (1985). Stress, social support, and the buffering hypothesis. *Psychological Bulletin, 98*, 310–357.

Cole, P. M. (2014). Moving ahead in the study of the development of emotion regulation. *International Journal of Behavioral Development, 38*, 203–207.

Concato, J., Shah, N., & Horwitz, R. I. (2000). Randomized, controlled trials, observational studies, and the hierarchy of research designs. *New England Journal of Medicine, 342*, 1887–1892.

Cowan, C. P., & Cowan, P. A. (1995). Interventions to ease the transition to parenthood: Why they are needed and what they can do. *Family Relations, 44*, 412–423.

Cowan, P. A., Cohn, D. A., Cowan, C. P., & Pearson, J. L. (1996). Parents' attachment histories and children's externalizing and internalizing behaviors: Exploring family systems models of linkage. *Journal of Consulting and Clinical Psychology, 64*, 53–63.

Crockenberg, S. B. (1981). Infant irritability, mother responsiveness, and social support influences on the security of infant–mother attachment. *Child Development, 52*, 857–865.

Cutrona, C. E., & Troutman, B. R. (1986). Social support, infant temperament, and parenting self-efficacy: A mediational model of postpartum depression. *Child Development, 57*, 1507–1518.

Donovan, M. K. (2011). Greater than the sum of its parts: An exploration of family home visiting programs involving both volunteer and paid visitors. Retrieved January 5, 2015, from *http://hdl.handle.net/10222/14400.*

Drummond, J. E., Weir, A. E., & Kysela, G. M. (2002). Home visitation programs for at-risk young families: A systematic literature review. *Canadian Journal of Public Health, 93*, 153–158.

Dunkel Schetter, C. (2011). Psychological science on pregnancy: Stress processes, biopsychosocial models, and emerging research issues. *Annual Review of Psychology, 62*, 531–558.

Feeney, J. A. (2002). Attachment, marital interaction, and relationship satisfaction: A diary study. *Personal Relationships, 9,* 39–55.

Feldman, R. (1998). *Coding interactive behavior manual.* Unpublished manuscript, Bar-Ilan University, Ramat Gan, Israel.

Fonagy, P., Steele, H., & Steele, M. (1991). Maternal representations of attachment during pregnancy predict organization of infant–mother attachment at one year of age. *Child Development, 62,* 891–905.

Fox, S. E., Levitt, P., & Nelson, C. A. (2010). How the timing and quality of early experiences influence the development of brain architecture. *Child Development, 81,* 28–40.

Gilkerson, L. (2004). Irving B. Harris distinguished lecture: Reflective supervision in infant–family programs: Adding clinical process to nonclinical settings. *Infant Mental Health Journal, 25*(5), 424–439.

Gilkerson, L., Hofherr, J., Heffron, M. C., Sims, J. M., Jalowiec, B., Bromberg, S. R., & Paul, J. J. (2012). Implementing the Fussy Baby Network® Approach. *ZERO TO THREE, 33,* 59–65.

Goldblatt, M., Yahav, R., & Ricon, T. (2014). Overview of intervention programs for parents of young children (0–6). *Open Journal of Pediatrics, 4,* 185–207.

Guterman, N. B. (2012). Promoting father involvement in home visiting services for vulnerable families: A pilot study (Final Report to Pew Center on the States). Retrieved January 5, 2015, from *www.pewtrusts.org/~/media/legacy/uploadedfiles/pcs_assets/2013/fatherinvolvementexecuti vesummarypdf.pdf.*

Haft, W. L., & Slade, A. (1989). Affect attunement and maternal attachment: A pilot study. *Infant Mental Health Journal, 10,* 157–172.

Harris, W. W., Lieberman, A. F., & Marans, S. (2007). In the best interests of society. *Journal of Child Psychology and Psychiatry, 48,* 392–411.

Hauer, K. E., ten Cate, O., Boscardin, C., Irby, D. M., Iobst, W., & O'Sullivan, P. S. (2014). Understanding trust as an essential element of trainee supervision and learning in the workplace. *Advances in Health Sciences Education, 19,* 435–456.

Hazan, C., & Shaver, P. (1987). Romantic love conceptualized as an attachment process. *Journal of Personality and Social Psychology, 52,* 511–524.

Heinicke, C. M., Ruth, G., Recchia, S. L., Guthrie, D., Rodning, C., & Fineman, N. R. (1999). Relationship-based intervention with at-risk mothers: Outcome in the first year of life. *Infant Mental Health Journal, 20,* 349–374.

Hiatt, S. W., Sampson, D., & Baird, D. (1997). Paraprofessional home visitation: Conceptual and pragmatic considerations. *Journal of Community Psychology, 25,* 77–93.

Hoffman, S., & Hatch, M. C. (1996). Stress, social support and pregnancy outcome: A reassessment based on recent research. *Paediatric and Perinatal Epidemiology, 10,* 380–405.

Isabella, R. A. (1993). Origins of attachment: Maternal interactive behavior across the first year. *Child Development, 64,* 605–621.

Jarrett, P., & Barlow, J. (2014). Clinical supervision in the provision of intensive home visiting by health visitors. *Community Practitioner, 87,* 32–36.

Kaitz, M., Bar-Haim, Y., Lehrer, M., & Grossman, E. (2004). Adult attachment style and interpersonal distance. *Attachment and Human Development, 6,* 285–304.

Kaitz, M., & Katzir, D. (2004). Temporal changes in the affective experience of new fathers and their spouses. *Infant Mental Health Journal, 25,* 540–555.

Karavasilis, L., Doyle, A. B., & Markiewicz, D. (2003). Associations between parenting style and attachment to mother in middle childhood and adolescence. *International Journal of Behavioral Development, 27,* 153–164.

Lakey, B., & Orehek, E. (2011). Relational regulation theory: A new approach to explain the link between perceived support and mental health. *Psychological Review, 118,* 482–495.

Landy, C. K., Jack, S. M., Wahoush, O., Sheehan, D., & MacMillan, H. L. (2012). Mothers' experiences in the Nurse–Family Partnership program: A qualitative case study. *BMC Nursing, 11*, 15–26.

Lieberman, A. F., & Van Horn, P. (2005). *"Don't hit my mommy!": A manual for child–parent psychotherapy with young witnesses of family violence.* Washington, DC: ZERO TO THREE.

Lieberman, A. F., & Van Horn, P. J. (2008). *Psychotherapy with infants and young children: Repairing the effects of stress and trauma on early attachment.* New York: Guilford Press.

Lutz, C. J., & Lakey, B. (2001). How people make support judgments: Individual differences in the traits used to infer supportiveness in others. *Journal of Personality and Social Psychology, 81*, 1070–1079.

McMahon, C., Trapolini, T., & Barnett, B. (2008). Maternal state of mind regarding attachment predicts persistence of postnatal depression in the preschool years. *Journal of Affective Disorders, 107*, 199–203.

Mikulincer, M., & Florian, V. (1998). The relationship between adult attachment styles and emotional and cognitive reactions to stressful events. In J. A. Simpson & W. S. Rholes (Eds.), *Attachment theory and close relationship* (pp. 143–165). New York: Guilford Press.

Mikulincer, M., & Shaver, P. R. (2016). *Attachment in adulthood: Structure, dynamics, and change* (2nd ed.). New York: Guilford Press.

Mikulincer, M., Shaver, P. R., & Pereg, D. (2003). Attachment theory and affect regulation: The dynamics, development, and cognitive consequences of attachment-related strategies. *Motivation and Emotion, 27*, 77–102.

Odgers, C. L., Caspi, A., Russell, M. A., Sampson, R. J., Arsenault, L., & Moffitt, T. E. (2012). Supportive parenting mediates widening neighborhood socioeconomic disparities in children's antisocial behavior from ages 5 to 12. *Development and Psychopathology, 24*, 705–721.

Olds, D. L., Sadler, L., & Kitzman, H. (2007). Programs for parents of infants and toddlers: Recent evidence from randomized trials. *Journal of Child Psychology and Psychiatry, 48*, 355–391.

Paris, R., & Dubus, N. (2005). Staying connected while nurturing an infant: A challenge of new motherhood. *Family Relations, 54*, 72–83.

Paris, R., Gemborys, M. K., Kaufman, P. H., & Whitehill, D. (2007). Reaching isolated new mothers: Insights from a home visiting program using paraprofessionals. *Families in Society: Journal of Contemporary Social Services, 88*, 616–626.

Pistole, M. C., & Watkins, C. E. (1995). Attachment theory, counseling process, and supervision. *The Counseling Psychologist, 23*, 457–478.

Raby, K. L., Lawler, J. M., Shlafer, R. J., Hesemeyer, P. S., Collins, W. A., & Sroufe, L. A. (2015). The interpersonal antecedents of supportive parenting: A prospective, longitudinal study from infancy to adulthood. *Developmental Psychology, 51*, 115–123.

Ruch, G. (2005). Relationship-based practice and reflective practice: Holistic approaches to contemporary child care social work. *Child and Family Social Work, 10*, 111–123.

Sackett, D. L., Rosenberg, W., Gray, J. A., Haynes, R. B., & Richardson, W. S. (1996). Evidence based medicine: What it is and what it isn't. *British Medical Journal, 312*, 71–72.

Segal, L., Opie, R. S., & Dalziel, K. (2012). Theory!: The missing link in understanding the performance of neonate/infant home-visiting programs to prevent child maltreatment: A systematic review. *Milbank Quarterly, 90*, 47–106.

Shonkoff, J. P. (2010). Building a new biodevelopmental framework to guide the future of early childhood policy. *Child Development, 81*, 357–367.

Slade, A. (2002). Keeping the baby in mind: A critical factor in perinatal mental health. *ZERO TO THREE, 22*, 10–16.

Slade, A., Belsky, J., Aber, J. L., & Phelps, J. L. (1999). Mothers' representations of their relationships with their toddlers: Links to adult attachment and observed mothering. *Developmental Psychology, 35*, 611–619.

Stern, D. N. (1995). *The motherhood constellation: A unified view of parent–infant psychotherapy.* New York: Basic Books.

Sweet, M. A., & Appelbaum, M. I. (2004). Is home visiting an effective strategy?: A meta-analytic review of home visiting programs for families with young children. *Child Development, 75,* 1435–1456.

Watkins, C. E., Jr. (1995). Psychoanalytic constructs in psychotherapy supervision. *Clinical Supervisor, 14,* 345–368.

Watkins, C. E., Jr., & Riggs, S. A. (2012). Psychotherapy supervision and attachment theory: Review, reflections, and recommendations. *Clinical Supervisor, 31,* 256–289.

Weiss, M. J., Bloom, H. S., & Brock, T. (2014). A conceptual framework for studying the sources of variation in program effects. *Journal of Policy Analysis and Management, 33,* 778–808.

Wolff, M. S., & van IJzendoorn, M. H. (1997). Sensitivity and attachment: A meta-analysis on parental antecedents of infant attachment. *Child Development, 68,* 571–591.

CHAPTER 12

Video-Feedback Intervention
for Parents of Infants at High Risk
of Developing Autism

JONATHAN GREEN

This chapter begins with a review of the developmental science of caregiver–infant interaction in the context of early autism. The evidence reveals an essentially normal range of attachment dynamics in autism, but suggests how perturbations of early interaction may act to amplify, in transactional fashion, the ongoing risk trajectories in these neurologically vulnerable infants. The chapter then describes how this developmental science provides the rationale for our adaptation of the infancy version of the Video-Feedback Intervention to Promote Positive Parenting (infancy VIPP; see Juffer, Bakermans-Kranenburg, & van IJzendoorn, Chapter 1, this volume), designed, with the agreement of the originators, for intervention with infants at high risk of developing autism (iBASIS-VIPP).[1] The nature of the intervention is described, and evidence is presented for its effect from a published case series and randomized controlled trial (RCT), in the context of other reports of very early intervention in the autism prodrome.

Attachment and Early Development in Autism

Autism as a condition is emergent over the first few years of life and fully manifest from age 3 years or so onwards. Core difficulties include a range of impairments in social understanding, expression, and social reciprocity; as well as a lack of

---

[1] iBASIS-VIPP is different than VIPP-AUTI, which is a separate adaptation of the VIPP-SD (Sensitive Discipline) model for intervention with older preschool children already diagnosed with autism (Poslawsky et al., 2014).

flexibility, leading to rigidity and inflexibility of behaviors, and often disturbances of sensory and perceptual processing. It is one of a range of neurodevelopmental disorders that often show overlapping elements, reflecting varying but fundamental disturbances in neurodevelopment and the neurodevelopmental substrate for social competency.

Although autism may at times confer adaptive advantages and specific skills, individuals are usually disadvantaged in their interpersonal and social life. There remain key questions about the origin of this disadvantage, how it is that early interpersonal processes in autism development become disrupted, and whether enhancement of early interactions could help optimize the child's social adaptation and reduce disability. This is the contemporary context in which early relationships within autism need to be considered. We are long past the idea that primary relational or attachment problems themselves *cause* autism; this was a conceptual error, posited in the mid-20th century, that for many years did harm by holding parents responsible and stigmatizing them for having provided deficient care for their children. Yet intimate affectional bonds are just as necessary in the development of a child with a neurodisability as for any other child, and are worthy of detailed theoretical understanding and clinical care.

Interpersonal disruption for a child with autism potentially starts early enough to be outside parental awareness, but later, parents of an infant or toddler with the emerging disorder may feel perplexed by the subtly different responsiveness of the young child to ordinary social cues and responses. Sometimes, for experienced parents, it will be clear that this is "different" from their experience with a neurotypical child; however, for others, including first-time parents, this can be bemusing. Parents may have a variety of responses including demoralization, frustration, self-blame, and/or active attempts to shape the social interactions themselves; clinical experience suggests that there is no more deeply complex child condition for parents to adjust to.

It seems logical that such difficulties might have an impact on early attachment dynamics, but illuminating empirical work has countered a simple notion of this kind. Early work (Capps, Sigman, & Mundy, 1994) was followed by a Society for Research in Child Development monograph (Vondra & Barnett, 1999) that addressed the important issue of how attachment measures need to be adjusted or calibrated when studying developmental atypicality. Much further work has confirmed that when autism-specific styles of social communication are taken into account, patterns of maternal sensitivity and early childhood attachment in autism show broadly similar variation to those in neurotypically developing children (Koren-Karie, Oppenheim, Dolev, & Yirmiya, 2009; van IJzendoorn et al., 2007). More child attachment insecurity has been associated with higher levels of autism severity and intellectual disability in some studies (Rutgers, Bakermans-Kranenburg, van IJzendoorn, & van Berckelaer-Onnes, 2004) but not in others (Koren-Karie et al., 2009; Willemsen-Swinkels, Bakermans-Kranenburg, Buitelaar, van IJzendoorn, & van Engeland, 2000). Greater cognitive and language impairment in autism may also increase attachment insecurity (Rutgers et al., 2004). Thus, although the presence of autism does not seem to have a substantial impact on the normative range of parental caregiving and infant attachment behaviors as measured in these studies, there may a degree of shift to "insecurity" in some circumstances.

These overall results, however, leave open the question of whether a developing child's difficulties in perception and social understanding might have subtle social interaction consequences that act to compound neurodevelopmental vulnerability. Theory and evidence suggest that much social competency in normative development flows from dyadic mutuality, shared intersubjectivity, and contingent early interactions: Disruption of these processes in children with autism might therefore amplify their social impairment beyond attachment. We are also now used to the idea that this difficulty may operate at the level of brain, as well as psychological development; the lack of contingent social inputs may affect aspects of development of "social brain" networks that are environment expectant. The "interactive specialization" hypothesis (Johnson, 2001; Elsabbagh & Johnson, 2010) gives one account from neuroscience of how this might take place in parallel to psychological aspects.

The possibility that the child with a neurodisability may in this way experience a "double risk" to his or her social development, both from the primary neurodevelopmental vulnerability and its interactive consequences, provides a theoretical rationale for interpersonal intervention in the very early stages of the disorder (Dawson, 2008). But it also raises a number of empirical questions than need to be answered:

1. Can developmental science detect these theoretically postulated, subtle early perturbations in parent–infant interaction?
2. If we find perturbations, what will be their nature? Will they be of the kind observed as precursors of disrupted social development or attachment in neurotypical development—or something different?
3. If we do find early perturbation, would it be possible to intervene to counter this and improve psychological and social outcome? As well as practical clinical benefit, could a successful intervention of this kind also illuminate developmental science by demonstrating causal effects in the interplay among early interaction, early intersubjectivity, and social outcome?

The remainder of this chapter pursues answers to these questions through developmental science and the implementation and testing of an adapted VIPP model (see Juffer et al., Chapter 1, this volume) for infants at risk of developing autism.

Parent–Infant Interaction in the Autism Prodrome

First, is the central question of whether there is any evidence of early perturbation in key aspects of parent–child interaction (PCI) during the autism prodrome. There is considerable support from the general research literature that atypical neurodevelopment (e.g., in Down syndrome, cerebral palsy, or learning disability) can be associated with effectively reduced parental sensitivity to infant behavioral signals and increased "intrusiveness" during interaction (Cardoso-Martins & Mervis, 1985; Crawley & Spiker, 1983). This may result from parents' difficulty in accurately interpreting atypical infant behaviors (Sorce & Emde, 1982; Dunst, 1985; Slonims,

Cox, & McConachie, 2006). Parental structuring of interactions is not necessarily "insensitive" (it might constitute a "sensitive scaffolding" of the vulnerable child), but it could at other times represent overdirectiveness within the interaction, acting to disrupt effective interpersonal reciprocity in infants who are particularly prone to this. Such a nuanced balance between scaffolding, sensitive responding, and directiveness exemplifies the complex task for parents in responding to children who may have intrinsic difficulties in social communication or attentional regulation (Legerstee, Varghese, & van Beek, 2002; Yoder & Warren, 2004; Walden, Blackford, & Carpenter, 1997). Supportive contingent or sensitive parental responsiveness is central to the development of joint attention social skills and language in both typical development (Landry, Smith, Miller-Loncar, & Swank, 1997; National Institute of Child Health and Human Development [NICHD] Early Child Care Research Network, 2001) and communication impairment (Yoder & Warren, 2004), but overcontrol or overdirectiveness without sensitivity risks disrupting contingent social reciprocity and social learning.

Initial retrospective studies of parental home videos of children later diagnosed with autism investigated some of these interaction patterns. Despite the inevitable methodological weaknesses of such a retrospective method, often focused on videotapes of birthday parties or special events, there was an initial suggestion (Saint-Georges et al., 2011) that specific directive behaviors (including longer stimulation and more use of touch to elicit attention) differentiated parents whose infants were later diagnosed with autism spectrum disorder (ASD; $N = 15$) from parents of typically developing infants and infants with intellectual disability.

Our own studies have been able to take advantage of the more rigorous prospective developmental method of studying infants at risk of developing autism by virtue of being siblings of autism probands (so-called "autism baby-sibling" studies). A number of prospective longitudinal, naturalistic baby-sibling studies of this kind have been conducted over the last decade particularly in the United States and the United Kingdom, and have revolutionized understanding of the early neurodevelopmental emergence of autism in the prodrome (Szatmari et al., 2016). Within the United Kingdom, this work has been conducted within the British Autism Study of Infant Siblings (BASIS; *basisnetwork.org*) led by Mark Johnson, a study that now includes over 200 infant siblings followed from early in the first year of life through middle childhood. The studies of early caregiver–infant interaction relevant to this discussion began in 2009 and included babies in the latter part of the first year of life from the first two phases of the BASIS study. We needed to have a measure of PCI suitable for this developmental age, and a review of the literature made clear that there was no such measure. My colleague Ming Wai Wan developed a new instrument, from original observational piloting of at-risk infants and drawing on relevant aspects of two previous instruments: (1) the Global Rating Scale (GRS; Murray, Fiori-Cowley, Hooper, & Cooper, 1996), developed for measurement of early PCI in the context of parental depression, but applicable to the first 6 months—at an earlier developmental age than we were going to study in our children; and (2) the Coding of Attachment-Related Parenting for Autism (CARP-A; Blazey 2007; Blazey, Leadbitter, Holt, & Green, 2008), an instrument adapted from the original CARP measure (Matias, Scott, & O'Connor, 2006; Matias, O'Connor, Futh, & Scott, 2013) and designed specifically as an observational coding of interaction between older preschool children with autism and their parents. Integration of observational study with relevant elements from these instruments formed the Manchester Assessment of Caregiver–Infant Interaction (MACI), a global rating instrument of parental sensitivity and directiveness, child responsiveness, and dyadic mutuality (Wan, Brooks, Green, Abel, & Elmadih, 2016).

Relevant for this context, MACI includes ratings of both parental Sensitive Responsiveness and Nondirectiveness. The latter scale is derived from GRS Acceptance: Nondirectiveness (framed positively) denotes a behavioral and mental acceptance of and focus on the infant's experience irrespective of whether this is sensitive or not, as opposed to Directiveness, which includes implicit or explicit demanding and intrusive parental behavior and negative comments. The two parental scales in MACI thus touch in turn on the notion of parental sensitivity and nonsensitive intrusiveness, with the latter particularly important to PCI dynamics in disability. Studying these two aspects in the early autism prodrome allows us to address how different theoretical frameworks may illuminate the social and relational development in the disorder.

There are in addition three scales in the MACI that focus on infant behavior and responses: Attentiveness to Caregiver, Affect, and Liveliness; and two dyadic scales, Mutuality and Engagement Intensity. The 7-point scales (with an anchor for each point) were refined out of extensive piloting in the specific infant-risk group at the ages to be studied (for scale details, see Wan et al., 2012, 2016). Validity studies applying the MACI to typically developing infants and their mothers ($N = 147$; Wan et al., 2016) showed a range of evidence for consistency, reliability and validity on the normative sample, particularly in relation to caregiver sensitivity. Overall, caregiver sensitivity and nondirectiveness were correlated, but, in caregivers showing low levels of sensitive responding, 80% also showed overcontrol (i.e., low in nondirectiveness), while 20% showed a more passive withdrawal (i.e., coded higher in nondirectiveness). These two ("active" and "passive") forms of insensitivity are relevant in early developmental atypicality. Also, a toddler version of MACI has been developed for the study of infants in their second and third years.

MACI was used to study parent–infant interaction in infants at 6 and then 12 months of age within the BASIS cohort study. *At-risk infants* were defined as having an older sibling with a clinical diagnosis of ASD (or in four cases, a half-sibling); *low-risk infants* had at least one older sibling but no family history of ASD or other neurodisability. The results (see Table 12.1) showed that differences between at-risk and low-risk infant–caregiver interactions could indeed be identified from 6 months (Wan et al., 2012). Caregiver *sensitivity* and *nondirectiveness,* were both lower in at-risk dyads compared to low-risk dyads. At 12 months (Wan et al., 2013), these group differences were amplified; the differences in caregiver *sensitivity* and *nondirectiveness* continued but, in addition, there were also group differences in the *infant* and *dyadic* scales (Table 12.1).

About 20% of at-risk infants in infant-sibling studies go on to develop identified ASD at 3 years (Ozonoff et al., 2011), and the Wan et al. study further showed for the first time that PCI status at 12 months independently predicted this ASD emergence at 3 years (Table 12.1). The predictions to later ASD related to infant behavior within the dyad rather than caregiver behavior: At-risk infants at 12 months who were later diagnosed with ASD at 3 years ($N = 14$) showed *less attentiveness* to

TABLE 12.1. Global Ratings of Parent–Infant Interaction by ASD/Risk Status at 6 Months and 12 Months

	Sibling group mean (*SD*)				
	At-risk ASD[a]	At-risk no-ASD[b]	Low-risk[c]	Unadjusted *F*	Adjusted *F* for infant age
6 months	(*N* = 14)	(*N* = 31)	(*N* = 45)	(*p* value)	(*p* value)
Parent scales					
Sensitive responsiveness	3.14 (0.95)	3.23 (1.23)	3.84 (1.33)	3.03 (0.05)*	2.58 (0.08)
Nondirectiveness	3.14 (1.35)	3.03 (1.28)	3.93 (1.36)	4.82 (0.01)**	4.25 (0.02)*
Infant scales					
Attentiveness to parent	3.71 (1.64)	3.90 (1.19)	3.91 (1.38)	0.12 (0.89)	0.14 (0.87)
Positive affect	4.36 (0.84)	3.77 (1.26)	3.80 (1.04)	1.60 (0.21)	1.71 (0.19)
Liveliness	3.69 (0.86)	3.42 (1.23)	4.21 (1.01)	5.01 (0.009)**	4.45 (0.02)*
Dyad scales					
Mutuality	3.00 (1.52)	3.03 (1.28)	3.18 (1.44)	0.14 (0.87)	0.09 (0.92)
Engagement intensity	3.86 (1.46)	4.93 (1.22)	3.96 (1.33)	0.09 (0.92)	0.11 (0.89)
12 months	*N* = 12	*N* = 31	*N* = 48		
Parent scales					
Sensitive responsiveness	2.92 (1.08)	3.58 (1.41)	3.98 (1.50)	2.86 (0.06)	2.83 (0.07)
Nondirectiveness	3.17 (1.34)	3.55 (1.52)	4.31 (1.43)	4.37 (0.02)*	4.03 (0.02)*
Infant scales					
Attentiveness to parent	3.17 (1.19)	4.37 (1.22)	4.67 (1.28)	6.79 (0.002)**	6.95 (0.002)**
Positive affect	3.00 (0.74)	4.06 (1.00)	4.04 (0.85)	7.26 (0.001)**	7.31 (0.001)**
Liveliness	5.33 (1.07)	4.77 (1.04)	5.00 (1.07)	0.91 (0.41)	0.75 (0.48)
Dyad scales					
Mutuality	2.25 (0.87)	3.61 (1.50)	3.92 (1.54)	6.27 (0.003)**	6.50 (0.002)**
Engagement intensity	3.42 (0.90)	4.40 (0.93)	4.21 (0.74)	4.45 (0.01)**	4.35 (0.02)*

Note. From Wan, M. W., Green, J., Elsabbagh, M., Johnson, M., Charman, T., Plummer, F., & the BASIS Team (2013). Quality of interaction between at-risk infants and caregiver at 12–15 months is associated with 3-year autism outcome. *Journal of Child Psychology and Psychiatry, 54,* 763–771. Copyright © 2013 John Wiley & Sons, Inc. Reprinted by permission.

[a]At-risk infants who developed ASD at 3 years.

[b]At-risk infants who did not develop ASD at 3 years.

[c]Infants not at familial risk of autism.

*p < .05; **p < .01.

their caregiver, *less positivity* of affect, and *less dyadic mutuality,* adjusting for developmental and behavioral status. Parental sensitivity and nondirectivness were not predictive. In addition, of the group of infants who were themselves already showing higher levels of atypical (preautism) behaviors at 12 months, those with lower quality MACI interaction scores were much more likely to go on to develop full ASD at 3 years—for instance, 50% with low mutuality had emergent ASD at 3 years compared to 17% with high levels of mutuality (Wan et al., 2013).

In parallel with the parent–infant interaction work, BASIS was studying early neurophysiological and neurodevelopmental precursors of emergent autism. One of the earliest predictive markers of later autism development at 3 years was found to be a comparative lack of visual event-related potential (ERP) response discrimination to direct versus averted gaze stimuli, especially at the P400 signal processing level, compared to low-risk and high-risk babies not developing autism (Elsabbagh et al., 2012). We tested whether the extent and nature of this ERP abnormality, measured in a laboratory environment with a computer simulation, was correlated with contemporaneously assessed parent–infant naturalistic interaction on MACI in 45 at-risk infants against 47 low-risk controls. There was evidence of some association: lower parental sensitivity associated with less infant discrimination in the P100 ERP signal in low-risk children and decreased infant affect and mutuality with lower P400 discrimination in at-risk infants (Elsabbagh et al., 2015). These empirical data are compatible with our theoretical hypotheses about early transactional effects on PCI in the development of autism trajectories.

In summary, early perceptual abnormalities in infants at risk of autism predict later autism emergence at 3 years and also show some association with perturbation of early dyadic PCI with their caregivers at 7 months. The interaction perturbation at 7 months is seen largely in lowered parental responsiveness and increased directiveness, but is amplified by 12 months to include also infant interaction and mutuality effects, suggesting an escalating process. The child interaction perturbation at 12 months then predicts later autism emergence, independent of infant presymptom behavior.

A number of other developmental precursors of later autism identified in this infancy period also have a theoretical risk of resulting in a similar (or additive) perturbation to early dyadic interaction (see Table 12.2), although relevant empirical studies to confirm this have not yet been done.

We are suggesting here, therefore, a transactional account (see Sameroff, 2009) whereby the infant's atypicality may be further sustained and amplified into an increasingly atypical trajectory during the autism prodrome (see Zeliadt, 2015). The interactional perturbation may lead the infant at risk to experience decreasing opportunities for high-quality social learning. Furthermore, infants with preexisting risk vulnerabilities for ASD might be particularly vulnerable to such decreased opportunity, leading to further behavioral avoidance and loss of environmentally socially expectant cognitive and brain growth in sensitive "social brain" areas (Dawson, 2008). This account provides logic for an early interaction-based psychosocial intervention. The 8- to 14-month period is notable for the earliest emergence of these social interaction and behavioral atypicalities, in advance of more definite symptom emergence from 18 months or so onward (Yirmiya & Charman, 2010), thus making the logical choice for the timing of an early intervention, to which this chapter now turns.

TABLE 12.2. Early Developmental Atypicalities in Prodromal Autism and Their Potential Interactive Effects

Differences in *visual preference and ERP response to gaze* (Elsabbagh et al., 2012)	Reduced social eye contact during reciprocal interaction and a limit to social reinforcement to reciprocal eye gaze. Other interactional consequences could include reduced shared affect, poor monitoring of turn taking, and a potential lack of understanding of facial signals.
Lack of *motivation toward reciprocal social interaction* described in high-risk sibs (Zwaigenbaum et al., 2005)	Disruption of finely tuned developing parent-infant reciprocity
Poor *affect matching and responsiveness to affect change* (Zwaigenbaum et al 2005)	Similar effect.
Poor *nonverbal communication,* including following an adult's gaze and/or head turn, protodeclarative pointing and communicative gestures (Parladé & Iverson, 2015)	The building blocks for shared meaning and later language comprehension. Parents' ability to recognize their child's focus of interest is important (Yoder & Munsen, 1995) and is assisted where infants are clearly engaged in joint attention behaviors; these are areas that may be at risk in children with prodromal ASD.
Inflexible attentional style	Difficulty in disengagement and smooth pursuit of attention between objects/topics is a consistent finding in the prodrome of autism (Zwaigenbaum et al., 2005). The dyadic consequences of this could be anticipated to be mistiming of adult response through adults "getting ahead" of the child and not waiting for the attention to disengage or for topics to shift. The adult may become intrusive and try and impose an intentional shift on the child, and this is likely to be counterproductive.
Reactivity and atypical sensory behaviors	High or low reactivity at the extremes are atypical ASD markers and have been shown to predict autism outcomes in longitudinal studies (Zaigenbaum et al., 2005). These similarly could have a disruptive effect on interaction.

Sensitivity-Based Intervention in the Autism Prodrome

The theoretical aim for the intervention was, as far as possible, to "normalize" the interactional perturbation, aiming to optimize the infant's dyadic affective and social learning over the early infancy period. ASD has a baseline population prevalence of about 1%, making a "universal" prevention intervention impracticable; instead, a "selective" strategy is more feasible, targeting a group of infants at relatively high risk of developing autism. The iBASIS study was based on this idea. A cohort of infants at familial risk within BASIS was randomly allocated to a 5-month intervention between the 7- and 14-month assessment points of the longitudinal study. Because there was no predictive marker of later ASD at this age validated at an individual-case level we decided on both ethical and pragmatic grounds not to select infants on the basis of other risk markers or early symptoms. Because around 20% of infants in longitudinal studies of this kind develop ASD at 3 years (Ozonoff et al., 2011), we needed, again both for ethical and pragmatic reasons, to select an intervention that could be applicable and acceptable to both families of babies who would go on to develop autism and families of babies who would not. The aim of the intervention was to intervene at the level of the naturalistic dyad, and in keeping with our previous work on parent-mediated treatment for children with diagnosed autism, we wanted a parent-mediated intervention also in this infancy period. An evidence review of sensitivity-based infancy interventions (Bakermans-Kranenburg, van IJzendoorn, & Juffer, 2003) suggested that a personalized, brief, video-aided intervention with parents is most effective in improving early parental responsiveness to infants and is best delivered in the latter part of the first year—our target period. We chose the VIPP program as the best studied and evidence-based of these intervention methods across a range of risk conditions (although VIPP at the time of the design of the study had not previously targeted autism). VIPP has a strong evidence base for good effect on relevant aspects of parental sensitive responding, along with some more modest downstream effects on child outcomes (Juffer, Bakermans-Kranenburg, & van IJzendoorn, 2008; and Juffer et al., Chapter 1, this volume). Using the original infancy VIPP model (for under 1 year) as foundation, we undertook adaptation of the original six core sessions for our group, then added on an additional six booster sessions focused on consolidation and management of any specifically arising atypicality.

The adaptations made to the VIPP model were informed by experience from the preschool autism communication therapy (PACT), a separate but conceptually similar parent-mediated video-aided intervention previously developed for children between ages 2 and 5 years already diagnosed with ASD. PACT has been evaluated in a series of RCTs (Aldred, Green, & Adams, 2004; Green et al., 2010; Pickles et al., 2015, 2016; Rahman et al., 2015). These studies have shown that this video-aided technique with parents has a strong impact to improve parental communicative synchrony behavior with the child with autism (effect size [ES] = 1.44 at 6 months; 1.22 at 13 months; Green et al., 2010) and that this improvement in parental synchrony mediates improvements in child dyadic communication (ES = 0.5 at 6 months, 0.44 at 13 months) and this change in child dyadic communication mediates reduction of autism symptom behaviors (Autism Diagnostic Observation Schedule combined severity score at 13 months; ES = 0.63; 0.02, 1.29). This reduction of autism symptoms from intervention is maintained at follow up 6 years after the end of intervention (Pickles et al., 2016). Such effectiveness and causal mediation evidence is consistent with other early autism intervention work (Kasari, Paparella, Freeman, & Jahromi, 2008) and with the developmental literature in that high early parental synchrony is associated with enhanced later language and social development in both neurotypical and autistic children (Siller & Sigman, 2002, 2008). A final level of evidence behind iBASIS comes from the empirical studies described earlier showing differences in parent–infant social interaction in the situation of infant siblings at high risk for autism compared to infant controls at low risk for autism both at 7–9 and 12–15 months, with the latter associated with later ASD diagnosis (Wan et al., 2013). The intervention included specific procedures to deal with any observed atypicality during the course of intervention.

The resulting intervention, called iBASIS-VIPP is therefore an adapted version of the original infant VIPP program (without the "sensitive discipline" element), and with an additional six sessions, giving a total possible of 12 home-based sessions over 5 months. Sessions are initially weekly, then reduced in frequency. The parent is encouraged to undertake 30 minutes of structured practice each day between sessions. The intervention is parent-mediated and video-aided, with no direct contact between infant and therapist. The method integrates video-aided techniques to enhance parent–infant interaction (Juffer et al., 2008; Wels, 1995) and includes (1) a focus on dyadic, communicative aspects of the relationship, with a high degree of adaptation for each particular parent–infant dyad; (2) video clips of "successful" interactions, providing positive examples of sensitive, competent parenting; and (3) involvement of a trained therapist to frame observations to assist parent's self-reflection, with focused discussion on behavioral change. Parents' sense of efficacy is enhanced by active participation and the support given for their intuitive knowledge of their child. Intervention content focuses initially on enhancing parental observation, the attribution of communicative intent to infant behaviors that may be difficult to interpret, and facilitating contingent parental responding and affective attunement. To this foundation is added related components to enhance early communication development. Future findings in relation to specific interaction perturbations associated with atypicalities may lead to the inclusion of other specific elements. The fact that, in neurodisability, the focus is less on parental vulnerability and more on child vulnerability resulted in some subtle changes of emphasis in both procedure and content.

   The initial core sessions of iBASIS-VIPP follow the VIPP model (see Juffer et al., Chapter 1, this volume), with adjustments for autism and neurodisability. A preliminary session (baseline/relationship building with parent) is followed by six intervention sessions (delivered weekly to fortnightly); each with a theme building on techniques and learning from the previous session.

Core Intervention Sessions

In Session 1 the parent and therapist watch together the play video taken at the previous home visit. The parent is encouraged to watch the baby's behavior, focusing on its pace and nature, while the therapist's feedback comments focus on the baby's behavior at this stage and *not* on parental responses. Collaborative observation and techniques of "speaking for the child" and behavioral commentary aim to sensitize the parent to the child's behavior and intentions. The focus in the original VIPP is on attachment and exploratory behaviors. In the context of children at autism risk, this "baby-watching" phase instead focuses mainly on the infant's social communication and the interactional consequences of any early atypicality (see Table 12.2). For instance, in this context, parents often communicate to young children at too rapid a pace or communicative level; the observational focus on child behavior naturally involves a gradual slowing of parental perception and response to the child's speed, a reduction in overdirectiveness, and improved meshing and timing. Infants in prodromal autism typically poorly integrate vocalization and gesture; use of eye gaze can be unpredictable and idiosyncratic, sometimes with gaze avoidance, but also with poorly modulated use of eye gaze, such as staring. By beginning to watch and wait, the parent will be able to take the time to decode these aspects of infant functioning, which require attentive observation. This will then help the parent to infer coherent communication intent in an infant whose signaling is poorly coordinated.

In Session 2 the parent builds on these observations to make inferences about intentionality. Given that the at-risk infant will communicate in a way that makes early inferences about intention more difficult, raising the capacity of the parent to make intention inferences should be a key component of generating synchronous and reciprocal interaction, as well as providing a platform for intersubjectivity. The technique within VIPP for facilitating this is "speaking for the baby," which has been found to be a powerful method for allowing focus and insight.

Sessions 3 and 4 build on the observations in the first two sessions but direct more focus on parental responses to the infant. The concept of "sensitivity chains" in VIPP is initially behavioral, identifying a sequence of infant signaling, parental sensitive response, then infant reaction. These reciprocal chains are the foundation of reciprocal interaction and relating. The achievement of sensitivity chains with the infant at neurodevelopmental risk is a good indicator of early success. In Session 4 the concept of sensitivity chains is generalized into practical activities in order to embed the concepts.

In Session 5 the focus shifts toward intersubjectivity and affect sharing. The video feedback emphasizes more subtle cues from the infant, including affect, and parents are encouraged to verbalize their understanding of the infant's facial expressions and nonverbal cues using a new technique of "baby talk." This is subtly different from the previous "speaking for the baby" technique, in that it is more immersive and experiential. The parent is encouraged to interpret the baby's physical and emotional communication *as if he or she is actually the infant*—for example: "I like showing how well I can do this" or "I'm trying to figure out how this works." This kind of immersive interpretation in relation to a child who is showing atypical communication represents a high-level skill in the parent. It may well also stimulate deeper insights as he or she identifies with the child's confusion or struggle to communicate. Retrospective accounts of individuals with autism as adults recalling their infancy or childhood experience (e.g., Bemporad, 1979) risk being unrepresentative, since individuals able to articulate in this way are relatively uncommon in the autism community; nevertheless, a common theme running through many of them is a sense of disorientation and perceptual disturbance in experiencing the world. There are distortions of time and space, and unpredictable sensations of intrusion of the perceptual world at a sensory level. These accounts illustrate how a child with autistic sensitivity may find complex social contact difficult to manage and be more comfortable with restricted inanimate and mechanical inputs. Such sensory disruption has potential impact on early reciprocity and development of internal representation of a relatively predictable and secure interpersonal world; developmentally vulnerable children might therefore be particularly dependent on a well-tuned environmental response. In the "baby talk" exercise, the parents are being asked to attempt to enter this world empathically: They will inevitably have to slow down in order to understand this, and the child may benefit from such a slower pace. Key for the intervention is how successful such adjustment may be.

In Session 6 the focus shifts to communication, and aims to enhance semantically contingent responses from the parent to early communication from the baby. Use is made of a "funny sound game" in which the parent mirrors and echoes funny sounds made in the course of reading a book. The therapist will also have identified clips from the videotape in which the parent may have responded in a contingent way to communication initiations of any kind from the baby. Early communication in prodromal autism is often characterized by repetitive, stereotyped phrases or repetition of heard talk that is not generative—so-called immediate or delayed echolalia. A challenge for the parent is to find ways of contingent responding that can distinguish repetitive from generative language in the child (there is usually a mixture). "Speaking for the baby" and "baby talk" techniques may be helpful here, since they provide a way for the parent to intuit the child's intentionality behind the communication and therefore identify which communications are truly generative and which are not.

Booster Sessions

In booster sessions following the six core sessions, the therapist continues to work with the parent to reinforce learning and enhance progress in parent–infant synchrony, attunement, and communication. We considered that this extension to the core VIPP program was necessary in this situation given the potential complexity of intervention task in the autism context. The therapist may select video clips from the previous sessions to work on with the parent. The precise content of the booster sessions will be based on parental concerns (if any) discussed in previous sessions, therapist observations of the parent–infant dyad, video clips of parent–infant interaction taken in Session 6 and by progress identified in the profile of identified atypicalities. These sessions also provide an opportunity for other caregivers of the infant to be involved alongside the primary caregiver, which can also reinforce learning in the primary caregiver.

Identifying Atypicality

A checklist of potential atypicalities is completed by the therapist at the end of every session. Any identified atypicalities can be identified in conversation with the parent as part of the range of the infant's behavioral repertoire *without labeling them as prodromal signs*. They can be identified as potential barriers to the processes of reciprocity and communication that have been a more general focus in previous sessions. Therapist and parent take a collaborative and exploratory approach to identify effective techniques to minimize these atypicalities. However, mindful of the maxim "less is more" in this period (Bakermans-Kranenburg, van IJzendoorn, & Juffer, 2003), if the sessions seem to be getting repetitive, then they can be spaced more apart and the total number limited by mutual agreement with the parent. In this preemptive intervention it is very important not to assume atypicality (in a client group that may not show it) and adapt naturally to the range of situations that will be encountered. The generic parental enhancement techniques in VIPP have demonstrated applicability across a range of normative parenting styles; the additional components more specific to prodromal autism identified here build on the close attention to behavior advocated by VIPP in ways that support parents of infants with developmental difficulties. *Remediation strategies for atypicality* are designed to (1) focus on the "interactional perturbations"/dyadic consequences of the atypicality on the parent–infant interaction and encourage more typical interactions where possible or (2) provide the infant with the optimal PCI to improve the atypicalities in the child (see Table 12.3).

TABLE 12.3. Developmental Atypicalities and Potential Remediation Strategies

Observed atypicalities in infant	Potential dyadic consequences	Remediation	
		Core iBASIS strategies to emphasize	Additional strategies
Gaze behaviors			
• Reduced/unusual use of eye contact in face–face interactions • Reduced ability to follow parent gaze • Reduced joint attention behaviors	• Parental disengagement • Reduction in gaze initiations/length by parent		• Enhance parental observation and monitoring of their infant's use of eye gaze. • Assist parents to recognize episodes in which eye contact may occur and to respond immediately and contingently with a response that is appropriate to their infant's tolerance.
Attention behaviors			
• Overlong staring at toy • Reduced level of gaze switching during play	• Mistiming of parent responses through adults getting ahead of the child • Parent may become intrusive and attempt to impose an attentional shift on the infant	• Enhance further the parent's skill in observing and matching the infant's focus and the pace of the interaction	• Shifting attention to a range of toys/situations or transitions in routine care. • Encourage parents to sensitively experiment with strategies for shifting attention (e.g., touch, sound, using the baby's name, moving objects to face level).
Atypical play behaviors			
• Low interest in sharing toys • Tendency to play alone, removed from parent	• Parent may become intrusive and direct/take control of play in an attempt to interact with the infant.	• Encourage parent to allow infant to explore the environment and toys, and attend to infant's focus of interest without interfering	• Encourage parent to observe what types of play their child enjoys most and what opens up opportunities for interaction (e.g., rough-and-tumble/physical games). Encourage parent to learn through observing their child's individual signals that indicate the child is ready to join in.
Atypical reciprocity			
• Reduced reciprocal social smile • Reduced response to social talk from parent • Reduced response to parents' attempts to engage infant in play • Reduced affective response to social touch	• Disruption of finely tuned reciprocity that typically develops between parent and infant	• Emphasize core iBASIS procedures that promote reciprocity (e.g., affect matching, imitation)	• Encourage a balance of response and the introduction of novel information that is developmentally appropriate.

(continued)

TABLE 12.3. *(continued)*

Observed atypicalities in infant	Potential dyadic consequences	Remediation	
		Core iBASIS strategies to emphasize	Additional strategies
Affect			
• Reduced expression of affect • Reduced affect matching	• Parent may miss subtle expressions of affect and not respond appropriately • Lack of response to affect from infant may have led to parents reduction in sharing their own affect.	• Emphasize the "talking for the child" technique to enhance the parent's skills in inferring intentionality and affect in the infant. • Encourage the parents to respond to infant's affect as communicative, interpreting meaning based on contextual cues • Encourage the parents to mirror affect sensitively whilst monitoring the infant's response. Establish ways for the parents to reflect back to the infant their understanding; "feeling for them"	• Encourage parents to share their affect responses with the infant. However, avoid overexaggeration—work with the parents' natural style. • Encourage parents to ensure that the baby has a good view of their faces. • Encourage parents to use facial expression when interacting with their baby. • Encourage parents to use expression in their voices when speaking to the baby.
Emerging atypical communication			
• Reduced response to communicative gesture • Reduced use of communicative gestures • Reduced use of protodeclarative pointing • Delays in sound production • Reduced simple and complex babbling • Delays in early word production	• Parents may miss some of the infant's weaker communicative signals and not respond reciprocally • Parents may become more didactic in their approach to communication	• Emphasize iBASIS procedures for close observation of the focus and intent of the infant • Help parent respond to any vocalizations in a social context that recognizes the infant's intent and underlying affect	• Encourage parents to use simple natural gestures and pointing; to introduce sound games; to use symbolic sounds; to provide the infant with developmentally appropriate language models. • Help parents to recognize their child's attempts at early word approximations and provide the relevant word (e.g., "oh," "dog").

(continued)

TABLE 12.3. *(continued)*

Observed atypicalities in infant	Potential dyadic consequences	Remediation	
		Core iBASIS strategies to emphasize	Additional strategies
Atypical reactivity and sensory behaviors			
• Sensitivity to foods, textures, sounds, and so forth • Extremes of temperament—overly reactive or overly passive	• Extreme and unexpected reactions may adversely affect interaction if parents fail to recognize the reasons for the reaction • Extreme passivity may result in parents becoming less motivated to interact with their child		• Help parent to recognize when atypical reactions are affecting the interaction and to identify possible causes. • Parents will be assisted to experiment with ways to respond to atypical reactions.
Repetitive behaviors			
• Atypical motor mannerisms	• Parents may monitor for presence of mannerisms and if signs emerge, this may lead to parental anxiety that impacts on interaction with child • Parents may copy mannerisms in a nonsocial way and/ or may use them to initiate interaction		• Encourage parents to consider what the mannerism indicates (e.g., over- or understimulation) and respond accordingly. • Where possible, encourage parent to comment on child's perceived emotional state (e.g., hand flapping through excitement): "Oh it's exciting!" • Encourage parent to experiment with using imitation as a means of engagement. • Encourage parents to adapt mannerisms into meaningful actions (e.g., shaking a shaker, tapping a drum).

Note. See *http://research.bmh.manchester.ac.uk/ibasis/protocol/*.

Evaluating the Intervention

The iBASIS-VIPP intervention was evaluated within BASIS, a prospective longitudinal study of infants at risk of autism and low-risk controls, including a range of measurement and assessments from brain imaging, neurophysiological studies such as evoked potentials and laboratory-based tasks of attentional flexibility, face recognition, eye tracking, and motor development to measures of development and behavior. It includes detailed evaluation of emerging autism-related atypical behaviors, with a final consensus-based diagnostic ascertainment when the infants and have reached age 3 years. The intervention was conducted between the 7- and 14-month assessment points of the study. An initial case series study of seven infants (Green et al., 2013) served to refine the intervention and the measurement protocol. Since the context of this intervention was that families were already managing a child diagnosed with autism, in addition to the new infant and possibly other children, it was important to establish that the home-based intervention of this kind was both feasible and acceptable. Overall the data were positive; five of seven families attended all 12 sessions; one family ceased after 10 sessions (by mutual agreement, since they felt they had achieved their goals); and another family completed 11 sessions. Families were asked to undertake 30 minutes of focused practice per day; family members sometimes said this was difficult to achieve, but none of the seven families in the series considered this to be impossible. All seven parents strongly agreed that the intervention was enjoyable and had led to a greater understanding of their infant's behaviors; two of seven reported that the intervention had exceeded their expectation of benefit. All parents either strongly agreed (6) or agreed (1) that the intervention was helpful; and all either strongly agreed (3) or agreed (4) that sessions were of appropriate number and duration. All parents either strongly agreed (5) or agreed (2) that they had modified aspects of their parenting as a result of the program, that the home environment for intervention was suitable, and that they now spent more quality time with their child. No parents identified negative effects from participating, and four parents indicated they had been able to share some of their learning and/or some of the video from sessions with partners or the infant's older siblings. In supplementary interviews parents reported increased awareness of interaction with their infant and of their infant's communication with them:

> "It makes you look really closely at what your interaction with your child is and there is much more in it than you really thought."

> "It's amazing watching back how much she understands and how much she's taking in and communicating with you and you just don't notice it."

Three parents commented that they had found reviewing the videos the most helpful thing in terms of session content. Additional benefits of taking part included increased recognition of the infant's emotionality and intentionality:

> "It made me aware he does have feelings and he gets them across. Before I ignored it and thought it was just baby grunting."

"I was like—maybe he hasn't yet developed emotions. . . . But through the sessions I found out that actually, no, it was just the way that you do things and now he's full of energy."

The intervention was then formally studied in a parallel group RCT of 54 families (28 receiving an iBASIS-VIPP intervention, 26 receiving no intervention, with infants at familial risk of autism but not otherwise selected for developmental atypicality (Green et al., 2015, 2017). Intervention was given from infant ages 9–14 months; one family randomized to intervention failed to begin treatment due to personal commitments, but all 27 families beginning treatment completed the six core sessions over 5 months, with mean sessions attended per family of 9.5/12 possible (*SD* = 1.6; range = 6–11). Assessments were made at infant age 9-month baseline, 15-month treatment endpoint, and 27- and 39-month follow-up. Prespecified intention to treat analysis combined estimates from these repeated measures to estimate the overall effect of the infancy intervention over time, and these were summarized in analysis of the area between the trajectory curves for each group (Green et al., 2017; Figure 12.1).

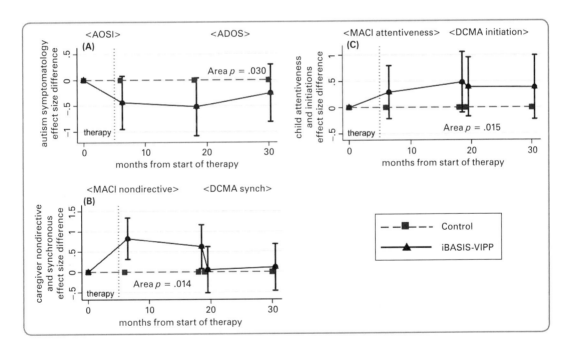

FIGURE 12.1. Time profile of treatment effects on autism symptoms and caregiver–child interaction ("area" = area between curves estimation; see text). The effect size difference is shown by holding TAU as zero. (A) primary outcome, autism prodromal symptoms (negative effect size reflects a reduction in symptom severity in iBASIS-VIPP relative to TAU). (B) parental dyadic social interaction. (C) child dyadic social interaction. From Green, Pickles, Pasco, Bedford, Wan, et al. (2017). Reprinted with permission from Creative Commons, at *https://creativecommons.org/licenses/by/4.0.*

Primary outcome was the severity of emerging autism prodromal symptoms, blind-rated on Autism Observation Schedule for Infants (AOSI) or Autism Diagnostic Observation Schedule (ADOS–2) over the four assessment points (see Figure 12.1A). The results show point estimates of reduced symptom severity which were close to individual significance at 15-month endpoint and 27-month follow-up, with the area between curves estimation from start of therapy to 24 months after end of therapy showing a significant effect size in favor of intervention over this time of 0.32 (95% CI 0.04, 0.60; p = 0.03).

Effect on parent–child dyadic social interaction was assessed on the MACI infant at 9, 15 months; MACI toddler at 27 months, and the conceptually related Dyadic Communication Measure for Autism (DCMA) (Aldred, Green, Emsley, & McConachie, 2012), as age appropriate for the 27- and 39-month follow-up (Figures 12.1B, 12.1C). For parental behaviors, intervention showed strong effects at endpoint on parental nondirectiveness (MACI; Figure 12.1B), but this had begun to reduce by 27 months and showed further reduction on switching from the MACI to the DCMA measure at 27 months. Nevertheless, the area-under-curve analysis still shows a significant overall positive treatment effect size on parental interactive behavior over time of 0.33 (95% CI 0.04, 0.63; p = 0.013). For child dyadic social behaviors in the dyad, the intervention showed consistent modest positive effects but sustained over time after the end of intervention (Figure 12.1C), giving an overall significant positive effect size over time of 0.36 (95% CI 0.04, 0.68; p = 0.015).

The study was not powered to detect an effect on autism diagnostic outcomes at age 3 years, and none was seen: 4 from the intervention group and 2 from the nonintervention group developed ASD (2 by 3 Fisher's exact p = 0.846; ordinal logistic OR = 0.83, p = .726). There were no overall significant intervention effects on structural language development or on other developmental measures such as Mullen or parent-reported Vineland (Green et al., 2017).

Conclusions

Subtle details of caregiver–child reciprocal interactions within the first year are foundational for the development of not only early attachment but also intersubjectivity and social competency. Early neurodisability, including autism, can disrupt early reciprocal interactions in specific ways that can be empirically established. Emerging patterns of atypicality in prodromal autism in the first year include disrupted interaction, and this perturbation may amplify over time, further disrupting fragile social learning and relational experience in the neurodevelopmentally vulnerable baby. On the other hand, attachment aspects of interaction appear to be largely preserved, suggesting differing mechanisms underlying attachment and these aspects of social competency.

We have adapted the infancy VIPP model into an intervention aiming to reduce this interaction perturbation in the first year and enrich infant social learning—in the hope of ameliorating atypical trajectories toward later autism. The intervention (iBASIS-VIPP) was tested in an RCT, which was the first randomized treatment trial of a preemptive intervention in the autism prodrome; previous similar studies were small case series or single-case designs plus a recent report on relevant neurophysiological markers from a further infancy RCT (see Table 12.4).

TABLE 12.4. Previous Studies of Interventions for Infants at Risk for Autism in the First Year of Life

Author	Design	Main reported results
Jones et al. (2017)	Parallel group RCT, $n = 33$.	Some improvements in electrophysiological and habituation markers of social attention
Green et al. (2015)	Two parallel group RCTs, intervention vs. regular care, $n = 54$.	Improvement in caregiver non-directiveness (ES = 0.81, CI = 0.28 to 1.52); 4.15 mean reduction in AOSI scores (ES = 0.5; CI = −0.15 to 1.08)
Rogers et al. (2014)	Case series, $n = 7$, observational study of intervention for symptomatic infants	Overall 2-point reduction in AOSI scores
Green et al. (2013)	Case series, $n = 7$, case–control observational study	Good feasibility/acceptability; signal of improvement in parental interactive behavior
Steiner et al. (2013)	Case series, $n = 3$, multiple-baseline design	Increased functional communication
Koegel et al. (2013)	Case series, $n = 3$, multiple-baseline design	Increased social engagement

The findings of the iBASIS RCT show a pattern of broadly positive effect estimates across a range of measures, and are consistent with an intervention with moderate effects on several ASD risk markers, including atypical presymptom behaviors. Follow-up study of the babies at 24 and 36 months suggests significant overall sustained change in emerging autism symptoms and parental and child dyadic behaviors, over the course of therapy and follow-up period. Such follow-up data are salient, since they have been sparse in the intervention literature of this kind (with no other follow-up studies to my knowledge of VIPP interventions at any length of time after the intervention itself).

There have been some conceptually related intervention studies for older children with the diagnosed condition. Thus, the VIPP model was also adapted by the originators of the model for use in older children following an autism diagnosis (VIPP-AUTI), and an RCT of this intervention (Poslawksy et al., 2014) showed good effect on parental sensitivity but no effect on child functioning. The group of which I am a part has also developed and studied a similar video-feedback staged intervention for preschool children diagnosed with autism, described earlier.

Tests of a targeted developmental intervention in this way using an RCT can be designed so as to illuminate developmental processes, as well as demonstrate effectiveness of the intervention (Green & Dunn, 2008). In this case, the results of the study serve to support the transactional development model of autism described—since changing targeted parental behavior leads to improvement in emergent symptoms for later autism. This is encouraging for further treatment development and testing in this area, and promises a potential window onto the complex dynamics of the precursors of social competency and relationships in neurodevelopmentally vulnerable young children.

ACKNOWLEDGMENTS

I gratefully acknowledge the colleagues who undertook with me the work described in this chapter, which was a highly rewarding collaboration between developmental psychologists and psychiatrists, developmental neuroscientists, interventionists, and methodologists. In alphabetical order: Rachael Bedford, Rhonda Booth, Tony Charman, Mayada Elsabbagh, Teea Gliga, Clare Harrop, Samina Holsgrove, Mark Johnson, Emily Jones, Janet McNally, Andrew Pickles, Vicky Slonims, Carol Taylor, Ming Wai Wan, along with the British Autism Study of Infant Siblings (BASIS) Team of Patrick Bolton, Amy Brooks, Kay Davies, Janet Fernandes, Jeanne Guiraud, Helen Maris, Greg Pasco, Helen Ribeiro, Leslie Tucker, and Pat Iverson.

I also acknowledge with great thanks the generous collaboration from the originators of the original VIPP intervention (Femmie Juffer, Marian Bakermans-Kranenberg, Marinus van IJzendoorn) in allowing and enabling our adaptation of the core model and making this work possible.

The enthusiasm and engagement of the families in the BASIS project were central to the work, which was made possible by awards from the charities Autistica, Waterloo Foundation, Autism Speaks in the United States, and the U.K. Economic and Social Research Council and Medical Research Council, as well as the BASIS funding consortium led by Autistica (*www.basisnetwork.org*).

The views expressed in the chapter are my own.

REFERENCES

Aldred, C., Green, J., & Adams, C. (2004). A new social communication intervention for children with autism: Pilot randomised controlled treatment study suggesting effectiveness. *Journal of Child Psychology and Psychiatry, 45*(8), 1420–1430.

Aldred, C., Green, J., Emsley, R., & McConachie, H. (2012). Brief report: Mediation of treatment effect in a communication intervention for pre-school children with autism. *Journal of Autism and Developmental Disorders, 42*(3), 447–454.

Bakermans-Kranenburg, M. J., van IJzendoorn, M. H., & Juffer, F. (2003). Less is more: Meta-analyses of sensitivity and attachment interventions in early childhood. *Psychological Bulletin, 129*(2), 195–215.

Bemporad, J. R. (1979). Adult recollections of a formerly autistic child. *Journal of Autism and Developmental Disorders, 9*(2), 179–196.

Blazey, L. (2007). *Attachment in autism: An investigation into parental sensitivity, mutuality and affect.* Master's thesis, University of Manchester, Manchester, UK.

Blazey, L., Leadbitter, K., Holt, C., & Green, J. (2008). *Attachment behaviours and parent child interaction in pre-school autism.* Poster presentation at the International Meeting for Autism Research (IMFAR), London, UK.

Capps, L., Sigman, M., & Mundy, P. (1994). Attachment security in children with autism. *Development and Psychopathology, 6,* 249–261.

Cardoso-Martins, C., & Mervis, C. B. (1985). Maternal speech to prelinguistic children with Down syndrome. *American Journal of Mental Deficiency, 89*(5), 451–458.

Crawley, S. B., & Spiker, D. (1983). Mother–child interactions involving 2-year-olds with Down syndrome: A look at individual differences. *Child Development, 54*(5), 1312–1323.

Dawson, G. (2008). Early behavioral intervention, brain plasticity, and the prevention of autism spectrum disorder. *Development and Psychopathology, 20,* 775–803.

Dunst, C. J. (1985). Communicative competence and deficits: Effects on early social interactions. In E. T. McDonald & D. L. Gallagher (Eds.), *Facilitating social–emotional development in multiply handicapped children* (pp. 93–140). Philadelphia: Home of the Merciful Savior for Crippled Children.

Elsabbagh, M., Bruno, R., Wan, M., Charman, T., Johnson, M. H., Green, J., & BASIS Team. (2015). Infant neural sensitivity to dynamic eye gaze relates to quality of parent–infant interaction at 7-months in infants at risk for autism. *Journal of Autism and Developmental Disorders, 45*(2), 283–291.

Elsabbagh, M., & Johnson, M. H. (2010). Getting answers from babies about autism. *Trends in Cognitive Science, 14,* 81–87.

Elsabbagh, M., Mercure, E., Hudry, K., Chandler, S., Pasco, G., Charman, T., . . . BASIS Team. (2012). Infant neural sensitivity to dynamic eye gaze is associated with later emerging autism. *Current Biology, 22*(4), 338–342.

Green, J., Charman, T., McConachie, H., Aldred, C., Slonims, V., Howlin, H., . . . PACT Consortium. (2010). Parent-mediated communication-focused treatment in children with autism (PACT): A randomised controlled trial. *Lancet, 375*(9732), 2152–2160.

Green, J., Charman, T., Pickles, A., Wan, M. W., Elsabbagh, M., Slonims, V., . . . BASIS Team. (2015). Parent-mediated intervention versus no intervention for infants at high risk of autism: A parallel, single-blind, randomised trial. *Lancet Psychiatry, 2,* 133–140.

Green, J., & Dunn, G. (2008). Using intervention trials in developmental psychiatry to illuminate basic science. *British Journal of Psychiatry, 192*(5), 323–325.

Green, J., Pickles, A., Pasco, G., Bedford, R., Wan, M. W., Elsabbagh, M., . . . Johnson, M. H. (2017). Randomised trial of a parent-mediated intervention for infants at high risk for autism: Longitudinal outcomes to age three years. *Journal of Child Psychology and Psychiatry.*

Green, J., Wan, M. W., Guiraud, J., Holsgrove, S., McNally, J., Slonims, V., . . . BASIS Team. (2013). Intervention for infants at risk of developing autism: A case series. *Journal of Autism and Developmental Disorders, 43*(11), 2502–2514.

Johnson, M. H. (2001). Functional brain development in humans. *Nature Reviews Neuroscience, 2*(7), 475–483.

Jones, E. J. H., Dawson, G., Kelly, J., Estes, A., & Webb, S. J. (2017). Parent-delivered early intervention in infants at risk for ASD: Effects on electrophysiological and habituation measures of social attention. *Autism Research.*

Juffer, F., Bakermans-Kranenburg, M. J., & van IJzendoorn, M. H. (2008). *Promoting positive parenting: An attachment-based intervention.* New York: Taylor & Francis Group.

Kasari, C., Paparella, T., Freeman, S., & Jahromi, L. (2008). Language outcome in autism: Randomized comparison of joint attention and play interventions. *Journal of Consulting and Clinical Psychology, 76,* 125–137.

Koegel, L. K., Singh, A. K., Koegel, R. L., Hollingsworth, J. R., & Bradshaw J. (2013). Assessing and improving early social engagement in infants. *Journal of Positive Behavior Interventions, 16,* 69–80.

Koren-Karie, N., Oppenheim, D., Dolev, S., & Yirmiya, N. (2009). Mothers of securely attached children with autism spectrum disorder are more sensitive than mothers of insecurely attached children. *Journal of Child Psychology and Psychiatry, 50,* 643–650.

Landry, S. H., Smith, K. E., Miller-Loncar, C. L., & Swank, P. R. (1997). Predicting cognitive-language and social growth curves from early maternal behaviors in children at varying degrees of biological risk. *Developmental Psychology, 33,* 1040–1053.

Legerstee, M., Varghese, J., & van Beek, Y. (2002). Effects of maintaining and redirecting infant attention on the production of referential communication in infants with and without Down syndrome. *Journal of Child Language, 29*(1), 23–48.

Matias, C., O'Connor, T., Futh, A., & Scott, S. (2014). Observational attachment theory-based parenting measures predict children's attachment narratives independently from social learning theory-based measures. *Attachment and Human Development, 16*(1), 77–492.

Matias, C., Scott, S., & O'Connor, T. (2006). *Coding of attachment-related parenting (CARP): Coding scheme specifically designed for direct observation of parent–child interaction.* Unpublished manuscript, Kings College London, London, UK.

Murray, L., Fiori-Cowley, A., Hooper, R., & Cooper, P. (1996). The impact of postnatal depression and associated adversity on early mother–infant interactions and later infant outcome. *Child Development, 67,* 2512–2526.

NICHD Early Child Care Research Network. (2001). Child care and children's peer interaction at 24 and 36 months: The NICHD study of early child care. *Child Development, 72,* 1478–1500.

Ozonoff, S., Young, G. S., Carter, A., Messinger, D., Yirmiya, N., Zwaigenbaum, L., . . . Stone, W. L. (2011). Recurrence risk for autism spectrum disorders: A Baby Siblings Research Consortium study. *Pediatrics, 128*(3), E488–E495.

Parladé, M. V., & Iverson, J. M. (2015). The development of coordinated communication in infants at heightened risk for autism spectrum disorder. *Journal of Autism and Developmental Disorders, 45,* 2218–2234.

Pickles, A., Harris, V., Green, J., Aldred, C., McConachie, H., Slonims, V., . . . PACT Consortium. (2015). Treatment mechanism in the MRC preschool autism communication trial: Implications for study design and parent-focussed therapy for children. *Journal of Child Psychology and Psychiatry, 56*(2), 162–170.

Pickles, A., Le Couteur, A., Leadbitter, K., Salomone, E., Cole-Fletcher, R., Tobin, H., . . . Green J. (2016). Long term symptom reduction following preschool autism intervention. *The Lancet, 388,* 2501–2509.

Poslawsky, I. E., Naber, F. B. A., Bakermans-Kranenburg, M. J., van Daalen, E., van Engeland, H., & van IJzendoorn, M. H. (2015). Video-feedback intervention to promote Positive Parenting adapted to Autism (VIPP-AUTI): A randomized controlled trial. *Autism, 19*(5), 588–603.

Rahman, A., Divan, G., Hamdani, S., Vajaratkar, V., Taylor, C., Leadbitter, K., . . . Green, J. (2016). The effectiveness of the Parent-mediated intervention for Autism Spectrum disorders in South Asia (PASS): A randomised controlled trial in India and Pakistan. *Lancet Psychiatry, 3*(2), 128–136.

Rogers, S. J., Vismara, L., Wagner, A. L., McCormick, C., Young, G., & Ozonoff, S. (2014). Autism treatment in the first year of life: A pilot study of infant start, a parent-implemented intervention for symptomatic infants. *Journal of Autism and Developmental Disorders, 44,* 2981–2995.

Rutgers, A. H., Bakermans-Kranenburg, M. J., van IJzendoorn, M. H., & van Berckelaer-Onnes, I. A. (2004). Autism and attachment: A meta-analytic review. *Journal of Child Psychology and Psychiatry, 45,* 1123–1134.

Saint-Georges, C., Mahdhaoui, A., Chetouani, M., Cassel, R. S., Laznik, M.-C., Apicella, F., . . . Cohen, D. (2011). Do parents recognize autistic deviant behavior long before diagnosis?: Taking into account interaction using computational methods. *PLOS ONE, 6,* 1–13.

Sameroff, A. (Ed.). (2009). *The transactional model of development: How children and contexts shape each other.* Washington, DC: American Psychological Association.

Siller, M., & Sigman, M. (2002). The behaviours of parents of children with autism predict their subsequent development of their children's communication. *Journal of Autism and Developmental Disorders, 32,* 77–89.

Siller, M., & Sigman, M. (2008). Modeling longitudinal change in the language abilities of children with autism: Parent behaviors and child characteristics as predictors of change. *Developmental Psychology, 44,* 1691–1704.

Slonims, V., Cox, A., & McConachie, H. (2006). Analysis of mother–infant interaction in infants with Down syndrome and typically developing infants. *American Journal on Mental Retardation, 111*(4), 273–289.

Sorce, J. F., & Emde, R. N. (1982), The meaning of infant emotional expressions: Regularities in caregiving responses in normal and Down's syndrome infants. *Journal of Child Psychology and Psychiatry and Allied Disciplines, 23*(2), 145–158.

Steiner, A. M., Gengoux, G. W., Klin, A., & Chawarska, K. (2013). Pivotal response treatment for infants at-risk for autism spectrum disorders: A pilot study. *Journal of Autism and Developmental Disorders, 43*, 91–102.

Szatmari, P., Chawarska, K., Dawson, G., Georgiades, S., Landa, R., Lord, C., . . . & Halladay, A. (2016). Prospective longitudinal studies of infant siblings of children with autism: Lessons learned and future direction. *Journal of the American Academy of Child and Adolescent Psychiatry, 55*, 179–187.

van IJzendoorn, M. H., Rutgers, A. H., Bakermans-Kranenburg, M. J., Swinkels, S. H. N., van Daalen, E., Dietz, C., . . . van Engeland, H. (2007). Parental sensitivity and attachment in children with autism spectrum disorder: Comparison with children with mental retardation, with language delays, and with typical development. *Child Development, 78*, 597–608.

Vondra, J. I., & Barnett, D. (1999). Atypical attachment in infancy and early childhood among children at developmental risk. *Monographs of the Society for Research in Child Development, 64*(3, Serial No. 258), 119–144.

Walden, T. A., Blackford, J. U., & Carpenter, K. L. (1997), Differences in social signals produced by children with developmental delays of differing etiologies. *American Journal on Mental Retardation, 102*(3), 292–305.

Wan, M. W., Brooks, A., Green, J., Abel, K., & Elmadih, A. (2016). Psychometrics and validation of a brief rating measure of parent–infant interaction: Manchester assessment of caregiver–infant interaction. *International Journal of Behavioral Development.*

Wan, M. W., Green, J., Elsabbagh, M., Johnson, M., Charman, T., Plummer, F., & BASIS Team. (2012). Parent–infant interaction in infant siblings at risk of autism. *Research in Developmental Disabilities, 33*, 924–932.

Wan, M. W., Green, J., Elsabbagh, M., Johnson, M., Charman, T., Plummer, F., & BASIS Team. (2013). Quality of interaction between at-risk infants and caregiver at 12–15 months is associated with 3-year autism outcome. *Journal of Child Psychology and Psychiatry, 54*, 763–771.

Wels, P. M. A. (1995). *Measuring the effects of Video Home Training.* Presented at the 5th EURSARF Congress, London, UK.

Willemsen-Swinkels, S. H. N., Bakermans-Kranemburg, M. J., Buitelaar, J. K., van IJzendoorn, M. H., & van Engeland, H. (2000). Insecure and disorganised attachment in children with a pervasive developmental disorder: Relationship with social interaction and heart rate. *Journal of Child Psychology and Psychiatry and Allied Disciplines, 41*, 759–767.

Yirmiya, N., & Charman, T. (2010). The prodrome of autism: Early behavioral and biological signs, regression, peri- and post-natal development and genetics. *Journal of Child Psychology and Psychiatry, 51*, 432–458.

Yoder, P. J., & Warren, S. F. (2004). Early predictors of language in children with and without Down syndrome. *American Journal on Mental Retardation, 109*(4), 285–300.

Zeliadt, N. (2015). How everyday interactions shape autism. Retrieved from *http://spectrumnews.org/features/deep-dive/the-social-network-how-everyday-interactions-shape-autism.*

Zwaigenbaum, L., Bryson, S., Rogers, T., Roberts, W., Brian, J., & Szatmari, P. (2005). Behavioral manifestations of autism in the first year of life. *International Journal of Developmental Neuroscience, 23*(2–3), 143–152.

CHAPTER 13

Child–Parent Psychotherapy
Theoretical Bases, Clinical Applications, and Empirical Support

SHEREE L. TOTH, LOUISA C. MICHL-PETZING,
DANIELLE GUILD, and ALICIA F. LIEBERMAN

This chapter describes Child–Parent Psychotherapy (CPP), a relationship-based, trauma-responsive, multitheoretical intervention through which joint sessions between the parent and the young child center on spontaneous interactions and play as vehicles to promote protective caregiving and secure attachment, target maladaptive mutual attributions between parent and child, and help the parent understand and respond in developmentally supportive ways to the child's signals of need (Lieberman & Van Horn, 2005, 2008). CPP has been shown to be effective with infants, toddlers, and preschoolers, and with families from a range of socioeconomic and cultural backgrounds, but its development was prompted primarily by the urgent need to address the disproportionate exposure of poor and minority children from birth to age 5 to traumatic events and other adversities (Chu & Lieberman, 2010). In the sections below we describe the dual attachment- and trauma-lenses informing CPP interventions, highlighting the relevance of attachment theory and maltreatment concerns to the development of CPP. We then present CPP core principles, followed by results from randomized controlled trials (RCTs) that demonstrate the efficacy of CPP for fostering attachment security and decreasing behavior problems and posttraumatic stress disorder in infants and young children who have been reared in maltreating families or by a caregiver struggling with depression, or exposed to domestic violence. Additionally, we provide illustrative examples of integrating CPP into community settings and discuss the current state of dissemination and training efforts. We conclude by considering the implications of this body of work for public policy.

The Dual Attachment- and Trauma-Informed Lens in CPP

The central organizing theme of CPP involves the importance of using both a trauma- and an attachment-informed lens in the assessment and treatment of infants and toddlers with mental health disturbances, exposed to trauma, and showing problems with attachment. The quality of attachment that children carry into and out of traumatic events deeply influences their ability to recover from the impact of traumatic events. However, parents are often traumatized by the same events that have traumatized their child, either due to the objective features of the event (e.g., a natural disaster, family or community violence, a life-threatening accident) or because the danger to the child represents a traumatic event for the parent (e.g., grave child illness or injury). These traumatic events can then disrupt even a previously secure attachment by inducing strong emotions in the parents that interfere with their ability to remain attuned to the child's needs. These emotions may include guilt, fear, overprotectiveness, and/or affective dysregulation. In parallel, traumatic events may damage the child's age-appropriate belief that the parent can be unconditionally protective in all circumstances and may give rise to psychogenic beliefs that the parent instigated the traumatic event or was unwilling to protect the child from it. In response, CPP focuses simultaneous attention to real-life traumatic stressors and to the internal experience of these stressors both in the child and the parent figures. This allows the therapist to assess the interplay between external and subjective realities, in accord with Bowlby's (1973, 1980a, 1980b, 1982) revolutionary insights on the role of primary emotional relationships as mediators and moderators of the impact of adversity on personality formation.

CPP is also guided by the organizational perspective, which addresses how development proceeds over time by identifying a progression of reorganizations within and among biological, psychological, and social systems (Werner & Kaplan, 1963). This perspective is a natural fit with Bowlby's attachment theory as elaborated on by Sroufe and Waters (1977). Development is conceived as consisting of a series of age- and stage-relevant tasks that, although ascendant at certain periods of development, continue to influence the emergence and resolution of subsequent tasks that remain important across the lifespan of the individual (Cicchetti, 1993). The successful resolution of an early stage-salient issue increases the likelihood that subsequent issues also will be resolved successfully (Sroufe & Rutter, 1984). As infants and toddlers are confronted with new demands at transitional periods of development, they encounter opportunities for growth and resolution, as well as challenges associated with new vulnerabilities. Dynamic transactions between internal and external factors can therefore result in either competent or maladaptive outcomes over the life course. Consistent with a developmental psychopathology perspective, this model imparts hope in the potential for change and highlights the importance of providing interventions that can prevent or ameliorate negative outcomes, particularly during the early years of life, before unresolved early stage-salient issues set in motion a negative cascade of failed developmental attainments.

Attachment considerations and the organizational perspective both inform the multilevel approach of developmental psychopathology, particularly relevant to understanding the impact of early traumatic experiences on the course of development (Toth & Cicchetti, 2011). CPP attends to the transactional influences among cultural values and practices, sociodemographic factors, parental mental health and functioning, the quality of the parent–child relationship, and the child's individual characteristics. These transactions emerge as important considerations in the development of effective interventions for traumatized children (Cicchetti & Lynch, 1993; Lieberman, Chu, Van Horn, & Harris, 2011).

Theoretical Foundations of CPP

The negative consequences accompanying trauma and early adversity highlight the importance of providing interventions to assist young children in coping with the sequelae of trauma and helping them learn to regulate affect and normalize responses to potential traumatic triggers, develop or maintain secure attachments, repair trust in relationships, and explore and learn in age-appropriate ways. CPP is a trauma-focused, relationship-based treatment that has been evaluated with racially and ethnically diverse infants, toddlers, preschoolers, and their mothers. The intervention has been utilized to promote attachment security and address behavioral and emotional problems in children with histories of trauma and early adversity, including exposure to domestic violence (Lieberman, Van Horn, & Ghosh Ippen, 2005), the experience of child maltreatment (Cicchetti, Rogosch, & Toth, 2006), and being reared by a depressed caregiver (Cicchetti, Rogosch, & Toth, 2000).

CPP has its origins in infant-parent psychotherapy (IPP), a psychoanalytic treatment developed by Selma Fraiberg (1980) to interrupt the intergenerational transmission of maladaptive patterns of relating. The metaphor "ghosts in the nursery" was used to describe the repressed affective experiences that were originally associated with terrifying childhood events and reemerge in the present in response to the urgent needs and demands of a new baby. The baby becomes a transference object onto whom the parent projects or displaces unresolved conflicts and unacknowledged impulses and feelings from the past. Fraiberg's work, firmly rooted in her social work and psychoanalytic background, emphasized the importance of attending to the reality-based hardships that compound the emotional burdens of abusive and neglecting parents who unwittingly reenact painful childhoods in their relationships with their children. It is in this shared understanding of the impact of external circumstances on the inner world that psychoanalysis and attachment theory meet to elucidate the emotional space between parent and child.

The goal of IPP is to help the parent examine negative or maladaptive feelings toward the baby in light of his or her childhood experiences. This process, guided with tact and emotional support by the therapist, enabled the parent to retrieve and reexperience the full force of the unremembered affect from the past in order to redirect it to its legitimate targets—frightening and neglecting parents, siblings, or other important figures from the parent's childhood. As negative affect was integrated with the past events that gave rise to it, the parent was freed to perceive and respond to his or her baby's needs and emotional signals in the developmental context where they belong. IPP helped to uncover and make conscious the childhood sources of unconscious, damaging parental impulses, so the baby might be protected from them and regain his or her individuality (Lieberman et al., 2005).

CPP continues to incorporate these psychoanalytic concepts and formulations, but it has become more multitheoretical in response to new knowledge about the impact of trauma on the anatomy and physiology of the brain (Frodl & O'Keane, 2013; McCrory, De Brito, & Viding, 2010); the emergence of trauma theory, research, and clinical practice (Cohen, Mannarino, & Deblinger, 2006; Pynoos, Steinberg, & Piacentini, 1999; van der Kolk, 2003); the clear diagnostic evidence that toddlers and preschoolers may develop posttraumatic stress disorder following traumatic events (Scheeringa & Zeanah, 2001); and the urgent need to provide effective intervention to traumatized toddlers and preschoolers who cannot wait while their parent figures uncover the sources of their maladaptive parenting patterns (Lieberman, 2004). In its current formulation, CPP places its psychoanalytic origins in the context of developmental psychopathology and attachment theory. Within this theoretical framework, clinicians may flexibly adapt behavioral interventions contributed by cognitive-behavioral therapy and other approaches in order to guide parental and child behavior toward more adaptive manifestations, never losing sight of the emotional meanings of the behaviors targeted for change.

A thorough initial assessment of the child, the parent, and their relationship is an integral component of CPP. This initial period of treatment is described as the "Foundational Phase: Assessment and Engagement" because it provides the cornerstone for establishing a working relationship with the parents and developing a shared narrative of the clinical needs that becomes the basis for case formulation and treatment planning. The foundational phase culminates in a feedback session where the clinician and parent discuss what they learned during this process and how to introduce the treatment to the child. One important component of this session involves the co-creation with the parents of a "triangle" that clarifies the causal connections possibly linking the child and family stressors and traumatic experiences with the child's presenting problems and the parents' difficulties in supporting the child's healthy development, and describing the goals of treatment. The "triangle" is also used to describe the reason for treatment to the child, using developmentally appropriate language and toys to illustrate the narrative. The foundational phase enables the therapist to gain knowledge of the concrete circumstances of the family, including risk and protective factors in their socioeconomic conditions and environmental context, as well as culturally rooted values and caregiving practices. It also enables the clinician to ascertain child and parent exposure to traumatic events, evaluate the parent and child mental health needs and emotional resources, and the quality of their relationship. The foundational phase also provides an opportunity to create a treatment plan in collaboration with the parent, an essential first step in treatment, because the establishment of corrective attachment experiences in the therapeutic relationship is conceptualized as the mechanism of change. Therapeutic change is theorized to occur via the process of learning and practicing reciprocal, mutually satisfying exchanges that give positive emotional valence to the network of meaning being constructed between the parent and the child (Lieberman et al., 2005). Such a corrective attachment experience acts as a vehicle for change in what once may have been a constricted or disorganized internal representation of the self in relation to major attachment figures (Lieberman, 1991). Although a consideration of the self and relationships in the context of attachment is an organizing focus, CPP considers the specific attachment categories as useful ways of organizing information for research purposes, but does not formally utilize them to guide treatment planning. Treatment guidelines are instead constructed in a collaborative fashion by the participants and the therapists on the basis of the foundational phase findings, and tailored to the specific characteristics and needs of the child and caregiver(s) (Lieberman et al., 2005).

The goals of the CPP model are summarized in Table 13.1.

As indicated in Table 13.1, there are four principal goals of CPP: (1) creating safety in the parent–child relationship and in the environment by identifying and addressing sources of objective danger, and by identifying and modulating responses to traumatic triggers that create affective dysregulation and frightened/frightening behavior in the parent, the child, and the parent–child interactions; (2) expanding the parent's empathic responsiveness, sensitivity, and attunement to the child's signals of need; (3) promoting the parent's ability to foster his or her child's autonomy while negotiating both his or her own and the child's needs positively; and (4) modifying parental and child distorted or maladaptive perceptions of each other and inappropriate parental reactions to the child that stem from the parent's representational models of his or her relationship history. Therapists implementing CPP foster positive interactions between child and parent and use spontaneous play and/or conflict as an opportunity to explore areas for growth in the child–parent relationship. Through observation of dyadic interactions, therapists facilitate improvements in parents' sensitivity to children's emotional needs and responsivity to children's verbal and nonverbal communication, as well as promoting children's development and appropriate expression of their needs and feelings. As part of their training, therapists gain knowledge in stage-salient developmental issues for infants, toddlers, and preschoolers. Discussions of normative development are

TABLE 13.1. Principal Goals of CPP

Goal	Description
1. Create safety in parent–child relationship and surrounding environment	• Identify and address sources of objective danger • Detect and modulate responses to traumatic triggers that create affective dysregulation and frightened/frightening behavior in the parent, child, and parent–child interactions
2. Expand parental responsiveness/attunement	• Develop parent's empathic responsiveness, sensitivity, and attunement to his or her child's signals of need
3. Promote parental capacity to balance parent and child needs	• Encourage the parent's ability to foster her child's autonomy • Promote parent's capacity to simultaneously negotiate his or her own and the child's needs in a positive manner
4. Modify maladaptive perceptions of parent and child for both members of dyad	• Adjust both parental and child distorted/maladaptive perceptions of each other • Modify inappropriate parental reactions to child influenced by the parent's representational models that stem from his or her own relationship history

introduced at clinically appropriate moments, while encouraging parents to support the developmental gains that their children make over time. This developmental guidance focuses on supportive exploration, recognition of strengths, and encouragement to practice new interaction patterns rather than didactic instruction in specific parenting skills. Although considerable flexibility is a hallmark of CPP, the treatment manual (Lieberman & Van Horn, 2005; Lieberman, Ghosh Ippen, & Van Horn, 2015) describes various strategies and provides examples to address the following domains of functioning: play; sensorimotor disorganization and disruption of biological rhythms; fearfulness; reckless, self-endangering and accident-prone behavior; aggressive, punitive, and critical parenting; the relationship with the perpetrator of violence and/or absent father/mother; and separation issues related to treatment termination.

CPP has been used with children from birth through age 5 years and their caregivers. It is typically implemented in weekly hour-long sessions over a period of approximately 10–12 months, although treatment length may vary depending on the severity and chronicity of the child and/or parent's mental health problems. The intervention can be provided in a variety of contexts, with the goal of allowing child and parent to interact as they typically do. In this way, one of the merits of the model is its flexibility. CPP may be conducted in homes, offices, or clinic settings, provided that there are age-appropriate toys for the child to play with. Individual sessions with the caregiver also may be scheduled as needed. This may be particularly important if a caregiver is struggling with trauma associated with sexual assault or material that would prove to be too distressing to address with the child present. Moreover, the CPP model allows for flexibility with respect to the inclusion of multiple caregivers (e.g., mother and father or grandparent) and siblings.

In the CPP intervention, the caregiver's relationship with the therapist is considered central to the process of therapeutic change. Therefore, it is important to establish a therapeutic relationship that is framed as a collaborative endeavor between the caregiver and the therapist. This collaboration sets the tone for future therapeutic work, as the caregiver's active role in CPP is needed in order to achieve positive results. The therapeutic relationship is the basis for exploring the parent's history of caregiving and addressing past experiences of trauma, loss, or maltreatment that may exert negative influences on parenting. The therapist strives to create an emotionally corrective experience for parents by acknowledging their wishes, needs, and fears, especially those relating to parents' past experiences with their own caregivers. Within the supportive environment of therapy, sessions with the parent, child, and therapist gradually begin to alter the relationship between the parent and the child. In the course of parent–child interactions, opportunities occur to explore the parent's internal representational world as it relates to his or her perceptions of and responses to the child. In session, the therapist also provides a voice for the child to help build the parent's awareness of the child's means of communicating his or her emotions, needs, and fears. Additionally, gentle modeling of appropriate behavior in relation to the child is implemented during child–therapist interactions so that parents may begin to internalize more effective ways to communicate with their offspring. Importantly, when provided, the modeling is done so as to be sensitive to the caregiver's perspective. As the intervention is not targeted toward an individual, but rather toward the *relationship* that exists between parent and child, CPP utilizes the corrective emotional experience in the context of the therapeutic relationship as a means to improve the parent–child attachment relationship.

Cultural sensitivity is essential for the success of this model, because "intimate relationships are regulated by cultural norms, which dictate if, how, and when feelings can be displayed" (Lieberman & Van Horn, 2005, p. 38). Thus, understanding and exploring cultural factors with the family is essential to the provision of empathic and nurturing therapeutic services. Due to the model's emphasis on cultural sensitivity, CPP has been successfully applied with several different cultural groups. Next, we direct our attention to the research base supporting CPP.

Randomized Controlled Trials

Numerous studies, summarized in Table 13.2, have demonstrated the therapeutic efficacy of CPP across multiple domains.

To examine the effects of CPP on quality of attachment and socioemotional functioning, Lieberman, Weston, and Pawl (1991) assigned anxiously attached 12-month-olds and their mothers to either CPP or a nonintervention condition. Securely attached mother–infant dyads comprised a second control group. The CPP intervention lasted 1 year and ended when children were 24 months old. Postintervention findings revealed that children in the CPP condition were significantly less likely than those in the anxiously attached control condition to avoid proximity to their mothers or to resist maternal contact. Furthermore, children who received the intervention evidenced a reduction in aggressive behavior, including yelling, kicking, hitting, or biting their mothers. CPP was also effective in enhancing maternal empathy and interaction with the child, as well as increasing the dyad's *goal-directed partnership*, or the degree of eagerness and reciprocity for interaction on behalf of both mother and child. No differences were found in postintervention outcome measures between the securely attached controls and those in the CPP condition.

Subsequent work by Cicchetti, Rogosch, and Toth (2006) demonstrated that CPP is compellingly effective at reorganizing early attachment patterns from insecure to secure. The authors randomized 1-year-old infants from maltreating families and their mothers to one of three conditions—CPP, a psychoeducational parenting intervention (PPI), or a community standard (CS) comparison group. A fourth group of infants from nonmaltreating families and their mothers were also included as a nonmaltreated comparison (NC) group. Mothers and infants in the intervention conditions received weekly therapy sessions for approximately 1 year. While CPP focused on the dyadic relational dynamics between mother and infant, the PPI intervention was more didactic in nature, with the goal of providing parent skills training and psychoeducation relevant to child development, reducing maternal stress, and fostering social support. Families in the CS and NC conditions were free to seek services in the community that are typically available.

All participants were from low-income (mean yearly salary = $17,151), urban neighborhoods, and the majority (74.1%) were of minority race/ethnicity. Infant attachment security was measured via the Strange Situation Procedure (Ainsworth,

TABLE 13.2. Empirical Support for CPP

Study	Study design	Group comparisons	Sample characteristics	Number of subjects	Age of child at outcome	Outcome
Lieberman et al. (1991)	RCT	CPP vs. no intervention vs. securely attached controls	Anxiously attached 12-month-olds and their mothers; securely attached mother–infant dyads	59 anxiously attached mother–infant dyads; 34 securely attached dyads	24 months	Offspring in the CPP group were significantly lower than anxiously attached controls in avoidance, resistance, and anger. They were significantly higher than anxious controls in partnership with mother. There were no differences on the outcome measures between the CPP and secure control groups.
Cicchetti et al. (2006)	RCT	CPP vs. psychoeducational parenting intervention (PPI) vs. community standard (CS) vs. nonmaltreated controls (NC)	12-month-old infants from maltreating families and their mothers; nonmaltreated infants and their mothers	137 maltreated infants and their mothers; 52 nonmaltreated controls	26 months	Offspring in the CPP and PPI groups showed significant increases in secure attachment, whereas those in the CS and NC groups did not.
Pickreign Stronach et al. (2013)	RCT; 1-year follow-up of Cicchetti et al. (2006)	CPP vs. PPI vs. CS vs. NC	12-month-old infants from maltreating families and their mothers; nonmaltreated infants and their mothers	137 maltreated infants and their mothers; 52 nonmaltreated controls	38 months	Offspring in the CPP group had significantly higher rates of secure attachment compared to those in the PPI or CS conditions.
Cicchetti et al. (2011)	RCT; 1-year follow-up of Cicchetti et al. (2006)	Early intervention (CPP or PPI) vs. CS vs. NC	12-month-old infants from maltreating families and their mothers; nonmaltreated infants and their mothers	137 maltreated infants and their mothers; 52 nonmaltreated controls	38 months	Morning cortisol levels of offspring who received intervention (CPP or PPI) were normalized over time, such that they were indistinguishable from the NC group, whereas maltreated offspring in the CS condition showed increasingly dysregulated cortisol rhythms over time.
Cicchetti et al. (2011)	RCT; same sample as Cicchetti et al. (2006)	Early intervention (CPP or PPI) vs. CS vs. NC	12-month-old infants from maltreating families and their mothers; nonmaltreated infants and their mothers	137 maltreated infants and their mothers; 52 nonmaltreated controls	24 months	Genetic variation in the *5-HTTLPR* and *DRD4* genes significantly affected attachment in *nonmaltreated* infants, but not maltreated infants. Early intervention (CPP or PPI) for maltreated infants was effective irrespective of genetic variation.

(continued)

TABLE 13.2. Empirical Support for CPP

Study	Study design	Group comparisons	Sample characteristics	Number of subjects	Age of child at outcome	Outcome
Toth et al. (2002)	RCT	CPP vs. psychoeducational home visitation (PHV) vs. CS vs. NC	4- to 5-year-old maltreated preschoolers and their mothers; nonmaltreated preschoolers and their mothers	87 maltreated preschoolers and their mothers; 35 nonmaltreated comparisons and their mothers	5 years	Maltreated offspring who received CPP showed significantly greater declines in maladaptive maternal representations than offspring in the PHV or CS groups, and a greater decrease in negative self-representations over time than offspring in the PHV, CS, or NC conditions. Offspring in the CPP condition developed significantly more positive expectations of the mother–child relationship over the course of the intervention than those in the PHV or NC groups.
Lieberman et al. (2005)	RCT	CPP vs. case management + individual therapy	3- to 5-year-old children exposed to domestic violence (DV) and their mothers	75 mother–child dyads	4–6 years	Offspring in the CPP group showed significant reductions in behavioral problems postintervention, whereas those in the comparison group did not.
Lieberman et al. (2006)	RCT; 6-month follow-up of Lieberman et al. (2005)	CPP vs. case management + individual therapy	3- to 5-year-old children exposed to DV and their mothers	75 mother–child dyads	4.5–6.5 years	The significant reduction in total behavioral problems seen for offspring in the CPP condition was sustained at 6-month follow-up.
Toth et al. (2006)	RCT	CPP vs. nonintervention depressed controls (DC) vs. normal controls (NC)	20-month-old toddlers and their depressed mothers; toddlers and their nondepressed mothers	130 toddlers and their depressed mothers; 68 toddlers and their nondepressed mothers	36 months	Offspring in the CPP group showed significantly higher rates of secure attachment postintervention than those in the DC or NC groups.
Cicchetti et al. (2000)	RCT; same sample as Toth et al. (2006)	CPP vs. DC vs. NC	20-month-old toddlers and their depressed mothers; toddlers and their nondepressed mothers	130 toddlers and their depressed mothers; 68 toddlers and their nondepressed mothers	36 months	Offspring in the CPP group showed equivalent levels of cognitive functioning at postintervention to those in the NC group. However, offspring in the DC condition showed significant declines in IQ over time.

Blehar, Waters, & Wall, 1978). At baseline, infants from maltreating families evidenced significantly higher rates of insecure attachment than infants from the nonmaltreated group. However, at postintervention, children in the CPP and PPI groups showed significant increases in secure attachment, whereas those in the CS and NC groups did not evidence such changes.

The same mother–child dyads were followed 1-year postintervention to examine the sustained efficacy of CPP (Pickreign Stronach, Toth, Rogosch, & Cicchetti, 2013). Findings indicated that children in the CPP condition evidenced higher rates of secure attachment and lower rates of disorganized attachment than children in the PPI or CS conditions. Furthermore, the rates of disorganized attachment for children in the CPP condition did not differ from those in the demographically matched NC group. These results suggest that while psychoeducational parenting interventions may be equally as efficacious as CPP in the short-term, only CPP was efficacious in maintaining attachment security over time.

Another follow-up of Cicchetti, Rogosch, and Toth's (2006) original sample indicated that CPP and PPI may normalize the development of cortisol regulation among maltreated infants. Children exposed to maltreatment encounter numerous stressful experiences that exert harmful impacts on their developing neurobiological systems (Heim, Shugart, Craighead, & Nemeroff, 2010; McCrory, De Brito, & Viding, 2012). In particular, the regulation of cortisol, a glucocorticoid involved in the body's stress response system, is often disrupted (Tarullo & Gunnar, 2006; Strüber, Strüber, & Roth, 2014). Cicchetti, Rogosch, Toth, and Sturge-Apple (2011) examined daily cortisol rhythms in infants across the CPP, PPI, CS, and NC conditions at baseline (13 months), midintervention (19 months), postintervention (26 months), and 1-year postintervention follow-up (38 months). Due to sample size, the two intervention conditions, CPP and PPI, were combined into a single maltreated intervention (MI) group for statistical analyses.

At baseline, findings revealed no differences between groups in morning cortisol regulation. However, beginning at midintervention, divergence among groups had already emerged. While morning cortisol in the MI and NC conditions remained stable and indistinguishable over time, the CS group evidenced significantly lower levels of morning cortisol, which continued to decline through the 1-year postintervention follow-up. Morning cortisol levels of maltreated infants who received intervention were therefore normalized, while maltreated infants in the CS condition showed progressive cortisol dysregulation as they entered toddlerhood. Further research will be necessary to distinguish potential differences in cortisol regulation among children who receive CPP compared to those who participate in alternative interventions for maltreatment, such as PPI.

Another study with the same participants explored the effects of child maltreatment and polymorphisms of the serotonin transporter linked promotor region (*5-HTTLPR*) and dopamine receptor D$_4$ (*DRD4*) genes on infant attachment and intervention efficacy (Cicchetti, Rogosch, & Toth, 2011). *5-HTTLPR* and *DRD4* are genes that have been shown to relate to attachment patterns among nonmaltreated infants (for a review see Papageorgiou & Ronald, 2013). As with the aforementioned study, Cicchetti, Rogosch, and Toth (2011) combined participants in the CPP and PPI conditions into a single maltreated intervention group for the purpose of statistical analyses. Interestingly, the authors found that genetic variation significantly affected attachment in nonmaltreated, but *not* maltreated, infants. It was posited that the high rates of disorganized attachment among maltreated infants may overpower the genetic contribution of *5-HTTLPR* and *DRD4* to attachment. Finally, results also indicated that early intervention for maltreated infants was effective irrespective of genetic variation, suggesting that beneficial outcomes are likely to generalize to children of varying phenotypes (Cicchetti, Rogosch, Toth, & Sturge-Apple, 2011).

In light of the evidence that attachment plasticity is possible, even in children with divergent genetic polymorphisms, these studies suggest that many of the harmful sequelae of child maltreatment need not be permanent. As a trauma-informed attachment-based relational intervention, CPP is effective in promoting secure attachment that remains stable over time. Furthermore, the evidence base suggests that early intervention can alter neurobiological development, such that young maltreated children receiving CPP or PPI show a normalization of cortisol regulation over time.

In a separate sample, Toth, Maughan, Manly, Spagnola, and Cicchetti (2002) also evaluated the relative efficacy of CPP versus PPI to modify maltreated preschoolers' perceptions of self and of self in relation to other. Toddlers were administered a set of narrative story-stems from the MacArthur Story-Stem Battery (MSSB; Bretherton, Oppenheim, Buchsbaum, Emde, & the MacArthur Narrative Group, 1990) and the Attachment Story Completion Task (ASCT; Bretherton, Ridgeway, & Cassidy, 1990) at baseline and postintervention assessment periods. Each of the story-stem narratives depicted moral dilemmas and emotionally charged events in the context of parent–child and family relationships. The narratives were designed to elicit children's perceptions of the parent–child relationship, of self, and of maternal behavior in response to child accidents or transgressions and interfamilial conflicts. Children's completed narratives were coded according to the MacArthur Narrative Coding Manual–Rochester Revision (MNCM-RR; Robinson, Mantz-Simmons, Macfie, & MacArthur Narrative Working Group, 1996) and Bickham and Fiese's (1999) child narrative codebook.

Findings indicated that children who received CPP showed more of a decline in maladaptive maternal representations over time than those in either the PPI or CS groups. Children in the CPP condition also evidenced a greater decrease in negative self-representations over time than those in the PPI, CS, or NC conditions. Finally, children who received CPP also developed more positive expectations of the mother–child relationship over the course of the intervention than those in the PPI or NC groups. These results are consistent with those reported on the 1-year sustainability of attachment security and also suggest that as development proceeds, an attachment-informed model of treatment such as CPP is better at improving children's internal representations of self and of self in relation to caregivers than a didactic parenting intervention, such as PPI.

CPP also has been shown to be efficacious in decreasing behavior problems and symptoms of posttraumatic stress disorder in a culturally diverse group of low-income preschoolers exposed to domestic violence and their mothers (Lieberman, Van Horn, & Ghosh Ippen, 2005). Participants in this investigation included 3- to 5-year-old girls and boys and their mothers. Dyads were referred based on clinical concerns about the child's behavior or the mother's parenting after the child was exposed to marital violence. Participants were randomly assigned to CPP or to case management plus individual treatment comparison group. Weekly CPP sessions of approximately 60 minutes were conducted over the course of 50 weeks. In a 6-month follow-up investigation, the durability of CPP was supported, revealing decreases for children's total behavior problems and mothers' general distress (Lieberman, Ghosh Ippen, & Van Horn, 2006). These results highlight the importance of providing a relationship-based treatment for traumatized preschoolers. A reanalysis of the data also showed that CPP is effective even when children have experienced more than four traumatic/stressful life events (Ippen, Harris, Van Horn, & Lieberman, 2011).

Finally, studies also have demonstrated that CPP is effective in reorganizing attachment in toddlers of depressed mothers. Toth, Rogosch, Manly, and Cicchetti (2006) randomized mothers with a history of major depressive disorder (MDD) and their toddlers (mean age = 20.3 months) to one of two conditions—CPP depressed intervention (DI) or depressed controls (DC). A third group of nondepressed mothers and their toddlers were recruited for a nondepressed control (NC) condition. Mother–child dyads in the DI condition participated in CPP once weekly for an average of 45 weeks. To minimize co-occurring risk factors associated with maternal depression, participants in the study were of middle to upper socioeconomic status, and the majority of mothers were married and of European American ethnicity. Similar to previous studies, child attachment at baseline and follow-up were measured via the Strange Situation Procedure (Ainsworth et al., 1978).

Consistent with prior research, the authors found that maternal depression was associated with increased incidences of insecure attachment in offspring. At baseline, toddlers in the DI and DC groups evidenced significantly higher rates of insecure and disorganized attachment than those in the NC condition. Following the completion of CPP, however, toddlers in the DI condition showed higher incidences of secure attachment than those in both the DC *and* NC conditions. These results indicate that children of depressed mothers who received CPP were more likely to have secure attachments than were children of well mothers, highlighting the efficacy of this intervention for improving mother–child relationships in high-risk groups.

In addition to fostering secure attachment in offspring of depressed mothers, CPP may also protect cognitive functioning in children. Utilizing data from the study described above, Cicchetti, Rogosch, and Toth (2000) examined the cognitive development of toddlers of depressed mothers. At baseline, none of the three groups (DI, DC, or NC) differed on the Bayley Mental Development Index (Bayley, 1969), a measure of cognitive and motor development used in infants and toddlers up to 30 months of age. At post-intervention, when toddlers were 3 years old, the Wechsler Preschool and Primary Scales of Intelligence–Revised (WPPSI-R; Wechsler, 1989) was used to reassess their cognitive development. Findings indicated that toddlers in the depressed control condition demonstrated declines in IQ over time, whereas those who received CPP and those in the nondepressed control condition continued to show equivalent levels of cognitive functioning. CPP therefore appears to be effective at minimizing and preventing cognitive decline in offspring of depressed mothers. Given extensive evidence on the efficacy of CPP, efforts to make the model more widely available become increasingly important.

Translational Research

In order to develop, evaluate, and disseminate evidence-based models of intervention, the need for translational research has been increasingly highlighted. Translational research involves examining how basic behavioral and biological processes can inform the diagnosis, prevention, treatment, and delivery of services for individuals at risk for or who have developed a mental illness (National Advisory Mental Health Council on Behavioral Sciences, 2000). The era of translational research is affecting all fields of inquiry in the medical, physical, social, and clinical sciences (Gunnar & Cicchetti, 2009). The impetus to conduct translational research in the behavioral sciences was spurred by the recognition of the tremendous individual, social and economic burden associated with mental illness (National Advisory Mental Health Council, 2000). Given the emphasis of developmental psychopathology on understanding the reciprocal interplay between basic and applied research and between normal and atypical development (Cicchetti & Toth, 2006), the parameters of developmental psychopathology lend themselves to fostering translational research that has implications for society, policymakers, and individuals with mental disorders and their families.

Increasingly, efforts to disseminate CPP to community settings have occurred. Such initiatives have been supported by Learning Collaboratives offered through the Substance Abuse and Mental Health Services Administration (SAMHSA) supported National Child Traumatic Stress Network (*www.nctsn.org*). As communities have come to recognize the deleterious effects of early trauma, funders also have begun to support the provision and evaluation of evidence-based models, including CPP. We next highlight efforts to export CPP into community settings.

Dissemination and Training

CPP is taught through a clinical manual (Lieberman & Van Horn, 2005; Lieberman, Ghosh Ippen, & Van Horn, 2015) and other publications (Lieberman et al., 2003; Lieberman & Van Horn, 2008) in university settings that provide psychology predoctoral internships and postdoctoral fellowships, master's level social work placements, and residency rotations in adult, child and adolescent psychiatry. National dissemination is conducted by endorsed CPP trainers using the Learning Collaborative and Learning Community adult learning models adopted by the National Child Traumatic Stress Network (NCTSN), with the mission of increasing access to treatment and raising the standard of care for traumatized children, their families, and communities throughout the United States. The Early Trauma Treatment Network (ETTN) is an NCTSN center led by the University of California San Francisco (UCSF) Child Trauma Research Program and composed also of the Boston Medical Center, Louisiana State University Medical Center, and Tulane University. The vehicles for CPP dissemination are the Learning Collaborative and Learning Community models of adult training used by the NCTSN as the core long-distance dissemination modalities for evidence-based trauma treatments. Long-distance CPP training using these adult learning models have a duration of 18 months and comprise an initial intensive 3-day face-to-face introduction, two 2-day face-to-face booster sessions at 6 months and 12 months, and biweekly telephone case-focused consultations.

Since 2001, numerous system-level and agency-level trainings have been conducted in more than 30 states to more than 2,000 clinicians, and CPP has been adopted at the state-level in 14 states. Internationally, the Learning Community model has also been used to train 100 clinicians in Israel to use CPP in a variety of settings throughout the country, and the CPP manual has been translated to Arabic and Hebrew for joint training of Palestinian and Jewish clinicians in Israel and the West Bank. CPP Learning Communities are also currently underway in Sweden.

Policy Implications

The corpus of research demonstrating the adverse consequences of childhood trauma, in conjunction with growing evidence on the availability of evidence-based treatments such as CPP for preventing a negative developmental cascade across the life-course, highlight the critical need for funding to increase the dissemination and implementation of trauma- and attachment-informed treatments. However, despite what should be an almost seamless integration of research, practice, and social policy, reciprocally beneficial interactions among these arenas have been difficult to achieve (Shonkoff, 2000; Toth & Cicchetti, 2006). Difficulties that impede the widespread availability of evidence-based services for children who experienced trauma are particularly egregious because of the extensive evidence that children's mental health improves significantly when they have access to these services (Toth, Gravener, Guild, & Cicchetti, 2013). In order to reduce impediments to access, it is vital to establish partnerships among professionals working with traumatized children, elected officials, and public interest advocates (Harris, Lieberman, & Marans, 2007; Toth & Cicchetti, 2006).

A crucial first step in ensuring access to trauma-informed treatments such as CPP pertains to actually identifying the fact that a traumatic event has occurred. Chu and Lieberman (2010) discuss entry points to care for young children exposed to trauma. They point out the unfortunate reality that, all too often, individuals in systems responsible for initial contact with young children lack the training and skills required to inquire about possible trauma or to recognize signs that trauma has occurred. When the need for treatment is recognized, far too few professionals are available to provide evidence-based, trauma- and attachment-informed treatments, particularly for children from birth to 5 years old (Osofsky & Lieberman, 2011; Lieberman et al., 2011). Fortunately, systemic barriers to access care can be minimized through large-scale educationally-based initiatives that encourage collaborations among professionals from diverse disciplines such as that embodied in the National Child Traumatic Stress Network (*www.nctsn.org*). The NCTSN has been very successful in increasing the availability of evidence-based services for traumatized children and improving the quality of care for children and families throughout the United States.

Even as increased dissemination is made possible, barriers to actual uptake of CPP and other evidence-based infant mental health treatments remain. Issues with reimbursement for services, particularly for the birth through age 5 population, remain complex. In many instances, a young child who has been traumatized may not be exhibiting symptoms that allow for a diagnosis of mental illness. Unfortunately, in the absence of a diagnosis third party payers may not view CPP as an allowable expense. Children's symptoms of mental health disorders are often misinterpreted by parents, primary care providers, and other professionals as behavioral problems that are temporary or require strict discipline or punishment. Moreover, utilization of CPP in a preventive mode is unlikely to be covered by traditional insurance. Finally, many providers of CPP utilize home-based service delivery in order to be able to reach overwhelmed parents who may lack the financial means or wherewithal to travel to clinic settings, with the 'no-show' parent at clinic being replaced by the 'no-one-home' experience for the clinician doing the home-visit. In any case, as currently configured, insurers are unlikely to cover the costs accompanying the provision of home-based services.

In spite of these obstacles, the growing demand for early childhood evidence-based intervention has led large systems at the state and county levels to request CPP trainings for clinicians working in the public health system. The growing expansion of state- and county-wide CPP-informed agencies and systems is a promising sign that public officials are becoming responsive to the need for trauma-informed evidence-based interventions. One surmountable barrier to the uptake of CPP often emanates from distrust among community providers about any "evidence-based" model of treatment. Misconceptions contributing to provider reluctance include such erroneous beliefs as all evidence-based models have been developed only with non-diverse populations and the use of an evidence-based model is inflexible and does not allow for tailoring to individual family needs. To truly increase the availability of this proven intervention model, we must continue to advocate for the best interest of society (Harris, Lieberman, & Marans, 2007). Just as CPP is a relationship-based treatment, the dissemination of CPP must be a relationship-based effort. Cultivating long-term relationships with child-serving systems and agencies at the local, state, and national levels is essential to promote understanding of the needs of high-risk and traumatized young children and their families and to forge partnerships that address those needs.

Community Implementation of Child–Parent Psychotherapy

Increasingly CPP is being implemented in community settings. One interesting example provided by the Florida Infant Mental Health Pilot Program is funded by the Florida state legislature (Osofsky et al., 2007). Participants included mothers with infants or young children (up to age 52 months) who had been investigated or substantiated for child maltreatment. The principal treatment was CPP. Notably, during and immediately after 25 CPP sessions, there were no further maltreatment reports for participants. In addition, there were also positive changes in observed maternal and child behaviors. Building on these findings, the national advocacy organization Zero-to-Three established the Safe Babies Court Teams Project, which provides similar court teams in five other states (Zero-to-Three, 2014). One study has indicated that children served by the Court Teams achieved a permanent placement sooner than comparison children, and that Court Team children were more likely to reach permanency with a member of their biological family (McCombs-Thornton & Foster, 2012).

Another example of community-based implementation of CPP is provided by a 2009 initiative in which CPP was one of three interventions integrated into a wrap-around foster care program for a diverse population of 216 three- to 18-year-olds (Weiner, Schneider, & Lyons, 2009). CPP was provided to children 6 years old and younger who had experienced a moderate or severe trauma and who had a caregiver willing to participate in the program. Pre-post analyses revealed significant effects in terms of reducing children's traumatic stress symptoms and behavioral and emotional disturbances for African American, Hispanic, and biracial children. White children improved on life domain functioning, but did not decrease in symptoms of traumatic stress and behavioral/emotional disturbances.

Child FIRST (Child and Family Interagency, Resource, Support, and Training) also is a community application involving a comprehensive, home-based, therapeutic intervention model for multi-risk young children and their families. Child FIRST has two core components: (1) a system of care intervention where the provider connects the family with comprehensive services such as early education, housing, substance abuse treatment, or other interventions tailored to the family needs; and (2) CPP as the therapeutic intervention to enhance nurturing and responsive parent–child interactions (Lowell et al., 2011). A randomized study was conducted with 157 mother–child dyads with children aged 6–36 months. At the 12-month assessment, Child FIRST children showed significant improvements compared with the Usual Care group in child language and externalizing symptoms. Mothers in the Child FIRST group showed less parenting stress at 6 months and lower psychopathology at 12 months, as well as less protective service involvement at a 3-year follow up. In addition, families in the intervention group accessed 91% of wanted services, while the Usual Care group accessed 33% of the services. This study demonstrates the synergy that may be achieved when integrating CPP with active assistance to families to improve concrete life circumstances, a core concept in Fraiberg's (1980) approach that has been incorporated in CPP.

The Building Healthy Children program, another community-based program, is an ongoing multi-pronged initiative for high-risk families that includes CPP as one component (Paradis, Sandler, Manly, & Valentine, 2013; Toth & Gravener, 2012). The program, funded by the Monroe County Department of Human Services and the United Way of Greater Rochester, focused on low-income young mothers who had their first child prior to age 21 and who have two or fewer children under the age of 3. Eligible families are identified through pediatric practices and enrolled into a randomized trial in which CPP is one of three home-based interventions provided to families depending on a baseline needs assessment conducted by a trained outreach worker. Therapists are cross-trained on all interventions to facilitate a seamless integration across models and to ensure continuity of the therapist providing services. Comparison families receive annual assessments and referrals for community services as needed. The program includes active, culturally sensitive outreach and careful coordination between the outreach worker and the therapist providing the evidence-based models. In 2014, the program had enrolled approximately 600 (treatment and comparison) families, provided CPP to 56 dyads (11%), and retained 85% of all families by the target child's third birthday. Initial findings from health and developmental assessments have been promising, revealing greater compliance with well-child visits (Paradis, Sandler, Manly, & Valentine, 2013). Preliminary data also are revealing positive outcomes for mothers, including decreases in depression and increases in perceptions of maternal efficacy.

A final successful model for community application consists of placing CPP postdoctoral fellows in community-based agencies that are geared to meeting multiple family needs. The Tipping Point Mental Health Initiative of the San Francisco Bay Area is a community extension of CPP where postdoctoral fellows are formally trained at the Child Trauma Research Program, where they attend didactic seminars and case review, and receive clinical supervision, but are based in community based agencies during much of the week to provide on-site CPP. The community-based agencies include a pediatric clinic, family resources centers, childcare centers, and a homeless family program. This initiative is funded by Tipping Point Community, a private foundation whose mission is to make poverty preventable and sees the hardships of parenting under adverse circumstances as a crucial obstacle in helping parents become self-sufficient. The collaboration between a private foundation devoted to eradicating poverty, community-based agencies providing a range of concrete services to meet family's problems of living, and mental health clinicians providing CPP as a trauma-informed evidence-based treatment model embodies the integration of Selma Fraiberg's concept of "psychoanalysis in the kitchen" (Fraiberg, 1980). The role of reality factors in attachment theory (Bowlby, 1980a), the ecological-transactional conceptual frame of developmental psychopathology (Cicchetti & Lynch, 1993), and a vital move toward what Freud imagined as an age when the urgent mental health needs of the poor would be addressed by a "psychotherapy for the people" (Freud, 1918, p. 168, cited in Aron & Starr, 2013) also are reflected in this initiative.

Concluding Remarks and Future Directions

In this chapter we have presented the theoretical framework, treatment strategies, and current evidence-base for CPP. This is an exciting time, as CPP is increasingly being embraced both nationally and internationally, thereby filling a critical gap in empirically-supported intervention for young victims of trauma. We also are particularly gratified that CPP is being exported into community settings and being evaluated to assess its effectiveness in those settings. This latter step is important as it will assist in ensuring that practitioners are able to maintain the fidelity of CPP in diverse settings.

In recent years, significant progress has occurred with respect to the maturation of CPP. Guidelines for therapist training have been distributed, a roster of CPP trained therapists has been developed, and instruments for measuring therapist competence and adherence to model fidelity have been made available. We conclude this chapter by reflecting on some important next steps.

One arena for continued growth emanates from the research domain. Although CPP has met the highest standards for designation as an evidence-based model, including RCT replication by independent research groups and evidence of continued benefit one-year post intervention, further evaluations with diverse populations and varied outcome measures will only serve to strengthen the empirical support of the model. Investigations designed to better understand the processes contributing to positive outcome and investigations that compare CPP with other evidence-based models such as Trauma-Focused Cognitive Behavioral Therapy (TF-CBT; Cohen, Mannarino, Berliner & Deblinger, 2000; Cohen & Mannarino, 2008; Deblinger, Mannarino, Cohen, Runyon, & Steer, 2011) or Alternative for Families Cognitive Behavioral Therapy (AF-CBT; Kolko, Iselin, & Gully, 2011) could be particularly valuable in beginning to identify which treatment model might be particularly effective with a given population. Given what we know about the adverse health consequences of trauma, RCTs that incorporate measures of psychophysiological functioning into outcome studies and investigations addressing epigenetics is an innovative new frontier. Of course, reasonably large cohorts would be necessary for the conduct of such studies and collaborations among research/clinical groups will most likely be necessary. From such efforts, we will draw closer to an understanding of the relevance of differential susceptibility theory, positing that some children and/or parents respond greatly, and others not much at all to an intervention (e.g. Ellis, Boyce, Belsky, Bakermans-Kranenburg, & Van IJzendoorn, 2011). Or, we may come to appreciate more fully the special and demanding case of trauma, where despite all range of psychophysiological and genetic variations that may be measured, children and parents benefit similarly from evidence-based trauma- and attachment-informed interventions (Cicchetti et al., 2011).

In concluding, we are encouraged by efforts that have contributed to refinements in the conceptual base and the development of empirical support for CPP. We are particularly enthusiastic about efforts that have been made to increase the availability and dissemination of CPP to community settings, thereby increasing access to this evidence-based model of treatment to greater numbers of children and families whose lives have been marred by exposure to trauma.

REFERENCES

Ainsworth, M. D. S., Blehar, M. C., Waters, E., & Wall, S. (1978). *Patterns of attachment: A psychological study of the Strange Situation.* Hillsdale, NJ: Erlbaum.

Aron, L., & Starr, K. (2013). *A psychotherapy for the people: Toward a progressive psychoanalysis.* New York: Routledge.

Bayley, N. (1969). *The Bayley Scales of Infant Development.* New York: Psychological Corporation.

Bickham, N., & Fiese, B. (1999). *Child narrative coding system.* Unpublished manuscript, Syracuse University, Syracuse, NY.

Bowlby, J. (1973). *Attachment and loss: Vol. 2. Separation: Anxiety and anger.* New York: Basic Books.

Bowlby, J. (1980a). *Attachment and loss: Vol. 1. Attachment.* New York: Basic Books. (Original work published 1969)

Bowlby, J. (1980b). *Loss: Sadness and depression: Vol. 3. Attachment and loss.* In *International Psycho-Analytical Library* (No. 109). London: Hogarth Press.

Bowlby, J. (1982). Attachment and loss: Retrospect and prospect. *American Journal of Orthopsychiatry, 52*(4), 664–668.

Bretherton, I., Oppenheim, D., Buchsbaum, H., & Emde, R. N., & the MacArthur Narrative Group. (1990). *MacArthur Story-Stem Battery*. Unpublished manual, University of Wisconsin–Madison.

Bretherton, I., Ridgeway, D., & Cassidy, J. (1990). Assessing internal working models of the attachment relationship. In M. T. Greenberg, D. Cicchetti, & E. M. Cummings (Eds.), *Attachment in the preschool years: Theory, research, and intervention* (pp. 273–308). Chicago: University of Chicago Press.

Chu, A. T., & Lieberman, A. F. (2010). Clinical implications of traumatic stress from birth to age five. *Annual Review of Clinical Psychology, 6,* 469–494.

Cicchetti, D. (1993). Developmental psychopathology: Reactions, reflections, projections. *Developmental Review, 13,* 471–502.

Cicchetti, D., & Lynch, M. (1993). Toward an ecological/transactional model of community violence and child maltreatment: Consequences for children's development. *Psychiatry, 56,* 96–118.

Cicchetti, D., Rogosch, F. A., & Toth, S. L. (2000). The efficacy of toddler–parent psychotherapy for fostering cognitive development in offspring of depressed mothers. *Journal of Abnormal Child Psychology, 28,* 135–148.

Cicchetti, D., Rogosch, F. A., & Toth, S. L. (2006). Fostering secure attachment in maltreating families through preventive interventions. *Development and Psychopathology, 18,* 623–650.

Cicchetti, D., Rogosch, F. A., Toth, S. L. (2011). The effects of child maltreatment and polymorphisms of the serotonin transporter and dopamine D4 receptor genes on infant attachment and intervention efficacy. *Development and Psychopathology, 23,* 357–372.

Cicchetti, D., Rogosch, F., Toth, S. L., & Sturge-Apple, M. L. (2011). Normalizing the development of cortisol regulation in maltreated infants through preventive interventions. *Development and Psychopathology, 23,* 789–800.

Cicchetti, D., & Toth, S. L. (2006). A developmental psychopathology perspective on preventive interventions with high risk children and families. In A. Renninger & I. Sigel (Vol. Eds.), *Handbook of child psychology: Vol. 4. Child psychology in practice* (6th ed., pp. 497–547). New York: Wiley.

Cohen, J. A., & Mannarino, A. P. (2008). Trauma-focused cognitive behavioural therapy for children and parents. *Child and Adolescent Mental Health, 13*(4), 158–162.

Cohen, J. A., Mannarino, A. P., Berliner, L., & Deblinger, E. (2000). Trauma-focused cognitive behavioral therapy for children and adolescents an empirical update. *Journal of Interpersonal Violence, 15*(11), 1202–1223.

Cohen, J. A., Mannarino, A. P., & Deblinger, E. (2006). *Treating trauma and traumatic grief in children and adolescents*. New York: Guilford Press.

Deblinger, E., Mannarino, A. P., Cohen, J. A., Runyon, M. K., & Steer, R. A. (2011). Trauma-focused cognitive behavioral therapy for children: Impact of the trauma narrative and treatment length. *Depression and Anxiety, 28*(1), 67–75.

Ellis, B. J., Boyce, W. T., Belsky, J., Bakermans-Kranenburg, M. J., & van IJzendoorn, M. H. (2011). Differential susceptibility to the environment: An evolutionary-neurodevelopmental theory. *Development and Psychopathology, 23,* 7–28.

Fraiberg, S. (1980). *Clinical studies in infant mental health*. London: Tavistock.

Frodl, T., & O'Keane, V. (2013). How does the brain deal with cumulative stress?: A review with focus on developmental stress, HPA axis function and hippocampal structure in humans. *Neurobiology of Disease, 52,* 24–37.

Gunnar, M. R., & Cicchetti, D. (2009). Meeting the challenge: Opportunities, roadblocks, detours. In M. R. Gunnar & D. Cicchetti (Eds.), *Minnesota Symposia on Child Psychology: Meeting the challenge of translational research in child psychology* (Vol. 35, pp. 1–27). New York: Wiley.

Harris, W. W., Lieberman, A. F., & Marans, S. (2007). In the best interests of society. *Journal of Child Psychology and Psychiatry, 48,* 392–411.

Heim, C., Shugart, M., Craighead, W. E., & Nemeroff, C. B. (2010). Neurobiological and psychiatric consequences of child abuse and neglect. *Developmental Psychobiology, 52*(7), 671–690.

Ippen, C. G., Harris, W. W., Van Horn, P., & Lieberman, A. F. (2011). Traumatic and stressful events in early childhood: Can treatment help those at highest risk? *Child abuse and Neglect, 35*(7), 504–513.

Kolko, D. J., Iselin, A. M. R., & Gully, K. J. (2011). Evaluation of the sustainability and clinical outcome of Alternatives for Families: A Cognitive-Behavioral Therapy (AF-CBT) in a child protection center. *Child Abuse and Neglect, 35*(2), 105–116.

Lieberman, A. F. (1991). Attachment theory and infant–parent psychotherapy: Some conceptual, clinical and research considerations. In D. Cicchetti & S. L. Toth (Eds.), *Rochester Symposium on Developmental Psychopathology* (Vol. 3, pp. 261–287). Rochester, NY: University of Rochester Press.

Lieberman, A. F. (2004). Traumatic stress and quality of attachment: Reality and internalization in disorders of infant mental health. *Infant Mental Health Journal, 25,* 336–351.

Lieberman, A. F., Chu, A., Van Horn, P., & Harris, W. W. (2011). Trauma in early childhood: Empirical evidence and clinical implications. *Development and Psychopathology, 23*(2), 397–410.

Lieberman, A. F., Compton, N. C., Van Horn, P., & Ippen, C. G. (2003). *Losing a parent to death in the early years: Guidelines for the treatment of traumatic bereavement in infancy and early childhood.* Washington, DC: ZERO TO THREE Press.

Lieberman, A. F., Ghosh Ippen, C., & Van Horn, P. (2006). Child–parent psychotherapy: 6-month follow-up of a randomized controlled trial. *Journal of the American Academy of Child and Adolescent Psychiatry, 45*(8), 913–918.

Lieberman, A. F., Ghosh Ippen, C., & Van Horn, P. (2015). *"Don't hit my mommy!": A manual for child–parent psychotherapy with young children exposed to violence and other trauma.* Washington, DC: ZERO TO THREE Press.

Lieberman, A. F., & Van Horn, P. (2005). *"Don't hit my mommy!": A manual for child parent psychotherapy with young witnesses of family violence.* Washington, DC: ZERO TO THREE Press.

Lieberman, A. F., & Van Horn, P. J. (2008). *Psychotherapy with infants and young children: Repairing the effects of stress and trauma on early attachment.* New York: Guilford Press.

Lieberman, A. F., Van Horn, P., & Ghosh Ippen, C. (2005). Toward evidence-based treatment: Child–parent psychotherapy with preschoolers exposed to marital violence. *Journal of the American Academy of Child and Adolescent Psychiatry, 44,* 1241–1248.

Lieberman, A. F., Weston, D. R., & Pawl, J. H. (1991). Preventive intervention and outcome with anxiously attached dyads. *Child Development, 62*(1), 199–209.

Lowell, D. I., Carter, A. S., Godoy, L., Paulicin, B., & Briggs-Gowan M. (2011). A randomized controlled trial of Child FIRST: A comprehensive home-based intervention translating research into early childhood practice. *Child Development, 82*(1), 193–208.

McCombs-Thornton, K. L., & Foster, E. M. (2012). The effect of the ZERO TO THREE Court Teams initiative on types of exits from the foster care system—A competing risks analysis. *Children and Youth Services Review, 34*(1), 169–178.

McCrory, E., De Brito, S. A., & Viding, E. (2010). Research review: The neurobiology and genetics of maltreatment and adversity. *Journal of Child Psychology and Psychiatry and Allied Disciplines, 51*(10), 1079–1095.

McCrory, E., De Brito, S. A., & Viding, E. (2012). The link between child abuse and psychopathology: A review of neurobiological and genetic research. *Journal of the Royal Society of Medicine, 105*(4), 151–156.

National Advisory Mental Health Council Behavioral Science Workgroup. (2000). *Translating behavioral science into action* (No. NIH 00–4699). Bethesda, MD: National Institute of Mental Health.

Osofsky, J. D., & Lieberman, A. F. (2011). A call for integrating a mental health perspective into systems of care for abused and neglected infants and young children. *American Psychologist, 66*(2), 120–128.

Papageorgiou, K. A., & Ronald, A. (2013). "He who sees things grow from the beginning will have the finest view of them": A systematic review of genetic studies on psychological traits in infancy. *Neuroscience and Biobehavioral Reviews, 37*(8), 1500–1517.

Paradis, H. A., Sandler, M., Manly, J. T., & Valentine, L. (2013). Building healthy children: Evidence-based home visitation integrated with pediatric medical homes. *Pediatrics, 132*(Suppl. 2), S174–S179.

Pickreign Stronach, E. S., Toth, S. L., Rogosch, F. A., & Cicchetti, D. (2013). Preventive interventions and sustained attachment security in maltreated children: A 12-month follow-up of a randomized controlled trial. *Development and Psychopathology, 254*(1), 919–930.

Pynoos, R. S., Steinberg, A. M., & Piacentini, J. C. (1999). A developmental psychopathology model of childhood traumatic stress and intersection with anxiety disorders. *Biological Psychiatry, 46*(11), 1542–1554.

Robinson, J. L., & Mantz-Simmons, L., Macfie, J., & the MacArthur Narrative Working Group. (1996). *The MacArthur Narrative coding manual–Rochester revision*. Unpublished manuscript, University of Rochester, Rochester, NY.

Scheeringa, M. S., & Zeanah, C. H. (1995). Symptom expression and trauma variables in children under 48 months of age. *Infant Mental Health Journal, 16*(4), 259–270.

Scheeringa, M. S., & Zeanah, C. H. (2001). A relational perspective on PTSD in early childhood. *Journal of Traumatic Stress, 14*(4), 799–815.

Shonkoff, J. P. (2000). Science, policy, and practice: Three cultures in search of a shared mission. *Child Development, 71*(1), 181–187.

Sroufe, L. A., & Rutter, M. (1984). The domain of developmental psychopathology. *Child Development, 55*(1), 17–29.

Sroufe, L. A., & Waters, E. (1977). Attachment as an organizational construct. *Child Development, 48*, 1184–1199.

Strüber, N., Strüber, D., & Roth, G. (2014). Impact of early adversity on glucocorticoid regulation and later mental disorders. *Neuroscience and Biobehavioral Reviews, 38*, 17–37.

Tarullo, A. R., & Gunnar, M. R. (2006). Child maltreatment and the developing HPA axis. *Hormones and Behavior, 50*(4), 632–639.

Toth, S. L., & Cicchetti, D. (2006). Promises and possibilities: The application of research in the area of child maltreatment to policies and practices. *Journal of Social Issues, 62*(4), 863–880.

Toth, S. L., & Cicchetti, D. (2011). Frontiers in translational research on trauma [Special issue]. *Development and Psychopathology, 23*, 353–355.

Toth, S. L., & Gravener, J. (2012). Bridging research and practice: Relational interventions for maltreated children. *Child and Adolescent Mental Health, 17*, 131–138.

Toth, S. L., Gravener-Davis, J. A., Guild, D. J., & Cicchetti, D. (2013). Relational interventions for child maltreatment: Past, present and future perspectives. *Development and Psychopathology, 25*(4), 1601–1617.

Toth, S. L., Maughan, A., Manly, J. T., Spagnola, M., & Cicchetti, D. (2002). The relative efficacy of two interventions in altering maltreated preschool children's representational models: Implications for attachment theory. *Development and Psychopathology, 14*, 877–908.

Toth, S. L., Rogosch, F. A., Manly, J. T., & Cicchetti, D. (2006). The efficacy of toddler–parent psychotherapy to reorganize attachment in the young offspring of mothers with major depressive disorder: A randomized preventive trial. *Journal of Consulting and Clinical Psychology, 74*(6), 1006–1016.

van der Kolk, B. A. (2003). The neurobiology of childhood trauma and abuse.*Child and Adolescent Psychiatric Clinics of North America, 12*(2), 293–317.

Wechsler, D. (1989). *WPPSI-R: Wechsler Preschool and Primary Scale of Intelligence.* San Diego, CA: Psychological Corporation.

Weiner, D. A., Schneider, A., & Lyons, J. S. (2009). Evidence-based treatments for trauma among culturally diverse foster care youth: Treatment retention and outcomes. *Children and Youth Services Review, 31*(11), 1199–1205.

Werner, H., & Kaplan, B. (1963). *Symbol formation: An organismic-developmental approach to language and the expression of thought.* New York: Wiley.

ZERO TO THREE. (2014). The safe babies court teams project. Retrieved from *www.zeroto-three.org/maltreatment/safe-babies-court-team.*

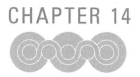

CHAPTER 14

The Attachment Video-Feedback Intervention Program

Development and Validation

ELLEN MOSS, GEORGE M. TARABULSY,
KARINE DUBOIS-COMTOIS, CHANTAL CYR,
ANNIE BERNIER, and DIANE ST-LAURENT

In this chapter, we describe an attachment-based, video-feedback intervention program, Attachment Video-Feedback Intervention (AVI), developed for vulnerable parents and their children ages 0–5 years. The program pilot tested over the course of many years with different high-risk groups of parents, was more recently validated with maltreating parents in collaboration with the Lanaudière Child Protection Services in Québec and replicated with maltreating parents in collaboration with the Montréal Child Protection Services. The 8-week program is of interest to researchers and clinicians because it is a practical, validated, short-term, attachment-based intervention program that has demonstrated efficacy in enhancing parental sensitivity, improving child attachment security, and reducing disorganized attachment for children and parents who have been reported for child abuse and/or neglect. We have published previous articles that describe the theoretical components and empirical bases of the intervention program and evidence for its efficacy (Dubois-Comtois, Cyr, Tarabulsy, St-Laurent, Bernier, & Moss, 2017; Moss, Dubois-Comtois, Cyr, Tarabulsy, St-Laurent, & Bernier, 2011; Tarabulsy et al., 2008), and have presented a detailed case study to illustrate its application (Moss et al., 2014). We provide in this chapter a summary of (1) the development and evolution of the program in the context of a university–community partnership; (2) the theoretical and empirical basis of the program and its relevance to clinical work when addressing attachment in the context of high-risk parenting; (3) implementation, testing of the program, and evidence for its efficacy; and (4) information regarding training.

Development and Evolution of the Strategy: A University–Community Partnership

The AVI was developed over the course of many years with different groups of high-risk parents. The rationale for elaborating this strategy was based on a number of critical observations that emanated from research involving high risk groups of parent–child dyads that characterized child welfare policy and intervention in the province of Québec in the late 1990s and early 2000s. At that time, despite the overwhelming evidence as to the long-term effects of maltreatment and otherwise high-risk parenting on infant and child social, emotional, and cognitive development (Cicchetti & Valentino, 2006), there existed relatively few empirically supported, developmentally informed intervention programs specifically intended for such families. As in much of the Western world at that time, Québec social services involved in either prevention or early intervention with maltreating or high-risk parents addressed many different aspects of the developmental ecology. Parental characteristics, such as mental health and knowledge of child development, were important intervention targets, as were social support and greater networking with social services and available community resources. The goal of these programs, similar to that of other community-based initiatives, was to improve the family environments that provide the context for child development, with the goal of improving parenting and related child outcomes. These efforts were inspired by research showing that problematic child development is associated with a constellation of risk factors that transcend child and family environments (see Rutter, 2012). Similarly, problems in parenting and, eventually, child development, are based in the proximal and distal developmental ecology. However, we and others have argued elsewhere that, in many cases, addressing the features of the developmental ecology that are more distal to the parent–child dyad does not meaningfully alter the primary aspect of the early environment that has a strong bearing on infant and child development—that is, the quality of parent–child interaction (Cyr, Moss, St-Laurent, Dubois-Comtois, & Sauvé, 2012; Spieker, Nelson, DeKlyen, & Staerkel, 2005; Tarabulsy et al., 2008). In social services-based intervention contexts, which are often delivered in groups or through parenting courses, it is possible to positively change the ecology or parental well-being. However, without appropriate changes in parent–child interaction, in many ways, child development remains at risk.

Moreover, within the specific context of child protection and welfare services, certain peculiar practices have emerged in some settings that may not be helpful to the child. In some cases, in order to help vulnerable parents deal with the challenges of parenthood, community organizations and child protection centers offer the possibility of providing parental relief by placing children in short-term foster care. This practice is viewed as providing much-needed parental support, without consideration for the potential developmental issues that are raised by repeated separations, and without considering the very real possibility that such parental support has no positive effect on parental sensitivity and interactive behavior. These practices are clearly based on good intentions and remain quite common in community and applied settings. However, given that they are rarely grounded in solid developmental theory and evidence based, it is not surprising that they may well leave children at high risk for experiencing important problems in adjustment.

High-risk families in general, and families in which maltreatment is documented in particular, have a greater proportion of children with insecure and disorganized attachment to their primary caregivers (van IJzendoorn, Schuengel, & Bakermans-Kranenburg, 1999). Cyr, Euser, Bakermans-Kranenburg, and van IJzendoorn (2010) report rates of disorganization ranging from 32 to 86% when maltreatment is documented, across different studies. Research has regularly shown that insecure and disorganized attachments constitute important risk factors that undermine normal socioemotional and cognitive developmental processes, especially when they take place in pathogenic environments (Fearon, Bakermans-Kranenburg, van IJzendoorn, Lapsley, & Roisman, 2010; Groh, Roisman, van IJzendoorn, Bakermans-Kranenburg, & Fearon, 2012; Lemelin, Tarabulsy, & Provost, 2006; Madigan, Atkinson, Laurin, & Benoit, 2013; Moss, Cyr, & Dubois-Comtois, 2004; Sroufe, Egeland, Carlson, & Collins, 2005). Furthermore, much independent and convergent evidence has demonstrated that attachment processes are related to early differences in emotion regulation during infancy (Fearon & Belsky, 2004; Tarabulsy et al., 2003), underlining the importance of early identification of high-risk families and the elaboration of effective intervention strategies. Our own work in these areas convinced us of this need and created the impetus for testing new strategies to help high-risk families. Intervention with such populations was not only warranted but also critical to prevent the emergence of adjustment problems during childhood, and to help redirect the course of development in more favorable directions. The fields of attachment research and developmental psychopathology firmly indicate the need for effective interventions with children from the most vulnerable families. Perhaps the greatest difficulty with vulnerable families is the assumed long-term intervention that is needed. If attachment-based intervention strategies are to be accepted and implemented in budget-constrained child protection settings, they must be effective with a shorter number of sessions. Otherwise, they will remain marginal within public service contexts, and difficult to incorporate into mainstream intervention and prevention work with the families most in need. Moreover, parents who participate in long-term treatment may become discouraged or experience stressful life events that continually interfere with the effectiveness of these intervention strategies. This is not to say that longer periods of prevention and intervention are unnecessary in meeting the diverse therapeutic needs of high-risk and maltreating families; indeed, there are circumstances in which ongoing care of parent and child (at least until the child enters school) is something that should not only be hoped for but also actively lobbied for. High-risk families, in general, and maltreatment populations, in particular, are faced with a number of major challenges that short-term intervention strategies cannot meet (Lieberman, 2007; Olds, Holmberg, Donelan-McCall, Luckey, Knudtson, & Robinson, 2014). However, in light of the Bakermans-Kranenburg, van IJzendoorn, and Juffer (2003; Bakermans-Kranenburg, & Bradley, 2005; also see Juffer, Bakermans-Kranenburg, & van IJzendoorn, Chapter 1, this volume) meta-analyses and other studies suggesting that short, highly focused interventions may be effective, even in high-risk contexts, we chose to work on modifying the quality of mother–infant interaction in maltreatment samples as a first step toward changing children's developmental trajectories. This combination of urgent clinical concerns and the desire to further develop and test an emerging attachment-based clinical model motivated the collaboration of the researchers and child welfare personnel in this project. Our objectives were to test the efficacy of a short-term, attachment-based intervention strategy in a rigorous fashion with respect to specific attachment-based outcomes, including caregiver sensitivity, and child attachment insecurity and disorganization. We also examined the efficacy of the program with respect to emerging child behavior problems.

Foundations of the Program in Attachment Theory

A central tenet of attachment theory is that early experiences linked to child behaviors, signals, and emotions, as well as caregiver responses taking place in the context of daily interactions, form the basis for the development of internal working models (IWMs; Bowlby, 1973; Bretherton, 1985). Parental responses to infant manifestations of distress have been hypothesized to be particularly important (Goldberg, Grusec, & Jenkins, 1999). IWMs are at the heart of child representations regarding the availability of the attachment figure to help organize and support exploration and expectations for emotional support in alarming situations (Bowlby, 1973; Bretherton, 1985, 2013). The IWM is also carried forward in other relationship contexts, as a kind of blueprint for the extent to which others are expected to be dependable and caring, as well as the extent to which oneself is worthy of others' care and attention (Pederson, Bailey, Tarabulsy, Bento, & Moran, 2014; Sroufe, 1986). Numerous studies have supported these ideas in showing longitudinal links between the quality of children's early attachment relationships and their socioemotional functioning in close relationships, peer, and educational contexts throughout development (Fearon et al., 2010; Groh et al., 2012; Madigan et al., 2013; Pallini, Baiocco, Schneider, Madigan, & Atkinson, 2014; Sroufe et al., 2005).

The development of children's IWMs is grounded in the sensitive responsiveness of the attachment figure to child signals, emotions, and behaviors (Ainsworth, Blehar, Waters, & Wall, 1978). *Sensitivity* has been defined in different ways, but most definitions include the idea that sensitive caregivers accurately perceive children's behaviors, emotional signals, and needs, and respond in an appropriate, consistent, and predictable manner (Moran, Pederson, & Tarabulsy, 2011; Pederson et al., 2014; Waters, Petters, & Facompre, 2013). These interactions form the primary postnatal experience of the child and the most proximal context for development. As others have pointed out (Belsky, 1993; Rutter, 2012), it is in these interactive contexts that children from high-risk or maltreating contexts first experience the challenges of their environments and it is here that, from the child's perspective, intervention becomes critical (Cyr et al., 2012; Rutter, 2000; Spieker et al., 2005; Tarabulsy et al., 2008). High-risk and maltreating parents are more likely to be insensitive during interactions, showing intrusiveness, coerciveness, lack of interactive synchrony or lack of response to child behaviors or signals (Borrego, Timmer, Urquiza, & Follette, 2004; Bousha & Twentyman, 1984; Burgess & Conger, 1978; Milot, St-Laurent, Éthier, & Provost, 2010; Wilson, Rack, Shi, & Norris, 2008). Moreover, these markedly insensitive parent behaviors expectedly lead to insecure and disorganized child–parent attachment relationships that are linked to impoverished child adjustment that is likely to be a reliably stable feature of their development in the absence of intervention (Moss, Cyr, Bureau, Tarabulsy, & Dubois-Comtois, 2005; van IJzendoorn et al., 1999). In other words, the presence of attachment insecurity and disorganization within a maltreating or high-risk environment confirms the risk to which the child has been exposed, and adds to this risk by placing the child on a problematic developmental pathway (Fearon et al., 2010; O'Connor, 2003).

In our intervention work, since we were dealing with a wide age range and a population with a high percentage of children with disorganized attachment patterns, we also incorporated ideas from our observations of mothers and preschool children with disorganized and controlling attachment patterns (Moss et al., 2004; Moss, Pascuzzo, & Simard, 2012). For example, there are widely noted associations between role reversal in parent–child relationship and disrupted affective communication characterized by failed reciprocity, low engagement, or hostile, conflictual interaction. Lack of parental responsiveness to children's distress often leads to children's attempts to regulate relationships on their own terms, as best as they are able. This will be accomplished by minimizing or maximizing proximity seeking through withdrawal and/or aggressive behavior, which, in turn, may increase parental hostility or withdrawal (Malik, Lederman, Crowson, & Osofsky, 2002). If a child is repeatedly confronted with parental distress and parental negative emotions when making requests of the parent, it is possible that the child will experience this pattern of interaction as an indication that emotion regulation is an autonomous task to be negotiated on one's own, rather than as a dyadic task on which the parent can be relied for help. This pattern of interaction during infancy may develop into a caregiving pattern in which the child continues to monitor parental emotions and behaviors to ensure through caregiving behavior (toward the parent) that the dyad remains regulated (Moss, Bureau, St-Laurent, & Tarabulsy, 2011). Throughout early development, the parent will support this pattern of interaction, valuing and reinforcing preschooler behavior that offers the parent comfort, via what the researcher and clinician label as *role reversal*. It is also possible for preschoolers who are faced with high levels of atypical or frightened/frightening parental behaviors, such as chronic dissociation accompanied with violent outbursts of anger, to attempt to control the relationship in a punitive manner—treating the parent as a bad child. Again, it is hypothesized that this type of control on the part of the child functions primarily to help the child regulate his or her own affect in different interactive circumstances to provoke parents to respond in ways that might defuse the distressing interactive situations that make up much of the child's experience. Such preschooler controlling attachment relationships, linked to dyadic interactive history, are highly predictive of the development of clinical externalizing and internalizing problems and suicidal thoughts in middle childhood (Dubois-Comtois, Moss, Cyr, & Pascuzzo, 2013).

When considering intervention during infancy and early childhood, the specific aspects of parental interactive behavior, so closely linked to the development of disorganized attachment, need to be meaningfully addressed. Thus, significant improvements in parental sensitivity and child attachment security, and decreases in child disorganization observed following intervention, suggest that children have increased their ability to regulate stressful emotional states during parent–child interactions. The significant decreases in child behavior problems following intervention further suggest that these positive changes in emotional regulation have contributed to interrupting the expected trajectory of maltreated children toward development of clinical behavior problems. As discussed by Toth, Cicchetti, and Kim (2002), emotional dysregulation has been shown to mediate the relation between maltreatment and development of internalizing and externalizing symptomatology.

From a clinical perspective, our perception was that to meaningfully address relationship dynamics that are manifested in the context of daily interactions, it was important for clinicians to gain a strong understanding of attachment relationship models, and to be trained in the home observations that are vital to develop working hypotheses for how best to address the difficulties and challenges that are observed. From this conviction, a specific video-feedback strategy, the AVI, was developed to help clinicians work with parents and children on a very practical level, helping parents to gain perspective on how to interact with their children in different circumstances. It is important to emphasize that clinicians are trained to address both interactive issues and other aspects that characterize high-risk environments, such as the experience of trauma, the coherence of maternal discourse, and the importance of other aspects of the family and home environment that may impinge on child development beyond the immediate parent–child relationship. However, the central focus of the AVI is to examine with parents the roles and functions of different kinds of interactions as they pertain to child development.

Topics to Address during Home Visits

When working with parent–infant dyads, the AVI emphasizes the development of interactive synchrony, shared positive affect, and balanced role structuring (Moss et al., 2014; Tarabulsy, Tessier, & Kappas, 1996). Throughout the early phase, an emphasis is placed not only on detecting and interpreting signals and emotions but also on specifically informing parents concerning the importance of responding to child distress as manifested at different ages in early childhood. An emphasis is also placed on shared pleasure during interaction and being supportive of the child's interests and exploratory behavior (Bernier, Matte-Gagné, Bélanger, & Whipple, 2014). Table 14.1 presents the different objectives pursued with parents during each phase of the 8-week cycle. With older children, increasing attention is given to verbal communication and addressing child emotional states, thoughts, and intentions with the help and support of the parent. Brief, structured discussions with the parent concerning child developmental issues, as well as parental developmental histories, complement the sessions. When working with toddlers and preschoolers, the same kinds of issues are addressed, but the focus is on the developing goal-corrected partnership, in the context of verbal negotiation and joint problem solving during play.

In summary, this intervention model has strong roots in attachment theory. Like other short-term attachment-based programs described in this handbook, our goals are to improve parental ability to detect and interpret child signals and

TABLE 14.1. Objectives Pursued with the Parents According to the Intervention Phases

Objectives	Session nos.:	Early phase: Familiarization			Middle phase: Integration			Ending phase: Generalization	
		1	2	3	4	5	6	7	8
• To develop working alliance/trust.									
• To help parents better detect and interpret their child signals, emotions, distress.									
• To recognize how changes in their response to these signals translate into child behaviors, emotions, attitudes. To see the importance of these changes across development.									
• To refer positively to their child, themselves, and their relationship.									
• To help parents reflect on their interactive difficulties and find solutions to relationship issues and to repair conflictual situations.									
• To take responsibility for intervention success.									
• To reinforce autonomy when taking decisions about the relationship (i.e., to find appropriate solutions).									
• To generalize new abilities to broader contexts.									
• To prepare for the end of the intervention and acknowledge anxieties this situation may raise.									

Note. The intensity of the shading indicates how important the objectives are according to the intervention phases.

respond appropriately and predictably in different interactive circumstances. This overarching goal is defined somewhat differently as a function of child age, as interactive sensitivity takes different forms across early childhood. However, certain principles transcend development: the importance of open emotional expression, interactive synchrony and parental monitoring of child exploration, as well as a general sense of the parent taking pleasure and enjoying the presence and the activities of the child. In this context, clinicians are trained to recognize the interactive patterns that lead to different forms of insecurity and to structure intervention activities that will give them the opportunity to validate appropriate parental behavior and affect, while emphasizing the importance of parental responses that form the basis of secure attachment.

Implementation and Testing of the AVI

To test some of our ideas concerning the possibility and the means by which intervention could focus on parental interactive sensitivity and child attachment security, we established collaborative relationships with different sectors of social services in the Province of Québec. Pilot work involved adolescent mother–infant dyads (Tarabulsy, Lacharité, & Hémond, 2000) and children placed in foster care (Moss, Dozier, Bernier, Tarabulsy, & St-Laurent, 2002). Specifically, different aspects of the strategies implemented by Moran, Pederson, and Krupka (2005) and Mary Dozier's group (Dozier et al., 2006) were examined. It became quickly evident that when parental conditions allowed them to be available for the AVI, effective mentoring relationships could be established that helped promote greater levels of interactive sensitivity and benefit child development. We then established a strong working relationship with the Lanaudière[1] Child Protection Centre to develop a structured intervention strategy that would help practitioners in their work with parents who, while followed by social services, nevertheless retained custody of their 0- to 5-year-old children. Here, our manualized, short-term intervention strategy, based on eight home visits by trained interveners was tested using a randomized controlled trial (RCT). In the first phases of implementation, we worked together with agency staff to structure the clinical model and research design, and to secure funding for the project.[2] The project became financially feasible when we were awarded a grant from a special Canadian research fund that supported collaborative community–university research projects focused on crime prevention.

Four clinical workers with experience in child welfare settings were trained by experienced attachment researchers to observe and understand attachment behavior in infants, toddlers, and preschoolers. Interveners had varied academic qualifications, ranging from bachelor's to master's degrees in psychology and psychoeducation. Training consisted of readings on attachment theory and viewing videotaped segments of infant and preschool attachment behavior and parent–child interactions with researchers, in order to identify relationship patterns and interpret both appropriate and problematic interactions and behaviors. To ensure treatment integrity, interveners were supervised on a weekly basis by a member of the project staff experienced with the intervention method. Intervention sessions generated video material that was used during supervision meetings.

Interveners collaborated with other child protection workers throughout the intervention setting. In this context, differences in knowledge of attachment theory and observation skills quickly became a major challenge. This issue manifested itself when recruitment procedures began. Social workers who were primarily responsible for recruiting families, and who had no training in attachment, did not perceive attachment issues to be problematic in the families with which they worked. Rather, they focused on issues related to poverty, parental adjustment, and mental health, as well as basic issues related to living arrangements and organization. When we first approached youth protection staff to refer maltreating families

---

[1]Lanaudière is a region of Québec.

[2]French-language versions of manuals, focused on attachment theory, observation and assessment, and intervention are currently available. English-language versions will be made available shortly.

for the attachment-based intervention program, only six parents and their children, from a possible list of several hundred, were referred. In response to this situation, our group spent the first months of the intervention project in discussions with staff aimed at raising awareness and deepening understanding of the fundamental role of parent–child interactive processes in the context of maltreatment. Moreover, many meetings were held with youth protection administrators to convince them of the usefulness of a short-term intervention strategy aimed at improving parental sensitivity and child attachment security. Following this basic groundwork, maltreating families were more systematically referred to the program. Of 135 families assessed for eligibility, 83 completed all phases of the research trial.

The design of the randomized trial included (1) pretest measures of different aspects of the parent–child dyad and family, including assessments of parent–child attachment, parental interactive sensitivity, and parental reports of child behavior problems; (2) assignment of dyads to intervention or control group; and (3) posttest evaluations of all pretest assessments. During the study, both groups received standard services from child protection services, that is, a monthly visit by a child welfare caseworker who monitored family conditions with respect to physical and psychological neglect and abuse. Caseworkers were also available to respond in crisis situations (e.g., separation or abandonment, episodes of violence perpetrated by the parent or someone else). The AVI was only introduced in the intervention group. Our hypotheses for the study were as follows: We expected that parents in the intervention group would show an increase in sensitivity following the 8-week intervention program. We also expected an increase in the proportion of children showing secure attachment and a decrease in the proportion showing disorganized attachment and behavior problems of an externalizing and internalizing nature.

Different teams of observers rated child attachment, based on pre- and posttest separation–reunion behavior, and maternal sensitivity, to ensure methodological independence of assessments. All raters were trained in the coding of infant or preschooler Strange Situation Procedure, and all visitors involved in assessments of parental interactive sensitivity were trained in conducting home observations and completing the Maternal Behavior Q-Sort (Pederson & Moran, 1995). Moreover, all coders were blind to participant group status (intervention or control) and to whether they were coding pre- or posttest procedures. Following pretest assessments, families were assigned to the intervention or control group using a simple 1:1 randomization procedure.

Structure of the Intervention Sessions

Participants in the intervention group took part in eight 90-minute intervention home visits. Each intervention visit comprised four segments:

1. A 20-minute discussion on a theme chosen by the parent. The selection was made from a list of themes given to the parent that are centered on either the child's needs or the parent–child relationship. Sometimes themes that were selected emerged from ongoing parental preoccupations regarding child behavior (e.g., "My child cries a lot and I am not sure how to handle him"). Among the

themes that were specifically programmed within the intervention visits were the following: interpreting infant signals and distress as a way to help foster a sense of security and confidence in the child; childrearing issues, such as supporting autonomy, monitoring; acting in predictable ways in different circumstances; the importance of warmth and affection; and developing alternative responses to problematic parent–child interactions.

2. A 10-minute videotaped interactive session. If toys were involved in the activity, they were provided by the intervener. The activity and instructions were individually chosen by the intervener as a function of child age and dyadic needs (e.g., imitation and turn taking; establishing face-to-face contact; building synchronous interactions; encouraging child proximity seeking; helping parents follow the child's interests in play or exploration; addressing parental ability to assume a parenting role).

3. A 20-minute video-feedback session during which the intervener played back the just-completed filmed sequence and addressed the parent's and child's feelings and observations of self and child during the interaction. The intervener's probes focused on positive sequences and providing feedback that reinforced parental sensitive behavior toward the child and its impact on child behavior.

4. A 10- to 15-minute wrap-up session during which progress was highlighted and the parent was encouraged to continue similar activities with the child during the coming week.

Unlike other short-term attachment-based intervention strategies, the AVI does not specify the order of themes and activities that must be accomplished in each intervention session. Rather, we adopt a flexible, individualized approach in which intervention goals are based on dyadic needs as they emerge. The general structure of the eight intervention visits allows for lengthy home-based observations that give interveners time not only to understand the relationship dynamics that characterize each dyad but also to adjust intervention objectives as a function of the dyad's evolution through the intervention process. With these observations, and in the context of close supervision, interveners identify some of the relationship challenges that confront each dyad. They structure both developmental discussions and play tasks to draw out interactions that they perceive to be important for the specific dyad with which they are working. Moreover, they establish intervention objectives with their supervisor and parents. In this context, the first session takes on particular importance as it sets the tone for the first intervention visits. Interveners conduct home observations, much like those proposed by Pederson and Moran (1996) when describing attachment relationships as they are manifested outside Ainsworth's Strange Situation (Ainsworth et al., 1978). However, it is important to underline that, as intervention visits progress and more observations are made, the intervener may choose to adjust the hypotheses that emerge from the first meeting with regard to relationship dynamics.

The intervener is always encouraged to validate parental strengths, including the presence of synchronous interactions, parental looks to the child and the establishment of eye contact, parental vocalizations that show interest in the child or otherwise structure his or her play, the organization that parents bring to more complex play, the manner in which they might carefully show a preschooler how a puzzle piece fits, support for exploratory behavior and interests, and so forth. All such behaviors are identified and encouraged. Interveners, trained to pick out such parental responses from the video, take time to explain how the child benefits from them both in the immediate context and, developmentally, in the long term. When this is indicated, interveners are encouraged to point to the child's appropriate response after being exposed to positive parental behavior. Such positive chains of behaviors serve as a support for feedback given to the parent, and are underscored while they view the video segment. Moreover, it is important to foster the idea for parents that they already possess certain abilities, in order to help them gain greater levels of perceived parental self-efficacy and confidence. High-risk and maltreating parents often carry helpless–hostile representations of their own caregiving experiences, sometimes associated with loss and abuse, as well as negative views of themselves and their child (Milot et al., 2014). When parents are able to discern that their sensitive responsiveness is important in helping children regulate emotions and guide behaviors, this becomes a powerful incentive to continue to be attentive to child signals and behaviors and manifest more predictable, warm, and coherent responses. Research that has examined the efficacy of this type of intervention with high-risk dyads has shown that significant, positive changes in parental behavior and the quality of mother–infant interactions are observable as early as the second intervention visit (Benoit, Madigan, Lecce, Shea, & Goldberg, 2001; Madigan, Hawkins, Goldberg, & Benoit, 2006). These positive changes become a key motivational factor for the parent to continue in the intervention process, to develop a trusting, working alliance with the intervener, and to continue to consolidate interactive strengths.

It is important to underline, however, that while most of the interactions with parents focus on positive parent–child interactions and the importance of parental sensitivity for child development, interveners note all behaviors and interactions. More problematic observations of insensitive or otherwise frightening/frightened or atypical parental behaviors are systematically addressed in the context of supervision and contribute to elaborating the intervention strategy for each specific dyad. A key element in the intervention program is the use of video to provide parents with targeted feedback. Video feedback is a clinical technique that involves viewing one's own interactive behavior while being guided by a sensitive clinician. During video feedback, interveners comment on parent and child emotion and behavior in the video segments in a way that encourages the parent to notice the positive impact of his or her own sensitive responsiveness to child behavior. The guide also uses probes, which help the parent conceptualize child needs and motivations. For example, it is possible that during a moment when positive affect is expressed by the child, the intervener may say, "That was a happy smile on your child's part. What do you think your child was thinking or feeling at that point? What do you think you did that caused that smile?" Probes serve to help parents address potentially distorted representations that they may have of their child, of his or her intentions regarding the parent, and also help parents see the connection between parental interactive behaviors and initiatives and child behaviors, emotions, and development.

One of the strengths of the video-feedback technique used in the AVI is that it is conducted immediately after the play session. It offers the opportunity to provide immediate feedback to the caregiver, based on interactions that have just taken place. The emotions and representations evoked during the experience are still easily accessible to parents. Especially for parents who have low insight or reflective capacity, this type of feedback may help them make more accurate associations between their own behavior and that of their child. This is in marked contrast to many clinical models in which events are often discussed after considerable delay. The use of video segments of the parent and child also allows tangible access to positive observations of self and child, which we believe are helpful in addressing parental representations for purposes of change. It is important to distinguish this approach from more long-term, traditional intervention strategies. Although in both approaches, the intervener and the caregiver explore attachment-based themes, the short-term use of video feedback focuses on more contained discussions related to the parent–child relationship and interaction, rather than on the caregiver's own developmental history.

Following the recorded interaction and feedback segment, the intervener has a short discussion with the parent to further address some of the issues raised during feedback. Sometimes these discussions focus on some of the same issues raised in the first segment of the intervention visit. Other times, the video segment raises new issues that parents would like to see addressed, such as emotion regulation or limit setting. The intervener systematically addresses the importance of carrying forward any positive elements from the video-feedback segment to help parents generalize positive interactions to contexts other than the intervention visits. Overall, we have found that these discussions are meaningful to parents, since they are connected to their own behavior rather than to more abstract principles and prescriptions.

In our study with maltreating parents, both the intervention and control groups received standard agency services, consisting of monthly visits by a child welfare caseworker. Agency standards for these meetings usually include monitoring family conditions with respect to neglect and abuse (e.g., nutrition and hygiene, use of coercive discipline), and rarely provide more structured clinical help. The pre- and posttest assessments were identical. The posttest meeting took place approximately 10 weeks following pretest assessments, at the end of 8 weeks of intervention.

AVI Outcomes

The RCT indicated that the AVI was quite successful, as shown in two studies conducted with two subsamples of young children (mean age = 3.35 months, SD = 1.38) and infants (mean age = 17.60; SD = 8.91). The full sets of results are available in Moss, Dubois-Comtois, et al. (2011) and in Dubois-Comtois et al. (2017), respectively, and summarized in Table 14.2. A detailed case study including session goals and progress is described in Moss et al. (2014).

Table 14.2 shows that the AVI was effective in helping maltreated and neglected children (substantiated or at high risk) and their parents. Specifically, results indicated increases in both parental sensitivity and child attachment security, cognitive

TABLE 14.2. Results of Studies Testing the Efficacy of the AVI Using Different RCTs

	N	Child age range	Sample	Parent outcome: Posttest *d*	Child outcome: Posttest *d*
Moss, Dubois-Comtois, et al. (2011)	67	12–71 months	Maltreated or high-risk children	• Sensitivity: *d* = 0.47	• Att security: *d* = 0.77 • Att disorganization: *d* = 0.80 • Externalizing prob[a]: *d* = 0.03 • Internalizing prob[a]: *d* = 0.11
Dubois-Comtois et al. (2017)	41	1–30 months	Neglected or high-risk children	• Sensitivity: *d* = 0.77 • Parenting stress: *d* = −0.86	• Cognitive develop: *d* = 0.74 • Motor develop: *d* = 0.95
Cyr et al. (2015)	106[b]	1–70 months	Maltreated children	• Quality of parent–child interaction: *d* = 0.53	• Att organization: *d* = 0.60 • Externalizing prob: *d* = 0.58
Baudry & Tarabulsy (2013)	64	4–8 months	High risk	• Sensitivity: *d* = 0.51	• Cognitive develop: *d* = 0.63
Dubois-Comtois et al. (2011)	40	7–49 months	Foster care	• Sensitivity: *d* = 0.57 • Parenting stress[c]: *d* = 0.35	

Note. Positive *d*'s indicate results in the expected direction. Att, attachment; Prob, problems; Develop, development.
[a]Intervention efficacy on child behavior problems was significantly moderated with child age.
[b]Only the randomized groups comparisons are reported here.
[c]Intervention efficacy on parental stress was significantly moderated with family SES and foster caregiver commitment.

development, and motor development. The AVI was also effective in reducing child attachment disorganization. In addition, the intervention led to greater reductions in parental reports of externalizing and internalizing behavior problems of older children in the sample. However, the intervention was not effective in reducing parenting stress; parents in the intervention group presented higher stress levels at posttest than did parents in the control group.

These research findings were replicated in an independent study by Cyr, Paquette, Lopez, and Dubois-Comtois (2015) based on a similar sample of maltreating parents and their children. In this second RCT, dyads in the AVI group showed increases in the quality of parent–child interaction and in child attachment organization, as well as decreases in child externalizing symptoms. Cyr et al. demonstrated the usefulness of AVI for children ages 0–5 years, pointing to the appropriateness of AVI from infancy to early school age.

In another study that involved simple random bloc assignment involving posttest measures only, we focused on testing the effectiveness of the AVI with very young infants between 4 and 8 months old. Outcomes that were considered involved maternal sensitivity and Bayley indices of infant cognitive development. In both cases, the intervention proved effective, with Bayley Mental Development Indices (which address issues linked to attention and emotion regulation) being more than 5 points higher for the intervention group (see Table 14.2; Baudry & Tarabulsy, 2013). As of this writing, we are also examining the feasibility of transferring training and expertise to child protection centers and local community social services that must work with vulnerable parents of 0- to 5-year-old children. This ongoing project, which involves an intervention and waiting-list comparison, will also assess the AVI's efficacy, with the difference that interveners are not university-based practitioners but standard child protection workers, trained by members of our research group (Tarabulsy, Baudry, Lemelin, Pearson, & Provost, 2015).

Finally, this intervention was also effective in promoting adaptation in a sample of 40 foster mother–child dyads (Dubois-Comtois, Cyr, Moss, St-André, & Carignan, 2011). In this study, foster mothers showed a marginal increase in sensitive behaviors following the intervention. This marginal result might be accounted for the already moderate level of sensitivity showed by foster mothers at pretest. It might also be accounted by the small sample size, considering the moderate to high effect size found for this result. The intervention was effective in preventing an increase in parenting stress for foster mothers considered to be at greater risk, that is, those having low socioeconomic status (SES) or poor commitment toward the child.

Training and Supervision

We have developed different levels of training, both short-term and more intensive, which are presented in Table 14.3. The short-term training model is an entry-level experience for practitioners in many disciplines who wish to become more familiar with AVI techniques. These, 3-day intensive sessions (a total of 24 hours) cover identification of infant and preschool attachment patterns, understanding of adult attachment states of mind, and AVI intervention techniques. Clinical psychologists, social workers, occupational and speech therapists, child care workers, psychiatrists, pediatricians, and nurses have used this training to learn more about coaching parental sensitivity, to distinguish between functional and dysfunctional types of attachment relationships through video examples, and to run the AVI program with their clients. The program is accredited by the Corporation of Québec Psychologists for continuing education. Those wishing to develop greater expertise in identifying early childhood attachment patterns for research or clinical purposes can participate in an 8-day training program leading to certification.

A second, long-term model for training includes a more intensive supervision component. Training involves about 64 hours of work with conceptual and video-based material, and focuses on understanding theory, conducting accurate observations, and learning the different procedures that are part of the AVI. The first 2 days focus on attachment theory and video observations. Two days are devoted to the AVI protocol itself. Four days of training involve interveners working with families who have accepted help to learn the AVI and have consented to use of their videotaped sessions in group supervision. Group supervision takes the form of video observations and discussion regarding dyadic and interactive issues, pointed feedback, and formative training on structuring subsequent visits using AVI techniques. Reflections on how to address obstacles to the intervention process are addressed.

TABLE 14.3. Training and supervision models with the AVI

	Training models		
	Short-term	Long-term	Mentor-based
Prerequisite			
• Being a professional practitioner or a university student	Yes	Yes	Yes
• Having work experience with families	Yes	Yes	Yes
Training (C or U)			

• Child attachment
  o Attachment theory
  o Video observations
	8 hours	16 hours	16 hours

• AVI
  o Intervention techniques
  o Video observations
	16 hours	16 hours	16 hours

Supervision (C or U)			
• Semimonthly supervision for the first two families	—	16 hours	16 hours
• Monthly supervisions for the three subsequent families	—	16 hours	16 hours
Mentor-based supervision (U)			
• Two meeting sessions to discuss intervention and training issues	—	—	Availability over 1 year
• Observation of a training session performed by the trained supervisor	—	—	Mandatory

Note. C, performed by intervener from the clinical setting; U, performed by researchers and trained personnel from the university setting.

Next, interveners are exposed to mentor-based supervision sessions with researchers and trained personnel from the university setting, who remain available throughout intervention following initial training. Typically, this availability on the part of researchers has covered the year following training. These sessions involve video conferencing that includes intervention session material (all families agree to share this video material with mentors). Many of those who participate in this training program work for settings that intervene with high-risk or maltreating families and continue to implement the AVI strategy within their settings. After demonstrating an appropriate skills level, these interveners become supervisors in their settings and are involved in training new interveners and establishing intervention communities that work with the AVI in their geographical areas. An important part of the supervision strategy involves continued training for the core group of interveners who have the responsibility to develop expertise in the AVI, support their colleagues, and maintain contact with the university setting as needed.

A central feature of training is to provide tools for interveners that allow them to make targeted observations and to recognize the strengths and weaknesses that characterize interaction patterns of parents and their children. Although many experienced clinicians working with maltreating populations are familiar with behaviors such as child avoidance, opposition and defiance, and parent–child role reversal, few have framed these within an attachment perspective. During training, many hours are spent viewing video segments that provide examples of infant and preschool attachment patterns—secure, insecure, and disorganized—and, in many cases, dyads are viewed in situations outside Ainsworth's Strange Situation Procedure to allow interveners to gain an appreciation for the manner in which patterns develop and present themselves in daily interactions. Examples of secure child–parent relationships provide concrete models for interveners to use when coaching parents in the use of more sensitive behavior. Examples of insecure–organized (*avoidant or ambivalent*) and disorganized/controlling attachment patterns illustrate how children adapt to caregivers who are repeatedly rejecting of their attachment behavior, inconsistent in responding to child distress, or even frightening. For detailed discussion and description of disorganized and controlling attachment and preschool manifestations see Moss and colleagues (2012; Moss, Bureau, et al., 2011).

Training also involves the use of case studies of parents and children (e.g., Moss et al., 2014) exposed to the AVI. Case studies provide a model of how to think and expect change, and how to evaluate the relational dynamics underlying maltreatment from an attachment perspective. Using case studies, participants are exposed to different types of interactions and different forms of parental sensitivity, and are encouraged to be attentive to interaction dynamics that are affected by the intervention process. Here, we emphasize that sensitivity and insensitivity are not parental traits (though they are related to a number of parental factors), but rather involve levels of predictable, warm, and appropriate responses on the part of the parent to child behaviors and initiatives.

This strategy does not purposefully try to modify adult attachment states of mind through psychotherapy, as individual work with parents might aim for. However, considerable training time is spent sensitizing interveners to be attentive to parents' discourse about themselves, their child, and their own developmental histories, because states of mind about attachment are important predictors and determinants of maternal interactive behavior. We discuss how parents' attachment experiences influence their perceptions of their child and can interfere with their ability to respond to child emotional signals. This increases the intervener's ability to empathize with the parent and to develop a therapeutic alliance, as well as a complete model of how parent and child representations of attitudes, goals, and feelings organize and regulate dyadic functioning.

Conclusion

Clinically, much child welfare practice in the West is moving toward being attentive to attachment issues. However, in many ways, the urgency of child protection cases makes it difficult for caseworkers to remain focused on child developmental needs, even though development is very much at risk. The AVI provides a structured, evidence-based, manualized approach that helps the intervener understand parental behavior and interactions with the child, and provides guidance in structuring a short-term intervention focusing on parental sensitivity. No doubt, intervention with such high-risk families requires that interveners focus on many other intervention targets. However, the AVI provides for interveners an important tool that addresses one of the determinants of infant and child development—the parent–child attachment relationship.

Finally, the AVI is the result of a high level of collaborative work between several community-based intervention settings and university researchers, all committed to enhancing the quality of social intervention for the most vulnerable children in our communities. The collaboration with child protection agencies and community services that has yielded the AVI is important, but it will be even more so to the degree that this knowledge and expertise can be effectively transferred back to those who work most closely with children in need.

ACKNOWLEDGMENTS

Several funding agencies supported the research reported in this chapter: Canada's National Crime Prevention Centre, the Québec Ministry of Public Security, the Lucie and André Chagnon Foundation, the Québec Fund for Research on Society and Culture, and the Social Sciences and Humanities Research Council of Canada. We thank all of the families who have so generously participated in our research. We also thank research assistants and workers from the different child protection centers, local community health centers, and community organizations who have collaborated in this work, with special thanks to the Lanaudière, Montréal, Québec, and the Mauricie-Centre-du-Québec Child Protection Centres.

REFERENCES

Ainsworth, M. D. S., Blehar, M. C., Waters, E., & Wall, S. (1978). *Patterns of attachment: A psychological study of the strange situation.* Hillsdale, NJ: Erlbaum.

Bakermans-Kranenburg, M. J., van IJzendoorn, M. H., & Bradley, R. H. (2005). Those who have receive: The Matthew effect in early childhood intervention in the home environment. *Review of Educational Research, 75,* 1–26.

Bakermans-Kranenburg, M. J., van IJzendoorn, M. H., & Juffer, F. (2003). Less is more: Meta-analysis of sensitivity and attachment intervention in early childhood. *Psychological Bulletin, 129,* 195–215.

Baudry, C., & Tarabulsy, G. M. (2013, April). *A critical examination of the link between the quality of mother–infant interactions and infant cognitive development.* Poster presentation at the Biennial meeting of the Society for Research in Child Development, Seattle, WA.

Belsky, J. (1993). Etiology of child maltreatment: A developmental–ecological analysis. *Psychological Bulletin, 114*(3), 413–434.

Benoit, D., Madigan, S., Lecce, S., Shea, B., & Goldberg, S. (2001). Atypical maternal behavior toward feeding-disordered infants before and after intervention. *Infant Mental Health Journal, 22,* 611–626.

Bernier, A., Matte-Gagné, C., Bélanger, M.-E., & Whipple, N. (2014). Taking stock of two decades of attachment transmission gap: Broadening the assessment of maternal behavior. *Child Development, 85*(5), 1852–1865.

Borrego, J., Timmer, S. G., Urquiza, A. J., & Follette, W. C. (2004). Physically abusive mothers' responses following episodes of child noncompliance and compliance. *Journal of Consulting and Clinical Psychology, 72,* 897–903.

Bousha, D. M., & Twentyman, C. T. (1984). Mother–child interactional style in abuse, neglect, and control groups: Naturalistic observations in the home. *Journal of Abnormal Psychology, 93,* 106–114.

Bowlby, J. (1973). *Attachment and loss: Vol. 2. Separation.* New York: Basic Books.

Bretherton, I. (1985). Attachment theory: Retrospect and prospect. *Monographs of the Society for Research in Child Development, 50*(1–2, Serial No. 209), 3–35.

Bretherton, I. (2013). Revisiting Mary Ainsworth's conceptualization and assessments of maternal sensitivity–insensitivity. *Attachment and Human Development, 15,* 460–484.

Burgess, R. L., & Conger, R. D. (1978). Family interaction in abusive, nelgectful, and normal families. *Child Development, 49,* 1163–1173.

Cicchetti, D., & Valentino, K. (2006). An ecological–transactional perspective on child maltreatment: Failure of the average expectable environment and its influence on child development. In D. Cicchetti & D. J. Cohen (Eds.), *Developmental psychopathology* (2nd ed., Vol. 3, pp. 129–201). Hoboken, NJ: Wiley.

Cyr, C., Euser, E. M., Bakermans-Kranenburg, M. J., & van IJzendoorn, M. H. (2010). Attachment security and disorganization in maltreating and high-risk families: A series of meta-analyses. *Development and Psychopathology, 22,* 87–108.

Cyr, C., Moss, E., St-Laurent, D., Dubois-Comtois, K., & Sauvé, M. (2012). Promouvoir le développement d'enfants victimes de maltraitance: L'importance des interventions relationnelles parent–enfant fondées sur la théorie de l'attachement [Facilitating the development of maltreated children: The importance of parent–child attachment-based interventions]. In M.-H. Gagné, S. Drapeau, & M.-C. Saint-Jacques (Eds.), *Les enfants maltraités: De l'affliction à l'espoir* [Abused children: From affliction to hope] (pp. 41–70). Québec: Les Presses de l'Université Laval.

Cyr, C., Paquette, D., Lopez, L., & Dubois-Comtois, K. (2015, April). *An attachment-based intervention protocol for the assessment of parenting capacities in child welfare cases.* In M. Bakermans-Kranenburg (Chair), Symposium presented to the Society for Research in Child Development, Philadelphia, PA.

Dozier, M., Manni, M., Gordon, M. K., Peloso, E., Gunnar, M. R., Stovall-McClough, K., . . . Levine, S. (2006). Foster children's diurnal production of cortisol: An exploratory study. *Child Maltreatment, 11,* 189–197.

Dubois-Comtois, K., Cyr, C., Moss, E., St-André, M., & Carignan, M. (2011, April). *Is attachment-based intervention with foster parents effective in enhancing sensitivity and reducing parental stress?* Poster presented at the biennial meeting of the Society for Research in Child Development, Montréal, Canada.

Dubois-Comtois, K., Cyr, C., Tarabulsy, G. M., St-Laurent, D., Bernier, A., & Moss, E. (2017). Testing the limits: Extending attachment-based intervention effects to infant cognitive outcome and parental stress. *Development and Psychopathology, 29,* 565–574.

Dubois-Comtois, K., Moss, E., Cyr, C., & Pascuzzo, K. (2013). Behavior problems in middle childhood: The predictive role of maternal distress, child attachment, and mother–child interactions. *Journal of Abnormal Child Psychology, 41*(8), 1311–1324.

Fearon, R. M. P., Bakermans-Kranenburg, M. J., van IJzendoorn, M. H., Lapsley, A., & Roisman, G. I. (2010). The significance of insecure attachment and disorganization in the development of children's externalizing behavior: A meta-analytic study. *Child Development, 81,* 435–456.

Fearon, R. M. P., & Belsky, J. (2004). Attachment and attention: Protection in relation to gender and cumulative social-sontextual adversity. *Child Development, 75*(6), 1677–1693.

Goldberg, S., Grusec, J., & Jenkins, J. M. (1999). Confidence in protection: Arguments for a narrow definition of attachment. *Journal of Family Psychology, 13,* 475–483.

Groh, A. M., Roisman, G. I., van IJzendoorn, M. H., Bakermans-Kranenburg, M. J., & Fearon, R. M. P. (2012). The significance of insecure and disorganized attachment for children's internalizing symptoms: A meta-analytic study. *Child Development, 83,* 591–610.

Lemelin, J.-P., Tarabulsy, G. M., & Provost, M. A. (2006). Predicting preschool cognitive development from infant temperament, maternal sensitivity, and psychosocial risk. *Merrill–Palmer Quarterly, 52*(4), 779–806.

Lieberman, A. F. (2007). Ghosts and angels: Intergenerational patterns in the transmission and treatment of the traumatic sequelae of domestic violence. *Infant Mental Health Journal, 28,* 422–439.

Madigan, S., Atkinson, L., Laurin, K., & Benoit, D. (2013). Attachment and internalizing behavior in childhood: A meta-analysis. *Developmental Psychology, 49,* 672–689.

Madigan, S., Hawkins, E., Goldberg, S., & Benoit, D. (2006). Reduction of disrupted caregiver behavior using modified interaction guidance. *Infant Mental Health Journal, 27,* 509–527.

Malik, N., Lederman, C., Crowson, M., & Osofsky, J. (2002). Evaluating maltreated infants, toddlers, and preschoolers independency court. *Infant Mental Health Journal, 23,* 576–592.

Milot, T., Lorent, A., St-Laurent, D., Bernier, A., Tarabulsy, G. M., Lemelin, J.-P., & Èthier, L. S. (2014). Hostile–helpless state of mind as further evidence of adult disorganized states of mind in neglecting families. *Child Abuse and Neglect, 38*(8), 1351–1357.

Milot, T., St-Laurent, D., Éthier, L. S., & Provost, M. A. (2010). Trauma-related symptoms in neglected preschoolers and affective quality of mother–child communication. *Child Maltreatment, 15,* 293–304.

Moran, G., Pederson, D. R., & Krupka, A. (2005). Maternal unresolved attachment status impedes the effectiveness of interventions with adolescent mothers. *Infant Mental Health Journal, 26,* 231–249.

Moran, G., Pederson, D. R., & Tarabulsy, G. M. (2011). Becoming sensitive to sensitivity: Lessons learned from the development of the Maternal Behavior Q-Sort. In D. W. Davis & C. Logdson (Eds.), *Maternal sensitivity: A critical review for practitioners* (pp. 259–281). Haupauge, NY: Nova.

Moss, E., Bureau, J. F., St-Laurent, D., & Tarabulsy, G. M. (2011). Understanding disorganized attachment at preschool and school age: Examining divergent pathways of disorganized and controlling children. In J. Solomon & C. George (Eds.), *Disorganized attachment and caregiving* (pp. 52–79). New York: Guilford Press.

Moss, E., Cyr, C., Bureau, J. F., Tarabulsy, G. M., & Dubois-Comtois, K. (2005). Stability of attachment during the preschool period. *Developmental Psychology, 41*(5), 773–783.

Moss, E., Cyr, C., & Dubois-Comtois, K. (2004). Attachment at early school age and developmental risk: Examining family contexts and behavior problems of controlling-caregiving, controlling-punitive, and behaviorally disorganized children. *Developmental Psychology, 40,* 519–532.

Moss, E., Dozier, M., Bernier, A., Tarabulsy, G. M., & St-Laurent, D. (2002). *Évaluation d'un programme d'intervention visant à optimiser la sécurité affective et l'autorégulation chez les enfants places en famille d'accueil: Rapport soumis au Conseil québécois de la recherche sociale* [Evaluation of an intervention program intended to favour the development of affective security and emotion regulation in a sample of foster-children: Report submitted to the Québec Council for Social Research]. Montreal: University of Quebec at Montreal.

Moss, E., Dubois-Comtois, K., Cyr, C., Tarabulsy, G. M., St-Laurent, D., & Bernier, A. (2011). Efficacy of a home-visiting intervention aimed at improving maternal sensitivity, child attachment, and behavioral outcomes for maltreated children: A randomized control trial. *Development and Psychopathology, 23,* 195–210.

Moss, E., Pascuzzo, K., & Simard, V. (2012). Treating insecure and disorganized attachments in school-aged children. In K. Nader (Ed.), *School rampage shootings and other youth disturbances: Early preventive interventions* (pp. 127–158). New York: Routledge.

Moss, E., Tarabulsy, G. M., St-Georges, R., Dubois-Comtois, K., Cyr, C., Bernier, A., . . . Lecompte, V. (2014). Videofeedback intervention with maltreating parent–child dyads. *Attachment and Human Development, 16,* 329–342.

O'Connor, T. G. (2003). Early experiences and psychological development: Conceptual questions, empirical illustrations and implications for intervention. *Development and Psychopathology, 15,* 671–690.

Olds, D. L., Holmberg, J. R., Donelan-McCall, N., Luckey, D. W., Knudtson, M. D., & Robinson, J. (2014). Effects of home visits by paraprofessionals and by nurses on children: Follow-up of a randomized trial at ages 6 and 9 years. *JAMA Pediatrics, 168*(2), 114–121.

Pallini, S., Baiocco, R., Schneider, B. H., Madigan, S., & Atkinson, L. (2014). Early child–parent attachment and peer relations: A meta-analysis of recent research. *Journal of Family Psychology, 28*(1), 118–123.

Pederson, D. R., Bailey, H. N., Tarabulsy, G. M., Bento, S., & Moran, G. (2014). Understanding sensitivity: Lessons learned from the legacy of Mary Ainsworth. *Attachment and Human Development, 16*(3), 261–270.

Pederson. D. R., & Moran, G. (1995). A categorical description of infant–mother relationships in the home and its relation to *Q*-sort measures of infant–mother interaction. *Monographs of the Society for Research in Child Development, 60*(2–3), 111–132.

Pederson, D. R., & Moran, G. (1996). Expressions of the attachment relationship outside of the Strange Situation. *Child Development, 67,* 915–927.

Rutter, M. (2000). Resilience reconsidered: Conceptual considerations, empirical findings, and policy implications. In J. P. Shonkoff & S. J. Meisels (Eds.), *Handbook of early childhood intervention* (2nd ed., pp. 651–682). New York: Cambridge University Press.

Rutter, M. (2012). Resilience as a dynamic concept. *Development and Psychopathology, 24,* 335–344.

Spieker, S. J., Nelson, D., DeKlyen, M., & Staerkel, F. (2005). Enhancing early attachment in the context of Early Head Start: Can programs emphasizing family support improve rates of secure infant–mother attachments in low-income families? In L. J. Berlin, Y. Ziv, L. Amaya-Jackson, & M. T. Greenberg (Eds.), *Enhancing early attachments: Theory, research, intervention, and policy* (pp. 250–275). New York: Guilford Press.

Sroufe, L. A. (1986). Bowlby's contribution to psychoanalytic theory and developmental psychology: Attachment: Separation: Loss. *Journal of Child Psychology and Psychiatry, 27*(6), 841–849.

Sroufe, L. A., Egeland, B., Carlson, E., & Collins, W. A. (2005). *The development of the person: The Minnesota Study of Risk and Adaptation from Birth to Adulthood.* New York: Guilford Press.

Tarabulsy, G. M., Baudry, C., Lemelin, J.-P., Pearson, J., & Provost, M. A. (2015). *Évaluation d'une approche fondée sur les principes de l'attachement: Implantation et efficacité au niveau des parents et des enfants* (Association des Centres jeunesse du Québec). [Evaluation of an attachment-based intervention strategy: Implementation and knowledge transfer and efficacy on the level of parents and children (Association for Child Protection Centers of Québec)]. Quebec: University of Laval.

Tarabulsy, G. M., Lacharité, C., & Hémond, I. (2000, June). *Effects of a short-term, home-based intervention for adolescent mothers and their infants: Preliminary results.* Presentation at the Congress of World Association for Infant Mental Health, Montréal, Canada.

Tarabulsy, G. M., Pascuzzo, K., Moss, E., St-Laurent, D., Bernier, A., Cyr, C., & Dubois-Comtois, K. (2008). Attachment-based intervention for maltreating families. *American Journal of Orthopsychiatry, 78,* 322–332.

Tarabulsy, G. M., Provost, M. A., Deslandes, J., St-Laurent, D., Moss, E., Lemelin, J. P., . . . Dassylva, J.-F. (2003). Individual differences in infant still-face response at 6 months. *Infant Behavior and Development, 26,* 421–438.

Tarabulsy, G. M., Tessier, R., & Kappas, A. (1996). Contingency detection and the contingent organization of behavior in interactions: Implications for socioemotional development in infancy. *Psychological Bulletin, 120*(1), 25–41.

Toth, S. L., Cicchetti, D., & Kim, J. (2002). Relations among children's perceptions of maternal behavior, attributional styles, and behavioral symptomatology in maltreated children. *Journal of Abnormal Child Psychology, 30,* 487–501.

van IJzendoorn, M. H., Schuengel, C., & Bakermans-Kranenburg, M. J. (1999). Disorganized attachment in early childhood: Meta-analysis of precursors, concomitants, and sequelae. *Development and Psychopathology, 11,* 225–249.

Waters, E., Petters, D., & Facompre, C. (2013). Some reflections in a special issue of *Attachment and Human Development* in Mary Ainsworth's 100th year. *Attachment and Human Development, 15*(5–6), 673–681.

Wilson, S. R., Rack, J. J., Shi, X., & Norris, A. M. (2008). Comparing physically abusive, neglectful, and non-maltreating parents during interactions with their children: A meta-analysis of observational studies. *Child Abuse and Neglect, 32,* 897–911.

CHAPTER 15

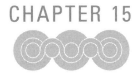

B.A.S.E.—Babywatching

An Attachment-Based Program to Promote Sensitivity and Empathy, and Counter Fear and Aggression

KARL HEINZ BRISCH and JEANNETTE HOLLERBACH

We describe in this chapter an attachment-based intervention, B.A.S.E.®–Babywatching (hereinafter referred to as "BASE"[1]), developed initially for preschool-age children in day care center settings, but with potentially wide applications across settings and across the lifespan. We first provide a background to the urgent need for attachment-based interventions in day care settings in which children have their first prolonged social experiences outside their homes, then describe the goals of the intervention, the theoretical foundations of the program, the training process and core questioning activities that comprise the intervention, and the empirical evidence in support of BASE.

The Day Care Context

Day care centers undoubtedly face major challenges today. Many staff members are becoming increasingly critical of their working conditions, which are a source of great stress—even though it is now well understood how important the quality of early childhood care is. At the same time, day care centers are being asked to fulfill numerous educational roles by parents, who, for one reason or another,

---

[1]B.A.S.E.®–Babywatching is a registered trademark of Dr. med. Karl Heinz Brisch in the United States of America and all member states of the European Union.

339

feel pressured to turn over important childrearing tasks to others. In addition, cultural contexts and language barriers confront day care staff with ongoing challenges.

The results of psychological, neuropsychological, and brain research have demonstrated that the quality of early childhood emotional attachment plays an important role in the cognitive development of the child and in the child's emotional resilience in the face of all forms of stress. In addition, acquiring and maintaining attachments is a crucial factor enabling the later ability to learn successfully, and contributes to the growth of the child's own capacity for empathy. Day care centers and their personnel are extrafamilial institutions within which attachment may take place, and as such play an important role in early childhood development (Bowlby, 2007; Hüther, 1998).

Then again, the public has over the past decade become increasingly aware of the problem of aggressive and violent children and adolescents. According to recent statistics compiled by the police in Germany, approximately 27,000 young people between ages 14 and 18 were involved in violent crimes in 2012. Although the overall rates of youth violence have decreased by 15% over the past several years, the violence itself seems to have become more brutal and the causes of it more complex (Schwenner, 2014).

These facts by themselves should make it clear why we must develop more effective strategies for working with children in a way that takes into account their need for sensitivity and the fulfillment of their basic attachment strivings. It is crucial that we help them in their emotional and socioemotional development, so that they may become more sensitive and empathetic as they grow into older children, adolescents, and eventually adults (Hollerbach & Brisch, 2015).

Because the various forms of aggressive and fearful behavior increase and become more complex with age, it is important to begin preventive strategies in early childhood. Day care centers and schools are the ideal places to encourage sensitive attachment experiences that can act as corrective emotional experiences, foster socioemotional strengths, and give children inner guideposts by which to steer as they navigate their way through the difficult situations that they will undoubtedly encounter (Brisch, 2012).

It is the goal of BASE to provide early assistance in dealing with problematic behavior in 3- to 12-year-old children and to help them to develop sensitivity and empathy. BASE expands the attachment-based spectrum of prevention. The program starts with a young target group, while at the same time providing skills enhancement to teachers through BASE training and intervention. In addition, BASE provides a framework within which each child in the target group may gain experience with sensitive attachment that may have corrective social and emotional (also cognitive) functions in interpreting the emotions and intentions of others. The goal, which has been supported in numerous settings, is to encourage children to enter into cooperative, prosocial, and creative relationships, so that problematic behaviors such as aggression, inattention, hyperactivity, and opposition are more likely to recede, while frustration tolerance, and conflict-resolution skills increase (Brisch, 2008).

Goal of the Intervention

Observing Interaction as a Way of Promoting Sensitivity and Empathy, and Countering Fear and Aggression

The BASE prevention program is aimed at young children as they start attending day care or preschool. BASE is compatible with the overall educational mission of schools. It can be integrated into day care centers, schools, family education centers, youth work, and into continuing education of staff. It can also be usefully integrated into social work and psychotherapy. BASE has a positive effect on not only the target groups mentioned but also group facilitators and mothers or fathers who take part in the program. Overall, the effect is to sharpen participants' ability to observe and to respond with empathy. These abilities can then be generalized to all forms of interaction in daily life. Initial research results are from a prospective study of BASE in a pretest–posttest matched-pair design conducted in Frankfurt on the Main (Brisch & Hollerbach, 2016). Support had various effects on mothers and children who took part in the BASE program (published findings pending at *www. base-babywatching.de*).

As an attachment-based prevention program, BASE enables all participants to observe and often experience secure attachment, generalize new hopeful and trusting interactions with others and, in the process, modify old attachment patterns (Brisch, 2010).

Implementation

A parent (mother or father) attends a nursery school group or school class with a recently born infant once a week for an entire year. The children, who sit in a circle, observe how the baby and parent develop their relationship from week to week, until she is able to walk by herself. The group facilitators, who have been given special training, guide the children through the weekly observational sessions and help them to put themselves into the emotional and motivational state of the parent and the baby. For many single children, this will be the first and often the only opportunity to observe such a relationship developing, as well as to note the milestones in the development of a baby continuously over the entire first year of life.

Goals of BASE

The main goal of BASE is to prevent aggressive and fearful behavior, and to foster sensitivity and empathy. Children who lack empathy, either partly or completely, often behave aggressively toward their peers in conflict situations (Parens, 1993b). Children who have suffered early deprivation or trauma may have a hard time identifying with the emotions and thoughts of others. These children in particular may vicariously experience positive attachment as they start to understand through the guided observation of interactions between the parent and his or her baby. This can improve their capacity for empathy and self-reflection, which in turn can help them gradually to moderate their aggressive or fearful behavior, or even prevent the development of these behaviors in the first place.

Observing, perceiving, and communicating about the intentions and feelings of others promotes an increasingly nuanced understanding of the parent and baby. Children who have gone through the Babywatching program have been shown to exhibit more cooperative, prosocial, creative, and attentive behavior, while aggressive, inattentive, hyperactive and oppositional behaviors tend to fade into the background (Brisch, 2007).

BASE Areas of Application

The BASE prevention program may be used in a variety of settings and with different age groups. Even though the target group here consists of children between ages 3 and 12, the intervention may be adapted for other ages and client groups.

Group facilitators must be trained in the theory and practice of the BASE program during a daylong session before it can be offered in schools or other settings. Training is primarily aimed at teachers, social workers, and therapists who already have practical experience with the target group. A trained group facilitator may offer BASE immediately after completing the training session, supervised and supported by a trained BASE Babywatching Mentor as he or she begins practice. Institutions with a constant client or child base are especially suitable.

Further Potential Applications

The BASE prevention program may be adapted for use in other settings and with different age groups. The age range extends from day nurseries with children of different ages to implementation during inpatient treatment of severely traumatized children ages 6–14 years (Brisch, Hollerbach, & Quehenberger, 2016). But it has even proved effective with residents in old age homes. Municipalities or independent sponsors of day care centers or other youth institutions can integrate BASE into their offerings. Institutions for which inclusivity is a priority and family education centers that work with a varied clientele are especially apt to benefit from the program. Pregnant women and their partners may also benefit from Babywatching, as they learn how to empathize with a baby and may feel especially motivated to increase their sensitivity in anticipation of their own baby. Interestingly, senior citizens living in old age homes are often very open to Babywatching, because it resonates with their own experience of parenting and childhood. It allows them access to their own emotional world and can encourage positive interactions. It also affords them a good time, a reason to smile, and a welcome change to their daily routine. At the same time, it encourages empathy and sensitivity in the institutional staff, who are very important to their older adult patients.

The program may under certain circumstances also be implemented in correctional facilities, especially with youth offenders.

Both the contents of the program and the hands-on experience are especially suited to teacher training. For example, the bishopric of Limburg, Germany, sponsored teacher training at the Marienschule, a school for day care center staff. In a pilot program, BASE group facilitator training is being integrated into the general curriculum of these institutions.

In addition to the educational and therapeutic professions, BASE can also be used as a form of coaching with supervisory staff to promote empathy and the ability to communicate and interact. Because it is so easy to implement, the costs are very low, and large target groups may be addressed simultaneously, BASE can be a very attractive program for many types of institutions.

BASE may also be used effectively to enhance the skills of teaching or therapeutic staff members. Sensitivity and the capacity to interact and intervene with assuredness are basic competencies in all helping, teaching, and therapeutic professions. In comparison to other preventive programs, BASE offers direct experience and practice in developing these competencies. In the BASE program, the focus is on the observation of the mother– or father–infant dyad and on the mentalizing process. The baby is not touched by either the children who observe, or by the teacher or other adults in the room.

From the perspective of attachment theory, it is important that the Babywatching group be conducted under constant conditions, in a regular sequence, and by sensitive facilitators who have sufficient experience and self-confidence to lead such a group.

Field Testing to Date

BASE has been field-tested in numerous countries. Projects are currently under way in Germany, Austria, Switzerland, Great Britain, Australia, New Zealand, Israel, and on the Isle of Man (Brisch, 2016). A year-and-a-half-long BASE pilot project was initiated in Frankfurt on the Main, in 2012, as part of a collaboration between the school department of that city and the University of Munich. Up to 40 day care centers and their staff members received BASE training. Funding from the Frankfurt School Department enabled mentors to guide and support the group facilitators during the pilot phase. The mentors received special training in their function as supervisors. Both the group facilitators and the mentors were supervised by a BASE trainer at special supervision evenings with the trainer. Such supervision may take place once a month or whenever it is requested by the group leader or the mentors. The supervision may take the form of live supervision, in which the supervisor takes part in the next BASE session and gives feedback to the teachers immediately after the session. Or supervision may take place by telephone, if a particular question can be dealt with quickly.

In settings where performance and cognitive abilities are trained, such as in day care centers and schools, BASE provides an opportunity for children and educational staff to encounter each other on neutral ground. By examining their own feelings and those of others, the entire atmosphere within a group changes, and group members come to relate to each other on a more caring basis. The questioning that goes on over the course of BASE sessions can be generalized to other situations and help to resolve conflicts.

Babywatching can be a positive emotional experience for all participants, producing positive results in both boys and girls; it has been shown to decrease problematic externalizing and internalizing behaviors by deepening children's capacity for empathy. During Babywatching sessions, boys and girls not only observe how the baby develops but also learn a great deal about their own emotions, because they feel their way into the emotional state of both parent and infant. Over time, they begin to generalize this capacity to everyday situations with their friends, because they have begun to internalize more sensitive and prosocial patterns and behave less fearfully (Brisch, 2007).

The parents involved also enjoy spending time with their baby in this setting, because once a week they set aside time and devote themselves entirely to their relationship with their child. Babywatching appears to relieve the stresses of everyday life, allowing parents to enter into a quiet space for a time. As the young BASE participants comment and ask questions, the parent automatically focuses on the needs of his or her developing infant. Because of the calm nature of the setting, parents' more relaxed and sensitive responses to their infants promote secure attachment.

BASE also provides group facilitators or teachers the opportunity to encounter each child in the circle in a new way. The children's conflicts and needs, which had perhaps previously been hidden, are brought to light by BASE, which functions as a sort of early warning system. The group facilitators can then offer parents (of children in the circle) early support, which helps them to notice their children's distress and cues them to respond before more serious behavioral problems emerge.

Theoretical Foundations and the Development of the Program

History of BASE

The program is based on the work of the psychiatrist and psychoanalyst Henri Parens, who was born in Lodz, Poland, in 1928. In 1940, he and his mother fled the Nazi onslaught, first to Bruxelles, Belgium, then to France, where they ended up in the Rivesaltes internment camp. In 1942, his mother was deported from Rivesaltes to Auschwitz, where she was murdered. But before that, she had helped her 12-year-old son escape, and at the age of 13, 3 months before his mother was sent to Auschwitz, he arrived by a circuitous route in the United States. These experiences and the separation from his mother galvanized his desire to become a child analyst and to counter racism, war, and hatred in whatever way he could. His attempts to understand the causes of destructive aggression and malignant prejudice led to the conceptualization of preventive measures (Parens, 2012). In Philadelphia in the 1970s and 1980s, Parens and coworkers conducted studies aimed at preventing experience-derived emotional disorders in children, including especially aggressive behavior disorders, which became the foundation of his interventions. The insight that children eventually become parents led him to work creatively with children and adolescents.

If one's strategy is to avoid emotional disorders in children early on, it becomes clear that they must be prepared for parenthood. With that in mind, Parens developed materials that could be used with nursery- and school-age children (Parens, Scattergood, Duff, & Singletary, 1995). The materials were received enthusiastically. He simultaneously developed a curriculum for schools and a series of workshop for parents and educators. The primary goal was to optimize childrearing, thereby improving emotional development and health. Emotional health is intimately linked to the ability to achieve, to empathize, to solve problems, to engage in productive and creative activities, to enter into positive relationships with other people, and to adapt to change. Parens envisioned that by using the insights that had crystallized from his studies he might be able to decrease the emotional disorders in society as a whole. But for this to occur, both parents and educators would have to play a major role (Parens, 2008a). Children are primed to identify with their parents and their role models, and as a result, they absorb their beliefs, their capacity for aggression—and the trauma that they suffered as well.

Parens's insights and experiences were the inspiration for the development of the BASE prevention program. Dr. Brisch conducted the first pilot project in the small Bavarian town of Gilching near Munich in 2004. BASE is now well established in a number of European countries and beyond Europe as well, as indicated earlier in this chapter.

Research on Aggression

As a Holocaust survivor, Parens felt the need to engage with the development and prevention of aggression, prejudice, and racism. The Early Child Development Program that he and his coworkers founded at the Eastern Pennsylvania Psychiatric Institute in Philadelphia was designed around early childhood development to prepare children for adulthood. In the context of a mother-centered intervention, which was designed to improve the mother–child interaction, Parens conducted a longitudinal study from 1970 on, in which 16 mother–child pairs were closely observed twice a week. The study began in infancy and continued in its original design for 7 years. As early as 18 months, he and his team observed how certain of the mothers' behaviors that had undermined the children's growth were transformed into behaviors that optimized their development. Follow-up measurements after 19, 32, and 37 years found a correlation between the secure and positive quality of the early observed relationship between mother and toddler and the child's later favorable aggression profiles (Parens, 2008).

Parens's Theory of Aggression

Parens developed his theory of aggression from the insights gained from his psychoanalytical observational studies. But his results were no longer compatible with the psychoanalytic theory that every human being is inherently destructive and strives for destruction as a result of an innate death drive (Parens, 1993a). He found that not all aggressive behavior is destructive. The origins of destructive aggression are not to be found in the death drive; rather, human beings become hostile and destructive when emotional pain and psychological or physiological distress gain the upper hand.

This insight led to his "multi-trends theory of aggression" (Parens, 2008b/1979). His observations led him to catalogue the children's aggressive behaviors into four categories:

a. Unpleasure-related discharge of destructiveness (e.g., the rage reaction of infancy);

b. Nonaffective discharge of destructiveness (e.g., feeding activity);

c. Discharge of nondestructive aggression (e.g., pressured sensorimotor activity); and

d. Pleasure-related discharge of destructiveness (teasing and taunting activity) (Parens, 2008b/1979, p. 147).

The characteristics of these four categories were further analyzed and conceptualized into three categories:

1. *Hostile aggression (HA; categories a and d).* The overarching trend from annoyance to anger, and on to hostility and to rage.

2. *Hostile destructiveness (HD; a subtrend of HA).* From hostility to hate and rage, HA, and therefore HD, is not inborn and it is not biologically activated. However, the mechanism for the generation of HA (and HD) is inborn; this mechanism is activated by an experience of psychic pain ("unpleasure"). Psychic pain is required for the generation of HA: "PP → HA." Excessive psychic pain generates HD: "EPP → HD."

   Psychic pain gives to aggression the affective quality characteristic of annoyance to anger, and increasingly Excessive psychic pain does so for hostility, hate, and rage. Most critically, HA and HD can be moderated or heightened by experience.

3. *Nonaffective destructiveness (category b).* Nonaffective destructiveness corresponds to what is identified in ethology as "prey aggression." Every living creature destroys other living creatures and plants for the purpose of feeding oneself to survive. The need to destroy in the service of alimentation is not driven by anger, hostility, or hate. It is affectively "neutral"—except for the pleasure that comes with gratifying a physiological need such as hunger.

4. *Nondestructive aggression (category c).* Nondestructive aggression is inborn, biologically generated, and essential for adaptation. It fuels mastery of self and environment, assertiveness, and goal achievement.

Note that, regarding the HA/HD trend, the multitrends theory of aggression proposes that experience is the foremost generator of HA and HD. The overarching hypothesis defining this trend of the MTTA holds that "Psychic pain (experience) generates HD." Underlying this hypothesis is that "irritability of the protoplasm" is the biological basis of "EPP → HD" (Parens, 2008b/1979). Thus, the cardinal hypothesis, "excessive psychic pain generates high-level HD": "EPP → HL–HD" informs that, most critically, HD can be moderated and it can be heightened by experience.

Parens's account of the diverse roots and consequences of aggression is consistent with the attachment perspective advanced by Bowlby (e.g., 1982a, 1982b, 1988) and Ainsworth, Blehar, Waters, and Wall (1978). For Bowlby and Ainsworth, with their alternative model of human motivation based on evolutionary theory and the concept of behavioral systems in the service of survival, aggression was seen as an unmediated response to activation of the fear behavioral system, a self-protective gesture displayed in response to a perceived threat. When attachments are secure, perceived threats may be examined and responded to with consideration of the source, and conflict-resolution strategies become available, making aggression a less needed option.

Attachment

Against this backdrop, it is clear that secure attachment to at least one attachment figure is a fundamental evolutionary need. If the primary attachment figure is not available, a secondary attachment figure may serve as a replacement for a time. Although secondary attachment relationships are not the same as the primary ones, they can be very helpful in imparting a sense of security by offering caring, stress reduction, and support in exploration (Bowlby, 2007). Secure attachment is the foundation of healthy emotional and physical development (Suess, Grossman, & Sroufe, 1992). If the educational staff members function as a secure base, children are more likely to develop into socially competent, empathetic, self-confident, and capable adults. The attachment relationship between the child and the staff member can be strengthened by BASE through sensitive questioning. At all age levels, the act of entering into a trusting and safe relationship has the effect of decreasing aggression and fear, and helps to socialize the child. At the physiological level, oxytocin is released during close contact with the attachment figure, which fosters attachment and has a calming effect. Oxytocin also decreases blood pressure and cortisol levels. Such close contact also decreases sensitivity to pain and supports the activity of systems that are involved in growth and recovery, as well as the absorption and storage of nourishment. In addition, it increases the ability to engage socially and to bond with others (Brisch, 2012).

Children who experienced trauma or deprivation early in their lives often attempt to stabilize by seeking closeness with one of the staff members during Babywatching. And children who are currently living through difficult situations are also more likely to seek out a comforting lap and friendly arms. Children with social, emotional, or physical deficits may stabilize in the presence of a person offering secure attachment and even catch up on missed developmental steps. Closeness to a trusted attachment figure who is able to offer prompt, sensitive, and reliable comfort strengthens the attachment relationship, and the child may come to feel the staff member as a safe haven. This should not be underestimated, because such a relationship can have a pronounced corrective effect.

Empathy and Attachment

The ways in which emotions, especially empathy, are expressed are acquired in the context of early experiences with the primary attachment figure. As attachment research has shown, a secure attachment between a child and his or her caregiver is an important protective factor in his or her further development. The quality of care has a demonstrable effect on behavior, attachment, stress regulation, and the emotional, socioemotional, and cognitive capacities of the child (Böhm, 2011). Baby-watching not only increases empathy in children, but it also encourages sensitivity in educational staff members, which in turn has a positive effect on their attachment relationships with each other. Babywatching entails the guided observation of the attachment relationship between a parent and infant. With the support of a sensitive group facilitator, children are given the opportunity in a protected observational setting to correct deficits in their own attachment patterns and become more adept at empathic and sensitive behavior, which in turn can decrease fearful and aggressive behavior. In addition, mothers and fathers who have taken part in the BASE program report that working through the questions that are raised and the responses from the children during the session increases their own sensitivity, especially sensitivity to the needs of their infant.

Corollary findings on the value of a secure couple relationship in adulthood have been observed by Mikulincer et al. (2001). They conducted a series of studies at Bar-Ilan University in Israel on the effect of latent and contextually activated attachment systems on the response to the needs of others. They found a connection between a secure attachment pattern and an increase in empathic responses, along with decreased stress responses to the neediness of others. An avoidant attachment pattern was associated with less empathy, and the anxious attachment pattern in particular was associated with stress in the face of others' needs. These studies demonstrate the relevance of attachment theory to adult couple relationships and of empathic reactions to the needs of others (Mikulincer et al., 2001), highlighting the lifelong relevance of attachment relationships.

Affective and Cognitive Empathy

Empathy, a multidimensional construct, consists of a cognitive (the interpretation of mental states, the theory of mind) and an affective (the emotional response to the emotional state of others) component.

The cognitive component of empathy has to do with the ability to switch perspectives, enabling a person to understand the position of someone else, and to evaluate that position abstractly. The affective component generates an emotional resonance in which the same neuronal networks are activated as when our own emotions are directly involved. This leads to a physical response (*embodied cognition*).

The capacity to empathize is hypothesized to be linked to the mirror neurons (Carr, Iacoboni, Dubeau, Mazziotta, & Lenzi, 2003). Neuronal systems vary greatly from person to person. These systems should be exercised in infancy, because the networks need to develop, and because unused systems tend to atrophy. This is where childrearing and learning processes play an important role. The questions that are posed during BASE sessions may increase activity in these crucial neuronal networks and promote their development, and the different emotions and intentions in the children in the group are discussed. This encourages them to learn in a neutral setting how to understand and even reinterpret their own thought patterns and perceptions. When people, including children, are fearful and stressed, their mirror neurons are adversely affected, as a result of which intuition (gut feelings) becomes unreliable and the ability to learn is reduced. The better children are at imagining themselves into the intentions of others, the less fearful they will be, and the more comfortable they will feel interacting. This has a positive effect on learning.

"Theory of Mind"

Lockl, Schwarz, and Schneider (2004) defined the "theory of mind" as an ability to ascribe to oneself and to other persons mental states such as desires, intentions, motivations, or convictions. The questioning technique used in Babywatching promotes these abilities, so that the children become ever more skilled at taking on the perspective of the mother or father and their baby, explaining their behaviors, then predicting them. This also enables the children to make sense of the actions of others. Hughes and Leekam (2004), Silbereisen and Ahnert et al. (2002), and Ferstl (2007) concluded that primary and secondary attachment figures can have a moderating effect on children's social-cognitive abilities and on development of a theory of mind.

In addition, various environmental conditions that come into play during Babywatching have also been identified, and these are viewed as especially favorable to the development of a complex theory of mind. The acts of observing interactions, having positive role models around, and the opportunity to converse with other engaged participants are viewed as especially effective. Situations in which the child and the (primary or secondary) attachment figure have each other's attention encourage the formation of a theory of mind (see, especially, Astington, 1996; Gopnik, 1996; Gopnik, Meltzoff, & Kuhl, 2001; Gopnik & Schulz, 2007; Harris, 1996; Tomasello, 2013).

Observing the interaction between a parent and an infant is precisely this sort of observation. The group facilitators use a questioning technique to engage the children. As a result, all of them observe the same situation together, which often results in animated discussion. Of course, these interactional moments are dependent on sensitive attachment figures, who are able to employ psychological language and talk about the causal connections between thoughts or feelings and events (Silbereisen & Eyferth, 1986). Hughes and Leekham (2004) have pointed out that conversations about feelings that involve causality are predictors of theory of mind tasks. However, this can be achieved only if the attachment figures (in the BASE program) ensure an emotionally supportive atmosphere (see Fonagy, Gergely, Jurist, & Target, 2002; Denker, 2012).

It has been shown that conversations between attachment figures and young children about the feelings and motivations behind actions are associated with the acquisition of a theory of mind (see Fonagy et al., 2002; Hughes & Leekam, 2004). Fonagy et al. (2002) assume that early acquisition may be attributed to the development of secure attachment, which allows a relaxed, task-oriented attitude between the partners to the interaction, which in turn increases the joy of exploration. As a result, these children are increasingly able to engage in cognitive processes. According to a study by Meins et al. (2002; Meins, 2013), a secure attachment relationship in a child cannot by itself explain the capacity for a theory of mind. Rather, it is the special way mothers communicate with their infants during the first year of life (so-called "mind-mindedness") that characterizes secure attachment relationships and that mediates the association between attachment and a theory of mind. It appears that specific forms of "mentalizing language" affect the ability to form a theory of mind. A theory of mind can be encouraged by interventions that employ mentalizing language and ensure the contingent and ongoing responsiveness of the attachment figure. The attachment figure makes transparent to the child the connection between his or her behavior or that of others and their associated mental states. This makes it possible for the child to integrate his or her behavior or that of others with linguistic perspectives about mental states (Denker, 2012). These are precisely the processes that underpin BASE and make it work. Using a special questioning technique, the group facilitators enter into dialogue with the children about their observations of how the parent and the baby interact. The questioning technique allows for the use of a specific form of mentalizing language that is especially conducive to developing theory of mind competence. During the entire process, the group facilitator responds sensitively to the children's answers and signals, and helps them to improve their mentalizing capabilities. The group facilitator helps them to understand their own motivations, behaviors, and mental states, making these transparent and enriching them with new vocabulary words that enable the children to integrate this information with linguistic perspectives on their own mental states and those of others.

It is immensely important to teach educational staff members about the concepts of attachment and sensitivity as they relate to early childhood development, and the methods used in mentalizing as they are applied in the BASE program (see also Fonagy et al., 2002). Staff members can use these internalized understandings to encourage children's ability to understand mental states. Secure educator–child attachment relationships can then be maintained into elementary school, where children continue to develop dialogue structures (mind-mindedness) that facilitate the understanding of mental states, which they need to successfully negotiate the challenges of the next stages in their development (see Meins et al., 2002; König, 2009). Looking beyond Babywatching, the contents and questioning technique may be used in day care centers and in the classroom generally. The BASE questioning technique (mentalizing language and perspective) is an ideal method for dealing with and resolving conflicts constructively wherever they occur, such as between children, in negotiations with staff members or parents, when looking at picture books together, in symbolic play, and in group interactions (see also Twemlow, Fonagy, Campbell, & Sacco, Chapter 16, this volume).

Secure attachment relationships facilitate educational interactions, form the foundations for exploration by creating a "safe haven," and support the child's adaptation to the world. Overall, sensitive, language-mediated interactions foster the development of a complex theory of mind (Denker, 2012).

Mirror Neurons

Mirror neurons form neuronal systems that exhibit the same activity pattern in the brain when viewing an action, emotion, or behavior in another as if it were one's own. The "emotional contagiousness" afforded by mirror neurons explains the calm and relaxed atmosphere that develops during BASE sessions, in that they enable people to resonate with the actions, emotions, and feelings of others.

Without mirror neurons it would be impossible to feel another person's happiness or pain. But because of this endowment, children observing a baby crying from hunger experience discomfort that allows them to empathize with the baby's physical and mental state. Conversely, children react with happiness when they observe a baby laughing. Babywatching allows us to observe how the children's mirror neurons become activated when they observe a parent–baby interaction. The emotional contagiousness is evidenced by the involuntary imitation of the feelings and actions of the parent and baby. The children perceive the feelings and actions, and respond to them with the appropriate facial expressions. If the baby smacks his or her lips, so will the children; if he or she laughs, so will they. A crying baby elicits concerned faces all around.

When researchers at the David Geffen School of Medicine at UCLA studied the neurobiological correlates of empathic behavior (Carr et al., 2003), they found that observing and imitating facial expressions elicit virtually the same activity patterns in the brain. They also identified the areas of the brain that are involved in empathy, and they clarified the neurobiological mechanisms underlying it.

Imitating and observing emotions activate virtually the same areas of the brain, the primary motor area and the premotor areas, respectively. Several regions are more strongly activated during imitation than during observation. Observation primarily activates the premotor area, which is responsible for coordinating complex movements (Carr et al., 2003). In contrast to the observation of facial expressions, the imitation of emotions has a much greater effect on the regions of the frontal lobe and temporal lobe, the amygdala, and the frontal insula than does pure observation.

Previous experience plays a considerable role in the functioning of the mirror neurons. For example, the mirror neurons of children who have experienced abuse at the hands of their parents respond differently than those of children who live in a loving and sensitive home. It has been shown that the experiences encountered in BASE sessions with the group facilitators and the parent and baby can have a corrective effect. If the ability to mirror is not developed or simply is not used, it may atrophy. This is why neuroscientists use the phrase "use it or lose it" to describe neuronal systems (Kaufmann, 2012). Elementary mirroring processes are present in newborns and commensurate with their fundamental emotional needs. But the ability to mirror another person does not develop by itself; it needs another person with whom this capability can be trained and expanded. Children must first learn to perceive the emotions of others, and this is where BASE can make an important contribution. Using the BASE questioning technique, the educational staff members can foster the ability of the children to empathize and mirror. Researchers theorize that mirror neurons are fully developed by age 3 or 4 years. Because BASE targets this young group, it is especially effective in helping children to develop empathy and, presumably, mirror neuron processes as well.

Training and Setting

While most of the training to become a BASE group facilitator is acquired through experience of running a BASE group with the support and supervision of a mentor, the preliminary 1-day BASE group facilitator training consists of three parts. The first part gives an overview of the program; the second examines its theoretical underpinnings and important aspects of attachment; and the third part prepares the group facilitator to translate theory into practice. Training sessions are conducted by accredited BASE trainers.

Part 1: Historical Overview

Parens's life story and his experiences with National Socialism elucidate the origins of his interest in discovering the causes of hostile and destructive aggression, and his determination to find preventive strategies. In the first part, the basic ideas behind Babywatching are clarified against a backdrop of Parens's scientific and therapeutic career.

Part 2: Theory

Theory provides the conceptual cornerstone of the preventive strategy. The origins of Parens's theory of aggression are explained, as are the ways it differs from Freudian conceptions. The idea that empathy and sensitivity (in word, language, rhythm, touch, and eye contact) can be learned is explained both theoretically and by example.

The BASE questioning technique, with its various levels of observation (of behavior, motivation, emotion, and identification), is central to training. The questioning technique is taught live, with a parent and baby visiting during the training day, so that a Babywatching session can be experienced by the trainees as a method to promote empathy, and is the cornerstone of the entire Babywatching intervention. Training also imparts practical tips. The results of research on BASE, which support both theory and method, are presented at the end of the daylong training session.

Part 3: Translating Theory into Practice

Videotaped examples and live demonstrations with a parent and baby are used to illustrate and practice the questioning technique, giving new group facilitators the experience to facilitate sessions of their own. The live demonstrations enable participants to become aware of their own emotional reactions, which in turn enables them to better imagine the reactions that may arise in the children. Training may not be appropriate for participants with an unfulfilled desire for children, an extremely negative experience of attachment, or a history of negative emotional enmeshment.

For children who have experienced great emotional trauma, observing the sensitive interaction during BASE may trigger reactions, and they may react with avoidance, agitation, or by seeking distraction. During training, participants learn how to intervene to support such children. The potential need for outside help is also discussed.

The B.A.S.E.—Babywatching Questioning Technique

The questioning technique with its five basic questions, detailed below, is the core of the intervention. It lends structure to the setting and is the strategy used to focus the children's attention. The facilitator guides the children through the Babywatching session using this questioning technique, which focuses the circular and reciprocal communications between the two partners upon the interaction (parent and baby), thereby encouraging empathy in the children (Brisch, 2010).

Spectrum of the B.A.S.E.—Babywatching Questions

The questioning technique is divided into an observation level and an identification level. The observation level concentrates on the behavior, motivations, and feelings of the parent and baby. In the identification level, the children are encouraged to identify with the actions and feelings of the parent and baby.

Observation Level

- Behavior level: What is the mother, father, or baby doing?
- Motivation level: Why is the mother, father, or baby behaving this way?
- Emotion level: How does this feel to the mother, father, or baby?

Identification Level

- Identification level (action): What would I do if I were the mother, father, or baby?
- Identification level (emotion): How would I feel if I were the mother, father, or baby?

These five questions may be asked from the level of behavior to the level of identification, or circularly, depending on the children's competencies. A circular question deals with the emotions and the behavior that develop in the parent as a result of the baby's behavior. The parent is not questioned directly, but rather the participating children in the circle are asked. For example, at the identification level, one might ask: "So Tommy, what do you think the mother is feeling when Jillie starts to cry?" The questions may also contain hypotheses that can expand the scope of the conversation and the range of possibilities within the BASE group (Simon & Rech-Simon, 2009). These hypotheses can be tested on the children and corrected as needed. In the process, the children learn that their observations do not necessarily have to be on target, and that there are perspectives that a particular child may not have initially considered. This can lead to fruitful exchanges among them.

The Duration of the Program

The number and duration of BASE sessions depend primarily on the type of target group, but sessions are usually conducted over the entire first year of a baby's life.

As soon as the parent and the baby have settled into a comfortable routine, they may come to the school, nursery school, or other facility once a week. The intervention should end at the beginning of the second year of life, because by then the baby will have entered a developmental stage in which he or she may wish to interact with the children in the group. At this point, the close proximity of parent to baby begins to recede somewhat as the infant gains locomotion skills.

BASE sessions should be limited to the time span mentioned earlier. Integration of the intervention into the daily routine of a facility should be planned well in advance. Vacations, personnel schedules, and daily routines need to be taken into account. All of the participants should understand clearly when the program will begin and when it will end.

Implementation with Other Target Groups

When implemented with other target groups, including professionals, BASE sessions can be conducted as a single guided session, offered as skill enhancement to those involved in the social, therapeutic, or educational professions. Even a single guided session can have a lasting effect, especially when staff members seek to expand their professional abilities. However, it has been shown that repetition deepens the effect. Single guided sessions may be repeated at frequent intervals (e.g., once a month) or in blocks (e.g., 5 days in a row). Experience has shown that the method and contents of BASE help trainees to develop their communication skills, and to become more sensitive and empathetic.

Empirical Foundations: Evaluation of the Acceptance and Efficacy of the Program

Three prospective longitudinal studies in a pretest–posttest control group design have been conducted to date on BASE— in the years 2004 (Brisch, 2010), 2011 (Haneder, 2011), and 2015 (Brisch & Hollerbach, 2016). The studies have demonstrated significant postintervention differences between the control groups and the intervention group (Brisch, 2010). The control groups were recruited in the same setting (nursery school, with children comparable in age and gender) and did not receive the intervention. Problematic behavior in children ($n = 50$) was evaluated by parents and teachers in a prospective, randomized, control-group design using the Child Behavior Checklist (CBCL; Achenbach, 1991). The evaluations were performed before BASE was implemented and 1 year afterward.

After the 1-year intervention, there was a significant improvement in the intervention group compared to the control group. The children in the intervention group exhibited a reduction in both externalizing and internalizing disorders. In terms of externalizing disorders, both the girls and the boys exhibited less aggressive and oppositional behavior and were generally more attentive. In terms of internalizing disorders, the children exhibited fewer fearful and depressive behaviors, were less socially withdrawn, and became more emotionally responsive. There were sex differences with regard to physical symptoms. After the intervention, only the girls exhibited fewer psychosomatic symptoms (Brisch, 2010).

In a study with a separate prospective control group design, Haneder (2011) evaluated the problematic behavior of 250 children of primary school age by both parents and educators using the Strengths and Difficulties Questionnaire (SDQ; Goodman, 1997). Behavior was evaluated before BASE and 9 months thereafter. To analyze group differences over time, children with zero scores for internalizing and externalizing behavior problems were excluded, as they were unlikely to show improvements. After the 9-month intervention, there were significant improvements in the intervention group compared to the control group in internalizing and externalizing behavior, whereby the decrease in internalizing behavior was higher. These effects were demonstrated in the areas of emotional problem behavior, behavior problems, peer problems, and hyperactivity (Haneder, 2011; Haneder, Quehenberger, Hollerbach, Landers, & Brisch, 2016).

A third longitudinal and matched-pair design study with two arms (intervention group, control group) has picked up where the previous studies left off and expands on them. The hypotheses concern empathy in the educational staff (Saarbücker Personality Questionnaire [SPF]; Paulus, 2012), the sensitivity of BASE mothers (SPF; Paulus, 2012; Emotional Availability [EA] Scales; Biringen et al., 1998), and the language competencies of children (Language Development Test for Children Ages 3–5 Years [SETK 3–5], Grimm, 2001; Language Level Test for Children between 5 and 10 Years [SET 5–10], Petermann, 2010). The sample consisted of 3- to 11-year-old healthy children ($N = 46$) from urban neighborhoods and different socioeconomic backgrounds.

BASE was implemented in preschools ($n = 2$) and schools ($n = 2$) of the intervention group over a time period of 8 months. To evaluate children's speech proficiency (SETK 3–5; Grimm, 2001; SET 5–10; Petermann, 2010), empathy (Griffith Empathy Measure [GEM]; Dadds et al., 2008), and aggression and anxiety level (CBCL 4–18; Achenbach, 1991) parents and professionals completed questionnaires at pre- and post-intervention time points.

Repeated-measures analyses of covariance (ANCOVAs) with baseline levels as the covariate show significant group * time effects, with an increase in children's affective and cognitive empathy (GEM), a decrease in aggression and anxiety (CBCL), and a marked increase in the ability to form singular–plural formations (SETK and SET) from pre- to postintervention in the intervention group. By contrast, there was a decrease in empathy (GEM) and rather stable aggression and anxiety levels (Achenbach & Rescorla, 2000; Caregiver–Teacher Report Form [C-TRF]) and a decrease in sentences and singular–plural formation in the control group. Mothers showed an increase in empathy (SPF) and less intrusiveness (EA Scales) compared to the control group (Brisch, 2016; Brisch et al., 2016) (*www.base-babywatching.de*).

Conclusion

The BASE prevention program is a simple program that provides participants—whether preschool children, their teachers, or very old adults in a retirement home—the sense of being part of a family with a baby and the baby's mother available with whom they may observe, empathize, and engage. Babywatching can be a positive emotional experience for all participants: the children, professionals, and parents with their babies. The BASE system thus provides what many in the postindustrialized world lack (Brisch, 2016), that is, quiet time to observe a parent and his or her infant over time, in a supportive context where wonder, questioning, and discussion about what is in the mind of the other is simply irresistible.

REFERENCES

Achenbach, T. M. (1991). *Manual for the Child Behavior Checklist/4–18 and 1991 profile*. Burlington: University of Vermont, Department of Psychiatry.

Achenbach, T. M., & Rescorla, L. A. (2000). *ASEBA preschool forms and profiles*. Burlington: University of Vermont, Research Center for Children, Youth and Families.

Ainsworth, M. S., Blehar, M. C., Waters, E., & Wall, S. (1978). *Patterns of attachment: A psychological study of the Strange Situation*. Hillsdale, NJ: Erlbaum.

Astington, J. W. (1996). What is theoretical about the child's theory of mind?: A Vygotskian view of its development. In P. Carruthers & P. K. Smith (Eds.), *Theories of theories of mind* (pp. 184–199). Cambridge, UK: Cambridge University Press.

Biringen, Z., Robinson, J., & Emde, R. (1998). Emotional availability (EA) scales. Available at *www.emotionalavailability.com*.

Böhm, R. (2011). Auswirkungen frühkindlicher Gruppenbetreuung auf die Entwicklung und Gesundheit von Kindern [Impact of early childhood care on the development and health of children]. *Kinderärztliche Praxis, 82*(5), 316–321.

Bowlby, J. (1982a). *Attachment and loss: Vol. 1. Attachment*. New York: Basic Books. (Original work published 1982)

Bowlby, J. (1982b). Attachment and loss: Retrospect and prospect. *American Journal of Orthopsychiatry, 52*(4), 664.

Bowlby, R. (2007). Babies and toddlers in non-parental daycare can avoid stress and anxiety if they develop a lasting secondary attachment bond with one carer who is consistently accessible to them. *Attachment and Human Development, 9*(4), 307–319.

Brisch, K. H. (2007). Prävention Bindungsstörungen [Prevention of attachment disorders]. In W. von Suchodoletz (Ed.), *Prävention von Entwicklungsstörungen* [Prevention of developmental disorders] (pp. 167–181). Göttingen, Germany: Hogrefe.

Brisch, K. H. (2008). Master Lecture 21: Attachment disorders, psychopathology, attachment therapy, and prevention. *Infant Mental Health Journal, 29*(3A), No. 487.

Brisch, K. H. (2010). *Bindung, Angst und Aggression. Theorie, Therapie und Prävention* [Attachment anxiety and aggression: Theory, therapy and prevention]. Stuttgart, Germany: Klett-Cotta.

Brisch, K. H. (2016, June 1). *A cross-cultural overview on an attachment based prevention program B.A.S.E.®–Babywatching. Symposium*. Presented at the 15th World Congress of the World Association for Infant Mental Health, Prague, Czech Republic.

Brisch, K. H., & Hollerbach, J. (2016, June 1). *B.A.S.E.®–Babywatching: Background of the program, research results on its effectiveness, and clinical application in in-patient treatment for severely early traumatized children*. Presented at the 15th World Congress of the World Association for Infant Mental Health, Prague, Czech Republic.

Brisch, K. H., Hollerbach, J., & Quehenberger, J. (2016, June 1). *Impact of an attachment-based prevention program B.A.S.E.®–Babywatching: A program to counter aggression and anxiety and to promote empathy and sensitivity*. Presented at the 15th World Congress of the World Association for Infant Mental Health, Prague, Czech Republic.

Carr, L., Iacoboni, M., Dubeau, M. C., Mazziotta, J. C., & Lenzi, G. L. (2003). Neural mechanisms of empathy in humans: A relay from neural systems for imitation to limbic areas. *Proceedings of the National Academy of Sciences USA, 100*(9), 5497–5502.

Dadds, M. R., Hunter, K., Hawes, D. J., Frost, A. D., Vassallo, S., Bunn, P., . . . & Masry, Y. E. (2008). A measure of cognitive and affective empathy in children using parent ratings. *Child Psychiatry and Human Development, 39*(2), 111–122.

Denker, H. (2012). *Bindung und Theory of Mind: Bildungsbezogene Gestaltung von Erzieherinnen-Kind-Interaktionen* [Attachment and theory of mind: Educational design from educator-child interactions]. Heidelberg, Germany: Springer-Verlag.

Ferstl, E. C. (2007). Theory-of-Mind und Kommunikation: Zwei Seiten derselben Medaille? [Theory-of-mind and communication: Two sides of the same coin?]. In H. Förstl (Ed.), *Theory of Mind: Neurobiologie und Psychologie sozialen Verhaltens* [Theory of Mind: Neurobiology and psychology of social behavior] (pp. 67–78). Heidelberg, Germany: Springer-Verlag.

Fonagy, P. (1997). Multiple voices vs. meta-cognition: An attachment theory perspective. *Journal of Psychotherapy Integration, 7*(3), 177–180.

Fonagy, P., Gergely, G., Jurist, E., & Target, M. (2002). *Affect regulation, mentalization, and the development of the self.* New York: Other Press.

Goodman, R. (1997). The strengths and difficulties questionnaire: A research note. *Journal of Child Psychology and Psychiatry, 38*(5), 581–586.

Gopnik, A. (1996). Theories and modules: Creation myths, developmental realities, and Neurath's boat. In P. Carruthers & P. K. Smith (Eds.), *Theories of theories of mind* (pp. 169–183). Cambridge, UK: Cambridge University Press.

Gopnik, A., Meltzoff, A. N., & Kuhl, P. K. (2001). *How babies think: The science of childhood.* London: Phoenix.

Gopnik, A., & Schulz, L. (Eds.). (2007). *Causal learning: Psychology, philosophy, and computation.* New York: Oxford University Press.

Grimm, H. (2001). *A test of language development for three-to-five-year-old children. Diagnosis of language processing skills and auditory memory performance.* Göttingen: Hogrefe.

Haneder, A. (2011). *B.A.S.E.®-Babywatching–ein Programm für Empathie und Feinfühligkeit und gegen Angst und Aggression: Implementierung und Evaluierung an Tiroler Volksschulen* [B.A.S.E.®—Babywatching–a program for empathy and sensitivity and against fear and aggression: Implementation and evaluation at Tyrolean schools]. Unpublished master's thesis, Innsbruck, Austria.

Haneder, A., Quehenberger, J., Hollerbach, J., Landers, S., & Brisch, K. H. (2016). Evaluation of B.A.S.E.®–Babywatching: A program to counter aggression and violence and to promote empathy and sensitivity. *Child and Adolescent Mental Health.* Manuscript under review.

Harris, P. (1996). Desires, beliefs, and language. In P. Carruthers & P. K. Smith (Eds.), *Theories of Theories of Mind* (pp. 22–38). Cambridge, UK: Cambridge University Press.

Hollerbach, J., & Brisch, K. H. (2015). Sekundäre Prävention von emotionalem Problemverhalten durch: B.A.S.E.®–Babywatching gegen Aggression und Angst zur Förderung von Sensitivität und Empathie [Secondary prevention of emotional problematic behavior: B.A.S.E.®–Babywatching against aggression and anxiety, for the promotion of sensitivity and empathy]. In I. Seifert-Karb (Ed.), *Frühe Kindheit unter Optimierungsdruck. Entwicklungspsychologische und familientherapeutische Perspektiven* [Early childhood under pressure for optimization. Perspectives of developmental psychology and famiy therapy] (pp. 165–174). Gießen, Germany: Psychosozial-Verlag.

Hughes, C., & Leekam, S. (2004). What are the links between Theory of Mind and social relations?: Review, reflections and new directions for studies of typical and atypical development. *Social Development, 13*(4), 590–619.

Hüther, G. (1998). Stress and the adaptive self-organization of neuronal connectivity during early childhood. *International Journal of Developmental Neuroscience, 16*(3), 297–306.

Kaufmann, S. (2012). *Spiegelneuronen* [Mirror neurons]. Available online at *www.planetwissen.de.*

König, A. (2009). *Interaktionsprozesse zwischen ErzieherInnen und Kindern:Eine Videostudie aus dem Kindergartenalltag* [Interaction processes between teachers and children: A video study from everyday kindergarten life]. Wiesbaden: Verlag für Sozialwissenschaften.

Lockl, K., Schwarz, S., & Schneider, W. (2004). Sprache und Theory of Mind [Language and Theory of Mind]. *Zeitschrift für Entwicklungspsychologie und pädagogische Psychologie, 36*(4), 207–220.

Meins, E. (2013). Sensitive attunement to infants' internal states: Operationalizing the construct of mind-mindedness. *Attachment and Human Development, 15*(5–6), 524–544.

Meins, E., Fernyhough, C., Wainwright, R., Das Gupta, M., Fradley, E., & Tuckey, M. (2002). Maternal mind–mindedness and attachment security as predictors of theory of mind understanding. *Child Development, 73*(6), 1715–1726.

Mikulincer, M., Gillath, O., Halevy, V., Avihou, N., Avidan, S., & Eshkoli, N. (2001). Attachment theory and reactions to others' needs: Evidence that activation of the sense of attachment security promotes empathic responses. *Journal of Personality and Social Psychology, 81*(6), 1205–1224.

Parens, H. (1993a). Neuformulierungen der psychoanalytischen Aggressionstheorie und Folgerungen für die klinische Situation [New formulations of the psychoanalytic aggression theory: Conclusions for the clinical situation]. *Forum der Psychoanalyse,* 9(2), 107–121.

Parens, H. (1993b). Does prevention in mental health make sense? In H. Parens & S. Kramer (Eds.), *Prevention in mental health* (pp. 103–120). Northvale, NJ: Jason Aronson.

Parens, H. (2007). *Heilen nach dem Holocaust: Erinnerungen eines Psychoanalytikers* [Healing after the Holocaust: Memoirs of a psychoanalyst]. Weinheim: Beltz Verlag.

Parens, H. (2008a). *The urgent need for universal parenting education–A documentary.* A DVD produced by H. Parens & P. Gilligan. Philadelphia: Thomas Jefferson University.

Parens, H. (2008b). *The development of aggression in early childhood* (2nd ed.). Lanham, MD: Aronson/Rowman & Littlefield. (Original work published 1979)

Parens, H. (2010). *Parenting for emotional growth: A textbook; two series of workshops; a curriculum for students in grades K through 12 (students 5 to 18 years old; and lines of Development.* Philadelphia: Thomas Jefferson University. (Original work published 1995)

Parens, H. (2011). *Handling children's aggression constructively–Toward taming human destructiveness.* Lanham, MD: Aronson/Rowman & Littlefield.

Parens, H. (2012). Attachment, aggression, and the prevention of malignant prejudice. *Psychoanalytic Inquiry, 32*(2), 171–185.

Paulus, C. (2009). *Der Saarbrücker Persönlichkeitsfragebogen SPF (IRI) zur Messung von Empathie: Psychometrische Evaluation der deutschen Version des Interpersonal Reactivity Index.* [The personality questionnaire from Saarbrücken SPF (IRI) for the measurement of empathy. Psychometric evaluation of the German version of the interpersonal reactivity index]. Saarbrücken: University of Saarland.

Petermann, F. (2010). *Sprachstandserhebungstest für Kinder im alter Awischen fünf und zehn Jahren* [Test of speech development for children 5–10 years of age] (SET 5-10). Göttingen: Hogrefe.

Petermann, F., & Lehmkuhl, G. (2010). Prävention von aggression und gewalt [Prevention of aggression and violence]. *Kindheit und Entwicklung, 19*(4), 239–244.

Schwenner, L. (2014). *Mädchen verprügeln 13-Jährige: Kennt Jugendgewalt keine Grenzen mehr?* [Girls beat up a 13-year-old: Does juvenile violence have any limitations?]. Available online at *www.focus.de/maedchen-verpruegeln-13-jaehrige-kennt-jugendgewalt-keine-grenzen-mehr_id_3530774.html*.

Silbereisen, R. K., & Ahnert, L. (2002). Soziale Kognition: Entwicklung von sozialem Wissen und Verstehen [Social cognition: Development of social knowledge and understanding]. In R. Oerter & L. Montada (Eds.), *Entwicklungspsychologie* (pp. 590–618). Weinheim: Psychologie Verlags Union.

Silbereiscn, R. K., & Eyferth, K. (1986). Development as action in context. In R. K. Silbereisen, K. Eyferth, & G. Rudiger (Eds.), *Development as action in context: Problem behavior and normal youth development* (pp. 3–16). Berlin: Springer.

Simon, F. B., & Rech-Simon, C. (2009). *Zirkuläres Fragen: Systemische Therapie in Fallbeispielen: ein Lernbuch* [Circular questions: Systematic therapy in case studies: A learning book]. Heidelberg: Carl-Auer-Verlag.

Suess, G. J., Grossmann, K. E., & Sroufe, L. A. (1992). Effects of infant attachment to mother and father on quality of adaptation in preschool: From dyadic to individual organisation of self. *International Journal of Behavioral Development, 15*(1), 43–65.

Tomasello, M. (2013). *Die kulturelle Entwicklung des menschlichen Denkens: zur Evolution der Kognition* [The cultural evolution of human thinking: The evolution of cognition]. Frankfurt: Suhrkamp Verlag.

CHAPTER 16

Creating a Peaceful
School Learning Environment

Attachment and Mentalization Efforts to Promote
Creative Learning in Kindergarten through Fifth-Grade
Elementary School Students with Broad Extension
to All Grades and Some Organizations

STUART W. TWEMLOW, PETER FONAGY, CHLOE CAMPBELL,
and FRANK C. SACCO

The model described here—Creating a Peaceful School Learning Environment (CAPSLE)—uniquely applies mentalization-based thinking combined with work on power and shame dynamics to create an institutional climate in which the student is better able to deal with bullying aggression and other critical psychodynamic climate factors.

The literature on mentalization-based interventions focuses largely on the treatment of individual psychopathology stemming from disrupted attachment experiences resulting, for example, in borderline personality disorder (Bateman & Fonagy, 2004). This thinking has been only scantily applied in schools.[1] The absence of mentalizing in thinking about the school context is particularly striking given the significance of mentalizing to issues of developmental psychopathology (Fonagy & Luyten, 2016). Childhood and adolescence is a period associated with dramatic changes in social cognition. A recent study (Dumontheil, Apperly, & Blakemore, 2010) of mentalizing in adolescence found that the capacity to adopt others' perspectives improves substantially between 12½ and 16½ years. The challenge of promoting mentalizing skills is formidable given that, like Piagetian formal operational thinking, most adults are not capable of consistently applying mentalizing

[1] In PsycINFO, mentalization had over 1,000 references, with fewer than 15 referring to the application of mentalization to schools, organizations, or other groups.

skills (Dumontheil et al., 2010). The intervention described here was originally implemented at elementary school, a phase of childhood in which children's attitudes toward aggression begin to crystallize as they advance in impulse control and peer relationship skills (Aber, Brown, Chaudry, Jones, & Samples, 1996). The CAPSLE program is designed to support mentalizing in children—and critically, all staff members in a school, by creating a social system that is able to retain its own capacity for balanced mentalizing and in so doing support the surrounding students to do the same.

We begin this chapter by setting out the basis of the Peaceful Schools Program in mentalizing and attachment theory, and explain how the program is organized and underpinned by these theoretical considerations. We then set out results of our evaluations of the Peaceful Schools Program, and finish by briefly describing how the program has evolved into a flexible approach that has been adapted internationally and in different settings.

Mentalizing School Communities with Balanced Power and Shame Dynamics: A Modern Synthesis

The theory of mentalizing is rooted in attachment. Indeed, *mentalizing*—the capacity to understand ourselves and others in terms of intentional mental states (i.e., needs, desires, feelings, beliefs, goals, and reasons)—in most normal developmental scenarios, develops within attachment relationships: In this sense, attachment and mentalizing are intimately connected both theoretically and at the level of developmental heuristic experience. An infant begins to grasp mentalizing through exposure to being mentalized by other people, through the experience of interacting with primary caregivers who attribute valid and separate mental states to the infant (Fonagy, Gergely, Jurist, & Target, 2002).

Secure attachment relationships, in which attachment figures are interested in the child's mind and the child is safe to explore the mind of the attachment figure (Fonagy, Lorenzini, Campbell, & Luyten, 2014), enable the infant to explore other people's perspectives. The infant's experience of being represented as a thinking and feeling, intentional being in the mind of his or her caregiver in turn strengthens the infant's own capacities for mentalizing. This ability then provides the requisite skills to navigate future social exploration and obstacles (Fonagy et al., 2002).

To do this effectively, however, it is vital that the child learns to master the four separate, but related, dimensions of mentalizing: (1) automatic versus controlled mentalizing, (2) mentalizing the self versus others, (3) internal versus external mentalizing, and (4) cognitive versus affective mentalizing. Effective mentalizing can take place when these dimensions are balanced. Different types of psychological and behavioral difficulties often arise when one is "stuck" at one end of these dimensions (Bateman & Fonagy, 2012).

When mentalizing fails (mostly in high stress contexts), individuals often start to operate in prementalizing modes—these have some parallels with the ways that young children behave before they have developed their full mentalizing capacities. These are psychic equivalence, teleological, and pretend modes. In the *psychic equivalence mode,* thoughts and feelings become "too real." It becomes difficult for the individual to consider alternative perspectives, and what is thought or felt is experienced as completely real and true, creating a kind of concreteness of thought. The *teleological mode* describes a state in which mental attitudes are only recognized if they are accompanied by a tangible signifier and lead to a definite outcome. The individual can recognize the existence and potential importance of states of mind, but this recognition is limited to very concrete, observable situations. For example, affection is only accepted as genuine if it is accompanied by a touch or caress (or, similarly, feelings of anger need to be accompanied by acts of violence or aggression). In *pretend mode*, thoughts and feelings are cut off from reality; in the extreme, this may lead to full dissociative experiences. Individuals in pretend mode can discuss experiences in pseudopsychological terms—with articulacy and apparent accuracy—without contextualizing these through reference to their lived physical or material reality. It is as if they are creating a pretend world (Bateman & Fonagy, 2012, 2016).

The theory of mentalizing, we argue, has valuable implications for understanding how institutions and organizations (or, indeed, any social group) may be supported in behaving in ways that are both more effective and more humane. In our terms, we describe this way of operating as reflecting the ability of the system to maintain balanced mentalizing without slipping into prementalizing modes, even when faced with challenges. The school environment, according to this thinking, is a system that creates its own climate, lending itself to the promotion of greater or lesser levels of mentalizing in both staff and students. The school, in generating an environment that models balanced mentalizing, thus minimizing power–shame dynamics, is capable of containing heightened affect and is of critical importance in preventing bullying and violence. The impact of mentalization/power dynamic-based techniques in reducing group violence may work in a similar way as interventions that focus on the mentalizing difficulties that lead to affect regulation problems in individuals who are chronically angry and impulsive (Bateman & Fonagy, 2016). A mentalizing individual is able to empathize with the self and others, modulate affect storms, set boundaries, have a strong sense of agency, and be reflective. Social groups operate on the same principle. Dysfunctional social systems cause the collapse of mentalizing and result in the highly reactive, tense, and defensive interactions that can lead to violence. Particular attention also needs to be given to the impact of shame and humiliation on children and adults in this context (Twemlow & Sacco, 2012; Gilligan, 1997; Gilligan, Guier, & Blumenfeld, 2001). When an individual is unable to mentalize, in particular, when he or she is operating in prementalizing modes, the experience of shame or humiliation is experienced as an overwhelming attack; it is a devastating experience, and violence or aggression may appear to be the only resolution.

Mentalizing theory proposes that those children and young people who have an adequate capacity for mentalizing (and linked capacities of effortful control, assisted by teacher modeling and attention) can develop their capacity to make sense of their own mind and the complexities of relationships during the elementary school period, leading to relatively stable and essentially positive feelings of identity (including sexual identity) and autonomy, and the capacity to enter into stable, differentiated interpersonal relationships (Blatt & Luyten, 2009; Fonagy & Luyten, 2011). This is not a linear process, however, and both research and clinical practice suggest that even in normal development, it is characterized by (1) much trial and error and (2) hypomentalizing–hypermentalizing cycles, features that may be typical indicators of psychosocial dilemmas that accompany the elementary and high school years (Erikson, 1963; Fonagy & Luyten, 2016).

Whereas these developmental phases present considerable challenges for those with normal developmental histories, children and adolescents with a history of poor mentalizing are at even greater risk when faced with social challenges. The exaggerated experience of affect and limited capacities for affect regulation because of impairments in effortful and attention control and mentalizing seriously impair the capacity to make sense of developmental changes in one's own mind, and in relation to others' minds. At the extreme, this may lead to feelings of identity diffusion and extreme hypomentalizing–hypermentalizing cycles (Sharp et al., 2011, 2013). Furthermore, the adults in a school—whether teachers, management, or support staff—all need support in maintaining their capacity to mentalize, particularly when they are confronted with highly anxiety-provoking, affect-driven or aggressive/hostile behavior from students. Mentalizing is a highly interactional process, and even adults with robust mentalizing capacities are highly challenged in stressful environments without support.

Mentalizing is developed and sustained by the social system we live in: Social systems that are compassionate have physical effects (e.g., in the production of oxytocin) and psychological effects that enhance self-awareness and awareness of the mental states of others. On the other hand, social systems that do not respect agency or subjectivity recreate the evolutionary environment that encodes for self-sufficiency and reduced empathy, creating an environment that is primed for bullying. We consider successfully mentalizing social systems to have certain features in common: They are relaxed and flexible rather than becoming stuck in one rigid point of view; they can use humor and be playful in a style that engages individuals, rather than in a way that is hurtful or distancing; they can resolve difficulties and problems through "give-and-take" that involves being able to take on others' perspectives; they advocate describing one's own experience rather than defining other people's experience for them; they convey a sense of ownership of behavior, showing agency and responsibility; and finally, they demonstrate openness and curiosity about others' perspectives.

Conversely, a nonmentalizing, disorganized social system creates fear and can hyperactivate attachment. This undermines the capacity for higher order cognition and forces the system into prementalizing modes. Such a nonmentalizing social system can be highly self-reinforcing, because it tends to undermine the social mechanism that could alter its character: human collaboration based on negotiation and creativity. To refer back to the prementalizing modes, a disorganized system operating in *pretend mode* shows few links between inner and outer worlds; the mental world is decoupled from external reality. Everyone in such a system can think and feel, but there is a sense of no real consequence, which creates a somewhat meaningless social landscape. It can lead to selfishness that arises from a sense of the unreality of everything other than one's own thoughts and feelings. Ultimately, this can permit aggression and harm, because other people's minds are not felt to really exist. Such a system is often characterized by endless communication, consultation, and searching for solutions, but little real change.

In a social system operating in *psychic equivalence* mode (and the different pre-mentalizing modes can operate simultaneously), mental reality and outer reality become blurred: thoughts are too real; hence, they must be controlled. There is only one possible solution, and alternative visions or perspectives cannot be tolerated. Given the power of thoughts, negative ideas become terrifyingly real threats on which one needs to act. Finally, in the *teleological* mode, only behavior that has a visible outcome is regarded as meaningful—aggression and acts of physical harm become more legitimate, and there can be a hunger for physical acts to reveal states of mind (e.g., acts of subservience or highly punitive acts).

Our experience has been that few, if any, schoolchildren caught in the blight of a nonmentalizing system can sustain mentalizing to any degree, whatever their age. Another conceptualization is that they (in the bullying school social system), have all lost their individuality in favor of a constrictive social role that fosters social stereotypes and perseverative group behavior that fails to recognize and mentalize the individual-in-the-group (Twemlow & Sacco, 2008, 2012). The unique individual presence of the other is negated by the requirements of a stereotyped social role that is part of the typical teaching pattern in children (the teacher is in charge) until puberty.

Mentalizing within a system, and the sense of self that emerges, is a complex process. As interpersonalist theories and other current relational theories hold, the person in the extreme situation feels completely defined by the social system, and his or her sense of reality is rooted in that reality being shared by others. We know that the world outside is real partly because others respond to us in ways that are consistent with our reactions, a form of social biofeedback started by the primordial mother who trains her infant with feedback such as "This is your thought, not mine," or "This is my thought, not yours." The extraordinary impact of social responses on the developing individual has also, for example, been illustrated by experiments with 6-month-old infants using the still-face paradigm (Weinberg & Tronick, 1996).

From a mentalizing and interpersonalist perspective, the personal consensus between two people may be seen as creating an external (social) reality, when they have balanced their power and shame dynamics. On a larger scale, when power dynamics influence that social reality, either through individual psychopathology—especially of leaders—or the overuse of coercion and punishment in legal institutions or codes of conduct, then victim, victimizer, and bystander mindsets are created in members of that system, who then function in the roles created by this nonmentalizing social system; that is, in violent environments, there is a chronic failure of mentalizing in the pure sense. When mentalizing fails, it also creates for the witness to the power struggle (the bystander) an avenue to the pleasure of sadism, illustrated by the child who gains vicarious pleasure by watching the bullying process. This is possible because the child distances him- or herself from the internal world of the other—and at the same time—benefit from using the other as a vehicle (part-object or part-person) for unwanted (usually frightened and disavowed) parts of the self projected into the victim. The perpetrator of violence, being the focus of so much attention (from the victim and from the bystanders), is able to experience him- or herself as more coherent and complete (though, of course, through a deeply pathological process) (Twemlow, 2012). For violent children or adolescents, mentalizing is deeply limited, such that the suffering and pain of the victim need never be fully represented as mental states in their consciousness.

The overarching goal of the CAPSLE approach is to create in the school (and in the community) a family in which secure attachments predominate. The more the school can operate as a large coordinated group and avoid being stuck in the victim role when bullies dominate, the more possible a creative secure outcome becomes. From our perspective, the security of attachment is reflected in the way in which people cooperate and become friends. In a local community, this might mean things like dealing with graffiti around schools. In schools operating under this model, there may be regular cleanup of the local area by school children, voluntary helping of older adults with the raking of leaves and so forth, and children who are ill for prolonged periods of time are kept in touch with class actions by telephone calls or by visits by students when appropriate. Children love to help others and greatly benefit from the experience; being allowed to help is an acknowledgment of agency (Twemlow, Fonagy, Sacco, Vernberg, & Malcom, 2011; Twemlow & Sacco, 2013).

When a school climate starts to change, and it takes about a year for this to happen, what one sees is episodes, such as the one we observed when a boy was waiting to be picked up by his father, who was a leader of a prominent gang. Beside this boy was a kindergarten child, crying because he couldn't tie his shoelaces; the older boy bent down to tie this child's shoelaces. This was the beginning of a change for him. He became a natural leader within the school environment, because there was no social status anymore for bullying power. Social status arose out of being reflective, having one's feelings under control, and helping others as much as possible (i.e., mentalizing). In summary, when mentalizing and power dynamics are well balanced within a group, the group members feel good and want to feel even better by helping others when a need is present.

The Peaceful Schools Approach

CAPSLE (as the initial randomized controlled trial [RCT] was named) is based on three major assumptions:

1. That to reduce violence in schools we need to systematically increase awareness of the mental states that underpin behavior.
2. That the whole school community contributes to unthinking, bullying-related dysfunction through an absence of mentalizing.
3. That peaceful collaboration with others requires prioritizing their subjective states, thus putting limits on the urge to violently control the behavior of less powerful members of the group.

Accordingly, CAPSLE is a whole-school approach that seeks to create a system-wide awareness of the omnipresence of power struggles, and how such struggles undermine and unbalance one's mentalizing capacities. By building emotional and cognitive skills in handling interpersonal power struggles, empathy and self-agency are improved, and the likelihood of violence is reduced. This is an approach that focuses on the school's whole-group functioning rather than on the behavior of individual problem children. It involves a move away from targeted, antibullying, mental health, and learning disability programs, and so forth, toward a focus on the wider school climate (Cohen & Brooks, 2014).

CAPSLE is a teacher-implemented, manualized program with four components, summarized below in Table 16.1.

As shown in Table 16.1, the first component of the CAPSLE model is a positive climate campaign, using learning methods and materials to create an awareness that allows for the identification and resolution of coercive power dynamics. The second component is a classroom management plan that helps teachers to discipline by focusing on the understanding and correction of problems rather than on punishment and criticism. The third component is a physical education program—the Gentle Warriors Program—derived from a combination of role playing, relaxation techniques, and defensive martial arts. This teaches children skills to self-regulate and control their emotions, mind and behavior, while also providing skills in how to handle victimization and bystanding behavior, thereby helping children to protect themselves and others with nonaggressive physical and cognitive strategies. Finally, the fourth component is one or two (or both) possible mentorship programs—using adults or older peers as mentors. This mentorship support provides additional containment and modeling to assist children in mastering the skills and language to deal with power struggles. The choice of whether to opt for adult or peer support (or both) is a practical one for the school, depending on the availability of appropriate outside adults or older children within the school.

What We Learned from the Pilot Study

This work evolved through collaboration with three schools over a 6-year process (between 1993 and 1999) in Topeka, Kansas. One was a K–5 elementary school in a poor area of the community with the poorest academic achievement, high levels of violence, and the highest out-of-school suspension rate in the Topeka school district. It had gained considerable notoriety as a result of the attempted rape of a second-grade girl by some second- and third-grade boys. The principal of the school had approached the first author (S. W. T.) for ideas that might help the school after he had heard about our work with a violent secondary school system in a city in Jamaica (Twemlow & Sacco, 1996).

The pilot first revealed what has been a consistent finding in our work: that sustained effective change depends on the enthusiasm and degree of buy-in shown by teachers, students, parents, and the surrounding community. The initial experimental school showed a marked increase in Parent Teacher Organization (PTO) attendance and teachers who were happy to administer and score instruments to test effectiveness, including teachers who did this in their own time, because they fully understood how this process would work and it made sense to them. This experience demonstrated the critical importance of community engagement and involvement in an intervention.

TABLE 16.1. The components of CAPSLE

Component	Goals	Techniques involved
A positive climate campaign	• Goals are to make awareness of power struggles, reflection, and modulation of feelings a regular part of the children's day, so that it eventually becomes part of their language and shifts the tone of the school. • Create awareness of the three roles: victim, bully, and bystander. • Motivate children to obtain social rewards and social status that come from helpfulness and consideration of others rather than from the power gained and retained with aggression. • Empower children to peacefully resolve issues with each other with minimal adult participation.	Use of a variety of "campaign" strategies including posters, magnets, bookmarks, buttons, class projects and discussions, the school peace flag, lectures, school assemblies, and integration of the program philosophy into the curriculum.
Classroom management plan	• Emphasize the effects of each class member's behavior on others to promote balanced mentalizing within the classroom. • Enhance understanding of the importance of insight into the meaning of behaviors, thereby reducing scapegoating.	Use of Reflection Time to facilitate class participation in setting class goals and in reflecting on progress toward those goals, encouraging students to use skills learned in Gentle Warriors Program training (e.g., Relaxation Response), conceptualizing a behavior problem in a single child as a problem for the whole class.
Gentle Warriors Program of physical education	• A structured set of activities that teach self-regulation and self-control, provide children with alternative actions to fighting, and teach children to be agents of positive social change in their school. • The program fulfils the school requirement for physical education, is easily implemented, requires no martial arts experience, and is well accepted by physical education teachers.	• Physical exercises include stretching, relaxing, self-defense, and role-playing activities such as the enacting of bully–victim–bystander roles. • Activities also include the reading of stories that emphasize ethical conduct including self-respect, respect for others, self-control, kindness, and generosity.
Peer and adult mentorship	• Adult and peer mentoring efforts, with a focus on the playground, lunchtime, and the school corridor. • To assist children in avoiding one of the three roles—bully, victim, and bystander—wherever they are in the school.	Peer Mentors spend time weekly with their assigned child at school and are closely supervised. In The Bruno Program, older adults are encouraged to help children manage unstructured school time such as recess and lunch hours, with mentors using creative ways to help children resolve problems, such as setting rules for basketball games, and playground disputes (e.g., sharing play equipment).

The original problem school had changed dramatically. First, this was noted on an observational level: For example, on one occasion when the first author (S. W. T.) attended the experimental school, he thought it must have been closed because it was so quiet. Second, black children began to outperform white children academically, which in the 1990s was quite unusual, and subject to a variety of studies by school districts. Third, teachers became happier in their professional work. The reduction in the number of disciplinary referrals and the improved achievement in test scores continued even when children left the peaceful school, if they had had 2 years' experience with CAPSLE. This pilot study warranted the expansion of the research into a fuller RCT (Twemlow et al., 2001).

A Multischool Cluster RCT

On the basis of the original pilot study and the theoretical work that evolved with it, we began an RCT in 1999. It was conducted over a 3-year period. Nine schools participated, and were assigned randomly to one of three conditions: (1) CAPSLE; (2) school psychiatric consultation (SPC), which involved the child psychiatrist visiting the school once a week, observing classrooms, meeting with mental health teams, and helping teachers in referring children for appropriate mental health treatment when necessary; and (3) no intervention but the promise of free access at the end of the study to whichever intervention was found most effective. The CAPSLE approach as implemented in this RCT contained all four components previously described in Table 16.1 and was actively implemented across 2 years. In Year 1, school staff members received a 1-day group training; students received nine sessions of self-defense training. In Year 2, school staff members received a half-day refresher group training; students received a three-session refresher self-defense course. Throughout active implementation, the CAPSLE team held monthly consultations with school staff. Table 16.2 shows how the CAPSLE program was implemented.

The study was based on the hypothesis that the bully and the victim are both symptomatic of a wider problem within the school system as a whole. This is made particularly pathological by the way in which teachers and police officers are left with the total responsibility for shaping the learning environment in U.S. school learning systems. We started to conceptualize the bully and victim as expressions of the group rage of the community (including abdicating bystanders) at those who were designated as leaders. Accordingly, the approach focuses on the power of bystanders in particular to change the climate. A school tends to have significant problems with bullying when designated leaders do not focus on the role of the bully/bystander in the evolution of school dynamics, and instead the institution becomes pathologically stuck in the victim role: The victim here in such situations is the school, and the bully is in informal charge. The bully would control the school, eventually to the extent that the school would in effect find it impossible to manage itself. Since these dynamics are often not obvious, actors in the drama may play their respective roles unknowingly, thus perpetuating the trauma across cycles of students (and teachers). More detail on the unconscious (or not recognized) elements are described elsewhere in our work (Twemlow & Sacco, 2012).

TABLE 16.2. Implementation of the CAPSLE Program

Active intervention		Maintenance intervention
Year 1	**Year 2**	**Year 3**
A CAPSLE team drawn from the school staff leads implementation using a training manual (Twemlow, Sacco, & Twemlow, 1999)		
• One-day introductory group training for teachers • CAPSLE intervention team consult with school staff monthly • Nine-session student self-defense program (formal training that is then continued in PE classes) • Biweekly supervision of CAPSLE intervention team with second author (P. F.)	• Half-day schoolwide refresher training for all staff at start of year • CAPSLE intervention team consult with school staff monthly • Three sessions self-defense refresher (formal training that is then continued in PE classes) • Biweekly supervision of CAPSLE intervention team with second author (P. F.)	• Inservice refresher training for staff • Three-session student self-defense program (formal training that is then continued in PE classes)

The results of the study are summarized in Table 16.3.

The table indicates that multiple positive outcomes followed from the CAPSLE intervention, and contrasts the treatment-as-usual (TAU) school and the SPC group.

Independently, we have evaluated the effectiveness of the Gentle Warriors Program, a traditional martial arts-based intervention addressing one of the core components of our model (see Table 16.1), aimed at reducing aggression in children. The Gentle Warriors Program involves nine 45-minute sessions in each of the first 2 years of the intervention, taught by a martial arts instructor. In the third year of the intervention, the maintenance phase, there were three further 45-minute sessions. Each session began with breathing and relaxation exercises designed to increase the children's awareness and control over their physiological arousal. Children were led through stretching exercises in preparation for the lesson. After stretching, children were taught defensive techniques, and they role-played common bully–victim–bystander situations and engaged in a question and answer discussion of philosophy with the martial arts instructor. Throughout the instruction, the basic philosophical foundations of nonaggression, self-awareness, respect for self and others, and self-control were reinforced through question-and-answer discussion. At the conclusion of the session, the lesson was reviewed, another brief period of relaxation was practiced, and stories depicting traditional martial arts values were shared. It was implemented in three elementary schools (CAPSLE schools). The sample consisted of 254 children in grades 3, 4, and 5. Results indicated that boys who participated in more Gentle Warriors Program sessions reported a lower frequency of aggression and greater frequency of helpful bystanding (i.e., helpful behavior toward victims of bullying) over time. The effect of participation on aggression was partially

TABLE 16.3. Results of the Cluster RCT for CAPSLE

Intervention	Active intervention years				Follow-up year	
	Baseline	Time 2	Time 3	Time 4	Time 5	Time 6
Aggression						
Peer report						
TAU	97.8 (.48)	99.6 (.61)	101.0 (.59)	102.7 (.72)	99.5 (.54)	103.2 (.63)
CAPSLE	98.2 (.43)	99.9 (.52)	99.8 (.46)	101.7 (.47)	97.7 (.41)	101.2 (.41)
SPC	97.5 (.44)	99.6 (.52)	100.2 (.55)	101.6 (.65)	98.4 (.48)	100.7 (.55)
Self-report						
TAU	98.2 (.56)	99.3 (.57)	99.0 (.55)	99.7 (.59)	99.3 (.49)	100.9 (.66)
CAPSLE	100.4 (.49)	99.7 (.50)	100.0 (.47)	100.2 (.49)	98.9 (.42)	100.3 (.46)
SPC	100.6 (.53)	100.2 (.52)	100.3 (.59)	101.1 (.61)	99.5 (.50)	101.0 (.63)
Victimization						
Peer report						
TAU	97.6 (.56)	99.1 (.73)	100.2 (.67)	102.8 (.74)	100.0 (.68)	102.8 (.75)
CAPSLE	98.7 (.41)	99.9 (.44)	100.1 (.39)	100.7 (.39)	98.0 (.44)	99.8 (.42)
SPC	97.8 (.55)	100.5 (.54)	100.3 (.56)	101.9 (.63)	99.3 (.46)	101.1 (.45)
Self-report						
TAU	99.70 (.61)	101.0 (.71)	98.7 (.53)	99.9 (.61)	99.8 (.56)	100.2 (.59)
CAPSLE	100.64 (.46)	99.4 (.46)	99.1 (.46)	99.2 (.44)	99.0 (.45)	99.4 (.43)
SPC	100.63 (.54)	101.0 (.58)	100.2 (.58)	100.6 (.61)	101.1 (.55)	100.7 (.60)
Aggressive bystanding						
TAU	97.6 (.50)	99.4 (.66)	100.3 (.58)	102.7 (.71)	100.2 (.56)	102.2 (.65)
CAPSLE	98.1 (.44)	100.1 (.55)	100.4 (.46)	101.2 (.45)	98.1 (.41)	100.2 (.50)
SPC	97.1 (.41)	100.0 (.49)	100.5 (.52)	102.2 (.63)	98.6 (.47)	101.5 (.57)
Helpful bystanding						
TAU	96.6 (.54)	100.2 (.64)	104.0 (.69)	104.0 (.60)	98.5 (.58)	102.3 (.64)
CAPSLE	99.4 (.48)	100.7 (.51)	100.5 (.43)	100.3 (.48)	100.2 (.48)	101.4 (.50)
SPC	96.7 (.53)	99.6 (.54)	98.8 (.51)	98.9 (.50)	98.2 (.45)	98.9 (.50)
Mentalizing empathy						
TAU	102.2 (.61)	101.3 (.63)	100.4 (.59)	98.8 (.59)	101.1 (.60)	98.8 (.59)
CAPSLE	100.4 (.47)	99.1 (.50)	100.0 (.47)	99.1 (.47)	100.3 (.47)	99.2 (.48)
SPC	101.5 (.53)	100.3 (.55)	99.0 (.55)	98.3 (.55)	101.3 (.51)	99.2 (.53)

(continued)

TABLE 16.3. *(continued)*

Intervention	Active intervention years				Follow-up year	
	Baseline	Time 2	Time 3	Time 4	Time 5	Time 6
Aggression is legitimate						
TAU	96.5 (.47)	98.1 (.56)	98.7 (.52)	99.0 (.50)	98.9 (.55)	100.4 (.59)
CAPSLE	99.1 (.50)	100.6 (.56)	100.7 (.47)	100.9 (.49)	98.4 (.42)	99.5 (43)
SPC	100.5 (.54)	99.9 (.53)	101.8 (.59)	102.1 (.60)	100.9 (.54)	102.0 (.64)

Note. Data from Fonagy, P. Twemlow, S. W. Vernberg, E. M., Nelson, J. M., Dill, E. J., Little, T. D., & Sargent, J. A. (2009). A cluster randomized controlled trial of child-focused psychiatric consultation and a school systems-focused intervention to reduce aggression. *Journal of Child Psychology and Psychiatry, 50*(5), 607–616.

mediated by empathy. The effect of participation on helpful bystanding was fully mediated by changes in student empathy. No significant results were found for girls (Twemlow, Biggs, Nelson, Vernberg, & Fonagy, 2008). The findings for girls are interesting and warrant further consideration. Significantly less aggression among girls was reported at outset. Previous research has suggested that relational aggression tended to predominate over physical aggression among girls, and such forms of aggression are targeted less by this aspect of the program. A further consideration is that the Gentle Warriors Program might benefit girls in different ways, not measured empirically in the study: for example, in increased assertiveness and self-esteem (Twemlow et al., 2008).

The impact of a schoolwide intervention seems to occur at multiple levels. This was indicated by prior research in this school district that showed a clear improvement in academic performance for children who spent 2 or more years in schools offering this program (Fonagy, Twemlow, Vernberg, Sacco, & Little, 2005). This improvement also continued into middle school for children who had been in the CAPSLE program at least 2 years.

Evolution into New Settings

Since 2000, the CAPSLE model has been used in all school grades and in many adult organizations as well, with a number of modifications based on iterative replications and clinical experience. The model has evolved not as a protocol to be carefully followed as originally formulated in the RCT for CAPSLE; it has developed into a very adaptable model. It has been highly successful in Australia, where the model focused on child control of the work with psychoanalytically trained assistants, and in North Carolina, where the actual interventions were designed by school staff members adhering to the framework design but using their own ideas about how to make it all happen. In Hungary, the work was adapted to a school for severely visually impaired children and children with major transplant recovery problems, and the book describing the approach (Twemlow & Sacco, 2008) was eventually translated to Hungarian. It evolved around the Samovar strength concept that enhanced children's feeling of self-determination.[2] Its use for a long period helped us create major cultural adaptations of the fundamental framework but still preserve the mentalizing/shame/power dynamics framework (Twemlow et al., 2011; Twemlow & Sacco, 1996). The 2011 article describes an extraordinary intervention in a school in Negril, Jamaica, which resulted in notable reductions in aggression and improvement in altruistic behavior especially by boys. We have projects in various stages of development in Brasilia and in Botswana, where a group of retired school principals are working together on the program, and with U.S. military personnel, who are looking for flexible approaches to supporting military families. Houston, Texas, has a 12-school program in its fifth year, focusing on communities of schools and how parents and teachers can help each other improve communication. This system has a monthly meeting of principals who share good ideas. When this process began, two schools across the road from each other had principals who had never met. Now it is a truly integrated community of schools.

Conclusion

CAPSLE is a mentalizing and attachment-based approach to developing a school climate that encourages students—and staff members—to hold the minds of others in mind. Seeking to extend attachment and mentalizing approaches to thinking about systems might appear to be a shift in emphasis from the dyadic focus on primary caregivers in developmental psychopathology. However, we argue that such an approach is highly congruent with John Bowlby's evolutionary conceptualization of attachment as a means of developmentally adapting according to the psychological and social environment in order to best navigate it. Attachment and mentalizing are both artifacts and drivers of the human capacity for social complexity. As such, they are highly suggestible to cues given by the social environment—this is what makes possible the flexibility and adaptability that is such a marked human capability. Humans evolved to parent in a far more collaborative and cooperative way than is currently practiced (Hrdy, 2011); as such, it is fitting that we give thought to transactional implications of the psychological cues—preeminently and ideally, mentalizing from a secure base—provided by the social system around the child.

ACKNOWLEDGMENTS

This research was supported by the Child and Family Program of the Menninger Foundation, Topeka, Kansas, and the Menninger Department of Psychiatry, Baylor College of Medicine, Houston, Texas. Peter Fonagy is in receipt of a U.K. National Institute for Health Research (NIHR) Senior Investigator Award (NF-SI-0514-10157) and was in part supported by the NIHR Collaboration for Leadership in Applied Health Research and Care (CLAHRC) North Thames at Barts Health NHS Trust. The views expressed are those of the authors and not necessarily those of the NHS, the NIHR, or the Department of Health.

---

[2]More on the Hungarian Peaceful Schools work can be found at *http://bekesiskola.hu/en*.

REFERENCES

Aber, J. L., Brown, J. L., Chaudry, N., Jones, S. M., & Samples, F. (1996). The evaluation of the Resolving Conflict Creatively Program: An overview. *American Journal of Preventive Medicine, 12*(Suppl. 5), 82–90.

Bateman, A. W., & Fonagy, P. (2004). Mentalization-based treatment of BPD. *Journal of Personality Disorders, 18*(1), 36–51.

Bateman, A. W., & Fonagy, P. (Eds.). (2012). *Handbook of mentalizing in mental health practice.* Washington, DC: American Psychiatric Publishing.

Bateman, A. W., & Fonagy, P. (2016). *Mentalization-based treatment for personality disorders: A practical guide.* Oxford: Oxford University Press.

Blatt, S. J., & Luyten, P. (2009). A structural–developmental psychodynamic approach to psychopathology: Two polarities of experience across the life span. *Development and Psychopathology, 21*(3), 793–814.

Cohen, J. W., & Brooks, R. A. (2014). *Confronting school bullying: Kids, culture, and the making of a social problem.* Boulder, CO: Lynne Rienner.

Dumontheil, I., Apperly, I. A., & Blakemore, S. J. (2010). Online usage of theory of mind continues to develop in late adolescence. *Developmental Science, 13*(2), 331–338.

Erikson, E. H. (1963). *Childhood and society* (2nd ed.). New York: Norton.

Fonagy, P., Gergely, G., Jurist, E., & Target, M. (2002). *Affect regulation, mentalization, and the development of the self.* New York: Other Press.

Fonagy, P., Lorenzini, N., Campbell, C., & Luyten, P. (2014). Why are we interested in attachments? In P. Holmes & S. Farnfield (Eds.), *The Routledge handbook of attachment: Theory* (pp. 38–51). Hove, UK: Routledge.

Fonagy, P., & Luyten, P. (2011). Die Entwicklungspsychologischen Wurzeln der Borderline-Persönlichkeitsstörung in Kindheit und Adoleszenz: Ein Forschungsbericht unter dem Blickwinkel der Mentalisieurngstheorie [The roots of borderline personality disorder in childhood and adolescence: A review of evidence from the standpoint of a mentalization based approach]. *Psyche: Zeitschrift für Psychoanalyse und ihre Anwendungen, 65*(9–10), 900–952.

Fonagy, P., & Luyten, P. (2016). A multilevel perspective on the development of borderline personality disorder. In D. Cicchetti (Ed.), *Development and psychopathology* (3rd ed., pp. 726–792). New York: Wiley.

Fonagy, P., Twemlow, S. W., Vernberg, E. M., Nelson, J. M., Dill, E. J., Little, T. D., & Sargent, J. A. (2009). A cluster randomized controlled trial of child-focused psychiatric consultation and a school systems-focused intervention to reduce aggression. *Journal of Child Psychology and Psychiatry, 50*(5), 607–616.

Fonagy, P., Twemlow, S. W., Vernberg, E., Sacco, F. C., & Little, T. D. (2005). Creating a peaceful school learning environment: The impact of an antibullying program on educational attainment in elementary schools. *Medical Science Monitor, 11*(7), CR317–CR325.

Gilligan, J. (1997). *Violence: Our deadliest epidemic and its causes.* New York: Grosset/Putnam.

Gilligan, J., Guier, A., & Blumenfeld, Y. (2001). *Preventing violence.* London: Thames & Hudson.

Hrdy, S. B. (2011). *Mothers and others.* Boston: Harvard University Press.

Sharp, C., Ha, C., Carbone, C., Kim, S., Perry, K., Williams, L., & Fonagy, P. (2013). Hypermentalizing in adolescent inpatients: Treatment effects and association with borderline traits. *Journal of Personality Disorders, 27*(1), 3–18.

Sharp, C., Pane, H., Ha, C., Venta, A., Patel, A. B., Sturek, J., & Fonagy, P. (2011). Theory of mind and emotion regulation difficulties in adolescents with borderline traits. *Journal of the American Academy of Child and Adolescent Psychiatry, 50*(6), 563–573.

Twemlow, S. W. (2012). The Columbine tragedy ten years later: Psychoanalytic reminiscences and reflections. *Journal of the American Psychoanalytic Association, 60*(1), 171–180.

Twemlow, S. W., Biggs, B. B., Nelson, T. D., Vernberg, E., & Fonagy, P. (2008). Effects of participation in a martial arts–based antibullying program in elementary schools. *Psychology in the Schools, 45*(10), 947–959.

Twemlow, S. W., Fonagy, P., Sacco, F. C., Gies, M. L., Evans, R., & Ewbank, R. (2001). Creating a peaceful school learning environment: A controlled study of an elementary school intervention to reduce violence. *American Journal of Psychiatry, 158*(5), 808–810.

Twemlow, S. W., Fonagy, P., Sacco, F. C., Vernberg, E., & Malcom, J. M. (2011). Reducing violence and prejudice in a Jamaican all age school using attachment and mentalization theory. *Psychoanalytic Psychology, 28*(4), 497–511.

Twemlow, S. W., & Sacco, F. C. (1996). Peacekeeping and peacemaking: The conceptual foundations of a plan to reduce violence and improve the quality of life in a midsized community in Jamaica. *Psychiatry: Interpersonal and Biological Processes, 59*(2), 156–174.

Twemlow, S. W., & Sacco, F. C. (2008). *Why school antibullying programs don't work.* Lanham, MD: Jason Aronson.

Twemlow, S. W., & Sacco, F. C. (2012). *Preventing bullying and school violence.* Arlington, VA: American Psychiatric Publishing.

Twemlow, S. W., & Sacco, F. C. (2013). How and why does bystanding have such a startling impact on the architecture of school bullying and violence? *International Journal of Applied Psychoanalytic Studies, 10*(3), 289–306.

Twemlow, S. W., Sacco, F. C., & Twemlow, S. W. (1999). *Creating a peaceful school learning environment: A training program for elementary schools.* Agawam, MA: T & S Publishing Group.

Weinberg, K. M., & Tronick, E. Z. (1996). Infant affective reactions to the resumption of maternal interaction after the still-face. *Child Development, 67,* 905–914.

CHAPTER 17

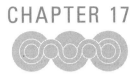

Connect

An Attachment-Based Program for Parents of Teens

MARLENE M. MORETTI, DAVE S. PASALICH,
and KATHERINE A. O'DONNELL

We begin this chapter with a brief discussion of the typical and atypical challenges that adolescence presents to parents and their growing children, both in contemporary and past societies. We do so with an emphasis on adolescence as a unique transitional period, one with important implications for the nature of the attachment relationship between parent and child. Next we describe Connect, an attachment-based intervention for parents and alternative caregivers of preteens and adolescents. We provide an overview of the program, including the attachment-related mechanisms and processes that are targeted during the intervention; key attachment principles that guide session content, reflection exercises, and role plays; and a model of therapeutic change. Training, implementation, and building capacity/sustainability across diverse communities are discussed, and the evidence of effectiveness is presented. We conclude by emphasizing the importance of knowledge translation in the field of attachment in expanding well-defined, feasible, and effective interventions to promote adolescent mental health and family functioning.

Adolescence in History and Contemporary Times: A Similar Story

Adolescence is one of the most intriguing periods of human development and the subject of considerable debate by parents, scientists, and philosophers alike. As children enter adolescence, most parents express bewilderment and concern about the volatility in their children's moods, their interests, and sensitivity to minor slights or disappointments. Some are astonished or offended by their teens' newly found oppositional stance and contemptuous attitude toward authority. Parents commonly lament about teens today. Yet these concerns are remarkably similar to those expressed some 2,500 years ago by early philosophers including Socrates (470–399 B.C.E.) and Aristotle (384–322 B.C.E.). Adolescence, it turns out, is not a fictitious developmental stage born of modern society as is commonly believed; it is a period of semi-immaturity that hangs between childhood and adulthood that has been recognized in virtually every human society across time and is also observable in nonhuman species (Crone & Dahl, 2012). In fact, the plasticity that occurs during this unique period of development may play an invaluable role in ensuring survival of the species across changing ecologies. Nonetheless, it is a frustrating time for nearly all parents and teens, and for some families it represents a period in which relationships become so strained that bonds are severely damaged or broken.

Only recently have we begun to understand the complex neurobiological and social-relational changes that occur during adolescence. It is now clear that the depth and scope of these changes makes adolescence a distinctive period of vulnerability for the development or exacerbation of mental health problems, problems that can have lasting implications for adult adjustment. By age 25, 20% of young adults suffer from serious mental health problems, and between 50 and 70% of these disorders emerge before age 18 (Aber, Brown, & Jones, 2003) and may be diagnosed by age 15 (McGorry, Purcell, Goldstone, & Amminger, 2011). But at the same time that adolescent neuroplasticity confers risk, it also offers immense opportunities for growth and adaptation. The capacity for complex representational thought expands tremendously during this period; teens begin to differentiate their own values from those of others and to set life goals, shaping their identity. Social learning occurs rapidly; structural changes in the "social brain network" sensitize teens to engage with and attend to others in new ways, and this corresponds to a rise in social understanding between ages 12 to 16 (Crone & Dahl, 2012). In short, the adolescent brain could not be more perfectly designed to ensure maximal fit with ever-changing social contexts (Crone & Dahl, 2012).

As we start to understand the complexities of adolescent development, it becomes easier to appreciate why adolescence can sometimes be a challenging period, one that tests the maturity and skills of teens and the patience of parents again and again. But just as infants benefit from secure attachment with parents, teens also fare much better when they can turn to their parents for the reliable provision of a safe haven and secure base. Nonetheless, many parents experience caregiving as more difficult during the teen years compared to earlier developmental periods. Most agree that, although exhausting at times, younger children are generally receptive to parental guidance and comfort, and they are expressive of their need for and love of their parents. In turn, parents typically experience caring for babies and young children as gratifying and enjoyable. Teens, on the other hand, need their parents for both comfort and support (Rosenthal & Kobak, 2010), but they are simultaneously compelled toward autonomy, preferring to solve problems on their own or to seek comfort and support from peers and romantic partners (Allen & Hauser, 1996). As a result, they can express their needs in ways that miscue or confuse their parents; parents in turn may respond using strategies on which they relied when their child was younger but which are no longer effective. As teens push for autonomy, parents are often stressed, and some try to take control; alternatively, others may experience their teen's push for autonomy as deeply rejecting and consequently pull away from their teen. To make matters worse, the stakes can run high; whether parents like it or not, teens have greater latitude than younger children in whether they follow the guidance of their parents, and the results of not doing so can have significant life consequences. In families struggling with complex challenges including family violence, maltreatment, and fragile relationships, risks incurred during adolescence can be immense and in some cases life threatening (Moretti, Bartolo, Odgers, Slaney & Craig, 2014; Moretti & Craig, 2013). Helping parents and other caregivers develop the skills to see, understand, and respond sensitively to the attachment nuances of their teens' behavior can be enormously beneficial, restoring parents and teens to a more secure path and shared partnership as they journey together to (and through) adulthood.

Adolescence, Attachment, and Intervention

The robust relationship among adolescent–parent attachment security, mental health, and socioemotional functioning is well known (e.g., Allen et al., 2002; Allen, Porter, McFarland, McElhaney, & Marsh, 2007; Benson, Buehler, & Gerard, 2008; Brown & Wright, 2003; Caspers, Cadoret, Langbehn, Yucuis, & Troutman, 2005; Greenberg, Speltz, DeKlyen, & Jones, 2001; Kobak, Zajac, & Smith, 2009; Rosenstein & Horowitz, 1996; Speltz, DeKlyen, & Greenberg, 1999). Furthermore, attachment security in adolescence predicts adaptive functioning and attachment in early adulthood and beyond (Collins, Cooper, Albino, & Allard, 2002; Pascuzzo, Cyr, & Moss, 2013).

Although there is agreement that attachment security is a robust predictor of adolescent well-being and good outcomes in early adulthood, remarkably few attempts have been made to develop treatments to promote security between teens and their parents. Two factors may play a role here. First, it is generally agreed that intervening earlier rather than later in child development is more effective; therefore, efforts should focus on prevention, before problems take hold and grow. Second, there is a common belief that certain facets of personality are concretized early in development, so that changes in thinking, feeling, and behavior become difficult and even impossible over time. For example, attachment theory dictates that the foundation and core components of internal working models are rooted in early childhood experiences; hence, change is more difficult in later development. Not surprisingly, then, attachment-based therapies (ABTs) have focused on parents of young children (witness the balance of content in this handbook). The critical question in undertaking the development of ABTs for teens is whether internal working models and attachment strategies are malleable during adolescence, and whether changes are meaningfully related to positive outcomes in functioning concurrently and prospectively.

There is good evidence to suggest that this is the case. Beijersbergen, Juffer, Bakermans-Kranenburg, and van IJzendoorn (2012) found that maternal sensitive support during adolescence promoted a shift toward attachment security among teens who were insecurely attached as young children. Similarly, Booth-LaForce et al. (2014) found that children shifted from insecurity in early childhood as a function of increased levels of maternal sensitivity to security in midadolescence during the intervening period and especially in early adolescence. Likewise, children who shifted from secure to insecure attachment experienced a parallel decrease in maternity sensitivity over the interim. Findings from these studies suggest that adolescent attachment is relatively fluid and meaningfully related to changes in quality of caregiving. Yet this work focused on normative populations, and results may not reflect narrowed plasticity that may characterize the attachment system in adolescents exposed to adversity and trauma. Launching ABTs requires evidence that attachment strategies and security are changeable and meaningfully related to caregiving even in these clinical populations. In this regard, the work of Joseph et al. (2014) points to the adaptive nature and continued plasticity of the attachment system despite exposure to adversity. In a study of teens with a history of maltreatment, in youth removed from home at 7 years of age on average and subsequently placed in foster care, half developed a secure attachment with their foster mother (46%) and foster father (52%). The proportion of secure attachment in this sample was remarkable, because virtually all teens were insecurely attached with their biological mothers (91%) and fathers (100%) and had experienced an average of three foster care placements. Foster mother positivity and sensitivity predicted attachment security in teens, and attachment security in turn predicted lower levels of behavioral problems. Clearly, attachment is pliable during adolescence, even among teens who have experienced significant trauma, although, as clinicians, we know that adversity can make the path to security a long one. ABTs hold much promise of promoting sensitive and positive care toward teens, and this in turn can increase levels of attachment security, buffering teens from risk inherent in the adolescent developmental period. In fact, one might argue that ABTs are particularly well suited to promoting attachment security in adolescence given the neural plasticity and acute sensitivity to social relationships and contingencies that occur during this developmental stage. In short, there are compelling reasons to rethink our assumptions that earlier is always better, and that early is enough. Developmentally, time intervention in the early years and in adolescence, in which plasticity is especially pronounced, may substantially expand the reach of programs and improve mental health outcomes for youth.

The Connect Program

The Connect Program evolved over decades of clinical work and research with adolescents with complex mental health problems and their families. These teens were referred for assessment and treatment planning in relation to serious delinquent and aggressive behavior, as well as myriad other mental health problems, including attention-deficit/hyperactivity disorder (ADHD), depression, anxiety, substance use and dependence, suicidality, and posttraumatic stress disorder (PTSD) symptoms. Families struggled with transgenerational trauma, parental mental health problems, family violence, child maltreatment and neglect, and parental abandonment. A high proportion of these families had not responded well to prior treatment and were not keen to engage in another program; they felt blamed, burnt out, and hopeless, and vacillated between feeling guilty and feeling angry and resentful.

Connect targets parents and caregivers; teens do not participate in the intervention. The program is primarily designed to shift how parents perceive, understand, and respond to their teens' behavior, promoting sensitivity to the attachment meaning of their teens' behavior and the development of parenting skills that ensure the provision of a safe haven and a secure base. The program is delivered by two certified, trained leaders who guide groups of 8–14 parents through ten 90-minute sessions, each focused on an attachment principle that is relevant to parenting teens and to relationships in general (see Table 17.1).

Connect adopts a trauma-informed approach, welcoming parents to treatment through a "preinclusion interview" that incorporates motivational interviewing, identifies parents' strengths, and collaborates with parents to reduce barriers to treatment engagement. Connect leaders are careful to acknowledge the very real frustrations and concerns expressed by parents. The concept of attachment is never introduced as the cause of parents' difficulties with their teen, but rather as something that they can strengthen together, with the potential to buffer their teen from stress and negative influences, and to reduce parental stress. Although leaders are careful not to offer promises of "Hollywood endings," they do communicate a message of hope.

Once enrolled, parents who miss a session receive a phone call or message from Connect leaders, who reach out to them, let them know that they were missed, and offer assistance to encourage their return to the program. The program is a strengths-focused intervention. Rather than dictate how parents should or should not respond to their teen, Connect focuses first on helping parents recognize,

TABLE 17.1. Connect Program Principles

Principle	Definition
1. All behavior has meaning.	Attachment is a basic human need that shapes behavior.
2. Attachment is for life.	The need for attachment continues from cradle to grave, but how it is expressed changes with development.
3. Conflict is part of attachment.	When expressed and responded to constructively, conflict offers new opportunities for growth.
4. Autonomy includes connection.	Secure attachment balances connection and independence.
5. Empathy is the heartbeat of attachment.	Empathy supports growth and strengthens our relationships.
6. Balancing our needs with the needs of others.	Relationships thrive when we have empathy and balance our needs with the needs of others.
7. Growth and change are part of relationships.	Growth and change involves moving forward while understanding the past.
8. Celebrating attachment.	Attachment brings joy and pain.
9. Two steps forward, one step back: Staying on course.	Trust relationships in turbulent times. Adversity is an opportunity for growth.

accept, and step back from the strong emotional reactions they may have to their teens' behavior. Doing so makes room for parents to become curious about their teens' challenging behavior and the implicit attachment needs expressed by their children. In no way does this approach suggest that parents should accept every behavior in which their teen engages (e.g., destructive or aggressive behavior), but it does encourage parents first to consider and respond to the parent–teen attachment issues at play before they turn to setting limits or consequences.

Connect promotes parental autonomy in understanding and responding to parent–teen problems by adopting a collaborative stance in which parents are supported as they develop skills to effectively identify and respond to problems that arise with their teen. This decreases parental sense of blame and increases their engagement in, and their sense of efficacy and ownership of, new learning.

Attachment-Relevant Intervention Targets

The program specifically targets four aspects of parenting that are linked with attachment security in adolescence: caregiver sensitivity, reflective function, dyadic affect regulation, and shared partnership/mutuality. *Caregiver sensitivity* is the capacity of the parents to attend to and remain engaged with their teen, their openness and interest in their teen's feelings and thoughts, and their ability to "read" behavior as an expression of underlying attachment needs. We use the terms *reflective function* (Fonagy, Steele, Steele, Moran, & Higgitt, 1991) to describe parents' openness and awareness of their feelings and thoughts, especially as they relate to their parenting behavior, while simultaneously considering the mind of the teen. *Dyadic affect regulation* is the ability of parents to step in and modulate the affective exchange between themselves and their teen, to regulate their own emotional experiences and provide support when their teen feels overwhelmed. Finally, *shared partnership and mutuality* is parents' openness to adopting a collaborative stance in their relationship with their teen, wherein they continue to be responsible for protection and safety of their child while working together toward solutions that are in their best interest. In doing so, they promote developmentally appropriate steps toward autonomy.

Session Structure:
Attachment Principles, Role Plays, and Reflection Exercises

The content and flow of each session has been shaped over several years. The final session of Connect provides parents with a structured process for reflecting and commenting on the program, and their feedback is essential for determining the best type and order of session content. We also watched hundreds of group sessions and consulted with Connect leaders and clinicians throughout the development phase. Each Connect session begins with the introduction of a key principle related to attachment, parenting, and adolescence. These principles are also applicable across all relationships (e.g., in friendships and romantic relationships), a fact that parents often note about halfway through the program. The sequence of attachment principles is designed to fit together, first helping parents to see behavior through an attachment lens and gradually building their understanding of their teen, themselves, and their parenting skills.

Our experience has been that many parents become lost and emotionally overwhelmed when they discuss the challenges regarding their relationship with their teen in a group context. Moreover, parents' frustration can be contagious, especially when discussing teen behavior that is viewed as oppositional, disrespectful, irresponsible, and dangerous. Instead of reaching new understandings and insights into their teens' behavior, parents may be at risk of forming even more extreme opinions and ideas of how to correct misdeeds. For this reason, and after some hard-learned lessons, we adopted an approach of using role plays that demonstrate common parent–teen challenges (e.g., parent–teen conflict; problems with chores, school or peers) in almost every Connect session. This approach provides a context in which parents can identify with the struggles depicted in the role play, but as observers, thereby giving them a little distance from their own struggles but sufficient emotional engagement essential for growth. Parents often note that the role plays are similar to their own situations, and offer comments such as "Were you at my house last night?"

The structure of the role plays is essential to the goals of the intervention. First, role plays highlight how teens often miscue their parents about their attachment needs through behaviors that may appear angry, rejecting, or withdrawn. Second, role plays illustrate the different ways in which parents may respond in the situation, contrasting an angry–controlling response with a hostile–abandoning response in two separate versions of the role play. Together parents engage in reflection exercises, described below, that help them consider new options for responding sensitively to their teen while still setting limits and ensuring their teen's safety. The third "reconstructed" version of the role play integrates parents' suggestions; however, Connect leaders are careful to avoid depicting an unrealistically rosy outcome. Instead, leaders demonstrate that the relationship is left open for communication and understanding. Leaders also reassure parents that even though they may feel it is challenging to respond to their teen with sensitivity in the moment, there are always opportunities to return to the discussion later, when they find their footing. In this way, parents are protected from forming unrealistic expectations that may set them up for disappointment.

Reflection exercises following the role plays are structured and follow a clear, step-by-step process to help parents practice skills that promote attachment security. This stepwise problem-solving framework is repeated across sessions to help parents consolidate new skills that can be used outside the group, in their interactions with their teens. First, parents are asked to temporarily step into the teen's mind and reflect on what the teen might be feeling and thinking. Then they are asked to think about what attachment needs their teen's behavior might be communicating. Next, parents step into the mind of the parent in the role play, reflecting on what he or she might be feeling and thinking. Connect leaders support parents during this process by expressing empathy for the difficult situation faced by both teen and parents, and the power that their feelings have in shaping their interaction. Finally, parents reflect on whether the parent in the role play was aware of the attachment needs expressed by his or her teen and where the interaction left their relationship (e.g., open or closed in terms of opportunities for further communication and/or repair). Very little emphasis is placed on distinguishing feelings and thoughts as might be done in a cognitive-behavioral approach. Nor is there an emphasis on identifying a specific parenting behavior that is needed to correct the problem, as might be the case in parenting intervention based on social learning theory. Instead the emphasis is on practicing reflection on the teen's and the parent's affective experiences, as well as linking behavior with attachment needs of the teen. From there, parents consider what options might exist for responding differently in the scenario.

The increasing level of parents' participation in performing role plays across sessions, and the role they are invited to play (i.e., the teen), is in line with central goals of Connect to promote parents' reflective functioning and empathy. Parents simply observe and reflect on role plays demonstrated by the leaders for the first three sessions, which helps promote their curiosity regarding the relational dynamics and their teen's underlying attachment needs. In the fourth session they are invited to step into the role of the teen. From this point forward, parents are invited to take the role of the teen in the reconstruction role plays in which Connect leaders integrate parents' suggestions and demonstrate parental sensitivity, provision of a secure base, and a safe haven. By stepping into the role of the teen, parents experience firsthand the powerful impact of parental sensitivity and support. Many parents are surprised by the experience, commenting, "The way you responded changed how I felt" or "I didn't understand how my teen might feel until now." Stepping into the teen's role offers a new and often surprising vantage point that helps ease harsh attributions for problem behavior and increase parents' empathy toward their teen.

Although we do not ask parents to step into the role of the parent in the role play, they do practice reflecting on the parent's experience with empathy and understanding. This is also critical to parents developing awareness, understanding, and acceptance of their own feelings and thoughts, which is essential to the development of their capacity for reflective thought. The value of *in vivo* role plays cannot be overstated; they are emotionally poignant, and parents easily identify with both the parent and child. Most importantly, role plays offer an immediate and powerful opportunity for parents to practice reflective thought and mindfulness as they step back and forth between the experience of the teen and the experience of the parent, something that can be extremely challenging when parents discuss their personal experiences and challenges. Additionally, if needed, role plays can be carefully tailored by the skilled Connect practitioner to touch on the challenges of group members, while still retaining the structure that allows parents to work on key therapeutic tasks. In the feedback provided at the close of each Connect group, parents almost universally identify the role plays as the most helpful component of the intervention program.

A wide range of other reflection exercises are integrated across Connect. Most notably, parents engage in exercises designed to promote their awareness of their experiences of attachment, particularly those experienced in their relationships with their parents during their own adolescence. Through such exercises, Connect toggles back and forth between reflecting on teens' experiences and those of the parents, without blame or prescriptive solutions, offering new ways for parents to experience themselves and their teen and in turn opportunities to revisit and revise their internal working models of themselves, their child, and the parenting relationship.

Finally, in each session of Connect, parents learn about the importance of verbal and nonverbal communication with their teen. These exercises are integrated with the core focus of Connect on attachment and parenting. Exercises help parents understand the importance of nonverbal and verbal cues to their teen; address the importance of finding the right time to discuss issues with teens; and understand that the normative developmental tasks of adolescence can lead to miscommunication in the parent–teen relationship.

Overview of Connect Sessions and the Model of Therapeutic Change

Sessions build progressively, helping parents identify and respond to attachment needs underlying their teens' problem behavior. The progression of intervention follows a three-phase model of therapeutic change (see Figure 17.1). Throughout Connect, leaders provide parents with a safe haven (to bring concerns to) and a secure base from which parents can explore new ways of thinking and feeling. In the first phase of Connect, leaders build trust within the group and provide sensitive support to parents in regulating their feelings of frustration, anger, anxiety, and despair. This phase introduces a clear framework and structured exercises that help parents begin to step back from their frustration and understand their teens' behaviors from an attachment perspective. The first phase of the intervention encompasses the first three sessions.

In Session 1, parents are guided by the attachment principle that *all behavior has meaning.* This principle is the cornerstone of parents' understanding that behavior is a language that expresses attachment needs. The group discusses the various ways in which teens may miscue their parents with challenging and confusing behavior, expressing simultaneously the need for comfort and soothing, and the need for autonomy and independence. Using a single role play, Connect leaders help parents understand how a wide range of attributions and emotional meanings can be attached to a very short and ambiguous demonstration of teen behavior. Parents explore their reactions to challenging behavior and learn how their emotional reactions can drive their parenting responses. For example, some parents see the teen in the role as defiant and disrespectful, but others wonder whether something might have happened for the teen—perhaps the teen's behavior is an expression of frustration and sadness. Parents discuss the fact that teen behavior can look very different one moment versus the next and from one day to another. Such variation may reflect a variety of influences, including normative changes related to adolescent neurological and socioemotional development, life stress and the social experiences of their teen, as well as trauma. Parents practice temporarily "stepping back" from strong feelings and thoughts and "stepping forward" into their teens' experience. Connect leaders introduce the idea of "cracking the code" of the attachment meaning of their teens' behavior. Throughout this process, Connect leaders respond to and reassure parents about common concerns. For example, leaders assure parents that expressing curiosity in and a desire to understand their teens'

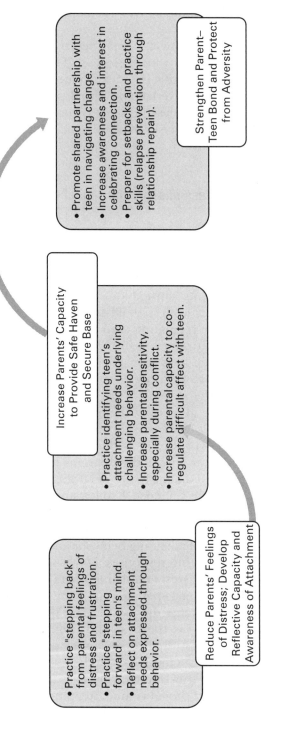

- Practice "stepping back" from parental feelings of distress and frustration.
- Practice "stepping forward" in teen's mind.
- Reflect on attachment needs expressed through behavior.

Reduce Parents' Feelings of Distress; Develop Reflective Capacity and Awareness of Attachment

Increase Parents' Capacity to Provide Safe Haven and Secure Base

- Practice identifying teen's attachment needs underlying challenging behavior.
- Increase parental sensitivity, especially during conflict.
- Increase parental capacity to co-regulate difficult affect with teen.

- Promote shared partnership with teen in navigating change.
- Increase awareness and interest in celebrating connection.
- Prepare for setbacks and practice skills (relapse prevention through relationship repair).

Strengthen Parent–Teen Bond and Protect from Adversity

FIGURE 17.1. A model of change in attachment-based parenting programs.

experiences does not condone problem behavior. Expectations and limit setting remain important but parents may have a choice of when to discuss this, and timing can make a difference. Leaders also emphasize that parents may never truly know the precise meaning and attachment needs expressed by their teens' behavior; what matters is not their accuracy but their interest in and openness to understanding. Similarly, parents are assured that the goal is not to drop everything in their life to meet each and every need expressed by their teen. Of greater importance is that the teen know that his or her parents are communicating genuine interest in, and respect for the teen's feelings and thoughts, even when differences between teen and parent are evident, as is often the case. With this footing in place, parents consider various options for responding to their teen in ways that recognize and respect their experience, strengthen their relationship, and gradually build a partnership for moving forward.

Session 2 builds on the concept that attachment needs are expressed through behavior by introducing the principle that *attachment is for life*. Parents learn that attachment needs are expressed differently across development; together, parents create a list of attachment needs, what children need to grow and develop. Exercises help parents reflect on how toddlers express attachment needs, cultivating a sense of empathy and tenderness in the group before tackling the question of how their teens are currently expressing their attachment needs. At the end of Session 2, parents begin to reflect on their own attachment history, revisiting how they expressed their attachment needs to their parents, how they felt when their parents seemed to understand them, and how they felt when this was not the case. This is a powerful and sometimes painful exercise for parents, because, not surprisingly, many come to Connect with a history of attachment injuries in their own families of origin.

By Session 3, parents are familiar with the concept that attachment needs are expressed through behavior, and they are aware that attachment needs are expressed differently over development. They have also practiced temporarily stepping back from their feelings and thoughts about their teen's behavior to consider the inner experiences of their teen. With these emerging competencies, Session 3 focuses on parent–teen conflict and introduces the principle that *conflict is part of attachment*. This is a challenging principle, because it is often one of the most pressing issues that leads parents to seek services. This session helps parents to reframe conflict as a part of all relationships and potentially as an opportunity for growth and understanding in relationships *when expressed constructively and responded to with sensitivity*. Parents consider how their history of conflict in past relationships may shape their expression and response to conflict in their current relationships. Two parent responses to conflict are depicted in role plays—one in which the parent reacts with hostility and aggression to their teen's anger, matching them toe-to-toe, and the other in which the parent avoids conflict and abruptly cut off the interaction with the teen, effectively abandoning the teen to deal with his or her own distress. In each case, parents follow a step-by-step sequence that begins with temporarily stepping back and reflecting on their teen's feelings, thoughts, and attachment needs; next they reflect on the parents' feelings and thoughts that drive their behavior; and finally they consider how the interaction affects the relationship with the teen. There is a wide range of responses of parents to each role play and much discussion within the group. Some parents feel that the teen's behavior warrants a strong response from the parent (e.g., "I understand how that parent feels; you need to nip it in bud" or "They can't get away with that—they need to learn a lesson"); others see the response of the parent as overly harsh and having more to do with the parent than the teen (e.g., "The parent got just as angry as the teen—it only made things worse" or "It was all about how the parents were offended—they didn't even seem to try to hear the teen"). Interestingly many parents identify the avoidant response of the parent as even more hurtful, because the teen seems invisible and irrelevant to the parent ("It's confusing for the teen—like the parent isn't even there" or "Well the parents tried to keep their cool—I get it—but I felt bad for the teen—like the teen didn't even matter"), but some praise the reaction of the parent ("I like what the parent did—I learned that we are supposed to ignore bad behavior"). Whatever the parents' reactions to the role play may be, they generally agree that the parent's emotional reaction made it difficult for them to be aware of the teen's attachment needs, and the interaction left the relationship closed.

Reflecting on the attachment needs of the teen, parents generate suggestions for how the parent might respond with sensitivity but also set limits. These suggestions are integrated into a reconstructed role play that is demonstrated by leaders and reflected on by parents. Parents generally agree that even though the reconstructed role play did not end perfectly, the parent seemed more aware and responsive to the teen's attachment needs, and the teen felt a little more understood. They also note that the parent probably felt better about the situation, too.

The second phase of the Connect program deepens parents' sensitivity and capacity to provide a safe haven and a secure base for their teens. Session 4 promotes parents' understanding of the importance of autonomy in adolescence. Autonomy strivings are framed as opportunities for parents to not only delight in their teen's experiences of joy in their growing independence but also to acknowledge and provide support around their teen's anxiety and needs for guidance and safety. Parents learn that their teen's autonomy strivings can provoke strong feelings of parental anxiety and anger if they interpret these behaviors as dangerous, rebellious, or rejecting of parental authority. Guided by the principle that *autonomy includes connection,* role plays and exercises help parents not only see their teen's delight in the world but also recognize that he or she still needs them as a secure base even though it may appear otherwise. Using a role play that depicts a teen who excitedly tells their parent they are going off with other teens unknown to the parent to an event that seems potentially dangerous, allows the observing parent reflect on the teen's thoughts and feelings and those of the parent. Two role plays, again depicting a hostile–controlling versus a hostile–abandoning parental response are presented. Parents are immediately drawn into concerns for the teen's welfare and the challenges of controlling and protecting them ("They don't have a brain in their heads—what's wrong with kids today?"; I wouldn't be letting my kid go—that spells trouble!"). On occasion, however, a parent will say the teen needs to learn a lesson ("Maybe they should learn on their own—figure it out the way I did"). Connect leaders help parents to see the teen's excitement and delight in the social invitation, as well as the parent's need to keep the teen safe. Together they discuss how the parent can share the teen's excitement about new social opportunities and how doing so provides the foundation for a partnership in setting limits to keep the teen safe. As the discussion unfolds, it is common for parents to begin to discuss feelings of sadness and loss as a result of the teen's growing autonomy ("I see he's growing up—it feels too fast for me"; "I worry that we will drift apart"). Together the group works on accepting change in the parent–teen relationship as part of growth and development, reassured by the fact that parents remain connected and important to their teen—especially in the sense of providing a secure base.

Session 5 focuses on empathy and is guided by the principle that *empathy is the heartbeat of attachment*. This is the first session in which parents are invited to participate in role plays, and in this and all subsequent role plays, parents are welcome to step into the role of the teen. The session opens with a discussion of empathy and how it may be expressed differently by different people. The group discusses the importance of listening and "being with" rather than sharing similar feelings, trying to cajole others into feeling better, or trying to fix whatever problem they might face. Empathy is presented as a skill that can be practiced and expressed very differently from one person to the next. The importance of attending to both verbal and nonverbal communication is emphasized.

The role play for this session depicts an angry and frustrated teen who announces he or she is quitting an activity of some importance to the parent and teen. Again, two different parental reactions are depicted. Parents are asked to focus only on the feelings of the teen and the parent. Reflection questions again follow the same sequence, reflecting on the teen and the parent, and encouraging curiosity about the teen's attachment needs and the parent's awareness. Parents work together to consider how the parent might express empathy to the teen. Subsequently, parents are invited to step into the role of the teen in the reconstructed role play. Parents often find this a surprising and disarming experience, with comments such as "You diffused the anger" or "I wanted to tell you whatever it was that made me feel bad— even if I didn't tell you I would probably talk to you later." Despite these insights, parents still discuss how easy it is to get pulled into the problem and how difficult it can be to practice empathy in the moment. The session also ends with parents reflecting on how they felt when others did or did not express empathy to them.

Session 6 turns to the needs of parents, which they often feel have been put on hold because of problems related to their teen. Guided by the principle *balancing our needs with the needs of others*, parents create a list of their own attachment needs, and in doing so recognize that there is considerable overlap between their needs and those of their child. They are encouraged to recognize their needs and to have empathy for themselves, reflecting on how best to balance their needs with those of their child. Session exercises encourage parents to consider developmentally appropriate expectations for teen behavior, providing an opportunity for parents to express their frustration at their teens' sporadic bouts of immaturity (Casey, 2015), the hallmark of adolescence, and a common flash point for parent–teen conflict. For example, leaders briefly note normative information on adolescent socioemotional and neurodevelopment, helping parents reframe behaviors that may appear inconsiderate, immature, and narcissistic. Role plays help parents explore different strategies to balance their needs with those of their teen and emphasize the importance of turning to adult relationships rather than their children to meet their needs. In reflection exercises following the role plays, parents tend to bring up a range of issues, from those that simply focus on finding time for themselves to complex feelings of anger and sadness as they discuss the responsibilities they carried prematurely during their own adolescence. They also worry that indulging their teen by failing to press responsibilities early upon them will leave their teen poorly equipped to survive and succeed in a world that they see as harsh and unforgiving. The focus of discussion ranges from the pragmatics of balancing everyday events to the challenges of balancing parents' complex and conflicting thoughts and feelings.

As parents enter the third and final phase of the Connect program, the focus shifts to deepening and consolidating the key parenting skills they have acquired that promote secure attachment (i.e., sensitivity; reflective function–mindfulness; dyadic affect regulation; and shared partnership and mutuality). Parents are now well versed in following a step-by-step framework for identifying, understanding, and responding to challenges in their relationship with their teen. With these skills well rooted in the group, sessions concentrate on building resilience in parents and within the parent–teen relationship to withstand anticipated challenges. Session 7 focuses on change and growth in terms of the inevitable and often rapid changes that occur within the parent–teen relationship and the frustration that parents can experience when they perceive their teen as reluctant, slow, and unwilling to move forward. The key principle in this session—*growth and change are part of relationships*—helps parents to understand that personal growth and change occurs within the context of relationships and requires understanding the past in order to move forward. Leaders introduce the notion that we all create stories about ourselves, and that these stories have a powerful influence on how we interpret and respond to events in our lives. They also learn that our stories are influenced by the stories that others have about us and have told to us, which we carry within ourselves at deep core level of which we are not necessarily aware. In effect, the session translates the notion of internal working models of self and other, and their effect on behavior and change, into terms that are easily understood by parents. Reflection exercises help parents think about their own stories and the stories that others hold for them. Leaders provide safe haven and a secure base for parents to reflect on their difficult stories, ensuring safety within the group. Parents consider whether the stories that others hold for them have helped or hindered their growth and change.

Role plays and reflection exercises help parents become aware of how their stories for their teen may make it difficult for them to see change and to support their children moving forward. Questions following the role play encourage parents to reflect on how they can let their teen know that their story about them is changing (e.g., noticing growth and change in their teen; remaining open to their teen's changing story about him- or herself). In response to the role plays, parents express how difficult it can be to see change in their teen when they are frustrated with problem behavior and their teen's slow pace of growth and change. They recognize the importance of not getting stuck in old stories about their teen and discuss how to remain open to their teen's changing story of him- or herself despite inevitable challenges in parenting. They also recognize that this entails changing their story about themselves as parents and how their lives are changing with their teen's growing autonomy. Some anticipate these changes with excitement, others with anxiety and a sense of loss; most feel a combination of the two.

Session 8 is organized around the principle that in *celebrating attachment, attachment brings joy and pain*; it is designed to encourage parents to take advantage of opportunities for positive interactions with their teen. Up to this point in the program, leaders and parents have focused heavily on problems in the parent–child relationship; in this session, they reflect on parents' thoughts, feelings, and concerns that get in the way of connecting with their teen. Not surprisingly, parents point to their teen's behavior as a significant barrier, but they also discuss the feelings and beliefs associated with problem behavior that make them reluctant to allow closeness with their teen. For example, parents express fear of being hurt or taken advantage of yet again; fear of losing parental authority; and the fear of allowing an emotional connection when they may lose their child through tragic circumstances. The teen may also cloak his or her desire for connection and closeness with the parents in behaviors that make this difficult for their parents to discern. As the session unfolds, parents frequently report feelings of sadness and loss as they come to realize how they have missed many overtures for connection expressed by their teen.

Leaders also raise the question of whether parents' past experiences in relationships may influence their feelings of safety and openness to connection with their teen. Through role plays and reflection exercises, parents consider whether there might be opportunities to join with their child and celebrate the relationship, even if these moments are brief and fleeting, and occur in a landscape dominated by parent–child conflict. They ponder the question of what they have to gain and what they have to lose by doing so. The session is closed by an exercise in which parents recall the special and often tender ways that they celebrate connection in their families, encouraging the understanding that small family rituals (e.g., watching a special TV program; enjoying a treat together) can have big attachment meanings.

Session 9 focuses squarely on relapse prevention. Guided by the principle *two steps forward, one step back: staying on course,* leaders weave all the principles together, integrating comments made by parents over the course of the therapy group and discussing the principles as a toolkit for weathering the inevitable storms that will occur as they move forward. Leaders encourage parents to anticipate that they will sometimes find it extremely difficult, if not impossible, to hang on to all they have learned. Rather than viewing setbacks as failure, parents are encouraged to step back and see them as opportunities to move forward by practicing repair in their relationship with their teens. They watch role plays in which the parent loses their footing and the parent–child interaction goes off track. Next they generate suggestions for repairing the relationship based on their consideration of all the principles covered in the program. Parents are invited to step into the role play as the teen, and they reflect on their experience of repair led by the group leader who plays the parent. Parents express both optimism and anxiety about weathering the storms ahead. They are reassured that revisiting the principles is akin to having a toolkit that they can apply to new and changing challenges as they go forward and booster sessions (see below) are discussed.

As previously noted, Connect also includes a feedback and integration session that encourages the parents to reflect on their experiences in the program, to discuss what was helpful to them and where they struggled. They provide feedback about the program that has been invaluable in its development. There are also two 120-minute booster sessions, each reviewing four principles and closing with relapse prevention exercises. Booster sessions are constructed to focus on progress made since the completion of Connect or the last booster session, retaining a strengths-focused and structured approach.

Training and Implementation Model

Connect was developed in partnership with government agencies and in conjunction with funding support from the Canadian Institutes of Health Research. Guided by principles of implementation science and recognizing broadly the need to reach families and youth in diverse communities, a structured training model and detailed program manual have been developed. Connect leaders are trained by completing an intensive 3-day workshop that provides them with a deep understanding of the clinical, research, and theoretical basis for the program, as well as hands-on training in the delivery of sessions. Once completed, leaders are well prepared to begin their first Connect group, and this provides the context for supervision to certification. Support is provided in how to conduct preinclusion interviews and group composition considerations. Program sessions are videotaped, focusing on the leaders, and these videotapes are reviewed weekly in teleconferences with in-person supervision. Supervision focuses both on adherence to the program structure and exercises, as detailed in the manual, as well as leaders' skills in facilitating group process and managing challenges. We adopt a reflective supervision model in which group leaders are encouraged to use the Connect principles to facilitate their understanding of the needs of parents in the group and group process issues. For example, Connect trainees are encouraged to consider the attachment meaning of parents' behavior in the sessions, reflecting on how best to provide safe haven and a secure base given the diversity of attachment strategies that parents adopt. Additionally, leaders consider the role of empathy and conflict as an opportunity for growth as parents' journey through the program. In parallel form, supervisors use the Connect attachment principles to understand and guide the practice of Connect trainees, helping them to understand the attachment meaning and dynamics of group process. In turn, Connect trainees promote parents' understanding and use of the attachment principles in responding to their teen. Supervision is strengths-focused with the goal of establishing autonomous practice as quickly as possible, most often based on the completion of the first group. Additional support is provided as needed. Recertification is required every 2 years or six groups and entails the review of two videotaped sessions and parent feedback from previously delivered Connect groups.

In short, the training model is guided by an appreciation of the need for a cost- and time-efficient strategy to support leaders in their development of program delivery skills, ensuring ease of program uptake and sustainability. Options are also available for seasoned leaders to train as Connect supervisors and Connect co-trainers, providing opportunities for communities to build capacity within their agencies. As a result, and in collaboration with partnering centers, well over 700 Connect leaders have been certified, and the program has been delivered to over 8,000 families in rural and urban communities across Canada and internationally.

Empirical Evidence for the Effectiveness of Connect and Mechanisms of Change

To date, studies evaluating Connect have focused on the effectiveness of the treatment as delivered in mental health and affiliated agencies by trained and supervised program leaders from a wide range of mental health professions (e.g., psychologists, social workers, counselors, child care workers, teachers, psychiatrists). Large-scale and continuous evaluation of Connect in community-based and institutional settings was achieved by embedding a standardized evaluation protocol into the treatment manual. This consists of standardized measures of parent, family, and child functioning that can be adapted to agency needs and modified to examine specific populations or clinical research interests. Additional qualitative and client satisfaction feedback is collected in the "Integration and Feedback" session at the close of each Connect group. Feedback is therefore available directly and quickly to each agency, providing information on the fit of the program with caregiver needs and implementation barriers such as problems with the location, timing, and availability of transportation or child care.

Our preliminary evaluations started with pilot studies of the Connect program in the setting in which the program was developed, which provided services to pre-teens and teens with serious behavioral and other mental health problems. These pilot studies provided promising evidence of the effectiveness. In the first open trial, Moretti, Holland, Moore, and McKay (2004) examined treatment-related changes in child behavior in 16 adolescents (mean age = 14.80 years, SD = 1.03, age range = 13–16 years) referred for severe antisocial behavior. Youth whose parents were included in the study had high rates of prior incarceration (31%), criminal convictions (47%), and placements outside their home (68%); a substantial proportion had threatened to seriously harm or kill another person (65%) or themselves (53%). Results showed significant decreases from pre- to posttreatment in caregivers' reports of youths' externalizing problems, such as aggressive, oppositional, and rule-breaking behavior.

A subsequent open trial (Obsuth, Moretti, Holland, Braber, & Cross, 2006) examined treatment outcomes with a larger sample (n = 48) of conduct-disordered youth (mean age = 14.51 years, SD = 1.33, age range = 12–18 years) and their parents. Parents reported significant increases in perceived parenting competence and satisfaction and decreases in controlling parenting practices. Parents also reported significant reductions in youth internalizing (e.g., depression and anxiety) and externalizing problems, and reduced levels of avoidance in the parent–adolescent relationship. In addition, youths' self-reports demonstrated improvements in their internalizing problems. Taken together, the results from these open trials provided preliminary support for the effectiveness of Connect. The absence of a comparison condition in these studies, however, limited confidence in the findings.

To build on these initial findings, we examined the effectiveness of Connect in a waiting-list control study (Moretti & Obsuth, 2009). A high-risk clinical sample of 20 antisocial youth (mean age = 14.50 years, age range = 12–18 years) and their parents was assessed at four time points: before a 4-month waiting-list control period, prior to beginning treatment, upon completion of treatment, and at a 12-month follow-up. There were no significant changes on any assessments across the waiting-list control interval. By contrast, significant pre- to posttreatment increases were found on parenting efficacy and satisfaction and reductions in externalizing and internalizing problems. Effect sizes (Cohen's d) ranged from medium to large. Importantly, the effects of treatment were maintained at 12-month follow-up, with additional significant declines observed in caregivers' reports of youths' externalizing and internalizing symptoms.

We next turned to the question of whether our initial findings could be replicated broadly across clinical settings. Our first portability study (Moretti & Obsuth, 2009) evaluated treatment outcomes in a large-scale effectiveness trial involving the implementation of Connect across 17 rural and urban Canadian communities. The sample included 309 adolescents (boys: mean age = 13.53 years, SD = 2.18; girls: mean age = 13.73 years, SD = 2.16, age range = 12–18) with antisocial behavior. To ensure treatment fidelity, Connect leaders completed a standardized training workshop and received weekly supervision based on a review of their videotaped group sessions. Consistent with findings reported earlier, significant pre- to prepost treatment changes were found on measures of youth and family functioning rated by caregivers; that is, improvements were evident in domains of parenting (e.g., perceived competence, caregiver strain), parent–adolescent relationship (e.g., reductions in verbal and physical aggression), and youth adjustment (e.g., reductions in aggressive and noncompliant behavior, depression, anxiety). Furthermore, results for youth with the most severe antisocial behavior were on par with those for youth with moderate antisocial behavior. Importantly, attrition was low, with 84% of caregivers attending at least 70% of Connect sessions. This attrition rate is very encouraging given the complex and chronic nature of youths' mental health problems and the fact that families were recruited from real-world services across different communities.

In addition to research in Canada, Connect has been evaluated in three published European studies. An RCT in Italy examined the feasibility and effectiveness of Connect as a preventive intervention for adolescent risky behavior (Giannotta, Ortega, & Stattin, 2013). Connect was considered to be a good fit for Italian parents, because they value building strong emotional family ties and may respond better to parenting programs that are not prescriptive (Claes, Lacourse, Bouchard, & Perucchini, 2003; Ortega, Giannotta, Latina, & Ciairano, 2012). Connect was delivered by psychologists who attended the standardized training workshop and received ongoing supervision. Participants included mothers of 147 youth (mean age = 12.46 years, SD = 0.72, age range = 11–14 years) recruited from one of nine middle schools. Using a quasi-experimental design, 40% of parents were assigned to receive Connect, and the others were included as a nonintervention control. In comparison to the control group, the treatment group demonstrated greater reductions in mothers' reports of coldness/rejection (trend level; d = 0.32) and in youths' self-reported alcohol use ($d = 0.55$ and 0.44 for beer and wine consumption, respectively). There were no significant group differences, however, in parents' reports of externalizing problems. This finding may be due to the low-risk nature of the community sample and the modest levels of antisocial behavior in youth at intake. These findings are consistent with other research showing that the effectiveness of prevention programs is typically most easily detected for youth who initially show elevated behavior problems (Conduct Problems Prevention Research Group, 2011). Importantly, this study showed good evidence of parent uptake and acceptance of Connect, as 90–95% as parents who attended at least 70% of the sessions reported that the components of Connect (e.g., knowledge attainment about attachment, role plays) were useful/very useful.

In a second European study, the effectiveness of Connect was examined in the context of a large RCT involving four group-based parenting programs for the treatment of child externalizing problems (Stattin, Enebrink, Özdemir, & Giannotta, 2015). Participants were 908 parents and their children (ages 3–12 years) randomized to one of four programs: Comet (Kling, Forster, Sundell, & Melin, 2010), Community Parent Education Program (COPE; Cunningham, Bremner, & Boyle, 1995), The Incredible Years (Webster-Stratton, 1984), or Connect. Comet and COPE included both younger (ages 3–8 years) and older (9–12 years) children; The Incredible Years only included younger children (ages 3–8 years); and Connect included only older children (9 to 12 years). Although similar in group format and the goal of improving child outcomes, Comet, COPE, and The Incredible Years differ from Connect in that they are grounded in social learning theory, focus on helping parents develop skills based on reinforcement principles of shaping behavior, and adopt a prescriptive approach in terms of providing parents with specific practices (e.g., "time out"; labeled praise) to manage child behavior (for further details, see Stattin et al., 2015, Table 1, for an outline of each program). In contrast, Connect focuses on understanding the child's attachment needs and their expression through reflective function and sensitivity, providing safe haven through dyadic affect regulation, and secure base through shared partnership and mutuality. Despite these differences in program content and focus, results showed that, compared with a waiting-list control, all four programs were effective in reducing externalizing problems at the end of treatment. However, the magnitude of these treatment effects was most pronounced on some measures for Comet, followed by COPE and The Incredible Years, and although significant differences were also found for Connect on a range of measures, these effects sizes were significantly smaller. It is possible that the smaller effect sizes for Connect were the result of the fact that older children (8- to 12-year-olds) were randomized to Connect, compared to younger children randomized to other interventions, and these increased problem behaviors often occur in the transition from preadolescence into the teen years. Smaller effect sizes may also reflect the lower dosage of Connect (i.e., fewer and shorter sessions) compared to that of other interventions. Nonetheless, treatment effects for changes in parenting behavior (e.g., use of rewards) and parental mental health (e.g., depression), were strongest for Connect and Comet and least evident for COPE and The Incredible Years.

Results at follow-up revealed a clearer and more clinically relevant set of findings. Högström, Olofsson, Özdemir, Enebrink, and Stattin (2016) found that at 1-year follow-up, programs differences were no longer apparent—all programs were equally effective. Importantly, from posttreatment to 1-year follow-up, only children in COPE and Connect continued to show trends toward further reductions in externalizing problems. Importantly, from 1- to 2-year follow-up, only children in Connect demonstrated additional significant declines in externalizing problems. Rarely are programs found to produce posttreatment and significant benefits, and such findings were particularly noteworthy given the fact that youth whose parents completed Connect were ages 11–13, at time at which problem behavior normatively increases rather than decreases. In summary, compared with parent training programs based on social learning theory (Comet, Incredible Years, and COPE), Connect showed a comparable level of potency in reducing externalizing problems at posttreatment assessment points, and benefits became more evident over the follow-up phase.

How does Connect improve youth outcomes, and why do the benefits of Connect in reducing problems become more pronounced following the completion of treatment? These questions have been the focus of two recent studies examining the mechanisms of change that underlie the Connect treatment model (see Figure 17.1). In the first study, Moretti, Obsuth, Mayseless, and Scharf (2012) examined shifts in parents' internal representations across treatment. Parents' representations were assessed using the Parenting Representations Interview—Adolescence (PRI-A; Scharf & Mayseless, 1997/2000, cited in Mayseless & Scharf, 2006). Consistent with prior results, significant pre- to posttreatment reductions in youths' internalizing and externalizing problems were noted. Furthermore, significant changes were observed in parents' representations of the parent, teen, and parent–teen relationship. Importantly, these shifts in parenting representations were significantly associated with reductions in youths' problem behavior. Thus, these findings support the suggestion that Connect has proximal effects on changing parenting representations, which in turn may influence parenting behavior and later child outcomes. Shifting parents' internal representations is arguably a more gradual process than training parents in behavior management practices; thus, these findings may help explain why therapeutic effects on child behavioral outcomes become increasingly apparent for Connect compared with behavioral management programs (Stattin et al., 2015).

Moretti, Obsuth, Craig, and Bartolo (2015) extended these findings by examining changes in parent–child processes that may underlie Connect treatment outcomes. In addition to assessing youths' problem behaviors, the study included parents' reports of youths' attachment avoidance and anxiety, and affect dysregulation. Results showed that reductions in attachment avoidance were linked to decreases in externalizing problems, whereas reductions in attachment anxiety were associated with decreases in internalizing problems. Furthermore, reductions in affect dysregulation were linked to decreases in both dimensions of problem behavior. This pattern of results was comparable for boys and girls, and for youth with clinical versus subclinical levels of externalizing problems at pretreatment. Overall, results from these two studies examining mechanisms of change support a model wherein Connect shifts parenting representations, changes parenting sensitivity, and reduces attachment insecurity and affect dysregulation (see Figure 17.1). Furthermore, preliminary results from a large-scale study of over 800 parents and 600 youth show that substantial reductions in youth internalizing (symptoms of depression and anxiety) and externalizing problems (symptoms of oppositional defiant disorder and conduct disorder) that are already evident by the fifth session of Connect can continue over the course of the remaining program sessions (Moretti & the Connect Team, 2016). Importantly, treatment effects are evident in reports from both parents and youth.

The effectiveness of mental health programs must be based on not only studies showing significant improvements but also on implementation indicators, including economic feasibility. Connect was designed to be inexpensive and portable; it is a brief (10 sessions), manualized program delivered in a group format. Sampaio, Zarabi & Feldman (2012) calculated the cost-effectiveness ratio (i.e., program cost minus cost saving) at posttreatment and 12-month follow-up across four parenting programs: Comet, COPE, The Incredible Years, and Connect. Participants included parents of 922 youth randomized to one of these programs. Three indices were estimated: training costs (training fees, travel costs, marketing), operating costs (practitioner's time, material, rent of venue) and total cost (training plus running costs). All cost estimates were the lowest for Connect compared with the other parenting programs (Comet, Cope, Incredible Years), which were 11 and 270% more expensive in terms of operating and running costs. These findings support the value of Connect from an economic standpoint, promoting the rapid uptake of Connect. We emphasize, however, that Connect should not be used as a stand-alone intervention for youth and families with clinically severe, chronic, and complex problems. Nonetheless, Connect could well be considered as part of a multifaceted treatment program tailored to address the unique needs of such families.

In summary, the existing evidence for the effectiveness of Connect comes from a range of studies involving different research designs (e.g., pilot trials, quasi-experimental, RCT) and distinctive groups of researchers. Although this body of work provides strong empirical support for the benefits of Connect in reducing problem behavior in at-risk youth, progress is still needed to ensure that the evidence base for Connect meets the rigorous standards of a "well-established treatment." This requires additional RCTs comparing Connect with alternative treatments to determine short- and long-term effectiveness. Additional studies are also needed to better understand mechanisms that underlie therapeutic outcomes and the factors that moderate effectiveness. To this end, our current research examines mechanisms of change and moderating factors at three points across treatment and at 6-, 12-, and 18-month follow-up (Moretti & the Connect Team, 2016). This study also investigates genetic markers that have been previously established as moderators of sensitivity to adversity and treatment, such as dopamine receptor D_4 (*DRD4*) and the serotonin transporter gene (*5-HTTLPR*) (Caspi et al., 2003; Bakermans-Kranenburg, van IJzendoorn, Mesman, Alink, & Juffer, 2008; Brody et al., 2014; Cleveland et al., 2015; Drury et al., 2012). In addition, we are investigating other factors that potentially moderate treatment effectiveness, including parental depression, parental attachment security, youth exposure to trauma, youth involvement in the justice system, foster care placement history, and the presence of callous–unemotional features in both parents and teens.

Closing Comments and Future Directions

The goal of the Connect program is to translate extensive research and clinical knowledge about attachment, development, and treatment into a structured, easy-to-grasp format that makes sense to parents and may also be readily implemented across diverse communities. Additionally, the program strives to support the greatest number of clinicians and families in the most efficient way, while retaining program adherence and integrity. These complex and often competing demands require close collaboration with the government systems and agencies responsible for providing mental health services for families and youth. As we move forward, we realize the need for continued research to ensure accuracy and completeness in the evaluation of program outcomes, as well as a better understanding of the processes that promote therapeutic outcomes.

Communities have also called for adaptations of Connect to address the special needs of various populations. In response to these requests, we have completed an adaptation of Connect for foster parents that provides training and support to help foster parents understand the impact of trauma on adolescent development, their attachment strategies, and their response to foster care. This adaptation also addresses the unique issues of foster care (e.g., loyalty conflict), and especially those related to teens who are placed in care ("aging out of care"). To date, it has been enthusiastically received by foster parents, who consistently note that it addresses a significant gap in foster parent training through its focus on issues of trauma and attachment among teens in care. Research is currently under way to determine whether Connect for foster parents indeed produces the types of outcomes we need to feel confident that it will promote better outcomes for teens in care.

Cultural diversity is also an important focus of our continuing work. Led by Aboriginal communities across British Columbia, we are in the process of reshaping the program to embody Indigenous history and the impact of colonialism, shared and unique cultural beliefs, parenting practices, and healing ceremonies. Universally Indigenous cultures understand individual, community, and global health through a relational lens in contrast to Eurocentric beliefs that focus on the importance of independence and self-sufficiency. Supporting Indigenous families, communities, and youth therefore requires significant shifts in understanding and collaboration across communities, as well as the development of culturally relevant and safe program content and delivery. Adopting the principle of "two-eyed seeing" (Marsh, Coholic, Cote-Meek, & Najavits, 2015), Reclaiming Connection represents an ongoing partnership across communities that has shaped and will reshape the program over time, with the goal of promoting the health and well-being of Indigenous families and their teens.

Contemporary culture frequently does teens and their families a great disservice. Teens are often assumed to be disinterested in their parents, disengaged from families, and dismissive of adults more generally. Their behavior is both feared and demeaned as the result of hormonal and neurobiological imbalances. Not surprisingly, few parents anticipate their child's adolescence with excitement and joy. Yet adolescence is a period of enormous opportunity, in which teens question conventional and social norms and come to new and creative insights. Although their behavior may suggest otherwise, teens continue to benefit from a secure base from which to explore. And while relationships with peers and romantic partners provide a safe haven, teens continue to turn to their parents in times of need. When parents can see, hear, and understand the attachment issues that remain paramount in their relationships with their teens, they are better equipped emotionally and relationally to sustain a strong partnership and to weather the journey ahead—a journey that can be surprisingly delightful, at least some of the time.

ACKNOWLEDGMENT

This research was supported by Grant Nos. 54,020 and 84567 from the Canadian Institutes of Health Research, Dr. Marlene M. Moretti, Principal Investigator.

REFERENCES

Aber, J. L., Brown, J. L., & Jones, S. M. (2003). Developmental trajectories toward violence in middle childhood: Course, demographic differences, and response to school-based intervention. *Developmental Psychology, 39*(2), 324–348.

Allen, J. P., & Hauser, S. T. (1996). Autonomy and relatedness in adolescent–family interactions as predictors of young adults' states of mind regarding attachment. *Development and Psychopathology, 8*(4), 793–809.

Allen, J. P., Marsh, P., McFarland, C., McElhaney, K. B., Land, D. J., Jodl, K. M., & Peck, S. (2002). Attachment and autonomy as predictors of the development of social skills and delinquency during midadolescence. *Journal of Consulting and Clinical Psychology, 70*(1), 56–66.

Allen, J. P., Porter, M., McFarland, C., McElhaney, K. B., & Marsh, P. (2007). The relation of attachment security to adolescents' paternal and peer relationships, depression, and externalizing behavior. *Child Development, 78*(4), 1222–1239.

Bakermans-Kranenburg, M. J., van IJzendoorn, M. H., Mesman, J., Alink, L. R., & Juffer, F. (2008). Effects of an attachment-based intervention on daily cortisol moderated by dopamine receptor D4: A randomized control trial on 1- to 3-year-olds screened for externalizing behavior. *Development and Psychopathology, 20*(3), 805–820.

Beijersbergen, M. D., Juffer, F., Bakermans-Kranenburg, M. J., & van IJzendoorn, M. H. (2012). Remaining or becoming secure: Parental sensitive support predicts attachment continuity from infancy to adolescence in a longitudinal adoption study. *Developmental Psychology, 48*(5), 1277–1282.

Benson, M. J., Buehler, C., & Gerard, J. M. (2008). Interparental hostility and early adolescent problem behavior: Spillover via maternal acceptance, harshness, inconsistency, and intrusiveness. *Journal of Early Adolescence, 28*(3), 428–454.

Booth-LaForce, C., Groh, A. M., Burchinal, M. R., Roisman, G. I., Owen, M. T., & Cox, M. J. (2014). Caregiving and contextual sources of continuity and change in attachment from infancy to late adolescence. *Monographs of the Society for Research in Child Development, 79*(3), 67–84.

Brody, G. H., Chen, Y. F., Beach, S. R., Kogan, S. M., Yu, T., Diclemente, R. J., . . . Philibert, R. A. (2014). Differential sensitivity to prevention programming: A dopaminergic polymorphism-enhanced prevention effect on protective parenting and adolescent substance use. *Health Psychology, 33*(2), 182–191.

Brown, L. S., & Wright, J. (2003). The relationship between attachment strategies and psychopathology in adolescence. *Psychology and Psychotherapy: Theory, Research and Practice, 76*(4), 351–367.

Casey, B. J. (2015). Beyond simple models of self-control to circuit-based accounts of adolescent behavior. *Annual Review of Psychology, 66,* 295–319.

Caspers, K. M., Cadoret, R. J., Langbehn, D., Yucuis, R., & Troutman, B. (2005). Contributions of attachment style and perceived social support to lifetime use of illicit substances. *Addictive Behaviors, 30*(5), 1007–1011.

Caspi, A., Sugden, K., Moffitt, T. E., Taylor, A., Craig, I. W., Harrington, H., . . . Braithwaite, A. (2003). Influence of life stress on depression: Moderation by a polymorphism in the 5-HTT gene. *Science, 301*(5631), 386–389.

Claes, M., Lacourse, E., Bouchard, C., & Perucchini, P. (2003). Parental practices in late adolescence, a comparison of three countries: Canada, France and Italy. *Journal of Adolescence, 26*(4), 387–399.

Cleveland, H. H., Schlomer, G. L., Vandenbergh, D. J., Feinberg, M., Greenberg, M., Spoth, R., . . . Hair, K. L. (2015). The conditioning of intervention effects on early adolescent alcohol use by maternal involvement and *DRD4* and *5-HTTLPR* candidate genes. *Development and Psychopathology, 27*(1), 51–67.

Collins, N. L., Cooper, M. L., Albino, A., & Allard, L. (2002). Psychosocial vulnerability from adolescence to adulthood: A prospective study of attachment style differences in relationship functioning and partner choice. *Journal of Personality, 70*(6), 965–1008.

Conduct Problems Prevention Research Group. (2011). The effects of the Fast Track preventive intervention on the development of conduct disorder across childhood. *Child Development, 82*(1), 331–345.

Crone, E. A., & Dahl, R. E. (2012). Understanding adolescence as a period of social–affective engagement and goal flexibility. *Nature Reviews Neuroscience, 13*(9), 636–650.

Cunningham, C. E., Bremner, R., & Boyle, M. (1995). Large group community-based parenting programs for families of preschoolers at risk for disruptive behaviour disorders: Utilization, cost effectiveness, and outcome. *Journal of Child Psychology and Psychiatry, 36*(7), 1141–1159.

Drury, S. S., Gleason, M. M., Theall, K. P., Smyke, A. T., Nelson, C. A., Fox, N. A., & Zeanah, C. H. (2012). Genetic sensitivity to the caregiving context: The influence of 5httlpr and BDNF val66met on indiscriminate social behavior. *Physiology and Behavior, 106*(5), 728–735.

Fonagy, P., Steele, M., Steele, H., Moran, G. S., & Higgitt, A. C. (1991). The capacity for understanding mental states: The reflective self in parent and child and its significance for security of attachment. *Infant Mental Health Journal, 12*(3), 201–218.

Giannotta, F., Ortega, E., & Stattin, H. (2013). An attachment parenting intervention to prevent adolescents' problem behaviors: A pilot study in Italy. *Child and Youth Care Forum, 42*(1), 71–85.

Greenberg, M. T., Speltz, M. L., DeKlyen, M., & Jones, K. (2001). Correlates of clinic referral for early conduct problems: Variable-and person-oriented approaches. *Development and Psychopathology, 13*(2), 255–276.

Högström, J., Olofsson, V., Özdemir, M., Enebrink, P., & Stattin, H. (2017). Two-year findings from a national effectiveness trial: Effectiveness of behavioral and non-behavioral parenting programs. *Journal of Abnormal Child Psychology, 45*(3), 527–542.

Joseph, M. A., O'Connor, T. G., Briskman, J. A., Maughan, B., & Scott, S. (2014). The formation of secure new attachments by children who were maltreated: An observational study of adolescents in foster care. *Development and Psychopathology, 26*(1), 67–80.

Kling, Å., Forster, M., Sundell, K., & Melin, L. (2010). A randomized controlled effectiveness trial of Parent Management Training with varying degrees of therapist support. *Behavior Therapy, 41*(4), 530–542.

Kobak, R., Zajac, K., & Smith, C. (2009). Adolescent attachment and trajectories of hostile–impulsive behavior: Implications for the development of personality disorders. *Development and Psychopathology, 21*(3), 839–851.

Marsh, T. N., Coholic, D., Cote-Meek, S., & Najavits, L. M. (2015). Blending Aboriginal and Western healing methods to treat intergenerational trauma with substance use disorder in Aboriginal peoples who live in Northeastern Ontario, Canada. *Harm Reduction Journal, 12*(1), 14.

Mayseless, O., & Scharf, M. (2006). Maternal representations of parenting in adolescence and psychosocial functioning of mothers and adolescents. In O. Mayseless (Ed.), *Parenting representations: Theory, research, and clinical implications* (pp. 208–238). Cambridge, UK: Cambridge University Press.

McGorry, P. D., Purcell, R., Goldstone, S., & Amminger, G. P. (2011). Age of onset and timing of treatment for mental and substance use disorders: Implications for preventive intervention strategies and models of care. *Current Opinion in Psychiatry, 24*(4), 301–306.

Moretti, M. M., Bartolo, T., Odgers, C., Slaney, K., & Craig, S. G. (2014). Gender and the transmission of risk: A prospective study of adolescent girls exposed to maternal versus paternal interparental violence. *Journal of Research on Adolescence, 24*(1), 80–92.

Moretti, M. M., & the Connect Team. (2016). *Effectiveness of a relational intervention in reducing violence and victimization in at-risk adolescent girls and boys.* Unpublished manuscript, Simon Fraser University, Burnaby, BC, Canada.

Moretti, M. M., & Craig, S. G. (2013). Maternal versus paternal physical and emotional abuse, affect regulation and risk for depression from adolescence to early adulthood. *Child Abuse and Neglect, 37*(1), 4–13.

Moretti, M. M., Holland, R., Moore, K., & McKay, S. (2004). An attachment-based parenting program for caregivers of severely conduct disordered adolescents: Preliminary findings. *Journal of Child and Youth Care Work, 19*(1), 170–178.

Moretti, M. M., & Obsuth, I. (2009). Effectiveness of an attachment-focused manualized intervention for parents of teens at risk for aggressive behaviour: The Connect Program. *Journal of Adolescence, 32*(6), 1347–1357.

Moretti, M. M., Obsuth, I., Craig, S. G., & Bartolo, T. (2015). An attachment-based intervention for parents of adolescents at risk: mechanisms of change. *Attachment and Human Development, 17*(2), 119–135.

Moretti, M. M., Obsuth, I., Mayseless, O., & Scharf, M. (2012). Shifting internal parent–child representations among caregivers of teens with serious behavior problems: An attachment-based approach. *Journal of Child and Adolescent Trauma, 5*(3), 191–204.

Obsuth, I., Moretti, M. M., Holland, R., Braber, K., & Cross, S. (2006). Conduct disorder: New directions in promoting effective parenting and strengthening parent-adolescent relationships. *Journal of the Canadian Academy of Child and Adolescent Psychiatry, 15*(1), 6–15.

Ortega, E., Giannotta, F., Latina, D., & Ciairano, S. (2012). Cultural adaptation of the strengthening families program 10–14 to Italian families. *Child Youth Care Forum, 41,* 197–212.

Pascuzzo, K., Cyr, C., & Moss, E. (2013). Longitudinal association between adolescent attachment, adult romantic attachment, and emotion regulation strategies. *Attachment and Human Development, 15*(1), 83–103.

Rosenstein, D. S., & Horowitz, H. A. (1996). Adolescent attachment and psychopathology. *Journal of Consulting and Clinical Psychology, 64*(2), 244–253.

Rosenthal, N. L., & Kobak, R. (2010). Assessing adolescents' attachment hierarchies: Differences across developmental periods and associations with individual adaptation. *Journal of Research on Adolescence, 20*(3), 678–706.

Sampaio, F., Zarabi, N., & Feldman, I. (2012). *Are parenting programs in Sweden cost effective in reducing child conduct problems?* Uppsala, Sweden: Uppsala University, Department of Women's and Children's Health, Social Pediatrics.

Speltz, M. L., DeKlyen, M., & Greenberg, M. T. (1999). Attachment in boys with early onset conduct problems. *Development and Psychopathology, 11*(2), 269–285.

Stattin, H., Enebrink, P., Özdemir, M., & Giannotta, F. (2015). A national evaluation of parenting programs in Sweden: The short-term effects using an RCT effectiveness design. *Journal of Consulting and Clinical Psychology, 83*(6), 1069–1084.

Webster-Stratton, C. (1984). Randomized trial of two parent-training programs for families with conduct-disordered children. *Journal of Consulting and Clinical Psychology, 52*(4), 666–678.

CHAPTER 18

Attachment-Based Family Therapy
for Adolescent Depression and Suicide Risk

E. STEPHANIE KRAUTHAMER EWING, SUZANNE A. LEVY,
SYREETA A. SCOTT, and GUY S. DIAMOND

Attachment-based family therapy (ABFT) is a manualized family therapy for depressed and suicidal adolescents and their families. It has been tested as a 12- to 16-week intervention, but it can be used as a longer intervention as well. It is a task-based model built around five key therapeutic tasks: (1) the relational reframe; (2) adolescent alliance; (3) parent alliance; (4) repairing attachment; and (5) promoting autonomy. The five tasks build on one another and guide therapists in their efforts to strengthen parent–teen relationships, build adolescent and family resilience, and buffer against future experiences of adolescent depression and despair. ABFT is strongly influenced by attachment theory and by empirical research in developmental psychology. Clinically, many of the model's components grew out of early innovations and thinking in the fields of family psychology and family therapy.

Four studies have shown that ABFT reduces adolescent depression and suicidal ideation more effectively than a waiting-list control or treatment as usual (Diamond, Reis, Diamond, Siqueland, & Isaacs, 2002; Diamond et al., 2010, 2012; Israel & Diamond, 2013). In these studies, ABFT was effective even with teens often categorized as "difficult to treat," including adolescents who were severely depressed, had a history of sexual abuse, identified as sexual minorities, or had parents who themselves were depressed. ABFT's efficacy with these patients is especially noteworthy, since these groups have frequently not responded well to other empirically supported treatments for adolescent depression (e.g., cognitive-behavioral treatment and/ or medication) (Asarnow et al., 2009; Barbe, Bridge, Birmaher, Kolko, & Brent, 2004; Curry et al., 2006). Based on this empirical work, ABFT was recognized as a "Proven Practice" by the Promising Practices Network (2011). In addition, the National Registry of Evidence-Based Programs and Practices has deemed ABFT to be a treatment with effective outomes for suicidal thoughts and behaviors and depression and depressive symptoms (*http://hrepp.smashsa.gov*). There are ongoing efforts to disseminate ABFT, both nationally and internationally. In 2013, the Attachment-Based Family Therapy Training Program (ABFT Training Program) was established at Drexel University in Philadelphia, Pennsylvania, to increase dissemination and implementation efforts. There is currently a formal training program for varied levels of training, ranging from introductory workshops to a more intensive ABFT therapist certification program.

The remainder of this chapter reviews the following in greater depth: (1) ABFT's theoretical grounding in attachment theory and the clinical model; (2) history of the development of ABFT; (3) ABFT in the context of other empirically supported treatments for adolescent depression and suicide risk, including efficacy and effectiveness study results; and (4) efforts to disseminate and implement the model, including information about ABFT training and certification.

Influence of Attachment Theory on the ABFT Model

ABFT is strongly guided by attachment theory and models of emotional development in childhood and adolescence. Attachment theory's central premise is that children have a basic evolutionary instinct to seek out parents for care and protection (Bowlby, 1982). When these needs are not met, children are at risk for developing insecure attachment. While insecure attachment predicts a range of maladaptive outcomes, including depression and suicide risk, secure attachment protects children and adolescents, and is related to a variety of adaptive outcomes (Kobak, Rosenthal, Zajac, & Madsen, 2007; Sroufe, 2005).

Research evidence strongly supports the protective role of secure attachments in early childhood, and there is also ample evidence for the continued importance of healthy attachment relationships in adolescence (Allen, 2008; Kobak, Cassidy, Lyons-Ruth, & Ziv, 2006; Steinberg, 1990; Stroufe, 2005). Secure attachment in adolescence, which is marked by confident expectations of a caregiver's availability to provide support, protection, and guidance enables more direct and effective parent–teen communication and better conflict negotiation (Allen, 2008). These dynamics are related to better adolescent emotion regulation and problem solving, qualities that predict better functioning and developmental outcomes in adolescents and young adults (Kobak et al., 2006; Kobak, Cole, Fleming, Ferenz-Gillies, & Gamble, 1993).

In contrast, insecure attachment in adolescence relates to poorer developmental outcomes (Allen, 2008). Insecure attachment confers a higher risk for the development of depression and suicidality. Specifically, preoccupied and unresolved states of mind (with respect to loss or abuse), as assessed by the Adult Attachment Interview (AAI; Main, Hesse, & Goldwyn, 2008), prospectively predict depressive symptoms and suicidality (Adam, Sheldon-Keller, & West, 1996; Allen, Porter, McFarland, McElhaney, & Marsh, 2007; Kobak & Sceery, 1988; Kobak, Sudler, & Gamble, 1991). In addition, insecure attachment in adolescence relates to higher levels of emotional avoidance, dysfunctional anger, and overpersonalization (Kobak et al., 1991; Marsh, McFarland, Allen, McElhaney, & Land, 2003). These processes can contribute to higher levels of parent–teen conflict. High levels of family conflict and negative interactional patterns can reinforce an adolescent's negative self-concept, causing or fueling depression (Yap, Allen, & Sheeber, 2007). In addition, Brent and colleagues (1988) found that 20% of adolescent suicides and 50% of nonfatal suicide attempts were directly preceded by conflict with parents.

ABFT was designed to revive an attachment-promoting family environment, in order to improve adolescents' sense of felt security in their relationship with their parent(s). To accomplish this, therapists meet with teens and parents separately, as well as together in joint family sessions. Therapists guide families through five specific treatment tasks: (1) relational reframe; (2) adolescent alliance; (3) parent alliance; (4) repairing attachment; and (5) promoting autonomy (see Table 18.1). In most sessions, conversations about family relationships and family interaction patterns, particularly during stressful times, are at the center of the therapeutic process.

In individual work with teens ("adolescent alliance," Task 2 sessions), therapists engage adolescents in reflective, attachment- and emotion-focused conversations targeting their right to be heard and cared for by parents and loved ones, particularly when confronting the deeply painful experiences of hopelessness and despair associated with depression and suicide. Specific attention is paid to what gets in the way of adolescents using their parent for comfort and help during times of depressive or suicidal crisis (e.g., lack of trust, fear of being a disappointment, lack of parental empathy).

TABLE 18.1. ABFT Process and Outcome Goals for Each Task

Task	Typical duration	Process goal	Outcome goal
Relational reframe	1 session	Attributional shift in how family members view the problem and solution	Agreement to participate in relational focused therapy
Adolescent alliance	2–4 sessions	Better understanding of attachment narrative (i.e., thoughts, feelings, memories)	Revived valuing of attachment and willingness to renegotiate it
Parent alliance	2–4 sessions	Shift in the parents' working model of the adolescent and their parenting role	Revived caregiving motivation; acquisition of emotion coaching, parenting skills
Repairing attachment	1–3 sessions	Engagement in conversations that work through attachment ruptures	Revised view of self and other, and renewed interpersonal trust
Promoting autonomy	4–8 sessions	Parents effectively help adolescents resolve non-family-based problems (school, job, depression)	Resumed negotiation of more normative issues related to adolescent development

Note: An in-depth description of the ABFT model can be found in Diamond, Diamond, and Levy (2013).

Many factors impact the likelihood that parents will provide sensitive and responsive care to children and teens, including stress levels (e.g., marital stress, occupational stress, health status, poverty), a parent's own attachment experiences and experiences of loss and/or trauma, and other parental psychological factors (e.g., parental depression or anxiety) (Belsky, 1984). Adolescent depression and suicidality can be stressful and challenging to even the most attuned and psychologically sound parents and caregivers. ABFT draws on empirical findings about attachment and caregiving in order to (1) improve attachment security in parent–child relationships that have likely always been challenging, and (2) revive security in parent–teen relationships that have primarily suffered under the enormous stress of teen depression and suicidality. Theoretical and empirical work on caregiving and attachment have consistently demonstrated that sensitivity and emotional attunement in parents fosters children's attachment security, while parenting that is rejecting, intrusive, emotionally unresponsive, or inconsistent increases children's risk for insecure attachment (van IJzendorn, 1995). ABFT incorporates this rich knowledge base into its therapeutic strategies and approaches aimed at helping parents become the best sources of support possible for their teens. ABFT also incorporates knowledge from the developmental literature on adolescence about the importance of parental flexibility with teenagers and the need for parents to responsively balance their adolescents' growing autonomy needs with continued attachment needs.

With this foundational knowledge, ABFT therapists work individually with parents to help build parents' reflectiveness about the important factors that may have impacted their approaches to parenting and their relationship with their teen in the past ("parent alliance," Task 3 sessions). Parents are often eager to talk with someone about the many challenges they have faced, and the helplessness, worry, and despair that accompanies parenting a teen struggling with depression and suicide risk. Whether the parent–teen relationship is tense and conflict filled, or the parents simply feel that they cannot reach their teen to help with recovery, parents are often intensely relieved to talk with a caring and empathic therapist about these struggles. With a good therapeutic alliance in place, therapists then work with parents to: (1) increase their empathy for their teen and renew their curiosity about the teen's experiences; and (2) revive parental motivation to try new approaches for engaging and talking about challenging topics with a teen whom they may have experienced as difficult, rejecting, or burdensome. Specifically, therapists coach parents to be more curious and validating, and less defensive and critical, elements grounded in empirical findings about attachment-promoting parenting and the benefits of an emotion-coaching parenting stance with children and teens (Gottman, Katz, & Hooven, 1996; van IJzendoorn, 1995).

With teens and parents prepared for joint family work, therapists proceed to bring them together for joint sessions ("attachment repair," Task 4 sessions). A primary goal of this next phase of therapy is to help structure and facilitate "corrective attachment experiences," in the form of attachment and emotion-focused therapeutic conversations between teens and their parents. During these conversations, adolescents are coached to talk openly and directly about interpersonal injuries and barriers in their relationships with their parents, particularly those barriers that have gotten in the way of them going to or using their parents for support around depression and suicide. Parents are coached to use emotion-focused approaches, nonjudgmental curiosity, comfort, support, and validation. Teens are able to work though past disappointments and hurts with their parents in these conversations, while having the opportunity to experience *in vivo* within-session exposure to more fulfilling and successful interpersonal interactions with them. Over time, and through repeated sessions such as this, adolescents come to feel more comfortable and trusting in their parents' availability, attunement, and responsiveness, while parents receive the reward of feeling closer to their teens and better able to help them.

With trust and feelings of safety on the mend, and a more secure foundation of relational closeness, therapy then takes a shift into the final phase ("promoting autonomy," Task 5 sessions) and begins to focus on (1) some of the other environmental, behavioral, and cognitive factors that may contribute to the adolescent's depression (e.g., lack of social support, depressotypic cognitive styles); (2) promoting teen autonomy and engagement in the more normative tasks of adolescence (e.g., school, employment, social life, dating); and (3) adolescent identity development (e.g., ethnic, sexual, religious identity). With a stronger parent–teen relationship as a secure base, teens are better able to use their parent(s) to help them in these endeavors and efforts (Allen, 2008).

Thus, ABFT aims specifically to target attachment processes between parents and teens, in order to strengthen the parent–teen bond. With stronger and more secure relational bonds, parents are able to serve as a better resource for their teens and help buffer against the feelings of isolation, hopelessness, and despair that characterize adolescent depression and suicide risk. ABFT depends on the premise that attachment and caregiving are open to revision, and that with consistently more attuned and supportive relational experiences, teens experience improvements in felt attachment security, relational trust, and internal working models of self and other (Bowlby, 1988; Main & Goldwyn, 1998).

History of the Development of ABFT

ABFT was developed in an urban hospital-based research center, beginning with the dissertation research of ABFT lead author, Dr. Guy Diamond. In his work, Diamond sought ways to manage the complexities and possibilities of therapeutic work with families of depressed and suicidal teens. He began by studying and thinking about a task-based approach to therapy. This approach grew out of process research methodology developed by Laura Rice and Les Greenberg (1984), aimed at helping investigators identify hypothesized key therapeutic change mechanisms or events in therapy that lead to growth of individuals and the family as a whole. The task structure identifies markers that indicate when the task has begun, the progression of steps or processes that should be evident within sessions, and some objective and observable indications that the task has been completed.

Dr. Diamond took this approach with him to postgraduate work at the Philadelphia Child Guidance Center. There, while working on the inpatient unit, he treated hundreds of depressed adolescents and their families. He and his clinical team began to ask themselves: When a case goes well, what are the essential clinical tasks that typically get accomplished? They worked together to begin to identify several factors that appeared consistent in successful treatment of depressed teens. First, it seemed that in many successful cases, therapists worked with families to move them toward a more relational view of the problem and potential ways to intervene (relational reframe). Second, and growing out of this family systems approach, successful therapists were able to build a strong therapeutic alliance with both the teens and their parents (adolescent alliance, parent alliance). Both a relational view of the adolescent's depression and the strength of the alliance with family members are common factors included in multiple family-based approaches. Dr. Diamond also turned to the developmental literature to understand better what might be changing in teens and families who made significant clinical progress. He increasingly observed and understood that successful clinicians were working to help families uncover, talk through, and resolve potential "ruptures" or "injuries" in parent–teen relationships. Specific to depressed and suicidal adolescents, it appeared that relational ruptures had occurred that had damaged and interfered with teens' feelings of safety and security with their parents, such that they did not feel that they could turn to their parent(s) for help, comfort, and support. The critical question that therapists asked teens became, "When you are feeling so down and in despair that you are thinking about hurting yourself, or even taking your own life, what gets in the way of you going to your parents for help and support?" It became evident that in the best cases, therapists were able to help teens effectively identify these core relational disappointments and hurts, and to talk through and process the emotional impact of these injuries, first with the therapist and ultimately in family sessions with parents. Thus, the next identified task was for clinicians to help teens and their families work through these issues in a way that would rebuild or earn back a more secure parent–teen relationship (repairing attachment). Finally, they observed that when parents and teens were able to work through the barriers and ruptures in their relationships successfully, therapists were often able to help guide them back with relative ease to the business and work of normative adolescent growth and development (academic achievement, dating, work, etc.).

With these five tasks identified (relational reframe, adolescent alliance, parent alliance, repairing attachment, and promoting autonomy), the team began to think about how to make them happen more systematically. Exploring the moment-to-moment changes within therapy sessions, they found that even within each task, there were patterns of conversation and exploration that seemed indicative of successful or unsuccessful change episodes. They began to further operationalize and study these tasks, leading to the very detailed road map of ABFT.

In addition to this detailed and careful task-based approach, much of ABFT's clinical sensibilities and intervention strategies grew from the thinking and models by pioneers in family psychology and family therapy, including structural family therapy (SFT; Minuchin, 1974), multidimensional family therapy (MDFT; Liddle, 2002), emotion-focused therapy (EFT; Goldman & Greenberg, 2015; Johnson, 2004), and contextual family therapy (Böszörményi-Nagy & Spark, 1973). ABFT is rooted in SFT. Minuchin proposed that "enactment" of new behavior (e.g., having families experience new ways of acting and relating) would be a more profound learning experience for families than just giving them "insight" or teaching them new skills (e.g., psychoeducation). Instead of enacting a behavioral change episode (e.g., controlling a rambunctious child, blocking an intrusive parent), ABFT enacts conversations about core attachment ruptures. The experiential learning focuses on affect regulation, direct communication, and trustworthy interactions between parents and adolescents.

MDFT emerged from SFT, but brought many innovations, upon which ABFT capitalized. Specifically, MDFT, like ABFT, recognizes the need to immediately and more actively engage adolescents and parents in family-based treatment in order to increase the odds of successful therapeutic outcomes (Liddle & Diamond, 1991). Similar to MDFT, ABFT advocates that getting families motivated for treatment is critical, multiple therapeutic alliances are required, and preparing everyone to interact in new ways is essential; thus, treatment occurs in stages.

EFT (Greenberg, 2011) also greatly influences ABFT. EFT was designed primarily for individual work with adults and then further developed by Sue Johnson as emotion-focused couples therapy (EFCT; Johnson, 2004) for work with couples. In EFCT work, as in ABFT, attachment and relational safety are primary organizing themes of therapy. An obvious difference in implementing EFCT for couples and ABFT for adolescents is that in the parent–teen relationship, the responsibility to provide safety and protection lies primarily with the parents as opposed to the equal balance of responsibility between partners in a couple. However, ABFT harnesses the principles of EFT and EFCT for identifying primary emotions, regulating the expression of emotional needs, and using softer, more vulnerable emotions to facilitate safe and open communication within a family.

Finally, ABFT has theoretical lineage to Ivan Nagy's contextual family therapy (CFT; Böszörményi-Nagy & Spark, 1973). Similar to CFT, ABFT views relational justice, fairness, and trust as the fundamental fabric of interpersonal relationships and understands that each family member's temperamental, historical, and circumstantial experiences explain difficulties and motivations that thwart or promote loving parent–child relationships. Additionally, as in CFT, forgiveness and exoneration become important topics of conversation when trying to repair attachment ruptures (Böszörményi-Nagy & Spark, 1973; McCullough, Pargament, & Thoresen, 2000). Rather than seeing each other as enemies, ABFT helps family members to use greater empathy and perspective taking to view one another more accurately as complex human beings with both incredible strengths and vulnerable weaknesses.

ABFT versus Other Empirically Supported Treatments for Adolescent Depression and Suicide Risk

To date, the majority of research and model development and evaluation of treatment of adolescent depression and suicide risk has focused on psychopharmacology and individual models of psychotherapy, primarily cognitive-behavioral therapy (CBT; David-Ferdon & Kaslow, 2008). While medication and CBT have both shown effectiveness in large-scales clinical trials, in the largest trial to date, the Treatment for Adolescents with Depression Study (TADS) study, the remission rates (symptom free) at posttreatment were only 37%, even with combined medication and psychotherapy treatment, indicating that over 60% of patients still had clinically significant symptoms at the end of treatment (March et al., 2004; Brent & Melhem,

2008; Goodyer et al., 2007; David-Ferdon & Kaslow, 2008). By 9 months, there were no differences in treatment outcomes between any of the treatment groups, and nearly 50% of patients who responded to treatment relapsed within a year. These results and other recent meta-analytic findings, in which CBT effect sizes were between 0.25 and 0.34, suggest that CBT and psychopharmacological interventions for depressed adolescents may not be as potent and/or lasting as hoped for or predicted (Bridge et al., 2007; Weisz, McCarty, & Valeri, 2006). Furthermore, far less work has been done to evaluate psychotherapeutic treatments specifically for depression complicated by adolescent suicidality. Many of the studies examining treatments for adolescent depression originally excluded participants with high levels of suicide risk and/or did not examine reductions in suicidality as primary or secondary outcomes. Existing data on CBT for adolescent suicidality suggests mixed results with only slight reductions in suicide attempts or ideation. (Spirito & Esposito-Smythers, 2006; Tarrier, Taylor, & Gooding, 2008; Brent, 2013). In light of these findings, leaders in mental health research have called for the exploration of alternative and supplemental treatments that might improve treatment potency and efficacy for both teen depression and suicide risk (Hollon et al., 2005).

Family treatments for youth depression and suicidality are promising for a number of reasons. First, adolescent depression and suicide risk have been consistently linked to family stress, conflict, and overall negative family functioning (Ehnvall, Parker, Hadzi-Pavlovic, & Malhi, 2008; Hardt et al., 2008; Salzinger, Rosario, & Feldman, 2007; Wagner, 1997; Wagner, Silverman, & Martin, 2003). Second, positive aspects of the family, such as family cohesion, warmth, and parental availability and monitoring are all protective factors against youth suicide and depression (Beautrais, Joyce, & Mulder, 1996; Brent et al., 1994; Fergusson, Woodward, & Horwood, 2000; Kurtz & Derevensky, 1993; McKeown et al., 1998; Resnick, Acierno, & Kilpatrick, 1997; Rubenstein, Halton, Kasten, Rubin, & Stechler 1998; Wagner et al., 2003; Zhang & Jin, 1996). Finally, and perhaps most important to efficacy studies, family conflict has frequently been a consistent negative moderator of treatment outcome (Asarnow et al., 2009; Birmaher et al., 2000; Brent & Melhem, 2008).

While some CBT researchers have added family psychoeducation components to treatment studies, the addition of parental psychoeducation has not led to increased CBT treatment efficacy (March et al., 2004; Wells & Albano, 2005). One reason for the absence in expected efficacy gains may be due to the fact that psychoeducation sessions do not typically incorporate time for families to work through problems together in sessions; rather, the sessions are primarily didactic, with patients encouraged to practice the skills at home, after the sessions. Adding more intensive relational approaches to clinical work with depressed and suicidal teens and their families may be needed to make impactful family and interpersonal relationship changes.

Indeed, depression (and suicide risk) has been well-conceptualized from an interpersonal perspective with the central tenet that regardless of the etiology of the depression (e.g., biological, environmental, cognitive etc.), depression affects relationships and relationships affect mood (Mufson, Dorta, Moreau, & Weissman, 2004). Interpersonal therapy (IPT) for depression and interpersonal therapy for adolescents (IPT-A) with depression grew out of this interpersonal conceptualization of depression. IPT therapists help clients to identify difficulties and sources of stress in their interpersonal relationships and to problem-solve potential solutions to these difficulties. IPT-A has yielded some promising results, outperforming CBT in some studies, including a 1999 study in which IPT-A showed better recovery rates (82%) than CBT (52%) (Mufson, Gallagher, Dorta, & Young, 2004; Mufson, Weissman, Moreau, & Garfinkle, 1999; Rossello & Bernal, 1999). However, although IPT-A focuses very specifically on improving the interpersonal functioning of adolescents, most of the interpersonal learning occurs between the teen and the therapist, and the adolescent–parent relationship is not necessarily the central focus of the work.

Indeed, aside from ABFT, no other model for adolescent depression and/or suicide risk places the parent–teen attachment relationship at the center of adolescent recovery and remission (Diamond, Asarnow, & Hughes, 2016). In contrast, in ABFT, the therapeutic processes around interpersonal and relationship problems begins with the premise that family relationships and dynamics are critical and foundational aspects of adolescent health, well-being, and recovery. Thus, ABFT was designed as a transactional process that directly targets and aims to improve family interactions. ABFT begins with a very specific focus on the interpersonal relationship between teens and their parent(s), and while some initial work is conducted individually with therapists, the majority of sessions are interactive family sessions that focus on facilitating enactments and *in vivo* therapeutic experiences between teens and their parents.

Four empirical studies provide evidence that ABFT reduces adolescent depression and suicide risk more effectively than waiting-list control or treatment as usual (see Table 18.2).

In the first study, adolescents (ages 13–17) were randomized to 12 weeks of ABFT or 6 weeks of waiting-list control. At posttreatment, patients treated with ABFT were less likely to be experiencing clinically significant symptoms of depression and were less likely to meet criteria for major depressive disorder (MDD), compared with waiting-list patients (Diamond et al., 2002).

In the next study, ABFT-treated teens were compared to teens treated with enhanced usual care (EUC) in the community (in addition to treatment in the community, EUC patients received weekly check-in calls from the study's clinical

TABLE 18.2. Overview of ABFT Empirical Studies

Study	N	Effect size: Depression at posttreatment	Effect size: Suicide at posttreatment	Effect size: Depression at follow-up	Effect size: Suicide at follow-up
Diamond et al. (2002)	32	1.21 (HAM-D)	0.52 (SIQ-JR)	*	*
Diamond et al. (2010)	66	0.37 (BDI-II)	0.95 (SIQ-JR)	0.22	0.97
Israel & Diamond (2013)	20	0.8 (BDI-II) 1.08 (HAM-D)	*	*	*
Diamond et al. (2012)	10	0.90 (BDI-II)	2.10 (SIQ-JR)	*	*

Note. *Data not collected for study; BDI-II, Beck Depression Inventory–II; HAM-D, Hamilton Depression Rating Scale; SIQ-JR, Suicide Ideation Questionnaire–JR.

team, access to a 24-hour crisis hotline run by the study therapists, and referrals to additional services if needed). Adolescents in the ABFT group demonstrated significantly greater reductions in suicidal ideation during treatment and significant differences at follow-up (6, 12, and 24 weeks) compared to the EUC group, with an overall large effect size ($d = 0.97$). This is one of the few studies that has demonstrated a research treatment was more effective than treatment as usual for reducing adolescent suicide ideation (Tarrier et al., 2008). Efficacy was also demonstrated with the most severely affected youth, including those who presented with comorbid anxiety, severe suicide ideation, a history of sexual abuse and multiple suicide attempts. Results also indicated that ABFT was associated with greater rates of significant clinical recovery, and clinical recovery benefits were maintained at follow-up. ABFT patients also experienced more rapid relief from depression than the EUC group, a critical consideration for depressed adolescents and their parents. Finally, retention was better in the ABFT group, even with the additional supports offered in the EUC model (e.g., frequent check-in calls and resource coordination) (Diamond et al., 2010). Indeed, retention was better than that in several research studies that have designed treatments specifically to enhance engagement and retention (Rotheram-Borus et al., 1996; Spirito et al., 2002).

In the third study, researchers conducted a pilot program to examine effectiveness and feasibility of training community-based therapists. Community-based therapists were able to be effectively trained, as demonstrated by supervisor ratings of treatment fidelity. Teens treated with ABFT had significantly lower self-reported depression ratings and higher rates of recovery than patients in treatment as usual (Israel & Diamond, 2013).

In the fourth study, ABFT was adapted to meet the unique needs of suicidal, openly lesbian, gay, bisexual, and transgender (LGBT) youth and their parents (Diamond et al., 2012). In this small pilot study, 10 suicidal and openly LGBT youth and their families received 12 weeks of LGBT-sensitive ABFT. Across the sample, suicidal ideation and depressive symptoms significantly decreased, as did anxiety and avoidance in relationships with mothers. These findings suggest that family-based treatments that focus on relational themes may be promising for suicidal openly gay youth (Diamond et al., 2012).

The empirical findings are promising, both for their general findings about efficacy and effectiveness, and for more specific findings regarding treatment of adolescents who often fall into "treatment-resistant" categories, including those who are severely depressed, who have a history of sexual abuse, or who have parents who themselves are depressed. ABFT's efficacy with these patients is especially noteworthy, since these groups have typically not responded well to CBT and/or medication (Asarnow et al., 2009; Barbe et al., 2004; Curry et al., 2006).

There is an ongoing programmatic line of process research exploring proposed change mechanisms in ABFT, a recently completed clinical trial, in which investigators are measuring potential changes in markers of secure attachment, as measured by pre- and postassessments with the AAI, observational parent–teen interaction coding, and self-report. Data from the AAI will be used to test changes in adolescent attachment, while data from the interaction task will be used to measure changes in the parent–teen communication around sources of conflict, a proxy for changes in the goal-corrected partnership. Preliminary results demonstrate treatment efficacy comparable to that from prior ABFT trials. Follow-up and mediation analyses will test the attachment-specificity of ABFT treatment mechanisms (Krauthamer Ewing, Diamond, & Levy, 2015).

ABFT Training and Dissemination Efforts

The ABFT Training Program was established at Drexel University in 2013 to increase national and international training and dissemination efforts. The formal training program includes a variety of training options, ranging from introductory workshops through a complete ABFT certification program.

Through experiences during the first decade of research and training efforts, it became clear that advanced training is often needed in order to become a competent ABFT therapist. It is not enough that therapists grasp the basic concepts of ABFT from reading the manual or attending an introductory workshop. Understanding the basic concepts does not necessarily translate into masterful or even competent practice. Therapists benefit greatly from close supervision, including discussions of attachment and emotions, elaborating on case conceptualizations presented to supervisors, tape review, and feedback. Without such guidance and supervision, ABFT supervisors have observed that novice therapists often continue to use methods and techniques that contradict core components of ABFT (e.g., remaining cognitive vs. emotion-focused in sessions, taking too much of an active role in family sessions, and subverting emotional processing and enactments). Through their training experiences, ABFT supervisors have developed a detailed therapist certification program that typically occurs over a 1-year period and consists of didactic work, video review, individual feedback, and group consultation. Therapists seeking certification participate in the 1-year program, which culminates in submission of approximately 10 of their own therapy videos for review and adherence ratings by certified ABFT trainers. Trainees must achieve average adherence ratings of 3.5 or better (on a 6-point scale), in order to successfully complete the certification process. Certification never expires.

With the establishment of the formal training center and a growing empirical evidence base, national and international interest in ABFT continues to grow. The ABFT Training Program works closely with agencies to tailor training to their needs (e.g., amount of training, funding available). Many agencies have also expressed interest in adaptations of ABFT for use with new populations (e.g., foster families, eating-disordered youth), and a number of research proposals have been developed in response to these interests (Wagner, Diamond, Levy, Russon, & Litster, 2016).

Internationally, ABFT trainers have conducted workshops in Australia, Belgium, Canada, England, Germany, Iceland, India, Ireland, Israel, Italy, Norway, and Sweden. Academic teams in five of these countries (Australia, Belgium, Norway, Sweden, Turkey, and Israel) are engaged in various ABFT-related research endeavors and are moving forward with plans to develop local ABFT centers to provide training opportunities for therapists in their native languages.

In Australia, Dr. Ingrid Wagner and her team at Queensland University of Technology are adapting ABFT for use with teens with eating disorders who have not had success using traditional family-based therapy (FBT; LeGrange & Lock, 2010).

They are also researching ABFT for use with specific pediatric populations (e.g., cystic fibrosis). In Belgium, Dr. Guy Bosmans, at Katholieke Universiteit Leuven, conducted a recent study evaluating the acceptability and feasibility of ABFT training and implementation in the Belgian Child Welfare System (Santens, Devacht, Dewulf, Hermans, & Bosmans, 2016). Ongoing clinical research projects include a trial examining the effectiveness of ABFT for young adults in inpatient settings, along with an innovative program to examine whether an ABFT framework can be a useful and accepted model of daily caregiving by nursing staff members on an inpatient unit. In Norway, Dr. Pravin Israel at Akershus University Hospital and the University of Oslo examined the feasibility of importing ABFT into a hospital-based outpatient clinic (Israel & Diamond, 2013). Dr. Israel is currently conducting a randomized controlled trial (RCT) with 100 families with depressed teens to test the effectiveness of 16 weeks of ABFT compared to routine clinical treatment.

In Sweden, Dr. Magnus Ringborg and his colleagues conduct introductory and advanced ABFT trainings, as well as clinical research. Hassling (2015) evaluated the use of ABFT among Swedish therapists who attended a 3-day introductory workshop. Results provided information about important supports for therapists that optimize training and certification, including cultural adaptations and supervision of therapists in their native language. As part of efforts to address language and cultural barriers to dissemination, a Swedish translation of the ABFT treatment manual has also been published.

Finally, in Israel, a co-developer of ABFT, Dr. Gary Diamond, in the Department of Psychology at Ben Gurion University, leads ABFT training and research efforts. Clinically, Dr. Diamond conducts ABFT workshops and supervision groups with graduate students and clinicians throughout Israel. In his research laboratory, Dr. Diamond conducts ABFT outcomes and process research studies, and has examined a number of processes hypothesized to be mechanisms in ABFT, including emotional processing, changes in parental acceptance, and changes in attachment (e.g., Feder & Diamond, 2016; Moran & Diamond, 2008; Shpigel, Diamond, & Diamond, 2012). Dr. Diamond recently completed an RCT examining emotional processing within and the resulting outcomes of ABFT versus individual EFT with young adults presenting with unresolved anger toward parents (Diamond, Shahar, Sabo & Tsvieli, 2016). Dr. Diamond also oversees the Family Connection Project, which is dedicated to helping parents and other family members struggling to accept their children's same-sex sexual orientation. ABFT is utilized in the program, as therapists work to help families to remain connected in a loving, supportive, and mutually respectful manner (Diamond & Shpigel, 2014; Samarova, Shilo, & Diamond, 2014). Researchers examine the outcomes of the treatment, including how the acceptance process unfolds in families.

Conclusion and Future Directions

ABFT is a family-based treatment aimed at strengthening parent–teen relationships to help teens recover from and buffer against depression and suicide risk. With attachment theory as a core foundation, ABFT therapists help families to repair relationship injuries and barriers to trust and open communication. Kobak, Zajac, Herres, and Krauthamer Ewing (2015) propose that attachment-based interventions for adolescents can focus on several different strategies to change internal working models of self and other, and revise negative expectancies about attachment relationships.

First, an intervention model can focus on implicit/procedural processes. A therapist can model and provide a safe, emotionally attuned, and responsive environment and style of communication, which may gradually help to revise a client's expectancies and feelings of felt security, and encourage greater emotional honesty and self-reflection. For example, in ABFT's Task 2 (adolescent alliance) and Task 3 (parent alliance), therapists work to create and communicate a safe and validating therapeutic environment for both teens and parents, encouraging open communication about emotions and exploration (Kobak et al., 2015). Without success in these tasks, the relationship repair work that comes later in the model is often not as potent.

Second, an intervention can focus on specific skills and strategies such as reflective dialogue and emotional deepening in an attempt to help a client revise internal working models. In ABFT, therapists use reflective dialogue and emotional deepening to help clients develop a better understanding of their individual attachment narratives and process the core emotions associated with these experiences. This work is done individually with both teens and parents, and culminates in skills building around effective communication and dialogue strategies for family communication (assertive communication vs. aggression or withdrawal for teens; emotion coaching for parents).

Finally, Kobak et al. (2015) distinguish between interventions that focus mainly on individual intrapsychic work to access and revise internal working models and those that focus on interpersonal interactive work. In this regard, ABFT takes a *both/and* approach. With its task-based building block model, ABFT incorporates important elements of *both* intrasychic *and* interactive work. Thus, ABFT is a multimodal treatment that combines an individual focus on revising internal working models of attachment with emotion-focused communication training and practice (Kobak et al., 2015; Carey, 2011).

Fifteen years of treatment development and empirical research provide evidence that ABFT is a promising evidence-based and empirically supported treatment for teens who struggle with depression and suicidality. However, there are still many questions to be answered (Krauthamer Ewing et al., 2015). Investigators are currently analyzing results from a 5-year National Institute of Mental Health (NIMH) RCT designed to answer a number of these questions:

1. Will ABFT efficacy hold up against a more rigorous control condition (i.e., supportive therapy instead of "treatment as usual")?

2. Does treatment with ABFT lead to measurable change in adolescent attachment security/state of mind as measured with the AAI?

3. Is treatment-related change in adolescent attachment a treatment mediator for reductions in adolescent depression and suicide risk?

The findings from this study will advance scientific understanding about purported mechanisms of change in ABFT. Additionally, this study, and other ongoing ABFT related research, should continue to help researchers and clinicians develop a better and more complete understanding regarding the relational nature of suicide, the feelings of isolation, helplessness and hopelessness that often drive it, and the best ways to effect positive change with clients and their families.

REFERENCES

Adam, K. S., Sheldon-Keller, A. E., & West, M. (1996). Attachment organization and history of suicidal behavior in clinical adolescents. *Journal of Consulting and Clinical Psychology, 64,* 264–272

Allen, J. P. (2008). The attachment system in adolescence. In J. Cassidy & P. R. Shaver (Eds.), *Handbook of attachment: Theory, research, and clinical applications* (pp. 419–435). New York: Guilford Press.

Allen, J. P., Porter, M., McFarland, C., McElhaney, K. B., & Marsh, P. (2007). The relation of attachment security to adolescents' paternal and peer relationships, depression, and externalizing behavior. *Child Development, 78,* 1222–1239.

Asarnow, J. R., Emslie, G., Clarke, G., Wagner, K. D., Spirito, A., Vitiello, B., . . . Brent, D. (2009). Treatment of selective serotonin reuptake inhibitor-resistant depression in adolescents: Predictors and moderators of treatment response. *Journal of the Academy of Child and Adolescent Psychiatry, 48*(3), 330–339.

Barbe, R. P., Bridge, J. A., Birmaher, B., Kolko, D. J., & Brent, D. A. (2004). Lifetime history of sexual abuse, clinical presentation, and outcome in a clinical trial for adolescent depression. *Journal of Clinical Psychiatry, 65*(1), 77–83.

Beautrais, A. L., Joyce, P. R., & Mulder, R. T. (1996). Risk factors for serious suicide attempts among youths aged 13 through 24 years. *Journal of the American Academy of Child and Adolescent Psychiatry, 35,* 1174–1182.

Belsky, J. (1984). The determinants of parenting: A process model. *Child Development, 55*(1), 83–96.

Birmaher, B., Brent, D. A., Kolko, D., Baugher, M., Bridge, J., Holder, D., . . . Ulloa, R. E. (2000). Clinical outcome after short-term psychotherapy for adolescents with major depressive disorder. *Archives of General Psychiatry, 57*(1), 29–36.

Böszörményi-Nagy, I., & Spark, G. M. (1973). *Invisible loyalties, reciprocity in intergenerational family therapy.* Hagerstown, MD: Routledge.

Bowlby, J. (1982). *Attachment and loss: Vol. 1. Attachment.* New York: Basic Books. (Original work published 1969)

Bowlby, J. (1988). *A secure base.* New York: Basic Books.

Brent, D. A., McMakin, D. L., Kennard, B. D., Goldstein, T. R., Mayes, T. L., & Douaihy, A. B. (2013). Protecting adolescents from self-harm: A critical review of intervention studies. *Journal of the American Academy of Child and Adolescent Psychiatry, 52*(12), 1260–1271.

Brent, D. A., & Melhem, N. (2008). Familial transmission of suicidal behavior. *Psychiatric Clinics of North America, 31*(2), 157–177.

Brent, D. A., Perper, J. A., Goldstein, C. E., Kolko, D. J., Allan, M. J., Allman, C. J., & Zelenak, J. P. (1988). Risk factors for adolescent suicide: A comparison of adolescent suicide victims with suicidal inpatients. *Archives of General Psychiatry, 45*(6), 581–588.

Brent, D. A., Perper, J. A., Moritz, G., Liotus, L., Schweers, J., . . . Balach, L. (1994). Familial risk factors for adolescent suicide: A case control study. *Acta Psychiatrica Scandinavica, 89*(1), 52–58.

Bridge, J. A., Iyengar, S., Salary, C. B., Barbe, R. P., Birmaher, B., Pincus, H. A., . . . Brent, D. A. (2007). Clinical response and risk for reported suicidal ideation and suicide attempts in pediatric antidepressant treatment: A meta-analysis of randomized controlled trials. *Journal of the American Medical Association, 297*(15), 1683–1696.

Carey, T. A. (2011). Exposure and reorganization: The what and how of effective psychotherapy. *Clinical Psychology Review, 31*(2), 236–248.

Curry, J., Rohde, P., Simons, A., Silva, S., Vitiello, B., Kratochvil, C., . . . March, J. (2006). Predictors and moderators of acute outcome in the Treatment for Adolescents with Depression Study (TADS). *Journal of the American Academy of Child and Adolescent Psychiatry, 45*(12), 1427–1439.

David-Ferdon, C., & Kaslow, N. J. (2008). Evidence-based psychosocial treatments for child and adolescent depression. *Journal of Clinical Child and Adolescent Psychology, 37,* 62–104.

Diamond, G. M., Diamond, G. S., Levy, S., Closs, C., Ladipo, T., & Siqueland, L. (2012). Attachment-based family therapy for suicidal lesbian, gay, and bisexual adolescents: A treatment development study and open trial with preliminary findings. *Psychotherapy, 49*(1), 62–71.

Diamond, G. M., Shahar, B., Sabo, D., & Tsvieli, N. (2016). Attachment-based family therapy and emotion focused therapy for unresolved anger: The role of productive emotional processing. *Psychotherapy: Theory, Research and Practice, 53,* 34–44.

Diamond, G. M., & Shpigel, M. (2014). Attachment-based family therapy for lesbian and gay young adults and their persistently non-accepting parents. *Professional Psychology: Research and Practice, 45,* 258–268.

Diamond, G. S., Asarnow, J., & Hughes, J. (2016). Optimizing family intervention in the treatment of suicidal youth. In D. A. Lamis & N. J. Kaslow (Eds.), *Advancing the science of suicidal behavior: Understanding and intervention* (pp. 111–134). Hauppauge, NY: Nova Science.

Diamond, G. S., Reis, B. F., Diamond, G. M., Siqueland, L., & Isaacs, L. (2002). Attachment-based family therapy for depressed adolescents: A treatment development study. *Journal of the American Academy of Child and Adolescent Psychiatry, 41*(10), 1190–1196.

Diamond, G. S., Wintersteen, M. B., Brown, G. K., Diamond, G. M., Gallop, R., Shelef, K., & Levy, S. (2010). Attachment-based family therapy for adolescents with suicidal ideation: A randomized controlled trial. *Journal of the American Academy of Child and Adolescent Psychiatry, 49*(2), 122–131.

Ehnvall, A., Parker, G., Hadzi-Pavlovic, D., & Malhi, G. (2008). Perception of rejecting and neglectful parenting in childhood relates to lifetime suicide attempts for females–but not for males. *Acta Psychiatrica Scandinavica, 117*(1), 50–56.

Feder, M., & Diamond, G. M. (2016). Parent–therapist alliance and parent attachment promoting behaviors in attachment-based family therapy for suicidal and depressed adolescents. *Journal of Family Therapy, 38*(1), 82–101.

Fergusson, D. M., Woodward, L. J., & Horwood, L. J. (2000). Risk factors and life processes associated with the onset of suicidal behaviour during adolescence and early adulthood. *Psychological Medicine, 30*(1), 23–39.

Goldman, R. N., & Greenberg, L. S. (2015). *Case formulation in emotion-focused therapy: Co-creating clinical maps for change.* Washington, DC: American Psychological Association.

Goodyer, I., Dubicka, B., Wilkinson, P., Kelvin, R., Roberts, C., Byford, S., . . . Harrington, R. (2007). Selective serotonin reuptake inhibitors (SSRIs) and routine specialist care with and without cognitive behaviour therapy in adolescents with major depression: Randomised controlled trial. *British Medical Journal, 335*(7611), 142.

Gottman, J. M., Katz, L. F., & Hooven, C. (1996). Parental meta-emotion philosophy and the emotional life of families: Theoretical models and preliminary data. *Journal of Family Psychology, 10*, 243–268.

Greenberg, L. S. (2011). *Emotion-focused therapy*. Washington, DC: American Psychological Association.

Hardt, J., Sidor, A., Nickel, R., Kappis, B., Petrak, P., & Egle, U. T. (2008). Childhood adversities and suicide attempts: A retrospective study. *Journal of Family Violence, 23*(8), 713–718.

Hassling, T. (2015). *Why don't you go to your parents when you are feeling so miserable?: On finding the courage and getting the opportunity to work with attachment-based family therapy (ABFT)*. Unpublished master's thesis, University of Gothenburg, Gothenburg, Sweden.

Hollon, S. D., DeRubeis, R. J., Shelton, R. C., Amsterdam, J. D., Salomon, R. M., O'Reardon, J. P., . . . Gallop, R. (2005). Prevention of relapse following cognitive therapy vs medications in moderate to severe depression. *Archives of General Psychiatry, 62*(4), 417–422.

Israel, P., & Diamond, G. S. (2013). Feasibility of attachment based family therapy for depressed clinic-referred Norwegian adolescents. *Clinical Child Psychology and Psychiatry, 18*(3), 334–350.

Johnson, S. M. (2004). *The practice of emotionally focused couple therapy* (2nd ed.). New York: Brunner-Routledge.

Kobak, R., Cassidy, J., Lyons-Ruth, K., & Ziv, Y. (2006). Attachment, stress, and psychopathology: A developmental pathways model. In D. Cicchetti & D. J. Cohen (Eds.), *Developmental psychopathology: Vol 1. Theory and method* (pp. 333–369). Hoboken, NJ: Wiley.

Kobak, R., Rosenthal, N., Zajac, K., & Madsen, S. (2007). Adolescent attachment hierarchies and the search for an adult pair-bond. *New Directions for Child and Adolescent Development, 117*, 57–72.

Kobak, R., Sudler, N., & Gamble, W. (1991). Attachment and depressive symptoms during adolescence: A developmental pathways analysis. *Development and Psychopathology, 3*, 461–474.

Kobak, R., Zajac, K., Heres, J., & Krauthamer-Ewing, S. (2015). Attachment based treatments for adolescents: The secure cycle as a framework for assessment, treatment and evaluation, attachment and human development. *Attachment and Human Development, 17*(2), 220–239.

Kobak, R. R., Cole, H. E., Ferenz-Gillies, R., Fleming, W. S., & Gamble, W. (1993). Attachment and emotion regulation during mother–teen problem solving: A control theory analysis. *Child Development, 64*(1), 231–245.

Kobak, R. R., & Sceery, A. (1988). Attachment in late adolescence: Working models, affect regulation, and representations of self and others. *Child Development, 59*(1), 135–146.

Krauthamer Ewing, E. S., Diamond, G. S., & Levy, S. (2015). Attachment-based family therapy for depressed and suicidal adolescents: Theory, clinical model, and empirical support. *Attachment and Human Development, 17*, 136–156.

Kurtz, L., & Derevensky, J. L. (1993). Stress and coping in adolescents: The effects of family configuration and environment on suicidality. *Canadian Journal of School Psychology, 9*(2), 204–216.

Le Grange, D., & Lock, J. (2007) *Treating bulimia in adolescents: A family-based approach*. New York: Guilford Press.

Liddle, H. (2002). *Multidimensional Family Therapy Treatment (MDFT) for adolescent cannabis users: Volume 5 of the Cannabis Youth Treatment (CYT) manual series*. Rockville, MD: Center for Substance Abuse Treatment, Substance Abuse and Mental Health Services.

Liddle, H. A., & Diamond, G. S. (1991). Adolescent substance abusers in family therapy: The critical initial phase of treatment. *Family Dynamics of Addiction Quarterly, 1*, 55–68.

Main, M., & Goldwyn, R. (1998). *Adult attachment classification system*. Unpublished manuscript, University of California, Berkeley, Berkeley, CA.

Main, M., Hesse, E., & Goldwyn, R. (2008). Study differences in language usage in recounting attachment history. In H. Steele & M. Steele (Eds.), *Clinical applications of the Adult Attachment Interview* (pp. 31–69). New York: Guilford Press.

March, J., Silva, S., Petrycki, S., Curry, J., Wells, K., Fairbank, J., . . . Severe, J. (2004). Fluoxetine, cognitive-behavioral therapy, and their combination for adolescents with depression: Treatment for Adolescents With Depression Study (TADS) randomized controlled trial. *Journal of the American Medical Association, 292*(7), 807–820.

Marsh, P., McFarland, F. C., Allen, J. P., McElhaney, K. B., & Land, D. (2003). Attachment, autonomy and multifinality in adolescent internalizing and risky behavioral symptoms. *Development and Psychopathology, 15,* 451–467.

McCullough, M. E., Pargament, K. I., & Thoresen, C. E. (2000). *Forgiveness: Theory, research, and practice.* New York: Guilford Press.

McKeown, R. E., Garrison, C. Z., Cuffe, S. P., Waller, J. L., Jackson, K. L., & Addy, C. L. (1998). Incidence and predictors of suicidal behaviors in a longitudinal sample of young adolescents. *Journal of the American Academy of Child and Adolescent Psychiatry, 37*(6), 612–619.

Minuchin, S. (1974). *Families and family therapy.* Cambridge, MA: Harvard University Press.

Moran, G., & Diamond, G. M. (2008). Generating nonnegative attitudes among parents of depressed adolescents: The power of empathy, concern and positive regard. *Psychotherapy Research, 18,* 97–107.

Mufson, L., Dorta, K. P., Moreau, D., & Weissman, M. M. (2004). *Interpersonal psychotherapy for depressed adolescents* (2nd ed.). New York: Guilford Press.

Mufson, L., Gallagher, T., Dorta, K., & Young, J. (2004). A group adaptation of interpersonal psychotherapy for depressed adolescents. *American Journal of Psychotherapy, 58*(2), 220–237.

Mufson, L., Weissman, M. M., Moreau, D., & Garfinkel, R. (1999). Efficacy of interpersonal psychotherapy for depressed adolescents. *Archives of General Psychiatry, 56,* 573–579.

Resnick, H. S., Acierno, R., & Kilpatrick, D. G. (1997). Health impact of interpersonal violence: 2. Medical and mental health outcomes. *Behavioral Medicine, 23*(2), 65–78.

Rice, L., & Greenberg, L. (Eds.). (1984). *Patterns of change: An intensive analysis of psychotherapeutic process.* New York: Guilford Press.

Rossello, J., & Bernal, G. (1999). The efficacy of cognitive-behavioral and interpersonal treatments for depression in Puerto Rican adolescents. *Journal of Consulting and Clinical Psychology, 67,* 734–745.

Rotheram-Borus, M., Piacentini, J., Miller, S., Graae, F., Dunne, E., & Cantwell, C. (1996). Toward improving treatment adherence among adolescent suicide attempters. *Clinical Child Psychology and Psychiatry, 1*(1), 99–108.

Rubenstein, J. L., Halton, A., Kasten, L., Rubin, C., & Stechler, G. (1998). Suicidal behavior in adolescents. *American Journal of Orthopsychiatry, 68*(2), 274–284.

Salzinger, S., Rosario, M., & Feldman, R. S. (2007). Physical child abuse and adolescent violent delinquency: The mediating and moderating roles of personal relationships. *Child Maltreatment, 12*(3), 208–219.

Samarova, V., Shilo, G., & Diamond, G. M. (2014). Changes over time in parents' acceptance of their Israeli sexual minority adolescents. *Journal of Research on Adolescence, 24,* 681–688.

Santens, T., Devacht, I., Dewulf, S., Hermans, G., & Bosmans, G. (2016). Attachment-based family therapy between Magritte and Poirot: Dissemination dreams, challenges, and solutions in Belgium. *Australian and New Zealand Journal of Family Therapy, 37,* 240–250.

Shpigel, M., Diamond, G. M., & Diamond, G. S. (2012). Changes in parenting behaviors in attachment-based family therapy. *Journal of Marital and Family Therapy, 38,* 271–283.

Spirito, A., Boergers, J., Donaldson, D., Bishop, D., & Lewander, W. (2002). An intervention trial to improve adherence to community treatment by adolescents after a suicide attempt. *Journal of the American Academy of Child and Adolescent Psychiatry, 41*(4), 435–442.

Spirito, A., & Esposito-Smythers, C. (2006). Attempted and completed suicide in adolescence. *Annual Review of Clinical Psychology, 2*, 237–266.

Sroufe, L. A. (2005) Attachment and development: A prospective, longitudinal study from birth to adulthood. *Attachment and Human Development, 7*, 349–367.

Steinberg, L. (1990). Autonomy, conflict, and harmony in the family relationship. In S. Feldman & G. Elliot (Eds.), *At the threshold: The developing adolescent* (pp. 255–276). Cambridge, MA: Harvard University Press.

Tarrier, N., Taylor, K., & Gooding, P. (2008). Cognitive-behavioral interventions to reduce suicide behavior: A systematic review and meta-analysis. *Behavior Modification, 32*(1), 77–108.

van IJzendoorn, M. H. (1995). Adult attachment representations, parental responsiveness, and infant attachment: A meta-analysis on the predictive validity of the Adult Attachment Interview. *Psychological Bulletin, 117*(3), 387–403.

Wagner, B. M. (1997). Family risk factors for child and adolescent suicidal behavior. *Psychological Bulletin, 121*(2), 246–298.

Wagner, B. M., Silverman, M. A. C., & Martin, C. E. (2003). Family factors in youth suicidal behaviors. *American Behavioral Scientist, 46*(9), 1171–1191.

Wagner, I., Diamond, G. S., Levy, S., Russon, J., & Litster, R. (2016). Attachment-based family therapy as an adjunct to family-based treatment for adolescent anorexia nervosa. *Australian and New Zealand Journal of Family Therapy, 37*, 207–227.

Weisz, J. R., Jensen-Doss, A., & Hawley, K. M. (2006). Evidence-based youth psychotherapies versus usual clinical care: A meta-analysis of direct comparisons. *American Psychologist, 61*(7), 671–689.

Weisz, J. R., McCarty, C. A., & Valeri, S. M. (2006). Effects of psychotherapy for depression in children and adolescents: A meta-analysis. *Psychological Bulletin, 132*(1), 132–149.

Wells, K., & Albano, A. M. (2005). Involving parents in CBT treatment of adolescent depression: Experiences in the TADS. *Cognitive and Behavioral Practice, 12*, 209–220.

Yap, M. B. H., Allen, N. B., & Sheeber, L. (2007). Using an emotion regulation framework to understand the role of temperament and family processes in risk for adolescent depressive disorders. *Clinical Child and Family Psychology, 10*(2), 180–196.

Zhang, J., & Jin, S. (1996). Determinants of suicide ideation: A comparison of Chinese and American college students. *Adolescence, 31*(122), 451–467.

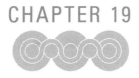

CHAPTER 19

Mentalization-Based Therapy for Adolescents

Managing Storms in Youth Presenting with Self-Harm and Suicidal States

TRUDIE ROSSOUW

This chapter details an evidence-based attachment-informed treatment for self-harming adolescents with suicidal states of mind, who typically live with highly adverse histories and threatening contemporary social contexts. The treatment is mentalization-based therapy for adolescents (MBT-A). The chapter is organized into seven sections: (1) a summary of recent research on the adolescent mind and experience; (2) the prevalence of self-harm during adolescence; (3) mentalization as a framework for understanding self-harm; (4) the structure of MBT-A; (5) specific techniques relied on in delivering MBT-A; (6) randomized controlled trial (RCT) results from a study comparing MBT-A to treatment as usual; and (7) a case example.

The Adolescent Mind and Experience

The original explorers of the Cape in South Africa described it either as the "Cape of storms" or the "Cape of good hope," which to some extent depicts the adolescent experience. As stormy as the seas can get, so can the days of clarity, calm, and hope. While being seen by their parents as risky, unstable, and unpredictable, adolescents describe themselves as passionate, capable, and craving responsibility, choice, and ownership. Why such a stark difference in perception? Is it in the brain?

Systematic research found that the logical–reasoning abilities of 15-year-olds are comparable to those of adults (Reyna & Farley, 2006). However, unlike logical–reasoning abilities, psychosocial capacities that improve decision making and moderate risk taking—such as impulse control, emotion regulation, delay of gratification, and resistance to peer influence—continue to mature well into young adulthood (Steinberg, 2004). The greatest mismatches in the development of these systems occur in adolescence. Additionally, adolescents show an increase in sensation seeking (Steinberg, 2004), which may in part be due to the remodeling of the dopaminergic system (Steinberg, 2008). These changes contribute to young people being more affected by their emotional context when they make decisions. In her neuroimaging studies, Yurgelun-Todd (2007) demonstrated that in reading about emotional material, adolescents showed brain activity in the limbic areas suggestive of subjective emotional experiences, whereas adults did not show the same. The latter finding might go some way in explaining why adolescents are so powerfully influenced by the feelings of others around them. Those of us working in inpatient units know very well how an emotional reaction in one adolescent create a ripple effect for others, triggering self-harming or acting-out behavior. This ripple effect can so easily be described by staff as "attention seeking," yet with neuroscience in mind, it is clear to see how a limbic discharge in one young person stimulates a similar discharge in another young person. Young people describe how they often feel at a loss to understand or explain their state and often describe themselves as being overtaken by overwhelming feelings that do not make sense. These states are often intolerable, and in order to cope, they just have to get rid of them through acting-out behavior, which usually results in immediate (albeit short-lived) relief.

Moving from the neuroscientific domain to the social and psychological domain of adolescence, both social and psychological domains comes together under an attachment umbrella, as it is indeed adolescents' attachment backgrounds that have been shown to have a considerable influence on their ability to cope with the developmental issues of this crucial transitional period (Dubois-Comtois et al., 2013). Cognitive and socioemotional changes lead to revisions and, at times, disturbances of the adolescent's internal working models of attachment. Adolescents with the highest risk of developing adaptation problems present with an insecure attachment profile (Dubois-Comtois, Cyr, Pascuzzo, Lessard, & Poulin, 2013). In their 11-year follow-up study, Allen, Hauser, and Borman-Spurrell (1996) demonstrated similar findings, in that a group of hospitalized adolescents who were followed up 11 years later all demonstrated insecure attachment organization. They suggested a strong connection between attachment organization and severe adolescent psychopathology, with attachment organization mediating some of the long-term sequelae of psychopathology. Similarly, resilience research demonstrated that the internal working model of attachment is a part of the adaptational system related to resilience (Truesdale, 2002).

The adolescent phase is a window period of vulnerability, but potentially also offers opportunities and hope. It is noteworthy, however that three quarters of mental health problems start before the age of 20 (Kessler et al., 2005). The most frequent difficulties in teenage years are anxiety, depression, self-harm, eating disorders, substance misuse and conduct disorders, as well as attention-deficit/hyperactivity disorder (ADHD). Although diagnosing personality disorder before age 18 has been a contentious issue, the onset of personality disorder before age 18 is now recognized in DSM-5 (American Psychiatric Association, 2013) and studies are beginning to show a clear link between those young people who presented with a personality disorder before age 18 and poorer global functioning at age 30 (Crawford et al., 2008). Clearly, interventions, which can be successful during this phase of life, can potentially turn around psychopathological trajectories that may otherwise have stretched into adult life with significant impact on global functioning. This chapter explores self-harm in adolescents and looks at mentalization-based therapy for adolescents (MBT-A) as a possible effective intervention.

Self-Harm in Young People

Alice, an attractive, 14-year-old young woman, comes from a loving home and has a close relationship with her mother and a good relationship with her father, who is divorced from her mother. Although she is quite beautiful and intelligent, Alice sees herself as ugly and stupid, and describes how she hates everything about herself. She does not have friends, because she easily feels misunderstood by people, which leads to her feeling angry and disappointed, and eventually pushing people away. She is easily overwhelmed with feelings of loneliness, anger, and anxiety, and her subjective experience of that is an overwhelming feeling of self-hatred. In this state, the only thing Alice can think of is a desire to cut herself, and she has fantasies of seeing her skin open deeply with the inside bulging out. She is clear that she does not want to kill herself, that her desire is only to cut herself. She is also clear that it has to be a deep wound, because only a deep wound would lead to a feeling of calm. In Alice's words, a deep cut makes her feel proud of herself, and that makes her feel calm. Seeing other young people with big purple scars on their arms overwhelms her with a desire to have the same.

All over the Western world, young people are harming themselves, and in some schools it has almost become a group-led gothic kind of fashion statement: a grungy display of hardness ("Look at the pain I can bear") and softness ("Look at the pain I am feeling inside"). Self-harm is often done outside the awareness of parents or teachers. It is not uncommon for young people to have a history of self-harm for a couple of years before their parents become aware of it. Self-harm is often featured in teenage magazines and teenage fiction. Like the example of Alice, self-harm is often a way of coping with overwhelming feelings, because it transforms mental pain into physical pain, which is far more bearable.

In an interview with *The Guardian,* Margot Waddell (Gerard, 2002) was quoted as saying: "Cutters . . . are not stupid or mad, but maybe they are trying to tell us something about their inner lives and can't find the words. So they unscrew the blade of their pencil sharpener and draw it over their skin. Blood flows. 'Look at me,' they're saying. 'Look how I hurt. Look.' And we should look."

The majority of people who self-harm are between ages 11 and 25 (Mental Health Foundation, 2006). A Scottish self report found that 14% of pupils between 15–16 claimed to have self-harmed (O'Connor, Rasmussen, Miles, & Hawton, 2009). The rates in girls were three times as high as those in boys. Rates of self-harm are on a steady incline every year. The rates of self-harm are higher in vulnerable groups, such as children in care and those in the juvenile justice system. Inpatient studies indicated self-harm rates between 60 and 80% of patients (DiClemente, Ponton, & Hartley, 1991; Nixon, Cloutier, & Jansson, 2008).

Self-harm refers to all acts of harm to oneself, including self-cutting, burning, self-poisoning, overdoses, attempted hanging, jumping from heights or bridges, and so forth. Self-harming acts can be with or without suicidal intent. Some studies suggested that there are distinct differences between a nonsuicidal self-harming group and a suicidal group, with the suicidal group presenting more with depression and posttraumatic stress disorder (PTSD) and the nonsuicidal group presenting more with personality disorder features (Jacobson, Muehlenkamp, Miller, & Turner, 2008). However, other researchers found that there is often a great overlap between the groups, with one-third of young people who engage in self-harm displaying suicidal feelings or intent during some of their self-harming acts (Brown, Comtois, & Linehan, 2002; Nock, Joiner, Gordon, Lloyd-Richardson, & Prinstein, 2006). Among adolescents in the United States, suicide is the greatest cause of death, and it is the second greatest cause of death in the rest of the developed world (Asarnow et al., 2011). Self-harm is the single greatest predictor of completed suicide (Gunnell & Frankel, 1994), with 40–50% of people who die by suicide having a prior history of self-harm (Hawton et al., 2003). Studies indicated that nonsuicidal self-harm in depressed adolescents prior to the onset of treatment was significantly linked with subsequent suicidal attempts (Wilkinson, Kelvin, Roberts, Dubicka, & Goodyer, 2011; Asarnow et al., 2011).

Increased rates of self-harm have been associated with family conflict (Bridge, Goldstein, & Brent, 2006), physical abuse (Hawton, Rodham, & Evans, 2006), sexual abuse (Fergusson, Horwood, & Lynskey, 1996), and parental mental health problems (Brent, 1995). Strong links were demonstrated with depressive disorders, hopelessness, and suicidal thoughts (Wilkinson et al., 2011; Haavisto et al., 2004). Cluster B personality disorders have been found to convey a greater risk for adolescent suicide, even after researchers control for the effects of mood, conduct, and substance disorders (Brent et al., 1993).

Adult outcomes of young people who harmed themselves indicate that over 30% of the sample harmed themselves repeatedly into adulthood (Harrington et al., 2006; Brezo et al., 2007). Mortality rates varied from 0.17% to 1.8% (Brezo et al., 2007; Hawton et al., 2008; Reith, Whyte, & Carter, 2003). Depression both in adolescence and in adulthood also almost always accompanies the suicidal attempt, and some studies indicate that the pathway to repeat attempts is through the link between depression and hopelessness creating suicidal ideation (Fergusson, Beautrais, & Horwood, 2003; Goldston et al., 2001). However, Fergusson et al. (2003) found that a much larger group of depressed young people did not harm themselves, which led them to explore vulnerability and resilient factors.

Mentalization as a Framework for Understanding Self-Harm

Allen (2004) describes that mentalizing is what renders behavior intelligible and that it is the basis of self-awareness and sensitivity to others.

Mentalization is the capacity to understand actions in terms of thoughts and feelings. Self-harm in adolescents occurs in response to relationship stress, when the individual fails to represent the social experience in terms of mental states (Bateman & Fonagy, 2004). When mentalizing is compromised, self-related negative cognitions are experienced with great intensity, leading to both intense depression and an urgent need for distraction. Furthermore, when nonmentalizing leads to social isolation (e.g., as with Alice), engaging in self-harm and manipulative behavior may restore reconnection (Zanarini, Frankenburg, Hennen, Reich, & Silk, 2006). When mentalization of social experience fails, impulsive (poorly regulated) behaviors and subjective states triggering self-harm become prominent.

Mentalization- based therapy (MBT) was originally developed by Peter Fonagy and Anthony Bateman for the treatment of adult patients with personality disorder. In their subsequent RCT comparing MBT and treatment as usual (TAU) for adult patients diagnosed with borderline personality disorder (BPD), they found that the group receiving MBT made significant improvements compared with the TAU group in terms of reduction in suicidality, borderline symptoms, and improvement in global functioning and vocational status (Bateman & Fonagy, 1999). These gains were maintained at the eight year follow-up (Bateman & Fonagy, 2008). Given the high prevalence of self harm in young people, as well as the close association between self harm and suicide, and the lack of any effective treatment intervention for this clinical group (Ougrin & Latif, 2011), Rossouw and Fonagy (2012) developed MBT-A, an adapted version of the treatment for use with adolescents. They conducted an RCT, comparing MBT-A and TAU for adolescent presenting with self-harm.

MBT is a psychodynamic therapeutic intervention that incorporates some elements of cognitive, interpersonal, systemic, and integrative therapies. Mentalization is a skill that renders subjective states and relationships intelligible. If you think about feelings you are mentalizing, if you empathize you are mentalizing, if you think to yourself, "Maybe he is doing that because he feels hurt, because I misunderstood him," you are mentalizing. We do this implicitly all the time without thinking, but when under stress, we fall prey to impairment in these automatic skills. When gripped by mentalization failure, we can confuse our own feelings with the feelings of others and in that way, instead of thinking they do what they do because of feelings *they* have inside them, we start to ascribe *our* feelings to them. The loss of capacity to mentalize in one person rarely exists in a vacuum; it often migrates into the interpersonal world, creating mentalization failures in those around the person; hence, one can see how this may frequently get hold of an entire team dynamic. This is especially true for those who work with complex patients or in inpatient units or complex teams. Once mentalization can be restored in teams or families, difficulties can be understood and ways to resolve the conflict become clearer.

Mentalization programs and training for teams (and families) and clinicians create a sense of curiosity about mental states in others. Like the mother who treats her infant as an intentional being whose communication can be understood, we, too, can treat others with whom we work with or whom we treat as if their intentionality has meaning that can be understood. As the baby becomes aware of itself based on the way the mother made sense of the baby's internal states, we, too, can help others to find meaning in themselves and in their interpersonal relationships. In the ward, where an acting-out patient causes chaos and great anxiety and staff members act out in response with knee-jerk, harsh responses, it is not hard to see how meaning and understanding get surpassed by action and reaction. However, the situation can very easily be turned around with a mentalizing approach—what happened before the acting out? What did the patient feel? What emotion was so overwhelming that it could not be mentalized? Did we as staff members do anything that contributed to the feeling?

In this way, mentalization puts action on hold in order to make room for time to engage in reflection: Who is feeling what and why? Are there any misperceptions? Did we say or do something or miss something that may have made the patient feel ignored or abandoned? Behavior can then be understood in the context of feelings and thoughts. Feelings and intentional states that are felt to be too overwhelming to bear can lead to acting out as described, but once shared with another, they can be metabolized and mentalized, and be given a different meaning that is more representative of reality and more bearable, reducing the need for acting out.

Mentalization is not a new skill, and neither is MBT a new intervention. It brings together aspects of developmental, analytic, and attachment theories to generate an understanding of how we all come to develop the capacity to understand others and to regulate our own internal states. As a treatment intervention, it brings together aspects of various interventions, with the ultimate aim to enhance the capacity to mentalize in our patients in the context of high emotional arousal. This will to turn passivity into mastery, and helplessness in families into greater connectedness and reciprocity.

Structure of Treatment Following the MBT-A Model

The capacity to mentalize is typically impaired when individuals are stressed. Adolescents in particular are prone to relapses in their ability to mentalize in the face of even mild interpersonal stress. During these moments, they experience an increasing sense that people do not make sense. They misrepresent others' motives, often seeing others as judging, attacking, or humiliating them. This may lead to acting-out behavior in an attempt to control the other or undo dysphoric internal states. Thus, strengthening the capacity of young people to mentalize, particularly under stress, may lead to an improved sense of agency and self-control, and protect against affect dysregulation and impulse control problems (Fonagy, 1998). In addition, by creating more accurate representations of the mind of the other, as well as forming a clearer understanding of one's own contribution to the behavior of others, enhanced mentalization facilitates self-compassion and empathy for others (Bleiberg, Roussow, & Fonagy, 2012).

Unlike models of cognitive-behavioral therapy with similar aims, the focus of MBT work is on affect, not cognition. This means forming an attachment relationship with the patient within which unmentalized affects—often comprising early feelings of being uncared for—can be explored (Bateman & Fonagy, 2004). A central assumption is that strong affective states derail the capacity to mentalize, and that distorted representations are secondary to the mentalization failure. To form more accurate representations, the capacity to mentalize needs to be restored. An overview of the structure of MBT-A is summarized in Table 19.1.

TABLE 19.1. Overview of MBT-A Structure

Outpatient treatment	Inpatient/day patient treatment
Weekly individual MBT-A therapy	Twice-a-week MBT-A individual therapy
Monthly or twice-monthly MBT family therapy	Weekly MBT family therapy
	Twice-a-week MBT group therapy

As shown in Table 19.1, treatment is a combination of individual and family MBT therapy. The frequency of sessions depends on the treatment program. Outpatient programs tend to offer individual therapy once a week and family MBT (MBT-F) once a month, whereas more intensive programs such as inpatient or day patient programs offer individual therapy twice a week, MBT-F once a week, and MBT group therapy twice a week. The duration of therapy also depends on the program. The therapy is manualized, and regular supervision with a mentalizing ethos is one of the posttraining requirements.

Treatment is divided into four phases, with expectations of what may be achieved in each. After the assessment phase, each MBT-A therapist offers a written formulation that contains a crisis plan for the young person and his or her family. The aim of subsequent sessions of the therapy is to enhance patients' capacity to represent their own and others' feelings more accurately in situations that tend to evoke intense emotions. The MBT-A sessions are generally unstructured but focus on the young person's current and recent interpersonal experiences, including the mental states evoked by these experiences. The aim of the family sessions is to improve family members' ability to mentalize, particularly in the context of family conflict that may involve either the designated young person or other family members. As in other models of psychodynamic psychotherapy that are based on ideas from attachment theory, the final phase of the therapy addresses separation issues, along with managing anticipated challenges in a mentalizing manner.

Specific Techniques of MBT-A

The MBT-A therapist is an active participant in the session, and his or her keen interest and curiosity in the patient should be evident throughout. The therapist prioritizes learning about the patient's feelings; if behavior is described, then the therapist's aim is to understand the mental state underneath it. The therapist sees him- or herself as a participant in the dynamic interaction between therapist and patient and takes responsibility for the fact that what he or she says or does can have an emotional impact on the patient. Similarly, misunderstandings on his or her part can evoke painful experiences in the patient, for which the therapist will need to take responsibility. This attitude by the therapist has been described as the *therapeutic stance* (Bateman & Fonagy, 2004).

Building a strong therapeutic alliance, making authentic emotional contact, and interacting in a supportive capacity are central to this work. These characteristics are of particular importance in working with adolescents, and even more so in working with young people with vulnerable self-esteem. It is important to remember that these youngsters may suffer from profound feelings of inadequacy associated with great difficulty in regulating self-experience and experiencing consistently positive self-regard. In fact, they are acutely sensitive to any experience that may exacerbate their sense of inadequacy or threaten their self-esteem. Thus, the first goal of MBT is to form an empathic and supportive alliance, then to try to improve mentalization.

Driven by early experiences of lack of attunement by caregivers—experiences that may lead to a sense of an "alien self" (Fonagy, Gergely, Jurist, & Target, 2002)—these young people have an expectation that those around them will fail them, leave them, or reject them. Furthermore, as a consequence of the effect of the sense of an alien self, these young people's sense of competence, and hence their confidence, is typically shattered, leading to a profound sense of failure. These young people usually have no sense of their own worth, skills, or talents, nor do they have any self-compassion. In MBT, the therapist sometimes embodies a counterpart to the sense of an alien self by being affirming, warm, compassionate, and validating—therapeutic elements that are, of course, also present in many other treatment modalities. In addition, to establish a therapeutic alliance with these youngsters and to maintain emotional contact, it is crucial for the therapist to be both authentic and explicit about his or her intentions, perceptions, and experiences in the session. An example of this is illustrated in the case discussion below.

These young people are typically so poor at perceiving their own and others' mental states that making thoughts explicit, especially in the beginning of therapy, is critical to the work. An example of this is the *written formulation,* which is a reflection of the therapist's mentalization of the difficulties that brought the patient to therapy. The formulation, given to the patient in the third session of therapy, is originally provided in draft form, then finalized jointly with the help of the patient. In this way it represents the therapist's thoughts but is based on a discussion with the patient.

Bateman and Fonagy (2004) coined the term *teleological thinking* to refer to a nonmentalizing state of mind in which there is a great reliance on literal facts and a great mistrust of anything in the absence of concrete "proof." For example, a patient will "know" you do not like him or her because you were 10 minutes late for a session—if you liked him or her, you would have been on time. Sometimes, too, individuals who struggle to mentalize overly rely on small bits of concrete evidence: Once during a session with me, a young man looked at his mobile phone, then shouted that his girlfriend was unfaithful. He said he knew this because he sent her a message to meet and she had not responded. It turned out he sent the message only a few minutes earlier.

Some adolescents treat thoughts, feelings, and memories not as mental content, but as concrete facts in reality, a phenomenon termed *psychic equivalence* (Bateman & Fonagy, 2004). This leads to an inability both to imagine a different perspective and to consider alternative possibilities. These states often lead to paranoid and anxious feelings that trigger affective storms, resulting in dysregulation and impulsive behavior. Therapeutic techniques, such as pausing and rewinding, help to slow the process down: "Hang on, can we slow down a bit? I want to make some sense and understand what is going on a bit." Exploration of what the young person feels, as well as clarification of what happened in the relevant interpersonal context, provides the building blocks of mentalizing the moment. Introducing the possibility of alternative perspectives, as well as some challenge to the fixed nonmentalizing state of mind, can restore mentalization abilities and reduce impulsive acting out.

The focus of the therapeutic work is in the here and now, especially detailed attention to the affective state of the patient. In the face of a mentalizing failure, the therapist tries to rewind to what happened before the failure, then attempts to establish both the affective and the interpersonal context in which the failure occurred. As noted earlier, the underlying therapeutic assumption is that such failures result from an unmentalized affect in an interpersonal context, and that once this has been identified and understood, mentalizing abilities will be restored (momentarily).

In fact, misperceptions and assumptions about the mental states and intentions of others often lead to extremely strong feelings that can tip into impulsive behavior, even before the feelings register consciously. By being fine-tuned to the dysregulation in these young people, therapists can help them slow down and try to make sense of what happened in that moment. By more accurately reflecting on their own internal states and developing greater curiosity about the mental states of others, these young people are less overwhelmed by abandonment anxieties and less vulnerable to self-esteem collapse, which protects them against affect storms and hence the need to act out.

In an attempt to mentalize the moment, the therapist uses various different techniques to identify the affect of the patient, such as affect elaboration, exploration, and clarification. Asking a patient to clarify his or her experiences by requesting specific details can open up intricate and subtle emotional tones. Similarly, affect elaboration and exploration refer to exploring affects in more detail, with the assumption that multiple affect states may be present rather than a single, easily focused upon affect. Consider, for example, a boy who stormed up a set of stairs and kicked the potted plants of his neighbors until they broke. Although his behavior may appear angry (and may be identified as such), detailed exploration of the preceding moments revealed feelings of hurt, humiliation, anxiety, and anger—all of which he experienced when he was attacked by a group of children minutes earlier. Therapists may also use themselves (i.e., refer to themselves) to connect with the patient's underlying affective state, such as saying, "I know I am not you, and we don't feel the same, but I think if that happened to me, I would have felt. . . ."

A formal paradigm of sitting in a chair in an office for nearly an hour talking to a stranger can be a terrifying experience for young people. I have conducted many sessions, particularly in inpatient contexts, while going for a walk with a patient or sitting outside. What seems crucial is that these patients experience the therapist's great interest in them and validation of them.

In addition to the task of helping them mentalize, therapists need to help these young people with the life tasks they fear and avoid, such as going to school. Concrete, practical help to address the difficulties they have is crucial to the recovery of their sense of mastery and hope and, ultimately, in restoring their self-esteem.

An RCT of the Effectiveness of MBT-A for Self-Harming Adolescents

Eighty patients presenting with self-harm to services in the northeast of London were recruited and randomly allocated to TAU or MBT-A (Rossouw & Fonagy, 2012). All treatments were outpatient treatments. MBT-A consisted of one session of individual MBT-A per week and one session of MBT-F per month. All therapists in the MBT-A arm of the study were trained in MBT-A and participated in weekly group supervision. The treatment program lasted 1 year. The case participants in the TAU group received the following: an individual therapeutic intervention alone (28%), consisting of counseling (with 38% of cases receiving an individual intervention), generic supportive interventions (24%), cognitive-behavioral therapy (19%) or psychodynamic psychotherapy (19%); a combination of individual therapy and family work (25%); or psychiatric review alone (27.5%).

The primary outcome was self-harm assessed by self-report at baseline and every 3 months until 12 months after randomization, using the self-harm scale of the Risk-Taking and Self-Harm Inventory (RTSHI; Vrouva, Fonagy, Fearon, & Rossow, 2010). Secondary outcomes included depression measured every 3 months by the 13-item Mood and Feelings Questionnaire (MFQ). (Crick, Murray-Close, & Woods, 2005). Two measures related to hypothesized mechanisms of change were also administered before and after treatment. Mentalization was assessed using the How I Feel (HIF) questionnaire (unpublished data, 2008). Attachment status was assessed using the Experiences in Close Relationships (ECR) scale developed by Brennan, Clark, and Shaver (1988). Patients presented with a variety of self-harm methods: 95% had a history of cutting or were currently cutting; 64% had taken an overdose at least once; and 80% reported attempting suicide either in the index episode or in the past. Results are summarized in Table 19.2.

The mean age of participants was 14 years, 7 months, and 85% of the sample was female. Although the TAU group was slightly younger, there was no difference between the groups in term of pubertal staging. In all, 75% of the sample were White, 10% were Asian, 5% were Black, 7.5% were of mixed race, and 2.5% were "other." Approximately half of the sample had started self-harming 5 months previously or more recently. There was a high level of mental disorder: 97% met criteria for depression, and 73% for BPD. Of the participants, 28% reported substance misuse, and 44% reported alcohol problems. A slightly higher proportion of the TAU group (53%) than the MBT-A group (30%) had a prior history of involvement with mental health services, but the difference was not statistically significant.

As indicated in Table 19.2, in terms of self-harm, those adolescents who received MBT-A fared relatively better than the TAU group, in that the MBT-A group demonstrated a recovery of 44% compared with 17% in the TAU group. Table 19.2 also indicates a reduction in depression scores on the MFQ, along with decreased self-harm. The standardized mean difference (SMD) between baseline and posttreatment depression scores for the MBT-A group was 1.12 (Cohen's $d = 0.49$), indicating moderate improvement. It has been suggested that depression is central in triggering self-harm, and the significant correlation between MFQ and self-harm scores ($r = .80$, $d = 0.41$, $p = .001$) may provide grounds for optimism that, at least in those adolescents whose depression remains improved, the decrease in self-harm may also be maintained beyond the end of the trial.

TABLE 19.2. Summary of the RCT

Continuous measure	Self-harm (RTSHI): log mean (SE)		Risk-taking (RTSHI): log mean (SE)		Depression (MFQ): mean (SE)	
	TAU (n = 40)	MBT-A (n = 40)	TAU (n = 40)	MBT-A (n = 40)	TAU (n = 40)	MBT-A (n = 40)
Baseline	3.08 (0.10)	3.12 (0.09)	1.92 (0.14)	2.29 (0.11)	16.32 (0.74)	17.46 (0.843)
3 months	2.19 (0.18)	2.02 (0.19)	1.45 (0.17)	1.69 (0.15)	12.89 (1.01)	12.11 (1.22)
6 months	2.21 (0.20)	1.98 (0.17)	1.59 (0.14)	1.67 (0.14)	12.79 (1.15)	12.34 (1.08)
9 months	2.04 (0.21)	1.37 (0.20)	1.46 (0.14)	1.25 (0.16)	11.66 (1.17)	7.76 (1.01)
12 months	2.01 (0.21)	1.33 (0.22)	1.66 (0.14)	1.6 (0.16)	11.54 (1.14)	9.26 (1.27)
	Coefficient (CI = 95%)		Coefficient (CI = 95%)		Coefficient (CI = 95%)	
Model: Wald χ^2(df = 5)	150.25***		70.37***		65.02***	
Linear change (both groups)	−0.92*** (−1.18 to −0.66)		−0.56*** (−0.75 to −0.37)		−4.12*** (−6.00 to −2.24)	
Quadratic change (both groups)	0.11*** (0.07 to 0.15)		0.08*** (0.05 to 0.11)		0.51*** (0.21 to 0.80)	
Differential linear change (MBT-A)	−0.19** (−0.32 to −0.07)		−0.13** (−0.21 to −0.04)		−0.93* (−1.82 to −0.05)	
Group differences at 12 months	−0.74** (−1.32 to −0.15)		−0.21 (−0.60 to 0.19)		−3.31* (−6.49 to −0.12)	

(continued)

TABLE 19.2. Summary of the RCT

Categorical measure	Self-harm (RTSHI): *n/N* (%)		Depressed (MFQ): *n/N* (%)	
	TAU	MBT-A	TAU	MBT-A
Baseline	40/40(100%)	40/40(100%)	38/40(95%)	39/40(98%)
3 months	33/37(89%)	29/35(83%)	29/37(38%)	22/35(63%)
6 months	31/36(86%)	33/39(85%)	25/34(74%)	27/38(71%)
9 months	28/34(82%)	22/35(63%)	23/33(70%)	14/34(41%)
12 months	29/35(83%)	20/36(56%)	25/37(68%)	19/39(49%)
	Odds ratio (CI = 95%)		**Odds ratio (CI = 95%)**	
Model: Wald χ^2(*df* = 5)	9.76*		22.17***	
Linear change (both groups)	1.20 (0.46 to 3.06)		0.18** (0.05 to 0.65)	
Quadratic change (both groups)			1.25* (1.04 to 1.52)	
Differential linear change (MBT-A)	0.29* (0.10 to 0.89)		0.68 (0.41 to 1.14)	
Group differences at 12 months	0.24** (0.08 to 0.76)		0.21* (0.05 to 0.98)	

Note. TAU, treatment as usual; CI, confidence interval.

*p; **p; ***p.

Although we (Rossouw & Fonagy, 2012) did not aim to recruit individuals with BPD, nearly three-fourths of those referred met DSM criteria for BPD. The rate of BPD in this sample is higher than rates of BPD found in community studies; however, higher rates of BPD in adolescents with self-harm have been reported in other clinical samples (Jacobson et al., 2008). As indicated in Table 19.2, we noticed a reduction in both BPD diagnoses and BPD traits in the MBT-A group at the end of treatment, in line with previous reports of MBT in moderating BPD symptoms (Bateman & Fonagy, 2008; Fonagy, 1998).

The study explored the impact of MBT-A on two potential mechanisms of change: attachment and mentalization. Self-rated attachment avoidance and mentalization, but not attachment anxiety, changed in the MBT-A group. The change in mentalizing did not account for attachment avoidance, and the regression including both terms suggested strong independent associations with self-harm. Mediation analysis confirmed that both paths remained significant, and that the direct effect of treatment condition was removed when changes in mentalizing and attachment avoidance were included in the path analysis. In terms of our theoretical framework, positive change in mentalizing and improvement in interpersonal functioning would be expected to bring about a reduction in self-harm. Bleiberg et al. (2012) suggest that anomalies of mentalizing in adolescents (Sharp et al., 2011) may be an appropriate target of intervention for those who self-harm.

Although these findings are promising, this study has several key limitations. The sample size was small. The effect sizes observed were statistically significant but modest, with effect sizes of the difference between groups never reaching 0.5. Despite being comparable in quantity, the comparison treatment was not manualized; it is possible that some of the difference may have arisen from the disorganizing impact of adolescents with self-harm on nonmanualized treatment planning and case management. It is also possible that the rigor of weekly supervision in the MBT-A group contributed to the outcome. Finally, these results were delivered by a single provider organization. Although three separate clinical teams were involved, the generalizability of the study is limited given that I was the supervisor of all three teams.

Given the lack of RCT evidence for successful therapeutic interventions for self-harm in adolescents, this initial demonstration of the usefulness of MBT-A in reducing self-harm, both as reported by adolescents and as assessed by blinded independent evaluators, indicates that larger-scale studies evaluating MBT-A for a population with comorbid depression and self-harm may be warranted.

Case Illustration

Background

Following admission to our unit, Sam, age 16 years, was anxious in the presence of others and initially preferred to spend her time withdrawn into her bedroom. She reported feeling depressed and hopeless, and certain that she would not be alive by the time she turned 17. Prior to admission she had dropped out of school and lived a reclusive life with ever-increasing social isolation, to the point that a few weeks before admission she even stopped online contact with friends.

She spoke of herself with extreme hatred, referring to herself and her body as horrible and ugly. She also expected hatred from those around her. She had an extensive history of self-harm, with a previous suicide attempt, mood fluctuations, and a lack of a sense of who she was and what she wanted from her life. Sam felt herself unable to perform academically but also expressed the wish to be a pediatrician one day. She was unable to travel on public transportation, describing every journey as an experience of being naked in front of a train full of people looking at her. Eating in front of others evoked similar horrors of mockery and ridicule; on further examination, this seemed to be linked to her experiencing a profound sense of shame when she was eating.

As we got to know her better, we noticed that she could be quick to criticize and to provide "supervision" to staff members about their interventions with other patients. She was sensitive about the way she was spoken to and frequently became very angry at staff members or her therapist for not using the right words or tone. Staff members increasingly felt as if they were "walking on eggshells" around her.

Sam's parents separated when she was 3 years old. She and her four siblings grew up with their mother; there was little contact with her father, who resided abroad. Her mother had suffered from depression throughout her childhood and could at times be humiliating and dismissive of Sam. Sam's descriptions of childhood experiences were filled with feelings of loneliness and shame. She felt inferior to everyone at school, and experienced herself as stupid and fat, even though she was in fact a very intelligent and beautiful young woman. She believed she was monstrous and unlovable. Self-harm became the outward expression of her internal state. Very deep cuts to her arms at times revealed the underlying fat tissue, and although those around her showed strong aversive responses to her wounds, she would dismissively state that she did not feel anything, and that the cuts were not deep enough.

The Therapeutic Intervention

The following clinical example is taken from Sam's third individual MBT-A session, which took place on the Monday after a weekend leave Sam spent at home with her mom. On Saturday, Sam had visited some old friends, and on Sunday she cut herself extensively. When she reported the self-harm in the session, the therapist tried to rewind to what happened before the self-harm in an attempt to try to identify the mental state and the unmentalized feelings underneath the self-harm.

THERAPIST: What happened before you cut yourself?

PATIENT: Nothing. I just wanted to cut myself.

THERAPIST: What was in your mind? What did you feel?

PATIENT: I just felt that I wanted to cut myself. I did not feel anything else. I just wanted to do some damage.

THERAPIST: Ah, but Sam, you know I believe that we always have deep feelings inside ourselves when we get desires like that.

PATIENT: I don't. I often just want to damage myself.

THERAPIST: You saw your friends the day before? When last did you see them?

PATIENT: Three months ago.

THERAPIST: What was it like to see them?

PATIENT: I could not connect to them. It gave me a lot of memories. [*silence*]

THERAPIST: What kind of memories?

PATIENT: I don't know, just memories from the time that I have very little memories. It is just kinda hazy.

THERAPIST: That sounds important. Could you try and take me there?

PATIENT: I don't know . . . I don't know.

THERAPIST: When you saw your friends, what feelings did you have?

PATIENT: I could not explain it. I don't have words for it. I get it sometimes that I have feelings that don't have a name. [This could be seen as a first indication of a flicker of improvement, as initially she indicated that she did not have feelings.]

THERAPIST: That is OK. I understand that. Could you describe them?

PATIENT: No, they are literally indescribable. They don't have names.

THERAPIST: Just listening to what you said, you said something about not feeling connected to them when you saw them? Maybe if I was in your shoes I would have felt as if I did not fit in, but I don't know if that is how you felt.

PATIENT: She smiles. Yeah, but this is not even worth saying anymore. That is just a permanent feeling.

THERAPIST: No, I don't agree with you. If you feel it, it is worth saying, and even if you feel it all the time, then it is still worth saying. What you feel is important, and it is important to me. Was there anything in particular that made you feel like that?

PATIENT: I don't know if there are layers to it.

THERAPIST: If we draw a picture on this page, we can draw you and then we draw your friends and we put bubbles above their heads. Then if we write in the bubble what feelings we think they may have in their heads, what do you think they felt on Saturday evening?

PATIENT: I don't know. I don't know what people think. I cannot tell. I am too scared to think.

THERAPIST: For you to be scared what they think already means you have an expectation, isn't it? What is your expectation?

PATIENT: That they look down on me.

THERAPIST: Shall we put that in the thought bubble?

PATIENT: Yes, and that I am not skinny and that I don't have the same clothes as them.

THERAPIST: OK, let's write that into the thought bubble as well. What should we write into your thought bubble?

PATIENT: I don't know. I feel bad about myself.

THERAPIST: Did they say or do anything that gave you the idea that they felt like that about you?

PATIENT: I don't know.

THERAPIST: Usually the way we behave can give people an idea of how we feel inside. How did they behave when they saw you?

PATIENT: They were friendly, but they did not mean it.

THERAPIST: Is there any way that you could perhaps confuse what was in your mind with what they felt?

PATIENT: I don't know. [It is hard for her to imagine the mind of the other, and perhaps the way the question was phrased did not help. Although the statement provided an alternative perspective, it did not include the necessary affective attunement.]

THERAPIST: If a friend of mine gets unwell and goes to hospital, I will feel caring feelings, I will feel concerned, and I will probably show that by being warm and friendly when I saw the friend. I just wonder, you know I may be wrong, but you said they were friendly—is it possible that they were having caring feelings?

PATIENT: I don't know. I don't know what people feel.

THERAPIST: Hmm, I may be wrong, but I wonder if you don't perhaps make assumptions about what people feel? And you know when we make assumptions, we could be wrong.

Sam's struggles with recognizing her own mental state and the mental states of those around her are clear in the example. The strength of the "alien self" in her mind, both subjectively and projected onto others, is clear, too. After Sam's description of self-harm, which can be seen as a manifestation of a collapse of mentalizing ability, the therapist rewinds to try to find the precipitating event that led to the unmentalized affective state; doing so allows it to be explored, understood, and ultimately mentalized. As Sam's account of what was in her mind prior to the self-harm remains devoid of emotional content, the therapist uses techniques such as exploration of affect, clarification, and elaboration of affect, by asking for more detail about the precipitating events. When Sam states that her feelings do not have words, the therapist uses herself to help with elaboration of affect, but the therapist poses this not as a statement of fact that Sam would feel the same, but more as a question. This enables Sam to share the intensity of these feelings, albeit in a very dismissive manner.

Then the therapist switched to another set of techniques. She stated that she felt Sam's feelings were important, and that they were important to her. She shared her own thoughts and feelings; that is, she expressed her interest in Sam's mind and experiences, and validated this as important to her despite it having been devalued and dismissed by Sam. This technique in particular is very important for this group of narcissistically vulnerable, self-harming patients, because they are notorious for expecting criticism and coldness, and for being unable to accurately judge the intentions of others. Declaring one's intentions explicitly and repeatedly provides the mentalizing scaffolding without which emotional closeness will not be possible. In addition, by stating, "What you feel is important to me," the therapist aims to provide a bridge of humanity for the patient as an escape from the cold, dehumanizing grip of the "alien self."

The next clinical vignette provides further examples of nonmentalizing, specifically, of thinking with psychic equivalence. This is demonstrated in Sam's descriptions of her conviction that the thoughts and feelings in her mind are exactly the same as those around her. The therapist uses active questioning and highlights alternative perspective to help Sam see the difference between her mind and the minds of others, and to facilitate her curiosity about the minds of others and to humanize others. The expectation is that the more Sam mentalizes, the more the world around her will become humanized, and the more compassion she will have for herself. Ultimately, it is hoped this will lessen the grip of the humiliating and shaming alien self.

A Further Session

PATIENT: People don't like me. I know that. I have learned to live with it.

THERAPIST: That sounds terribly painful. How do you know what people feel about you?

PATIENT: I know because of stuff they've said, like George here called me ugly the other day and I know he is right.

THERAPIST: That sounds like a terribly cruel thing to say and a very cruel thing to believe about yourself. It makes me wonder, do you think I have the same thoughts about you?

PATIENT: You won't tell because you are a professional, but I don't think you like me. I am just a patient and you are just doing your job. I hate myself and I cannot imagine people can feel differently about me.

THERAPIST: Well, I think that's the problem. Let me draw a picture of what I think and then you can tell me what you think about it. (*Draws a picture [Figure 19.1] to create a concrete portrayal of her idea*). [Drawing such pictures can enhance the impact of the intervention by providing an externalization of an underlying mental state. This is an example of a teleological intervention.]

THERAPIST: Let's imagine that is your mind. If we now look at what is in your mind, it seems there is something on your mind which is quite big, and it seems to have very strong feelings about you, in fact from where I stand, it seems to be a lot of hatred towards you and it constantly crushes you— would you agree? (*Sam agrees.*) This thing, I think, sometimes takes over your whole mind. I think sometimes it is all you can see.

PATIENT: That is all of me. There is nothing else.

THERAPIST: The sad thing is that there are other aspects to you, but with this thing in charge, you cannot see yourself and that is really sad.

PATIENT: That's just what it is. I have learned to live with it.

THERAPIST: But you see you don't only feel like that about yourself. If I draw myself next to you on the picture, what do you think is in my mind?

PATIENT: I don't know. I don't know what goes on in people's minds.

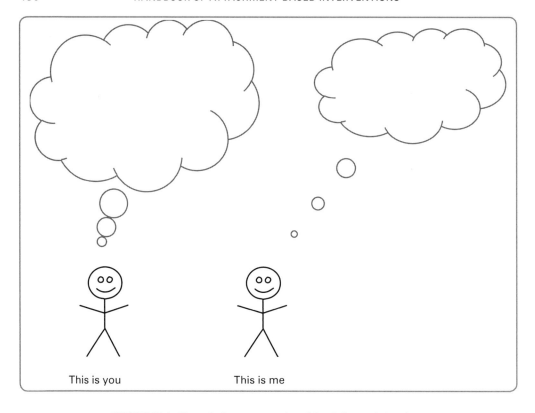

This is you   This is me

FIGURE 19.1. Therapist's representation of Sam's internal situation.

THERAPIST: I wonder if you think I have the same thoughts in my mind about you as what you are having?

PATIENT: Yes, I think that and I have had enough experience to know that people don't like me.

THERAPIST: I don't have the same feelings in my mind. I have my own feelings about you. I don't have your feelings about you. If someone else comes into the room now and they listen to our conversation and look at my facial expression and hear my tone of voice, what do you think they will think I feel about you? Will they think I dislike you?

PATIENT: I don't know. You could smile and not mean it.

THERAPIST: Or I could smile and mean it. And maybe other people coming in here may think I care about you. And to me it is really sad that this cold thing in your mind makes you have cold feelings about yourself and it makes you convinced that everyone around you also has cold feelings. And I just wonder whether you then tend to push people away a bit?

PATIENT: I don't allow anyone close to me. If people get close to you, they hurt you or take advantage. I don't want anyone to know what I feel inside.

THERAPIST: But if you keep people at such a distance, what do you think they feel?

Representing Sam's internal experience teleologically, by drawing it, not only illustrated it concretely but it also served to externalize it, offering her an opportunity to look at her internal state from a distance. By putting herself in the picture, the therapist tried to enable Sam to look at her relationship with her differently; she also tried to show Sam that her (the therapist's) mind was not the same as hers. By introducing other characters who could observe the interaction, the therapist tried to bring in the notion that others could have different feelings about Sam; at the same time, the therapist tried to embody compassion and a different attitude toward Sam than her (Sam's) internal one. Last, the therapist illustrated how Sam's internal conviction affects her relationships with others and the way that they feel about her.

Outcome and Prognosis

As therapy with Sam progressed, the therapeutic relationship was filled with struggles that the therapist had to reflect on in order that she not overreact or respond in an overly personalized fashion. As has been described, the therapist and other members of the team (and indeed Sam's family) had to walk a tightrope in terms of the views they expressed and the words they used. Carelessness in this regard could well lead to emotional injury. The therapist also had to battle against a strong sense of feeling useless or hopeless when every attempt to make emotional contact was rebuffed or devalued. Sam's dehumanizing approaches to herself when she was in the grip of rage driven by perfectionism could be relentless and serve as another source of anxiety in the therapist.

The working-through phase of therapy with Sam was a slow process of surviving strong countertransferential feelings, while attempting to make emotional contact with her feelings of anxiety, inadequacy, fears of rejection, and deep sense of shame. Nevertheless, as Sam became better able to tolerate emotional contact with those vulnerable states within her, and better able to allow herself to feel close to her therapist, she was more able to see her therapist as separate from her and capable of warmth toward her. She also became more curious about mental states of others, as well as her impact on others. She became more compassionate toward herself and expected a much less cold world around her. However, in meeting new people or forming new relationships, some of Sam's fragility reappeared and she remained vulnerable to shying away from contact. Her perfectionism remained a problem but was toned down into a strong ambition for her future. Moreover, she was able to reengage in her education.

Conclusion

Adolescence is a phase during which vulnerable young people may find themselves in a sea of fluctuating emotions, including a fluctuating sense of self. Their previous means of coping may be in danger of collapsing. They may be fearful of being alone but equally terrified of anxieties evoked when in relationships. In this stormy sea, people do not make sense and cannot be trusted. For these vulnerable adolescents, many of whom seem to embody multiple aspects of multiple personality disorders, often the only way of managing such extreme states is through self-harm.

MBT techniques make use of the therapeutic relationship in the here and now to examine some of the nonmentalized experiences of the patient to allow them to be understood and ultimately mentalized. This therapy also helps create a separation between the mind of the therapist and the patient. When patients increase their ability to mentalize, they become better able to be curious about their own minds, as well as the minds of others. They become better able to pause and take a reflective, observational stance, which helps with affect regulation and impulse control. These techniques, in addition to facilitating mastery, eventually lead to a more stable and robust sense of self, thus protecting against failure. This in turn enables the young person to proceed more appropriately along his or her developmental track and to be better able to master subsequent developmental challenges.

REFERENCES

Allen, J. G. (2004). *Coping with trauma: Hope through understanding* (2nd ed.). Washington, DC: American Psychiatric Publishing.

Allen, J. P., Hauser, S. T., & Borman-Spurrell, E. (1996), Attachment theory as a framework for understanding sequelae of severe adolescent psychopathology: An 11-year follow-up study. *Journal of Consulting and Clinical Psychology, 64*(2), 254–263.

American Psychiatric Association. (2013). *Diagnostic and statistical manual of mental disorders* (5th ed.). Arlington, VA: Author.

Asarnow, J. R., Porta, G., Spirito, A., Emslie, G., Clarke, G., Wagner, K. D., . . . Brent, D. A. (2011). Suicide attempts and nonsuicidal self-injury in the treatment of resistant depression in adolescents: Findings from the TORDIA study. *Journal of the American Academy of Child and Adolescent Psychiatry, 50,* 772–781.

Bateman, A., & Fonagy, P. (1999). The effectiveness of partial hospitalization in the treatment of borderline personality disorder–A randomised controlled trial. *American Journal of Psychiatry, 156,* 1563–1569.

Bateman, A. W., & Fonagy, P. (2004). *Psychotherapy for borderline personality disorder: Mentalization based treatment.* Oxford, UK: Oxford University Press.

Bateman, A., & Fonagy, P. (2008). 8-year follow-up of patients treated for borderline personality disorder: Mentalization-based treatment versus treatment as usual. *American Journal of Psychiatry, 165,* 631–638.

Bleiberg, E., Rossouw, T., & Fonagy, P. (2012) Adolescent breakdown and emerging borderline personality disorder. In A. W. Bateman & P. Fonagy (Eds.), *Handbook of mentalizing in mental health practice* (pp. 463–511). Washington, DC: American Psychiatric Publishing.

Brennan, K. A., Clark, C. L., & Shaver, P. R. (1998). Self-report measurement of adult romantic attachment: An integrative overview. In J. A. Simpson & W. S. Rholes (Eds.), *Attachment theory and close relationships* (pp. 46–76). New York: Guilford Press.

Brent, D. A. (1995). Risk factors for adolescent suicide and suicidal behaviour: Mental and substance abuse disorders, family environmental factors, and life stress, *Suicide and Life-Threatening Behaviour, 25*(Suppl.), 52–63.

Brent, D. A., Johnson, B., Bartle, S., Bridge, J., Rather, C., & Matha, J. (1993) Personality disorder, tendency to impulsive violence, and suicidal behaviour in adolescents. *Journal of the American Academy of Child and Adolescent Psychiatry, 32,* 69–75.

Brezo, J., Paris, J., Barker, E. D., Tremblay, R., Vitaro, F., Zoccolillo, M., . . . Turecki, G. (2007). Natural history of suicidal behaviors in a population-based sample of young adults, *Psychological Medicine, 37,* 1563–1574.

Bridge, J. A., Goldstein, T. R., & Brent, D. A. (2006). Adolescent suicide and suicidal behaviour, *Journal of Child Psychology and Psychiatry, 47,* 372–394.

Brown, M. Z., Comtois, K. A., & Linehan, M. M. (2002). Reasons for suicide attempts and nonsuicidal self-injury in women with borderline personality disorder, *Journal of Abnormal Psychology, 111,* 198–202.

Crawford, T. N., Cohen P., First, M. B., Skodol, A. E., Johnson, J. G., & Kasen, S. (2008). Comorbid Axis I and Axis II disorders in early adolescence. *Archives of General Psychiatry, 65,* 641–648.

Crick, N. R., Murray-Close, D., & Woods, K. (2005). Borderline personality features in childhood: A short-term longitudinal study. *Development and Psychopathology, 17,* 1051–1070.

DiClemente, R. J., Ponton, L. E., & Hartley, D. (1991). Prevalence and correlates of cutting behaviour: Risk for HIV transmission. *Journal of the American Academy of Child and Adolescent Psychiatry, 30,* 735–739.

Dubois-Comtois, K., Cyr, C., Pascuzzo, K., Lessard, M., & Poulin, C. (2013). Attachment theory in clinical work with adolescents. *Journal of Child and Adolescent Behavior, 1,* 111.

Fergusson, D. M., Beautrais, A. L., & Horwood, L. J. (2003). Vulnerability and resiliency to suicidal behaviours in young people. *Psychological Medicine, 33,* 61–73.

Fergusson, D. M., Horwood, L., & Lynskey, M. (1996). Childhood sexual abuse and psychiatric disorder in young adulthood: II. Psychiatric outcomes of childhood abuse. *Journal of the American Academy of Child and Adolescent Psychiatry, 34,* 1365–1373.

Fonagy, P. (1998). An attachment theory approach to treatment of the difficult patient. *Bulletin of the Menninger Clinic, 62,* 147–169.

Fonagy, P., Gergely, G., Jurist, E., & Target, M. (2002). *Affect regulation, mentalization and the development of the self.* New York: Other Press.

Gerard, N. (2002, May). Why are so many teenage girls cutting themselves? *The Guardian.*

Goldston, D. B., Daniel, S. S., Reboussin, B. A., Reboussin, D. M., Frazier, P. H., & Harris, A. E. (2001) Cognitive risk factors and suicide attempts among formerly hospitalized adolescents: A prospective naturalistic study. *Journal of the American Academy of Child and Adolescent Psychiatry, 40*(1), 91–99.

Gunnell, D., & Frankel, S. (1994). Prevention of suicide: Aspirations and evidence. *British Medical Journal, 308,* 1227–1233.

Haavisto, A., Sourander, A., Multimaki, P., Parkkola, K., Santalahti, P., Helenius, H., . . . Almqvist, F. (2004). Factors associated with depressive symptoms among 18-year-old boys: A prospective 10-year follow-up study. *Journal of Affective Disorders, 83*(2–3), 143–154.

Harrington, R., Pickels, A., Aglan, A., Harrington, V., Burroughs, H., & Kerfoot, M. (2006). Early adult outcomes of adolescents who deliberately poisoned themselves. *Journal of the American Academy of Child and Adolescent Psychiatry, 45*(3), 337–345.

Hawton, K., Hall, S., Simkin, S., Bale, E., Bond, A., Codd, S., & Steward, A. (2003). Deliberate self-harm in adolescents: A study of characteristics and trends in Oxford, 1990–2000. *Journal of Child Psychology and Psychiatry and Allied Disciplines, 44,* 1191–1198.

Hawton, K., Rodham, K., & Evans, E. (2006). *By their own young hand: Deliberate self harm and suicidal ideas in adolescents.* London: Jessica Kingsley.

Jacobson, C. M., Muehlenkamp, J. J., Miller, A. L., & Turner, J. B. (2008). Psychiatric impairment among adolescents engaging in different types of deliberate self-harm. *Journal of Clinical Child and Adolescent Psychology, 37,* 363–375.

Kessler, R. C., Berglund, P., Demler, O., Jin, R., Merikangras, K. R., & Walters, E. E. (2005). Lifetime prevalence and age-of-onset distributions of DSM-IV disorders in the National Comorbidity Survey Replication. *Archives of General Psychiatry, 62*(6), 593–602.

Mental Health Foundation. (2016). *The truth about self-harm for young people and their friends and families.* London: Author.

Nixon, M. K., Cloutier, P., & Jansson, S. M. (2008). Nonsuicidal self-harm in youth: A population-based survey. *Canadian Medical Journal, 178*(3), 306–312.

Nock, M. K., Joiner, T. E., Jr., Gordon, K. H., Lloyd-Richardson, E., & Prinstein, M. J. (2006). Non-suicidal self-injury among adolescents: Diagnostic correlates and relation to suicide attempts. *Psychiatry Research, 144*(1), 65–72.

O'Connor, R., Rasmussen, S., Miles, J., & Hawton, K. (2009). Self-harm in adolescents: Self report survey in schools in Scotland. *British Medical Journal, 194,* 68–72.

Ougrin, D., & Latif, S. (2011). Specific psychological treatment versus treatment as usual in adolescents with self-harm: Systematic review and meta-analysis. *Crisis, 32,* 74–80.

Reith, D. M., Whyte, I., & Carter, G. (2003). Repetition risk for adolescent self-poisoning: A multiple event survival analysis. *Australian and New Zealand Journal of Psychiatry, 37,* 212–218.

Reyna, V., & Farley, F. (2006). Risk and rationality in adolescent decision-making: Implications for theory, practice, and public policy, *Psychological Science in the Public Interest, 7,* 1–44.

Rossouw, T. I., & Fonagy, P. (2012) Mentalization-based treatment for self-harm in adolescents: A randomized controlled trial. *Journal of the American Academy of Child and Adolescent Psychiatry, 51,* 1304–1313.

Sandell, R., Andersson, M., Elg, M., et al. (2008). *A psychometric analysis of a new social–emotional maturity in adolescents.* Unpublished manuscript.

Sharp, C., Pane, H., Ha, C., Venta, A., Patel, A. B., Sturek, J., & Fonagy, P. (2011). Theory of mind and emotion regulation difficulties in adolescents with borderline traits. *Journal of the American Academy of Child and Adolescent Psychiatry, 50,* 563–573.e1.

Steinberg, L. (2004). Risk taking in adolescence: What changes and why? *Annals of the New York Academy of Sciences, 1021,* 51–58.

Steinberg, L. (2008). A social neuroscience perspective on adolescent risk taking. *Developmental Review, 28*(1), 78–106

Truesdale, C. E. (2002). Attachment organization and attributional style as predictors of resilience among adolescents in residential treatment. *Dissertation Abstracts International B: The Sciences and Engineering, 63*(1), 0419–4217.

Vrouva, I., Fonagy, P., Fearon, P. R., & Roussow, T. (2010). The Risk-Taking and Self-Harm Inventory for adolescents: Development and psychometric evaluation. *Psychological Assessment, 22,* 852–865.

Wilkinson, P., Kelvin, R., Roberts, C., Dubicka, B., & Goodyer, I. (2011). Clinical and psychosocial predictors of suicide attempts and nonsuicidal self-injury in the Adolescent Depression Antidepressants and Psychotherapy Trial (ADAPT). *American Journal of Psychiatry, 168,* 495–501.

Yurgelun-Todd, D. (2007). Emotional and cognitive changes during adolescence. *Current Opinion in Neurobiology, 17*(2), 251–257.

Zanarini, M. C., Frankenburg, F. R., Hennen, J., Reich, D. B., & Silk, K. R. (2006). Prediction of the 10-year course of borderline personality disorder. *American Journal of Psychiatry, 163,* 827–832.

CHAPTER 20

Promoting Responsiveness, Emotion Regulation, and Attachment in Young Mothers and Infants

An Implementation of Video Intervention Therapy and Psychological Support

CRISTINA RIVA CRUGNOLA, ELENA IERARDI,
ALESSANDRO ALBIZZATI, and GEORGE DOWNING

This chapter provides a detailed look at an intervention program aimed at fostering the development of a healthy secure relationship between adolescent mothers and infants starting from the infants' first months of life. A pilot program was conducted from 2006 to 2011 with a small number of cases. In 2011, a service for adolescent and young mothers was created, and the PRERAYMI (Promoting Responsiveness, Emotion Regulation, and Attachment in Young Mothers and Infants) intervention protocol was established (Riva Crugnola, Ierardi, Gazzotti, & Albizzati, 2013; Riva Crugnola, Ierardi, Albizzati, & Downing, 2016). The intervention was conducted in a consulting room of the San Paolo Hospital–University of Milan Infant Neuropsychiatric Unit with the collaboration of the Department of Psychology of the University of Milan–Bicocca, and was set up, drawing on a previous initiative in the same hospital, the Accompanying Your Baby's Growth Service, the aim of which was to provide support to new mothers by monitoring their relationship with their infants and the development of the infants during their first year. The PRERAYMI project was advanced by the collaboration with George Downing from the Pitié-Salpêtrière Hospital in Paris, allowing video intervention therapy to be integrated as a key component.

Being an Adolescent Mother

Various studies have underlined the fact that early motherhood is a significant risk factor for the establishment of an adequate relationship between mother and infant (Osofsky, Hann, & Peebles, 1993; Pomerleau, Scuccimarri, & Malcuit, 2003) and the subsequent developmental trajectories of both mothers and infants.

Problems relating to the transition to adulthood interfere with adolescent mothers' management of their parental role, creating individuation challenges for parent figures (Aiello & Lancaster, 2007). The central problem for adolescents who are parents stems from the fact that they themselves are still children yearning for love (and separation) from their own parents, which impedes their ability to easily embrace the parental role toward their infants. The newborn's strong need for physical and emotional care competes with the adolescent mother's needs, exacerbating feelings of vulnerability and low self-esteem (Reid & Meadows-Oliver, 2007). Adolescent pregnancy may also be considered, in many cases, to be an attempt to gain an independence that is difficult to achieve through more usual means (study, work, etc.). This often happens when the adolescent compares herself to her mother who, in turn, had a baby at a young age or experienced difficulty and failures in her own growing up process (giving up her studies, losing job opportunities, etc.), such that the adolescent mother may be repeating a familiar pattern she learned from observing her own mother. In other cases, pregnancy may be experienced as an attempt to restore or create *ex novo* maternal attention and care that either have been lost or were never given or, again, to receive from the infant the acknowledgment and love the adolescent never received from her own parents (Fraiberg, 1987; Waddell, 2009).

Motherhood in adolescence is often associated with other risk factors correlated to poor parenting, such as low socioeconomic status (SES) and low educational attainment. However, a number of studies have shown that even when the effect of such variables is controlled, adolescence per se is still a high-risk situation for a mother's parenting skills (Bornstein, Putnick, Suwalsky, & Gini, 2006; Rafferty, Griffin, & Lodise, 2011). Other well-known risk factors for maternal and child health are common for many adolescent mothers, such as postnatal depression (Brown, Harris, Woods, Buman, & Cox, 2012), being a single mother and perceived poor social support (Logsdon, Birkimer, Simpson, & Looney, 2005). A further important risk factor for mother–infant interaction (Riva Crugnola, Gazzotti, et al., 2013) and for the development of secure attachment in the infant (Main, 1995; H. Steele, Steele, & Fonagy, 1996) is the fact that adolescent mothers are more likely to have insecure attachment models than do adult mothers (Madigan, Moran, & Pederson, 2006; Riva Crugnola, Ierardi, Gazzotti, & Albizzati, 2014). Other factors, such as a supportive relationship with the partner and having adequate social support more generally may serve a protective function with respect to an adolescent mother's parenting ability (Logsdon et al., 2005), reducing levels of stress and depression (Roye & Balk, 1996).

A young age, together with the frequent presence of other risk factors, affect the responsiveness of adolescent mothers. In caring for their infants, adolescent mothers use more instrumental behavior (Krpan, Coombs, Zinga, Steiner, &

Fleming, 2005). They are also more likely to adopt harsh parenting, accompanied by both physical and verbal abuse (Lee & Guterman, 2010), and to use intrusive and neglecting styles (Dukewich, Borkowski, & Whitman, 1996). Adolescent mothers also attune themselves to a lesser degree with the emotions of their children compared to adult mothers, displaying poor emotional availability (Easterbrooks, Chaudhuri, & Gestsdottir, 2005; Osofsky, Eberhart-Wright, Ware, & Hann, 1992). Dyadic emotional regulation is also less adequate than it is between adult mothers and infants, with more negative affective states related to the difficulty of the mothers in regulating the negative emotions of their infants (Riva Crugnola et al., 2014). Compared to adult mothers, adolescent mothers are also less verbally stimulating (Lacroix, Pomerleau, & Malcuit, 2002) and their verbal comments are lower in mind-mindedness (Demers, Bernier, Tarabulsy, & Provost, 2010).

These characteristics of the responsiveness of adolescent mothers affect the development of their infants, who display less ability in affective communication (Osofsky et al., 1992), as well as a greater likelihood to develop insecure–avoidant and disorganized attachment ties than do the children of adult mothers (Broussard, 1995; Lounds, Borkowski, Thomas, Maxwell, & Weed, 2005). In the short term, the infants of adolescent mothers may also display delays in both their psychomotor development (Jahromi, Umana-Taylor, Updegraff, & Lara, 2012) and their cognitive and linguistic development (Morinis, Carons, & Quigley, 2013; Rafferty et al., 2011). In adolescence and adulthood, they display a range of adverse outcomes, such as poor academic achievement, unemployment, early parenthood, and violent offending (Hoffman & Maynard, 2008; Jaffee, Caspi, & Moffitt, 2001). Early motherhood, at the same time, limits the subsequent life opportunities of the young women (Jaffee et al., 2001), leading to low levels of education and underemployment, and giving rise to a higher probability of being involved in less stable relationships and of suffering depression (Boden, Fergusson, & Horwood, 2008; Horwitz, Bruce, Hoff, Harley, & Jekel, 1996).

Since the 1990s there have been various programs aimed at improving the relationship between adolescent mothers and their infants (Savio Beers & Hollo, 2009). Diverse approaches have included school-based programs aimed at preventing mothers giving up their studies (Strunk, 2008); clinical-based programs that focus on monitoring the health of the infant and the well-being of its parents, providing medical assistance and social support (Cox et al., 2005); and psychotherapeutic approaches for mothers who have particular problems linked to their difficult or traumatic infant experiences (e.g., Mayers & Siegler, 2004), including the approach detailed in this chapter (and others in this volume).

Some programs are more specifically attachment based, i.e. aimed at increasing the responsiveness of mothers and thus improving the quality of infant attachment. These include the pioneering program of Carter (Carter, Osofsky, & Hann, 1991) "Speaking for the Baby," which uses video feedback and aims to give a voice to infant communication, which often either not understood or is misunderstood by young mothers. The more recent attachment-based programs utilize different methods of intervention, combining, for example, the use of video feedback with the home-visiting approach (Slade, Sadler, & Mayes, 2005) or with a psychotherapeutic approach (Mayers & Siegler, 2004) drawing inspiration from parent–infant psychotherapy (Fraiberg, 1987) or from systemic therapy (McDonald et al., 2009), as reviewed recently by M. Steele et al. (2014).

Principles of the Intervention Program

The PRERAYMI intervention program is aimed at adolescent and young mothers (between ages 14 and 21), their partners, and their infants. It is an attachment-based intervention program in that its principal aim is to improve the mother–infant relationship in the first year of the infant's life, increasing maternal responsiveness and improving mother–infant dyadic emotional regulation, so as to establish secure attachment of the infant to the mother and other attachment figures. It is well known that secure infant attachment is predictive of adequate socioemotional development and, at the same time, serves a protective function with respect to psychopathological risk in the subsequent stages of development (Sroufe, Egeland, Carlson, & Collins, 2005). In the same way, maternal sensitivity and the absence of intrusiveness toward the infant in the first year have a long-term impact on the infant's socioemotional development (Mäntymaa, Puura, Luoma, Salmelin, & Tamminen, 2004). Arguably, a core element of this developmental process is the styles of emotional regulation that the infant constructs based on interactions with caregivers in its first year, indicated by infant attachment patterns (Cassidy, 1994; Riva Crugnola et al., 2011), in which emotion-regulation is dyadic, but over time these patterns become internalized as self-regulation patterns.

The second aim of the intervention program is to foster in the mother the process of integrating her experience of maternity and her relationship with the infant with her transition toward adulthood. In those most at-risk cases, an adolescent mother may distance herself from her experience of maternity, perceiving it as extraneous to her existential and developmental condition, delegating care of the infant to others both physically and emotionally, resulting in the infant's abandonment in the most problematic cases.

In order to achieve these objectives our intervention is based on three different approaches: Video Intervention Therapy, developmental guidance, and psychological counseling. Table 20.1 shows the main components and the principles of the intervention.

For what concerns the first objective—the creation of secure mother–infant attachment—the importance of keeping in mind the different factors that concur in the creation of this bond is well-known. Alongside maternal sensitivity (Malatesta, Culver, Tesman, & Shepard, 1989) the ability of the mother to regulate negative emotions and to share positive emotions is key (Lyons-Ruth et al., 2013), as is her ability to coordinate herself with the entire range of her infant's communication skills (gazing, vocalizing, seeking physical contact) (Beebe et al., 2010), and to keep in mind the infant and its mental and emotional states (Slade, Grienenberger, Bernbach, Levy, & Locker, 2005; H. Steele et al., 1996).

The video intervention therapy (VIT) method, developed by Downing (2005; Downing, Bürgin, Reck, & Ziegenhain, 2008), plays a key role in our program with regard to creating secure mother–infant attachment. VIT is a modified form

TABLE 20.1. Summary of the Principles and Form of Intervention

Aims	Method
Support the mother–infant relationship • Increase mother sensitivity and infant cooperation. • Improve dyadic emotion coordination. • Establish secure attachment of the infant to the mother.	• Video intervention therapy conducted in a two-way manner: analysis of videorecorded mother–infant interaction (outer movie) and of the feelings and representations of the mother in relation to the baby and to this interaction (inner movie) • Developmental guidance, a guide to the stages of the development of the infant, also conducted through discussion of the Bayley Scales results with the mother and the father
Increase well-being and reduce psychological distress of the mother.	Psychological counseling with the aims of fostering integration of adolescent mothers' experience of becoming a mother with their transition to adulthood; tackling adverse or traumatic aspects of the childhood experiences of the adolescents that could replicate themselves in their relationship with their infant; investigated also with AAI.

of cognitive-behavioral therapy, which also uses psychodynamic elements in its approach (M. Steele et al., 2014). It has long been used in psychiatric and other mental health settings, such as inpatient parent–infant units in which a psychiatrically disturbed parent and an infant can be hospitalized together (Downing, Wortmann-Fleischer, von Einsiedel, Jordan, & Reck, 2013).

VIT is conceived as a module methodology, intended to be inserted within a wider treatment program. Depending on treatment context, it may be used to help with parent–infant, parent–child, child–child, and/or couple relationships. Here we speak only of the parent–infant version. With VIT, a short video of parent–infant interaction is filmed. At some later point, once the therapist has had a chance to briefly scan it alone, the video is used in a session. The therapist (or therapists) and the parent (or parents) look at the filmed interaction together, and reflect on and discuss key moments and events.

VIT can be done in either individual or group therapy settings. In a group setting, this conversation about the video is at times widened to include other group members. A specific protocol is followed for any session in which video is used (Downing et al., 2013). Such a session might be "abbreviated" or "full." In an abbreviated session, the parent's initial observations about the interaction are discussed first. The therapist next highlights a certain number of specific events, commenting on what seems positive. Patient and therapist further reflect on these points. In a full session, additional steps are taken. When this pattern is not too far from the parent's conscious awareness, the therapist also points out, in a respectful and supportive manner, a negative interactional pattern. A more extensive therapeutic investigation of this pattern is then undertaken. Mentalization opportunities (i.e., the chance to think extensively about the inner states of the child) are emphasized. Beliefs, emotion, and modes of body organization relevant to the negative pattern are explored, and more functional alternatives are suggested and demonstrated. A plan for specific behavioral change is collaboratively determined.

VIT has proved particularly fitting for our therapeutic context. One reason is its flexibility. Our young mothers are highly divergent one from the other. Some are cooperative, whereas others are highly resistant. Some behave like young adults; others, like children. Some are ready for psychologically oriented exploration, whereas others need extensive prior work with motivation. One good answer to this need for flexibility is that with VIT, the therapist can focus more on either the "outer movie" (i.e., the objective behavior seen in the video) or the "inner movie" (i.e., the thoughts, feelings, and body experiences that were present in the patient during the interaction). In addition, with poorly motivated patients, it is possible to adopt abbreviated sessions, in which only positive patterns are explored, and more functional alternatives are found.

A second level of intervention provides mothers with developmental guidance (Papoušek, Schieche, & Wurmser, 2008), with the aim of increasing the mother's knowledge of her infant's stages of development. Developmental guidance is based on illustrating, through monthly sessions, the stages of development of the infant and its rhythms of regulation by psychomotor therapists.

A third level of intervention provides mothers with psychological counseling in order to increase her well-being and reduce her psychological distress. Just a few sessions are held in less problematic cases, and these are aimed at facilitating the mother's transition toward adulthood. However, counseling lasts longer and may be extended to the entire period of the intervention in cases (around 50%) in which the mothers have had traumatic experiences or are currently having problems with regard to their relationship with their infant, their family of origin, or their partner. In such cases, the mother is helped to reflect in depth on conflictual aspects of her past and/or current relationships with her own parents, and on how these now reflect her relationships with her infant (Lieberman & Pawl, 1993). The mother's elaboration of trauma is an important feature of the intervention also in the light of studies that have shown the difficulties encountered by researchers in attachment-based intervention programs for adolescent mothers who are disorganized with respect to abuse they have suffered (Moran, Pederson, & Krupka, 2005).

The Intervention Protocol

Intervention starts when the infant is 2 months old and takes place in a consulting room of the hospital. The aim is to provide mothers with a protected area they can inhabit as if it were their own. Adolescent mothers often find themselves living with their family of origin or with their partner's family in crowded conditions that offer them little chance to protect their individual relationship with the infant. Intervention is conducted by a team of psychologists, infant neuropsychiatrists, and psychomotor therapists, and is coordinated by a university professor of developmental psychology and by a doctor, an infant neuropsychiatrist. Operational organization is handled by a psychomotor therapist. Table 20.2 summarizes the intervention protocol.

TABLE 20.2. Summary of the Intervention Protocol

Team:	Psychologists, infant neuropsychiatrists, and psychomotor therapists		
Location:	Consulting room of the hospital		
Supervision:	Discussion and supervision of the cases in a group (monthly)		

Phases and tools		Instruments	Therapists
After baby's birth	First meeting to introduce the service and obtain informed consent		Psychologists, and psychomotor therapists
At infant age 2 months	Gathering sociodemographic data of the mother	Anamnestic form	Psychologists
	Assessment of maternal depression	Postpartum Depression Screening Scale	
	Assessment of parental stress	Parenting Stress Index—Short Form	
	Assessment of maternal attachment model	Adult Attachment Interview	
From 2 to 12 months	Assessment of dyadic interaction (monthly)	CARE-Index and ICEP	Psychologists
	Video intervention (monthly)	Video intervention therapy	Psychologists, psychomotor therapists
	Counseling (monthly)	Psychological support	Psychologists
	Developmental guidance (monthly)	Guide to the stages of infant development	Psychomotor therapists
At infant age 6 and 10 months	Assessment of the psychomotor development of the infant	Bayley Scales of Infant Development	Psychomotor therapists, infant neuropsychiatrists
Follow-up at infant age 14 months	Assessment of dyadic interaction and infant attachment	CARE-Index, ICEP, Strange Situation Procedure	Psychologists

The program begins with an initial meeting with the mother shortly after she has given birth, upon notification by the adolescent mothers-to-be service of the hospital. During this meeting an anamnestic form is compiled with the mother, and risk and protection factors (e.g., socioeconomic condition, relationship with the infant's father, social support, educational level, progression of pregnancy and adverse experiences) with respect to her relationship with the baby are therefore identified. Self-report questionnaires are used to assess levels of parental stress (Parenting Stress Index–Short Form [PSI-SF]; Abidin, 1995) and postpartum depression (Postpartum Depression Screening Scale [PDSS]; Beck & Gable, 2002). The "state of mind of the mother" with respect to attachment is also examined using the Adult Attachment Interview (AAI; Main, Goldwyn, & Hesse, 2002).

When possible, infants' fathers are also included in the intervention protocol. They are, however, often unavailable because of work commitments or current lack of engagement. Nonetheless, in order to foster collaboration between mothers and fathers, the more informative meetings that focus on developmental guidance are conducted at times compatible with the fathers' working hours. In the course of the intervention, we are also in contact with the parents of the adolescent mothers, albeit not systematically.

Monthly, from infant ages 2–12 months, video intervention is conducted through meetings led by a psychologist and a psychomotor therapist. During each meeting, the mother and the infant are videorecorded for 5–10 minutes in free-play situations in which suitable toys are available. In the following meeting, which occurs a few days after that of the videorecording, the recording is discussed with the mother, and another videorecording of her interaction with the infant is made.

The specific aim of using VIT in our program is to analyze microanalytically with the mother her communication with her infant at the level of affective state coordination, supporting mother–infant positive engagement, and the ability of the mother to regulate negative emotions. At the same time, there is a particular focus on supporting the mother in facilitating her infant's explorative activity, and episodes of joint attention are encouraged.

Specific importance is also attributed in the intervention to exploring with the mother her feelings upon viewing the video regarding both her own emotions and those attributed to her infant, with the aim of increasing her ability to keep her infant in mind (Slade, Sadler, et al., 2005). Self-observation of their interaction with the infant by means of the video is a particularly strong stimulus for parents, allowing them in a short space of time to render otherwise unexpressed emotions and representations explicit and therefore to activate specific resources (Downing, 2005; M. Steele et al., 2014). This proves to be particularly useful with adolescent mothers whose emotional awareness and ability to reflect are often limited and still in the course of development. At the same time, the possibility of using information drawn carefully and selectively from the AAI conducted with the adolescent mother at the beginning of the intervention is also of particular importance in the video intervention.

The interaction styles of mothers and infants are evaluated with the CARE-Index (Crittenden, 1998) and the interactive and emotional regulation of the dyads with the Infant and Caregiver Engagement Phases (ICEP; Weinberg & Tronick, 1999) in the version formulated by us (Riva Crugnola, Gazzotti, et al., 2013). The codified videorecordings give specific information for each mother–infant dyad, information that is important in both the discussion of the recordings with the mother and the assessment of the efficacy of the intervention.

Parallel to the video intervention, monthly meetings led by a psychomotor therapist focus on developmental guidance (Papoušek et al., 2008). In this context, the infant's motor and cognitive development is monitored using the Bayley Scales of Infant Development (Bayley, 2005) at 6 and 10 months. The results are discussed in specific meetings with the mothers and fathers in order to identify with them both the developing skills of the infant and any problems. In the event of delays in infant development, often due to communicative development, specific examinations are carried out by infant neuropsychiatrists and action is taken to recover psychomotor development.

The mothers are also given counseling sessions with psychologists; the sessions are usually monthly; in more problematic cases, they may be more frequent, even weekly. These aim to foster integration of the experience of becoming a mother with the transition toward adulthood. Should the mother have specific problems relating to the present, for example, the her relationship with her partner or family of origin, further pregnancies, difficulties with the infant, or the mother's past history, she may receive counseling during the entire intervention.

In order to ascertain the effectiveness of the intervention, at 14 months, the mother's and the infant's styles of interaction are evaluated once again with the CARE-Index and the ICEP, modified version. At the same time, the type of attachment developed by the infant to the mother is assessed using the Strange Situation Procedure (Ainsworth, Blehar, Waters, & Wall, 1978). In the protocol there is a final stage when mothers are given the Child Behavior Checklist (CBCL; Achenbach & Rescorla, 2001) at infant age 24 months, in order to evaluate the efficacy of the intervention with regard to the infant's psychopathological risk.

All the psychologists, infant neuropsychiatrists, and psychomotor therapists have already developed specific experience within the context of parent and child early infancy prevention programs. The experience of the infant neuropsychiatrists and psychomotor therapists is mainly clinical, while that of the psychologists is not only clinical but also research experience, drawn from studies of parent–infant interaction and attachment models in early infancy in conditions of normality and risk (Riva Crugnola, Gazzotti, et al., 2013; Riva Crugnola et al., 2011, 2014).

In the course of the program the cases followed by the team are discussed in a group, led by the coordinator of the project, with the aim of studying *in itinere* the best methods of intervention. The team attended a 6-day training seminar on video intervention supervised by George Downing, an expert in VIT.

One hundred seven adolescent mothers have so far been involved in the intervention, of whom 45 used the service for the first 4 months, and 30 for the entire period. The mothers were between ages 14 and 21 (mean = 18.36) and the fathers, between 17 and 39 (mean = 23.08). In the majority of cases the numerous risk factors included a family history of young parenthood (90%), a problematic social–family context (92%) characterized by early separation of parents (48%) and little social support (80%), low levels of education (88%), abandonment of studies (85%), and experiences of abuse and maltreatment (40%). Furthermore, although the partner, the father of the infant, was almost always present (90%), many of the mothers had an unstable relationship with this partner. In almost all cases, the mother's relationship with the infant, often the result of an unwanted pregnancy (73%), was, from the very first months, difficult, due in part to the mother's limited ability to "think of" the infant. Most of the mothers also had little awareness of their infants' stages of development, demonstrated in the way they cared for their infants, as if they wanted to speed up the infants' growth.

Efficacy of the Intervention

For the purposes of assessing the efficacy of the PRERAYMI intervention program we conducted a study to evaluate (1) whether the intervention was effective after 3 and 6 months for adolescent mother–infant dyads who received the intervention compared to a control group of adolescent mother–infant dyads who did not receive it, with respect to mother–infant styles of interaction and dyadic emotion regulation; (2) whether children in the intervention group were more likely to be securely attached to their mothers at 14 months compared to those of the control group. These outcomes are summarized in Table 20.3.

As indicated in Table 20.4, the participants were 50 adolescent mothers between ages 14 and 21 and their children, nonrandomly assigned to one of two groups: 34 dyads who received the intervention, and 16 dyads who received no intervention but did receive routine postnatal well-woman health visits and well-baby health care visits. The sociodemographic characteristics of the two groups are described in Table 20.4. It may be noted in particular that the two groups did not differ as to intake demographic characteristics, and both had high-risk profiles, including mothers who had a family history of young parenthood (about 90%), adverse childhood experiences (about 50%) and low SES (85%).

Due to dropouts from the program, by the time infants were age 9 months, the number of participants was much smaller: 16 in the intervention group and 10 in the control group.

At infant ages 3, 6, and 9 months, mother–infant interactions were video-recorded and coded with the CARE-Index (Crittenden, 1998), which evaluates the

TABLE 20.3. Summary of the Outcome

		Intervention group	Control group
After 3 months of intervention (3–6 months)	Increase	Mother's sensitivity Positive matches, total matches Ability to repair mismatches	Mother's controlling style
	Decrease	Mother's controlling style	Mother's sensitivity Total matches Ability to repair mismatches
After 6 months of intervention (6–9 months)	Increase	Mother's sensitivity Infant's cooperative style Positive matches, total matches Ability to repair mismatches	Infant's passive style Mismatches
	Decrease	Mother's controlling style Infant's passive style Mismatches	Infant's cooperative style Total matches Ability to repair mismatches
Follow-up 14 months		62% of children had a secure attachment to their mothers	All the children had an insecure attachment to their mothers

TABLE 20.4. Sociodemographic Characteristics

	Intervention group (*N* = 34)	Control group (*N* = 16)	Intervention vs. control
Mother			
Age: mean (*SD*; range)	18.34 (1.76; 14–21)	17.94 (1.94; 15–21)	NS
Marital status			
Single	24 (70%)	14 (87%)	NS
Married	10 (30%)	2 (13%)	
Living arrangements			
With a partner	12 (35%)	8 (50%)	NS
With parents/a parent	22 (65%)	8 (50%)	
Education			
No school diploma	0 (0%)	1 (6%)	
Less than secondary education	27 (79%)	14 (88%)	NS
Higher degree	7 (21%)	1 (6%)	
SES (mean; *SD*)	19.87 (5.79)	21 (5.99)	NS
Family history of young parenthood	31 (91%)	14 (87%)	NS
Adverse childhood experiences	16 (47%)	8 (50%)	NS
Unwanted pregnancy	23 (67%)	12 (75%)	NS
Infant			
Sex			
Female	21 (61%)	10 (62%)	NS
Male	13 (38%)	6 (38%)	

Note. N, number of subjects; *SD,* standard deviation; *NS,* nonsignificant.

styles of parent–infant interaction from infant ages 0–15 months. The categories for the parent are Sensitive, Controlling, and Nonresponsive, and for the infant, Cooperative, Compulsive–Compliant, Difficult, and Passive.

The interactions were also coded by the ICEP (Weinberg & Tronick, 1999) (see Tables 20.5), which we modified to analyze the interaction between mother and infant concerning objects (Riva Crugnola, Gazzotti, et al., 2013). The instrument evaluates the matching and mismatching of affective states between parent and child, the former being understood as moments in which mother and infant share the same affective states and the latter as moments in which they do not share the same affective states. It also permits assessment of the capacity of the dyad to move from states of mismatch to states of positive or neutral match, thus repairing communication.

TABLE 20.5. Definition of Affective States: Positive, Neutral, Negative, and Matches and Mismatches

Affective states	Codes
Infant positive	Social positive engagement, orientation to objects not offered by the mother, orientation to objects offered by the mother
Infant neutral	Social monitoring, orientation to the environment, allows caretaking, allows comforting
Infant negative	Negative engagement
Mother positive	Social positive engagement, offer of object, involvement in play
Mother neutral	Social monitoring, call for infant's attention, non-infant focused, caretaking, comfort
Mother negative	Negative engagement
Matches	Infant positive–mother positive, infant neutral–mother neutral
Negative match	Infant negative–mother negative
Mismatches	Infant positive–mother negative, infant positive–mother neutral, infant negative–mother positive, infant negative–mother neutral, infant neutral–mother positive, infant neutral–mother negative

We analyzed the changes in interactions and emotion regulation at 6 and 9 months after 3 and 6 months in the intervention group and in the control group. The intervention group after 3 months attended at least two sessions of video feedback, three psychological counseling sessions, and three developmental guidance sessions. After 6 months, the intervention group attended at least four sessions of video feedback, five psychological counseling sessions, and five developmental guidance sessions.

The AAI (Main et al., 2002) was administered to the mothers at infant age 3 months. In both intervention and control groups, 60% of adolescent mothers had an insecure attachment model. In the whole group, 37% were Dismissing, 29% were Preoccupied, 26% were Unresolved/Disorganized, and 8% were Cannot Classify, with a distribution similar to those of samples of at-risk and depressed mother groups (Bakermans-Kranenburg & van IJzendoorn, 2009).

At the preintervention assessment by the CARE-Index, the mean score of mother Sensitivity for both groups was 5, indicating the need for "further intervention," based on Crittenden's (1998) indications. Furthermore, the styles of interaction and emotion regulation of the intervention group and the control group at the 3-month baseline phase were very similar ($p > .05$).

Analysis with Linear Mixed Models showed significant interaction effects between groups (intervention/control) and time (3, 6, and 9 months). Adolescent mothers who participated in the intervention (compared to the control group) increased their Sensitivity after both 3 months of treatment, $b = 3.27$, $t(72) = 3.46$, *p* = .001, and 6 months of treatment, *b* = 4.20, t(79) = 3.69, *p* = .000 (see Figure 20.1), and reduced their Controlling style after both 3 months of treatment, *b* = −2.74, *t*(74) = −2.77, *p* = .007, and 6 months of treatment, *b* = −2.40, *t*(80) = −2.02, *p* = .047 (see Figure 20.2). The Sensitive style of the control group mothers, however, decreased, and their Controlling style remained high from infant ages 3–9 months. Infants who participated in the intervention increased their Cooperative style, *b* = 3.54, *t*(81) = 2.65, *p* = .010 (see Figure 20.3), and reduced their Passive style, *b* = −3.88, *t*(83) = −2.43, *p* = .017 (see Figure 20.4) from infant ages 3–9 months, compared to those of the control group, in which the Cooperative style at infant age 9 months was the same as it had been at 3 months and the Passive style increased from infant ages 3–9 months.

At the postintervention assessment by the CARE-Index, the intervention group improved its Sensitivity at infant age 9 months, with a mean score of 8.5, which indicates, according to Crittenden (1998), an adequate quality of mother–infant interaction, while the control group decreased its Sensitivity, with a mean score of 4.1, therefore placing it in the "needs further intervention" range.

The intervention group dyads (vs. control group dyads) spent more time in positive affective matches after 3 months of treatment, *b* = .15, *t*(66) = 2.78, *p* = .007, and after 6 months, *b* = .16, *t*(77) = 2.56, *p* = .012 (see Figure 20.5). With respect to affective state coordination, from infant ages 3–9 months, the intervention group dyads spent more time in affective matches after both 3 months of treatment, *b* = .10, *t*(70) = 1.95, *p* = .05, and 6 months of treatment, *b* = .15, *t*(81) = 2.47, *p* = .01 (see Figure 20.6), less time in affective mismatches after 6 months of treatment, *b* = −.14, *t*(72) = −2.17, *p* = .032 (see Figure 20.7), and had a greater ability to repair affective mismatches after both 3 months of treatment, *b* = 2.65, *t*(63) = 4.11, *p* = .000, and 6 months of treatment, *b* = 1.82, *t*(76) = 3.29, *p* = .001 (see Figure 20.8), compared to the control group. In the control group, the results were different, with an increase in mismatches and a reduction in matches and in the frequency of repairing communication errors from 3 to 9 months of treatment.

Last, from infant ages 3–9 months there was an increase in the amount of time spent by infants of the intervention dyads in involvement with objects offered by the mother, *b* = .17, *t*(94) = 2.45, *p* = .016 (see Figure 20.9), and an increase in the amount of time spent by mothers in participating in play with their infants both after 3 months of intervention, *b* = .09, *t*(74) = 2.94, *p* = .004, and after 6 months, *b* = .07, *t*(84) = 2.18, *p* = .032 (see Figure 20.10), compared to the control group in which reciprocal involvement in play with objects by mother and infant remained constant from 3 to 9 months.

At 14 months, preliminary analysis indicated that 62% of children (10 out of 16) who completed the intervention program had a secure attachment to their mothers. However, all children in the control group (5 out of 5) had an insecure attachment.

To sum up, the results indicate the intervention's efficacy considering at a global level the sensitivity of the mother and the cooperation of the infant, and at a microanalytic level, the affective matches, and the adolescent mothers' and their infants' ability to repair mismatch. Moreover, the results demonstrate the plasticity of mother–infant styles of interaction and dyadic regulation in the first year: The

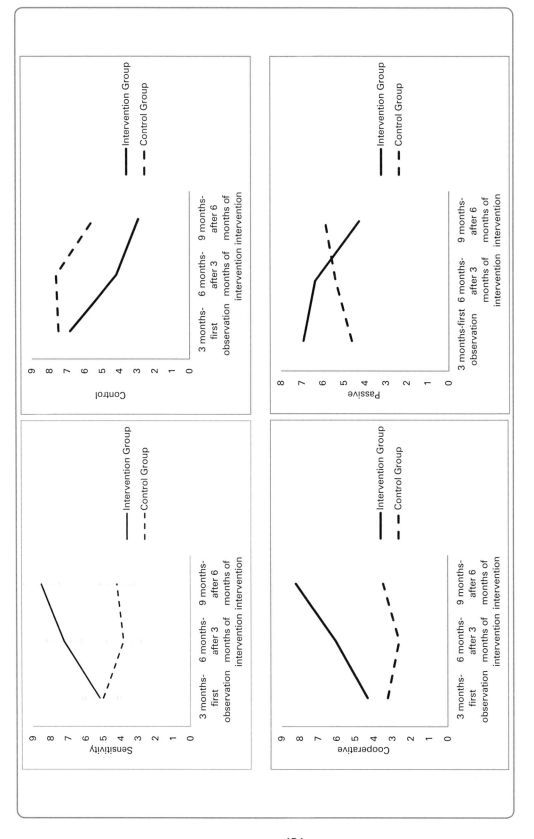

FIGURES 20.1–20.4. Differences in Sensitivity, Control, Cooperative, and Passive styles for the dyads who participated in the intervention and for the dyads of the control group from infant ages 3–9 months.

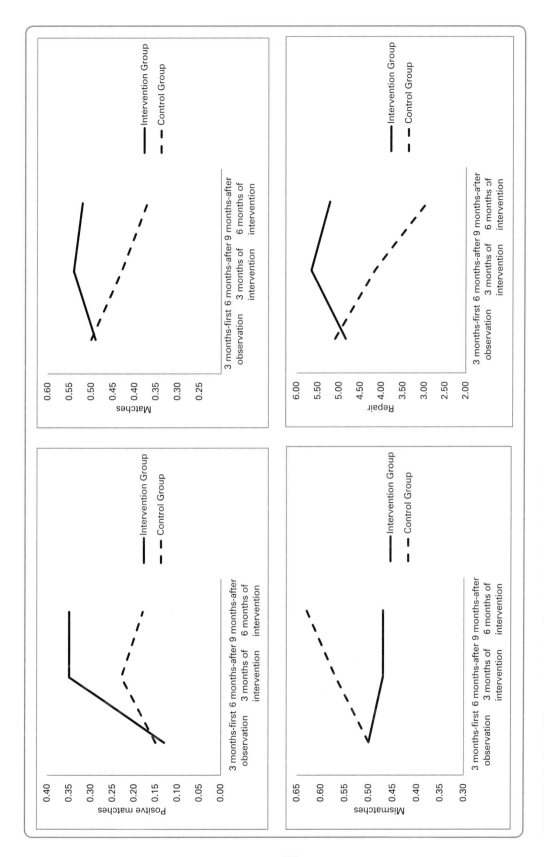

FIGURES 20.5–20.8. Differences in Positive Matches, Total Matches, Total Mismatches, and Repair for the dyads who participated in the intervention and for the dyads of the control group from infant ages 3–9 months.

455

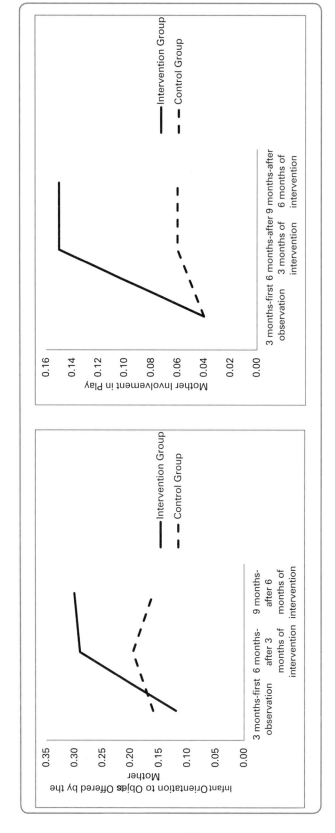

FIGURES 20.9 and 20.10. Differences in Infant Orientation to the Object Offered by the Mother and Mother Involvement in Play for the dyads who participated in the intervention and for the dyads of the control group from infant ages 3–9 months.

efficacy of the intervention with adolescent mothers and their infants can already be seen after 3 months, with better overall coordination and an increase in maternal sensitivity. On the other hand, the results show that without intervention, the inadequacy of adolescent mother–infant interactions remains the same or worsens, as demonstrated by the fact that in the control group, the capacity of the dyads to coordinate and to pass from mismatch to match tends to diminish and states of mismatch increase after 3 months. We may hypothesize that the use of different techniques—video intervention, counseling, and developmental guidance—aimed at increasing the sensitivity of the mother, her capacity to regulate the infant's emotions, and her capacity to reflect on her own mental states and on those of the infant, may explain this efficacy. Finally, the data, as shown by the preintervention evaluation using the CARE-Index at 3 months, indicate the advisability of early intervention for adolescent mothers and their infants in the first months given that maternal sensitivity is already inadequate at 3 months.

Supporting the Adolescent Mother–Infant Relationship: Growing as a Couple

We now illustrate our way of working from a closer perspective, describing the intervention with a mother–infant couple that we followed from infant ages 1–17 months.

Sofia was 20 when she arrived at our service with her 1-month-old infant, Marco. Right from the very first meeting we could see that Sofia's condition was characterized by multiple risk factors with regard to the establishment of a good parent–infant relationship, primarily due to her family history. Sofia had lived with both parents only until the age of 5, at which point she went to live with her father and his partner following her parents' separation and her mother's imprisonment. At the age of 13, Sofia left her father's home as a result of the physical and psychological abuse to which he subjected her. Her father was a drug addict and alcoholic. She went to live with her mother and found herself with her maternal grandparents and four younger siblings, three of whom were fathered with partners other than Sofia's father. From that time until the beginning of her pregnancy, Sofia had to substitute for her mother, who suffered from depression and spent some periods in prison, in looking after her siblings. She was obliged by her mother to care for them to the detriment of her own developmental needs and also had to stop going to school. Sofia told the personnel of the service that from the age of 15, she had suffered from acute anxiety and panic attacks, primarily when she attempted to "disengage" from caring for her siblings. During her pregnancy, which neither she nor her partner had expected, Sofia decided to stop looking after her siblings even though her mother was still in prison. However, she had to struggle with a marked sense of guilt, which she still had at the beginning of the intervention. Her siblings were therefore put in a children's home. After the birth, Sofia went to live with her partner and enjoyed good support from his family.

Drawing a map of risk and protection factors, the good relationship with her partner and the support of his family are protection factors with respect to Sofia's parenthood, while her family and personal history, together with the psychopathological traits of her parents, are risk factors. These risk factors are augmented by Sofia's precarious socioeconomic condition, abandonment of her studies, and by the fact that her mother became a parent at a young age—all risk factors that are often found in the histories of adolescent mothers participating in our intervention.

Of particular use in understanding how Sofia had processed these events was the analysis of the AAI conducted with her at infant age 3 months. Sofia's attachment model was preoccupied with aspects of anger (E2), according to the classification system (Main et al., 2002), even though Sophia's narration of her childhood appeared, at least in part, to be consistent and to display awareness of her experiences. Sofia seemed to be still involved in her attachment relationships, feeling anger toward her father and mother. She demonstrated, however, that she was aware of the experiences she had had, in particular the inversion of her role, which her mother had imposed on her: "I did everything on my own"; "I became an adult when I was still small"; "When I was 17, I was the mother of my siblings"; "Now that I'm about to become a mother I can't be responsible for all the children in the world." In this context, Sofia's pregnancy and Marco's birth had particular significance for her. She could at last look after her own needs and her life and not those of her siblings: "I had become the mother of three siblings: I hadn't lived my life. Now he's here I have to live my own life . . ."; she could claim her own space. However, this desire clashed almost immediately with Marco's needs: "It's difficult to disengage from him, too. He demands all the space for himself." When this happens, the anxiety and panic Sofia had experienced with her siblings reemerged.

The intervention with Sofia comprised the three levels indicated earlier. In the first level, the personnel used joint exploration of videos to help Sofia substantially change her interaction style with her infant. This work included improving her abilities to reflect on both her own inner states and those of her infant. In the second level, the personnel guided Sofia in discovering the infant's stages of development and his rhythms of regulation. In the third level, they accompanied Sofia through psychological counseling on her path of personal growth, helping her to get back in touch with her needs and to process the experiences of neglect she had suffered, in particular in her relationship with her mother. Sofia saw her mother as neglectful and as having little interested in her or her infant, even in the present.

In the first video sessions we could see immediately that interaction between Sofia and Marco was problematic: Sofia found it difficult to hold Marco in her arms in order to console him. The prevailing style of interaction oscillated between controlling/intrusive and nonresponsive, and Marco expressed distress by crying and avoiding contact with his mother. Observing their interaction microanalytically, we could see that negative matches and mismatches prevailed: Marco cried, Sofia offered him objects in an intrusive manner, and this caused Marco to express further distress. On the one hand, it was difficult for Sofia to regulate Marco's negative emotions; on the other hand, it was also difficult to have a dialogue with him based on visual and vocal contact and on holding at a physical level. In the video interventions, the team worked with Sofia on both the meaning of Marco's crying and his attempts at communication.

[Sofia uses a toy intrusively, repeatedly bringing it excessively close to Marco's face. Marco, after a few seconds, closes his eyes and cries.]

THERAPIST: Why is Marco crying?

SOFIA: I don't know.

THERAPIST: Try to imagine.

SOFIA: I've no idea.

THERAPIST: Try putting yourself in his place and imagine that someone is putting an object in your face. How would you feel?

SOFIA: I'd be irritated.

THERAPIST: Then try to imagine what Marco felt.

SOFIA: He'd be irritated. It wouldn't be very pleasant. He'd say, "Mom, stop it. I don't like it."

Sofia also expressed difficulty in interacting with Marco by playing and sharing positive emotions. She said that, in this regard, she had never really played with an adult. She had always played alone or with her younger brothers. In the course of the meetings, Sofia became progressively more able to dialogue with Marco, responding to his smiles and vocalization. Sofia was astonished by the fact that Marco responded to her and paid attention to her, for example, by laughing, vocalizing, and looking at her in the peekaboo game. Sofia got particular satisfaction from this: "It's lovely to see that he always needs me because I always need him." Reciprocal attachment slowly established itself.

In the second 6 months, however, new problems emerged for Sofia, particularly in following Marco's explorative activity and play with objects and carrying out an effective scaffolding role. Sofia seemed to find it difficult to understand and support Marco's desire to explore and play, to share games and activities with him. Marco often played alone, without his mother intervening. In this way, without the support of his mother, he tended continuously to direct his attention to new objects. Sofia, in turn, seemed to turn her attention elsewhere, without being able to follow Marco's activity. Thanks to the interventions with video, which highlighted these aspects, interaction improved, with significant moments of triadic interaction.

The assessment conducted with the CARE-Index and the ICEP at the beginning (2 months) and at the end of the intervention (12 months) confirmed the qualitative observations, showing, for Sofia, a significant increase in sensitivity and a decrease in nonresponsiveness and control, and for Marco, an increase in cooperative style and a decrease in passive and difficult style. There had also been a reduction in negative matches.

Together with the video intervention, the team also worked at the level of developmental guidance, discussing with Sofia her difficulties in caring for Marco whose sleep–wake rhythms and feeding rhythms were not very regular. Sofia tended to feed him continuously without pause.

The counseling conducted with Sofia in parallel with the video intervention also allowed her to process a number of issues that were key to her own growth and to her relationship with Marco. In the sessions, Sofia managed progressively to address the suffering and sense of solitude that she had experienced, and was still experiencing in the present, with respect to the neglect of her mother, managing to express her anger toward her mother, which she had previously suppressed and channeled into caring for her siblings. At the same time, Sofia managed to make sense of the panic attacks she had had as an adolescent when she was looking after her siblings, and which she still had from time to time caring for Marco. She had felt then, and sometimes now, overwhelmed by her own needs, which had scarcely been recognized by her parents, and which she herself still poorly understood.

At the end of the intervention, when Marco was 12 months old, Sofia began to make plans for herself, to start working again, and to consolidate her relationship with her partner, demonstrating that she had overcome her feelings of not being a good mother and her guilt due to her decision to stop looking after her siblings. The role of Marco's father in this regard was very important. Although he did not take part in the intervention, he constantly supported Sofia. At age 16 months, Marco's attachment to his mother, assessed with the Strange Situation, was secure, unlike that of Sofia, which was insecure–preoccupied at the beginning of the intervention. The chain of intergenerational transmission of attachment had therefore been broken. Likewise, the absence of neglect and abuse in Sofia's caring for Marco bear witness to the fact that there had been no transmission to Marco of the adverse and traumatic experiences suffered by Sofia.

To sum up, the intervention focused on enhancing Sofia's resources and supporting her fragile self-esteem. In particular, as a result of the video intervention, Sofia had more positive emotional engagement with Marco and shared more in his activities and interests. It helped her to think of Marco as a vital and communicative being, something which her parents had probably all too rarely thought with regard to herself. Helping Sofia, through psychological counseling, to think of herself as a "live" person with her own plans was also particularly important.

Conclusions and Suggestions for Future Directions

Sofia's case is typical. It is clear that the intervention with adolescent mothers is complex in that it aims to meet different objectives that at times are in conflict: to support the relationship between mother and infant and the development of the infant and, at the same time, to protect the growth process of the adolescent. Therefore, in line with other programs (Mayers & Siegler, 2004; Slade, Sadler, et al., 2005), the PRERAYMI intervention program uses different methods to monitor and support the double process of mother and infant growth—VIT, developmental guidance, and psychological counseling—as well as the different professional skills that support the process (those of the psychologists, infant neuropsychiatrists, and psychomotor therapists). The project, as it stands, has a number of limitations, due in part to the sheer complexity of work with adolescent mothers. We intend to take new steps concerning these limitations as the project continues. One is that fathers were not systematically involved. Likewise, the grandparents of the teenage mothers, in particular the maternal grandmothers, were involved only in a few cases.

Therefore, as the program continues we intend to use video intervention with fathers and grandmothers, too. The use of video is an especially promising avenue in our program. The following are some modes of video intervention we discovered to be important, and in certain cases almost essential, although we did not use them systematically.

- *Videos of the father with the infant.* To the extent the father has any continuing involvement with the infant, this is obviously useful. A father's influence on infant development can be considerable. To add work with father–infant videos is a natural extension. Depending on his and the mother's wishes, such sessions can be carried out either with him alone or with the mother present. These parent pairs vary enormously in their composition and living arrangements. The father may or may not also be an adolescent. They may or may not be living together. They may or may not see themselves as a couple, and be hoping for a future as a couple. Especially if they are living apart, the father may or may not be seeking a fatherhood role. Often he will feel turmoil and divided wishes in this respect. In such situations, work with video has the additional advantage of being likely to strengthen the father's bond with the infant. This in turn will help him clarify where he stands, what he wants, and how to plan for continuing involvement, if he so desires. His parenting skills will also increase, naturally. Such work, of course, assumes there are no contraindications to heightening his involvement (e.g., issues having to do with the infant's and/or the mother's safety).

- *Videos of both the mother and the father together with the infant.* The research of Fivaz-Depeursinge and Corboz-Warnery (1999) leaves no doubt that in the three-way setting, infants develop some interactional habits, benign or problematic, which are not the same as those prevalent when interacting with mother alone or father alone. Work with one or more videos of triadic interaction is definitely to be recommended in cases in which the mother and father live together, or intend to do so. Typically, both parents are present when the videos are explored.

- *Videos of the maternal grandmother with the infant.* In a good number of cases, the mother is living at home with her own mother, and caretaking is shared. Sometimes the maternal grandmother may even be, realistically, the principal caretaker. This is especially likely when either the mother herself is very young, and/or she has chosen to continue her school education (in itself a highly desirable decision). There can be a double payoff here. The grandmother will receive help for her own interactional capacities. But frequently this experience will also aid her more constructively to coach her daughter, an area fraught with conflicts in many cases. Work with video will in addition provide the grandmother and the mother with a shared conceptual framework for the parenting of an infant. These shared ideas will be linked with improved observational capacities for both. Needless to say, this work can be done with a grandfather, or an older sister of the mother who shares caretaking, and so forth.

- *Videos of the mother and the maternal grandmother together with the infant.* When the mother is living with her own mother, and caretaking is shared, this is to be recommended for the same reasons as those concerning mother–father–infant triadic interaction.

In conclusion, we find that work with adolescent mothers, though difficult, is fascinating. On the one hand, dealing with the needs of both sides of the dyad presents unusual challenges. On the other hand, current research continues to teach us more and more about the nature of interactional exchange and its influences on development. This in turn opens up new opportunities to make counseling and VIT for adolescent mothers and their infants increasingly effective.

ACKNOWLEDGMENTS

We would like to thank Professor Carlo Lenti, former Head of the Infant Neuropsychiatric Unit of the San Paolo Hospital and Professor Maria Paola Canevini, Head of the Infant Neuropsychiatric Unit of the San Paolo Hospital, who made it possible for the project to be set up and those people, other than the authors of this chapter, who took part in it: Laura Boati, Lorena Caiati, Elisabetta Costantino, Simona Gazzotti, Margherita Moioli, Laura Morè, Angela Silvano.

REFERENCES

Abidin, R. R. (1995). *Parenting Stress Index, Third Edition: Professional manual*. Odessa, FL: Psychological Assessment Resources.

Achenbach, T. M., & Rescorla, L. A. (2001). *Manual for the ASEBA School-Age Forms and Profiles*. Burlington: University of Vermont, Research Center for Children, Youth, and Families.

Aiello, R., & Lancaster, S. (2007). Influence of adolescent maternal characteristics on infant development. *Infant Mental Health Journal, 28*(5), 496–516.

Ainsworth, M. D. S., Blehar, M., Waters, F., & Wall, S. (1978). *Patterns of attachment*. Hillsdale, NJ: Erlbaum.

Bakermans-Kranenburg, M. J., & van IJzendoorn, M. H. (2009). The first 10,000 Adult Attachment Interviews: Distributions of adult attachment representations in clinical and non-clinical groups. *Attachment and Human Development, 11*(3), 223–263.

Bayley, N. (2005). *Bayley Scales of Infant Development* (3rd ed.). San Antonio, TX: Psychological Corporation.

Beck, C. T., & Gable, R. K. (2002). *Postpartum Depression Screening Scale (PDSS) manual*. Los Angeles: Western Psychological Services.

Beebe, B., Jaffe, J., Markese, S., Buck, K., Chen, H., Cohen, P., . . . Feldstein, S. (2010). The origins of 12-month attachment: A microanalysis of 4-month mother–infant interaction. *Attachment and Human Development, 12*(1–2), 3–141.

Boden, J., Fergusson, D., & Horwood, J. (2008). Early motherhood and subsequent life outcomes. *Journal of Child Psychology and Psychiatry, 49*(2), 151–160.

Bornstein, M. H., Putnick, D. L., Suwalsky, J. T. D., & Gini, M. (2006). Maternal chronological age, prenatal and perinatal history, social support and parenting of infants. *Child Development, 77*(4), 875–892.

Broussard, E. R. (1995). Infant attachment in a sample of adolescent mothers. *Child Psychiatry and Human Development, 25*(4), 211–219.

Brown, J. D., Harris, S. K., Woods, E. R., Buman, M. P., & Cox, J. E. (2012). Longitudinal study of depressive symptoms and social support in adolescent mothers. *Maternal and Child Health Journal, 16*(4), 894–901.

Carter, S. L., Osofsky, J. D., & Hann, D. H. (1991). Speaking for the baby: A therapeutic intervention with adolescent mothers and their infants. *Infant Mental Health Journal, 12*(4), 291–301.

Cassidy, J. (1994). Emotion regulation: Influences of attachment relationships. *Monographs of the Society for Research in Child Development, 59*(2–3), 228–249.

Cox, J., Bevill, L., Forsyth, J., Missal, S., Sherry, M., & Woods, E. (2005). Youth preferences for prenatal and parenting teen services. *Journal of Pediatric and Adolescent Gynecology, 18*(3), 167–174.

Crittenden, P. M. (1998). *CARE-Index: Revised coding manual.* Unpublished manual. Miami, FL: Family Relations Institute.

Demers, I., Bernier, A., Tarabulsy, G. M., & Provost, M. A. (2010). Mind-mindedness in adult and adolescent mothers: Relations to maternal sensitivity and infant attachment. *International Journal of Behavioral Development, 34*(6), 529–537.

Downing, G. (2005). Emotion, body, and parent–infant interaction. In J. Nadel & D. Muir (Eds.), *Emotional development: Recent research advances* (pp. 229–249). Oxford, UK: Oxford University Press.

Downing, G., Bürgin, D., Reck, C., & Ziegenhain, U. (2008). Interfaces between intersubjectivity and attachment: Three perspectives on a mother–infant inpatient case. *Infant Mental Health Journal, 29*(3), 278–295.

Downing, G., Wortmann-Fleischer, S., von Einsiedel, R., Jordan, W., & Reck, C. (2013). Video intervention therapy with parents with a psychiatric disturbance. In K. Brandt, B. Perry, S. Seligman, & E. Tronick (Eds.), *Infant and early childhood mental health: Core concepts and clinical practice* (pp. 261–280). Washington, DC: American Psychiatric Association.

Dukewich, T. L., Borkowski, J. G., & Whitman, T. L. (1996). Adolescent mothers and child abuse potential: An evaluation of risk factors. *Child Abuse and Neglect, 20*(11), 1031–1047.

Easterbrooks, M. A., Chaudhuri, J. H., & Gestsdottir, S. (2005). Patterns of emotional availability among young mothers and their infants: A dyadic, contextual analysis. *Infant Mental Health Journal, 26*(4), 309–326.

Fivaz-Depeursinge, E., & Corboz-Warnery, A. (1999). *The primary triangle: A developmental systems view of mothers, fathers, and infants.* New York: Basic Books.

Fraiberg, S. (1987). The adolescent mother and her infant. In S. Fraiberg & L. Fraiberg (Eds.), *Selected writings of Selma Fraiberg* (pp. 168–173). Columbus: Ohio State University Press.

Hoffman, S. D., & Maynard, R. A. (2008). *Kids having kids: Economic costs and social consequences of teen pregnancy* (2nd ed.). Washington, DC: Urban Institute Press.

Horwitz, S. M., Bruce, M. L., Hoff, R. A, Harley, I., & Jekel, J. F. (1996). Depression in former school-age mothers and community comparison subjects. *Journal of Affect and Disorder, 40*(1–2), 95–103.

Jaffee, S., Caspi, A., & Moffitt, T. E. (2001). Why are children born to teen mothers at risk for adverse outcomes in young adulthood?: Results from a 20-year longitudinal study. *Development and Psychopathology, 13*(2), 377–397.

Jahromi, L. B., Umana-Taylor, A. J., Updegraff, K. A., & Lara, E. E. (2012). Birth characteristics and developmental outcomes of factors. *International Journal of Behavioral Development, 36*(2), 146–156.

Krpan, K., Coombs, R., Zinga, D., Steiner, M., & Fleming, A. S. (2005). Experiential and hormonal correlates of maternal behavior in teen and adult mothers. *Hormones and Behavior, 41*(1), 112–122.

Lacroix, V., Pomerleau, A., & Malcuit, G. (2002). Properties of adult and adolescent mothers' speech, children's verbal performance and cognitive development in different socioeconomic groups: A longitudinal study. *First Language, 22*(2), 173–196.

Lee, Y., & Guterman, N. B. (2010). Young mother–father dyads and maternal harsh parenting behavior. *Child Abuse and Neglect, 34*(11), 874–885.

Lieberman, A. F., & Pawl, J. H. (1993). Infant–parent psychotherapy. In C. H. Zeanah (Ed.), *Handbook of infant mental health* (pp. 427–442). New York: Guilford Press.

Logsdon, M. C., Birkimer, J. C., Simpson, T., & Looney, S. (2005). Postpartum depression and social support in adolescents. *Journal of Obstetric, Gynecologic, and Neonatal Nursing, 34*(1), 46–54.

Lounds, J. J., Borkowski, J. G., Thomas, L., Maxwell, S. E., & Weed, K. (2005). Adolescent parenting and attachment during infancy and early childhood. *Parenting: Science and Practice, 5*(1), 91–118.

Lyons-Ruth, K., Bureau, J., Easterbrooks, M. A., Obsuth, I., Hennighausen, K., & Vulliez-Coady, L. (2013). Parsing the construct of maternal insensitivity: Distinct longitudinal pathways associated with early maternal withdrawal. *Attachment and Human Development, 15*(5–6), 562–582.

Madigan, S., Moran, G., & Pederson, D. R. (2006). Unresolved states of mind, disorganized attachment relationships, and disrupted interactions of adolescent mothers and their infants. *Developmental Psychology, 42*(2), 293–304.

Main, M. (1995). Recent studies in attachment: Overview, with selected implications for clinical work. In S. Goldberg, R. Muir, & J. Kerr (Eds.), *Attachment theory: Social, developmental and clinical perspectives* (pp. 407–470). Hillsdale, NJ: Analytic Press.

Main, M., Goldwyn, R., & Hesse, E. (2002). *Adult attachment scoring and classification systems (Version 7.1)*. Unpublished manuscript, University of California at Berkeley, Berkeley, CA.

Malatesta, C. Z., Culver, C., Tesman, J. R., & Shepard, B. (1989). The development of emotion expression during the first two years of life. *Monographs of the Society for Research in Child Development, 54*, 1–104.

Mäntymaa, M., Puura, K., Luoma, I., Salmelin, R. K., & Tamminen, T. (2004). Early mother–infant interaction, parental mental health and symptoms of behavioral and emotional problems in toddlers. *Infant Behavior and Development, 27*(2), 134–149.

Mayers, H. A., & Siegler, A. L. (2004). Finding each other using a psychoanalytic–developmental perspective to build understanding and strengthen attachment between teenaged mothers and their babies. *Journal of Infant, Child, and Adolescent Psychotherapy, 3*(4), 44–465.

McDonald, L., Conrad, T., Fairtlough, A., Fletcher, J., Green, L., Moore, L., & Lepps, B. (2009). An evaluation of a groupwork intervention for teenage mothers and their families. *Child and Family Social Work, 14*(1), 45–57.

Moran, G., Pederson, D. R., & Krupka, A. (2005). Maternal unresolved attachment status impedes the effectiveness of interventions with adolescent mothers. *Infant Mental Health Journal, 26*(3), 231–249.

Morinis, J., Carons, C., & Quigley, M. A. (2013). Effect of teenage motherhood on cognitive outcomes in children: A population-based cohort study. *Archives of Disease in Childhood, 98*(12), 259–264.

Osofsky, J. D., Eberhart-Wright, A., Ware, L. M., & Hann, D. M. (1992). Children of adolescent mothers: A group at risk for psychopathology. *Infant Mental Health Journal, 13*(2), 119–131.

Osofsky, J. D., Hann, D. M., & Peebles, C. (1993). Adolescent parenthood: Risks and opportunities for mothers and infants. In C. H. Zeanah (Ed.), *Handbook of infant mental health* (pp. 106–199). New York: Guilford Press.

Papoušek, M., Schieche, M., & Wurmser, H. (2008). *Disorders of behavioral and emotional regulation in the first years of life*. Washington, DC: ZERO TO THREE Press.

Pomerleau, A., Scuccimarri, C., & Malcuit, G. (2003). Mother–infant behavioural interactions in teenage and adult mothers during the first six months postpartum: Relations with infant development. *Infant Mental Health Journal, 24*(5), 495–509.

Rafferty, Y., Griffin, K. W., & Lodise, M. (2011). Adolescent motherhood and developmental outcomes of children in Early Head Start: The influence of maternal parenting behaviors, well-being, and risk factors within the family setting. *American Journal of Orthopsychiatry, 81*(2), 228–245.

Reid, V., & Meadows-Oliver, M. (2007). Postpartum depression in adolescent mothers: An integrated review of the literature. *Journal of Pediatric Health Care, 21*(5), 289–298.

Riva Crugnola, C., Gazzotti, S., Spinelli, M., Ierardi, E., Caprin, C., & Albizzati, A. (2013). Maternal attachment influences mother–infant styles of regulation and play with objects at nine months. *Attachment and Human Development, 15*(2), 107–131.

Riva Crugnola, C., Ierardi, E., Albizzati, A., & Downing, G. (2016). Effectiveness of an attachment-based intervention program in promoting emotion regulation and attachment in adolescent mothers and their infants: A pilot study. *Frontiers in Psychology, 7,* 195.

Riva Crugnola, C., Ierardi, E., Gazzotti, S., & Albizzati, A. (2013, August/September). *Emotion regulation and maternal attachment in adolescent mothers and their infants: Risk assessment and video feedback intervention.* Presented at the 6th International Attachment Conference, Medimond International Proceedings, Pavia, Italy.

Riva Crugnola, C., Ierardi, E., Gazzotti, S., & Albizzati, A. (2014). Motherhood in adolescent mothers, maternal attachment, mother–infant styles of interaction and emotion regulation at three months. *Infant Behavior and Development, 37*(1), 44–56.

Riva Crugnola, C., Tambelli, R., Spinelli, M., Gazzotti, S., Caprin, C., & Albizzati, A. (2011). Attachment patterns and emotion regulation strategies in the second year. *Infant Behavior and Development, 34*(1), 136–151.

Roye, C., & Balk, S. (1996). The relationship of partner support to outcomes for teenage mothers and their children: A review. *Journal of Adolescent Health, 19*(2), 86–93.

Savio Beers, L. A., & Hollo, R. E. (2009). Approaching the adolescent-headed family: A review of teen parenting. *Current Problems in Pediatric and Adolescent Health Care, 39*(9), 216–233.

Slade, A., Grienenberger, J., Bernbach, E., Levy, D., & Locker, A. (2005). Maternal reflective functioning and attachment: Considering the transmission gap. *Attachment and Human Development, 7*(3), 283–292.

Slade, A., Sadler, L., & Mayes, L. C. (2005). Maternal reflective functioning: Enhancing parental reflective functioning in a nursing/mental health home visiting program. In L. Berlin, Y. Ziv, L. Amaya-Jackson, & M. Greenberg (Eds.), *Enhancing early attachments: Theory, research, intervention, and policy* (pp. 152–177). New York: Guilford Press.

Sroufe, L. A., Egeland, B., Carlson, E. A., & Collins, W. A. (2005). *The development of the person.* New York: Guilford Press.

Steele, H., Steele, M., & Fonagy, P. (1996). Associations among attachment classifications of mothers, fathers, and their infants: Evidence for a relationship-specific perspective. *Child Development, 67*(2), 541–555.

Steele, M., Steele, H., Bate, J., Knafo, H., Kinsey, M., Bonuck, K., . . . Murphy, A. (2014). Looking from the outside in: The use of video in attachment-based interventions. *Attachment and Human Development, 16*(4), 402–415.

Strunk, J. A. (2008). The effect of school-based health clinics on teenage pregnancy and parenting outcomes: An integrated literature review. *Journal of School Nursing, 24*(1), 13–20.

Waddell, M. (2009). Why teenagers have babies. *Infant Observation, 12,* 271–281.

Weinberg, M. K., & Tronick, E. Z. (1999). *Infant and Caregiver Engagement Phases (ICEP).* Unpublished scoring manual, Boston Children's Hospital/Harvard Medical School, Cambridge, MA.

CHAPTER 21

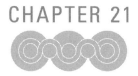

Supporting Father Involvement
A Father-Inclusive Couples Group Approach to Parenting Interventions

PHILIP A. COWAN, CAROLYN PAPE COWAN,
MARSHA KLINE PRUETT, and KYLE PRUETT

In this chapter we describe an evidence-based couples group intervention for parents of young children that has been conducted over many years, in several different contexts, under several different names. The first two authors' (P. A. C. and C. P. C.) first intervention program, Becoming a Family, was evaluated by following 96 working- and middle-class couples living in 28 cities and towns in the San Francisco Bay area who were making the transition to parenthood for the first time (C. P. Cowan & Cowan, 2000). The program followed couples from pregnancy, through 6 months of group meetings, and postintervention, until the children had made the transition to elementary school. They then evaluated the same intervention in the Schoolchildren and their Families program by following a similar sample of 100 couples with a first child about to make the transition to school—from prekindergarten until the children had entered high school (P. A. Cowan, Cowan, Ablow, Johnson, & Measelle, 2005; C. P. Cowan, Cowan, & Barry, 2011). In these first two longitudinal studies of working-class or middle-class families, approximately 85% of the participants were European American, and 15% were African American, Asian, or Hispanic. A third, much more extensive intervention trial, which is the main focus of this chapter, is the Supporting Father Involvement (SFI) program for primarily low-income families, developed in a collaboration among the four chapter authors (P. A. Cowan, Cowan, Pruett, Pruett, & Wong, 2009; P. A. Cowan, Cowan, Pruett, Pruett, & Gillette, 2014; K. D. Pruett, Pruett, Cowan, & Cowan, 2015). Over 10 years, using the couples group format created in the earlier two intervention studies, we offered the same curriculum to more than 800 low-income Mexican American, African American, and European American families in five California counties, who were considered at risk because of their poverty. Each successive iteration of these programs has involved climbing steps on a "ladder" representing increasing risk—from primary prevention groups for middle-class and working-class, mostly married couples making the transition to parenthood or with a child making the transition to school, to married and cohabiting couples at risk because of their poverty, to couples with young children referred to the child welfare system (CWS) because of concerns about domestic violence, child abuse, or neglect. Each iteration of the intervention followed a similar intervention format, curriculum, training of staff, and evaluation protocol. This chapter is organized into four broad sections: (1) important gaps in existing research on parenting and parenting interventions; (2) our couples groups approach to intervention with parents; (3) adult attachment and couple attachment in the family system; and (4) how attachment constructs help to explain our intervention outcomes. We note that at the outset, our intervention was not constructed on a *foundation* of attachment theory. We began in the 1970s with a guiding framework of family systems theory (e.g.,Watzlawick, Bavelas, & Jackson, 1967) and gradually incorporated new ideas from emerging research on couple relationships and emotion regulation (Levenson & Gottman, 1983). The development of the Adult Attachment Interview (AAI; George, Kaplan, & Main, 1985) opened up a new window on how attachment security or insecurity in terms of the parents' representations or working models of attachment were linked with their children's adaptation. We embraced this interview based on its promise to deepen our understanding of the relationship patterns in the families in our Schoolchildren and their Families program of work. We began with a set of correlational studies using data from the intervention participants, which included measures of mothers' and fathers' adult attachment and couple attachment (P. A. Cowan, Cowan, & Mehta, 2009), along with observations of couple and parent–child interaction. We use the results of this research to consider how attachment processes such as safe haven, secure base, affect regulation, and mentalizing help to explain the positive results of our couples group intervention approach to parents of young children. While we find attachment processes to be useful for understanding the findings from our intervention programs and for training the co-leaders who conduct the intervention groups, our initial family systems orientation led us to the conclusion that some key potential resources and targets of intervention are missing from the literature on attachment-based interventions, and indeed from the field of parenting interventions as a whole. Our analysis will show how resources and targets based on a family systems orientation have the potential to increase the positive effects of interventions with mothers and fathers on their children.

What's Missing from Current Research on Parenting and Parenting Interventions?

Fathers Are Missing

In the vast research literature on parent–child relationships, until very recently, most studies focused on mothers and children. The attachment literature exemplifies this pattern (P. A. Cowan & Cowan, 2007), with the exception of the pioneering work on father–child attachment by Karin and Klaus Grossmann (Grossman, Grossman, Kindler, & Zimmermann, 2008) and Miriam and Howard Steele (H. Steele, Steele, & Fonagy, 1996; M. Steele et al., 2003), and occasional mentions of fathers in the flagship journal *Attachment and Human Development*. In a recent worldwide survey of parenting interventions, Panter-Brick and colleagues (2015) reviewed more than 700 studies and found that only a small fraction included fathers or obtained information from them or about them. This is curious, since a careful review of the research literature makes it clear that men's positive involvement in their children's lives is associated with important advantages for children. For example, consistent correlations have been found between fathers' positive engagement with their children and the children's cognitive, social, and emotional development, and fewer behavior problems or DSM diagnoses (see comprehensive research summaries in Cabrera & Tamis-LeMonda, 2013; Lamb & Lewis, 2013; Parke, 2002; K. D. Pruett, 2000).

A more direct way of determining fathers' causal contribution to the development and well-being of their children is to examine the few studies that evaluate what happens when fathers are added to interventions usually administered to mothers. In three separate intervention programs (Brody & Forehand, 1985; Dadds, Sanders, Behrens, & James, 1987; Webster-Stratton, 1985), the developers became concerned about substantial numbers of boys reverting to baseline levels of aggression following their mothers' participation in a therapeutic intervention. Once the authors recruited the fathers to work on these problems and added a new focus on *co*-parenting, all three programs found that a combined parenting or co-parenting/ marital emphasis was more successful in reducing sons' problem behaviors than a parenting skills approach with mothers alone. Analyses of several different types of parent-training interventions in the United States and Europe by Lundahl, Tollefson, Risser, and Lovejoy (2008) and Bakermans-Kranenburg, van IJzendoorn, and Juffer (2003) came to the same conclusion about the potential advantages of including fathers in interventions designed to affect children's behavior.

The Relationship Between the Parents Is Missing

There is usually more than one parenting figure, even in so-called single-parent homes (Carlson, McLanahan, & Brooks-Gunn, 2008), so focusing on (1) the couple and (2) co-parenting is essential to develop strategies for resolving differences in parenting style and disagreements about parenting practices. Each of these two central aspects of parenting is elaborated below.

1. *The parents' relationship as a couple.* Studies of both middle-class (P. A. Cowan, Cowan, Ablow, Johnson, et al., 2005) and low-income families (Brody & Flor, 1997; K. J. Conger, Rueter, & Conger, 2000) reveal that when mothers and fathers are more satisfied with their relationship as a couple or are able to resolve disagreements without escalating the conflict between them, both parents are observed to be more effective in interaction with their children. In addition, their children are described by research staff and teachers as having fewer internalizing and externalizing behavior problems and scoring higher on academic achievement tests. In other studies of fathers' family involvement, one of the best predictors of whether fathers are engaged with their young children is the quality of the men's relationships with

their children's mothers (Carlson, Pilkauskas, McLanahan, & Brooks-Gunn, 2011), a finding that holds for married, cohabiting, separated, and divorced co-parents (M. K. Pruett & Johnston, 2004).

2. *The co-parenting relationship.* Beyond consideration of parent–child relationships, investigators have pointed to the need to consider whether parents are able to act as a team in their treatment of their children (Feinberg, Jones, Kan, & Goslin, 2010; Fivaz-Depeursinge, 2003; McHale & Lindahl, 2011; K. Pruett & Pruett, 2009). There is evidence that the quality of the couple and co-parenting relationships are overlapping but distinct domains of adult family life. In cohabiting, committed couples, for example, the quality of the intimate adult relationship and co-parenting collaboration are correlated, although certainly not perfectly (Krishnakumar & Buehler, 2000). In separated couples, by contrast, the dyadic romantic relationship is severed but the collaboration between the co-parents remains influential in child outcomes (M. Pruett, Insabella, & Gustafson, 2005). Parents in all family structures who maintain a positive alliance can protect their child against the expected negative impact of marital conflict or hostility on their parenting (Sturge-Apple, Cummings, & Davies, 2006).

Attention to the Intergenerational Transmission of Negative Parenting Is Missing

There is ample evidence that without intervention, parents are at high risk of repeating maladaptive interactions experienced in their families of origin (Elder, King, & Conger, 1996). This holds true whether we are talking about harsh parenting or serious forms of child abuse and neglect. While attachment-based parenting interventions usually pay attention to intergenerational patterns and difficulties in creating new and different parenting pathways, most other programs take a here-and-now approach by suggesting new behavioral alternatives for parents to adopt. This ignores the potential advantages of encouraging parents to reflect on early family patterns that did not serve them well, so that they can make conscious efforts to shift their behaviors in ways that are conducive to their children's optimal development.

How to Cope with Stressors Outside the Family and Find Supportive People and Agencies Is Missing

What affects children is not simply how parents behave toward them, but also how family members deal with external stressors that affect their own well-being and level of stress, and how their coping strategies affect their relationships as partners and parents. There is evidence that the impact of poverty and parental job loss on children occurs through an increase in mothers' and fathers' mental health symptoms and a resulting increase in couple distress, both of which lead to less effective parenting strategies (Conger & Donnellan, 2007; Masarik et al., 2016). While parenting interventions cannot directly alter challenges posed by society and culture, they can help parents to cope more effectively when they confront them. Spousal support is an especially powerful influence on parenting when other social supports are inadequate (Simons, Lorenz, Wu, & Conger, 1993). Couples can help each other in skills such as finding agencies and supportive influences in neighbors, extended family, and others, clarifying their common goals in the process.

How to Acknowledge Parents' Own Vulnerabilities Is Often Missing

In order for parents to provide nurturant and sensitive caregiving to their children, they need to feel that at least some of their own needs are being met, and that their own intrapsychic challenges are not shaping their parenting approach in debilitating ways. For example, depression and other forms of psychological distress can compromise mothers' and fathers' parenting, with unfortunate consequences for the children (Coyne, Low, Miller, Seifer, & Dickstein, 2007). Since the development of the AAI (George et al., 1985) and questionnaires that assess attachment style (Fraley & Shaver, 2000), a number of studies have revealed links between parents' insecure working models of attachment, parental insensitivity, and children's poorer developmental outcomes (van IJzendoorn, 1995). Most parenting programs do not take parents' internal working models of attachment into account. Parenting interventions for families at high risk because of poverty, the intergenerational transmission of trauma, identified problems in the child, or a parent's or child's mental illness are more likely to pay attention to helping parents recognize how their own parenting histories and psychological difficulties may be limiting their ability to nurture their child, but these interventions, too, are most often attended by mothers and not fathers, as can be seen in multiple chapters in this volume. Admittedly, when risk of child maltreatment is great, and the trauma burden upon parents is high, mothers are likely to be the ones who have or are awarded custody, while fathers are likely to be incarcerated or the known perpetrators of domestic violence, precluding their participation in the intervention. But even researchers of intimate partner violence are finding that couples treatments are often more effective than single-sex groups or more traditional treatment modalities (Miller, Drake, & Nafziger, 2013; Stith, McCollum, Amanor-Boadu, & Smith, 2012), affirming the power of the couple as a context for treating trauma in appropriate situations.

Implications of These Gaps for Our Couples Group Intervention

We have written elsewhere about evidence for a five-domain model of the risk and protective factors that affect individual family members and the quality of relationships among them (P. A. Cowan & Cowan, 2012). The research findings pushed us to widen our view of parenting interventions from the usual focus on mothers to include fathers, and to focus on (1) the psychological state of each parent; (2) the relationship between the parents, both as intimate partners and co-parents; (3) the quality of each parent's interactions with their child; (4) the difficulties involved in breaking intergenerational cycles of negative parenting; and (5) coping strategies for dealing with challenging external forces that influence the context in which couples and their children are developing. The curricula in each version of our couples group intervention included material that addressed these five domains of family life, in order to minimize risk and strengthen protective factors for the parents' and children's development and well-being. See Table 21.1 for a schematic presentation of the key aspects of our approach.

TABLE 21.1. Summary of Key Intervention Features

Intervention modality	Couples groups	4–7 couples	Male–female leader team
Target populations	Becoming a Family	Schoolchildren and Their Families	Supporting Father Involvement
	Primarily working-class and middle-class couples having a first baby: 85% European American; 15% Asian, African American, and Hispanic	Primarily working-class and middle-class couples with a first child entering school: 85% European American; 15% Asian, African American, and Hispanic	Low-income Mexican American, African American, and European American couples with young children (ages 0–11)
Hours	24 two-hour sessions	16 two-hour sessions	16 two-hour sessions
Leaders' role	Act as guides, helping couples to become the parents and partners they hope to be		
Curriculum topics	Sessions begin with open-ended check-in followed by structured curriculum material covering each of the five domains in our family risk/protective model.		

	Individual	Couple	Parent–child	Three generations	Life stress/ social support
Number of sessions	3	5	4	2	2

Group activities	Discussions, games, exercises, role plays, mini-lectures, videos, "homework" assignments

Theory of change	• Consistent with family systems theories, we assume that the couple or co-parenting relationship is a key influence on family members and their relationships. Improving the couple relationship will have positive reverberations in the family as a system.
	• In a safe environment, group leaders, couples, and the group itself provide a safe haven and a secure base. Group activities raise frequently avoided issues. Individuals and couples are able to
	  o normalize their experience of being partners and parents,
	  o explore areas of difference, disagreement, and conflict;
	  o provide more positively regulated emotion, create confiding and closeness rather than continued escalation of negative affect, and
	  o try new strategies of partnering and parenting.

Our Couples Group Approach to Parenting

The Groups

While the recruitment procedures and target populations for our couples group intervention have varied across five clinical trials, the curriculum structure and group process have remained relatively constant over the years. Four to six couples who are raising at least one young child together, and who are not recruited or mandated for treatment because of specific parent or child problems, meet weekly for 16 weeks (32 hours). In two of the 16 weeks, mothers and fathers meet separately with one of the co-leaders; the fathers bring their youngest child for a play session to highlight the men's parenting ideas and experiences without the women present, while the mothers meet to share their experience of encouraging the fathers' parenting, while honoring their own central parenting ideas.

Group leaders are male–female teams, with the equivalent of a master's level education or beyond and experience in therapy or counseling with couples or children, offered individually or in groups. Prospective leaders participate in 2–4 days of training and are followed weekly or bimonthly with consultation/supervision once their parent groups begin. After the first introductory meeting with the parents, each subsequent session starts with a half-hour check-in, during which couples can bring positive or negative issues that arose during the week or as they tried to do the "homework" suggested at the end of the previous session. The remaining time in each 2-hour session focuses on a topic from one of the five risk/protective aspects of family life: taking care of oneself or dealing with stress or depression; couple communication, conflict resolution, domestic violence, and co-parenting challenges; parenting styles (avoiding the continuation of negative patterns from one's family of origin) and finding help in dealing with external stresses and building additional support. Some topics are introduced by short presentations by the co-leaders that are then expanded by exercises that stimulate reflection and discussion. For example, after a presentation by the leaders defining authoritarian, authoritative, and permissive parenting (Baumrind, 1966; Larzelere, Morris, & Harrist, 2013), participants engage in role plays enacting different parenting approaches, which typically generate intense exchanges, especially as we focus on how both the parent and child might be feeling in these situations. Similar exercises focus on how couples handle their differences and conflicts as partners and parents with short video segments (about 10 minutes) from popular movies and presentations about communication styles of attacking, avoiding, or confiding, which stimulate discussions about couples' typical styles of resolving conflict, what they want to change, and how children typically react when they observe their parents' unresolved disagreements, frosty silences, or flaming arguments. In another example, a volunteer is given a small jug of water and asked to pour out the liquid that reflects his or her loss of energy when different ordinary and stressful life events are draining stamina or resourcefulness. The group members then discusses what they can do to "refill their jug," a metaphor that they often carry over from session to session as they describe their weekly challenges as parents and partners. To explore intergenerational issues, each person is given a set of family figures to place on a small board to represent how close or distant the members are relative to each other. In small subgroups, each parent then describes his or her family situation to the others. When the larger group reconvenes, a member of the small group who is not the partner describes to the larger group what he or she understood about another member's family situation. Many of these exercises foster reflection on the past and highlight the challenge of how to avoid repeating negative patterns from the families in which they grew up.

In the initial groups of working-class and middle-class couples making the transition to parenthood or with a first child starting school, most groups took place in the early evening and child care was not provided. The newborns in the first program became part of the groups as they were born and the preschoolers in the second program were put to bed at home before parents came to the groups. In the low-income communities in which the SFI intervention is offered, often immediately after work, the project has included three additional components: (1) food for the families before the meetings, (2) child care while the parents meet in their groups, and (3) the ongoing services of a case manager who monitors group attendance and is available to make referrals for other services as needed (housing, welfare, job training, mental health).

If we think of types of group process on a continuum ranging from open-ended group therapy on one end to didactic psychoeducational skills training on the other, our intervention is located in between: We use clinically trained co-leaders, unstructured time to discuss personal issues during the weekly check-ins, structured topics, and exercises and activities that make parts of the curriculum come alive. The aim of the group leaders is not to *teach* specific parenting or couple communication skills, but rather to provide a setting in which partners feel supported in examining their underlying ideas and goals, become more conscious of what upsets them and why, confide rather than attack or withdraw from each other when they confront challenges, and draw on each other, on other participants, and on the group leaders for help and support to try more effective strategies—all with the goal of trying to move closer to their conceptions of themselves as the partners and parents they hope to be. Although general topics are offered by the group leaders from the curriculum, much of the explicit content comes from parents themselves. We believe that this is why the program has been helpful to couples from varied economic and ethnic backgrounds—often in the same groups (see M. K. Pruett, Cowan, Cowan, & Pruett, 2009). These models, rather than being prescriptive, are open to individual and cultural interpretations imposed by the participants rather than the program developers.

Results

We present a brief summary of the results of our earlier studies with working-class and middle-class participants. We then focus on SFI, the latest version of our intervention with more vulnerable families, in part because it represents our most current thinking, and in part because we are finding that it is effective with an even broader range of families. A summary of these results is provided in Table 21.2.

The Earlier Studies

In the Becoming a Family intervention (C. P. Cowan & Cowan, 2000), couples were randomly assigned to a couples group intervention ($n = 28$) or a no-group condition ($n = 38$), and followed up regularly until the children had completed their first year of elementary school. A group of 24 comparable couples who had not yet decided to have a baby were followed over the same period of time, with the same personal interviews and questionnaires. The group intervention with the parents, conducted over 24 weeks before and after the babies' births (48 hours contact time over 6 months), had a long-term positive effect on maintaining couple relationship quality over 6 years (Schulz, Pape, & Cowan, 2006), demonstrating that working on challenging family issues *during* the transition to parenthood prevented

TABLE 21.2. Summary of Intervention versus Control Comparisons

Domain	Individual	Couple relationship quality	Parent–child	Three-generation relationships and patterns	Life stress/social support	Child outcome of intervention
Becoming a Family	Increase in investment in identity as parent	Stable satisfaction versus decline in satisfaction for controls	No intervention effects on father involvement (intervention and control fathers become more involved after the couple gave birth to a first child) Stable husband–wife satisfaction with level of father involvement versus decline for controls	Qualitative data indicated marked shifts, positive and negative, in relationships with family of origin	No intervention effects; life stress and social support remained stable	No intervention effects found 5 years after intervention
Schoolchildren and their Families (parenting emphasis versus controls)		Stable observed marital conflict versus increase in observed marital conflict for controls	No change in father involvement Increase in positive parenting (observed)	No intervention effects	No intervention effects; life stress and social support remained stable	Fewer internalizing behaviors rated by teachers 2 years postintervention Greater child-reported well-being
Schoolchildren and their Families (couple emphasis versus controls)		Less observed conflict versus no change for controls	No change in father involvement Increase in positive parenting (observed)	No intervention effects	No intervention effects; life stress and social support stable	Fewer externalizing behaviors 2 years postintervention Greater tested academic achievement
Supporting Father Involvement (SFI; fathers' groups versus controls)		Declining satisfaction for fathers' groups and controls	Greater father involvement	No intervention effects	No intervention effects; life stress and social support remained stable	Parent-reported behavior problems remained stable in children of fathers' group participants versus increased problems in controls
SFI (couples groups versus controls)	Reduction in depression scores in couples group participants	Stable satisfaction for couples group versus decline for fathers groups and controls Reduction in violent problem-solving in couples group versus controls	Reduction in parenting stress in couples group versus no change in controls	No intervention effects	No intervention effects; life stress and social support remained stable	Parent-reported child behavior problems remained stable in children of couples group participants versus increased problems in controls

Note. The results presented in this table include more findings than presented in the text. The results for the SFI intervention represent a composite of three separate clinical trials.

the documented normative decline in relationship satisfaction over time (Twenge, Campbell, & Foster, 2003). Whereas the couples who had babies but no special intervention showed the expected decline in marital satisfaction over the first 6 years of parenthood, the couples who participated in a couples group showed no decline in satisfaction as a couple—and neither did the couples who remained childless over the same 6 years.

In the Schoolchildren and their Families intervention (C. P. Cowan, Cowan, & Heming, 2005), 100 couples with a first child about to make the transition to school were randomly assigned to a low-dose consultation control condition (3 hours of voluntary contact time for each couple over 3 years) or to a couples group that met for 16 weeks before the children entered kindergarten (32 hours total contact time over 4 months). This time, group participants were randomly assigned to one of two variations of the couples group, all conducted by the same co-leader pairs with the same curriculum. During the introductory, open-ended part of each meeting, when parents were free to raise their own personal issues, the co-leaders helped parents in one set of groups focus more on parenting issues, and those in the other set of groups, more on issues in their relationships as a couple, to test whether an emphasis on parent–child or couple relationship issues made a difference to the outcomes of the intervention. The rest of the curriculum at each session was identical in both sets of groups. Two years after the couples groups ended, when the children had completed first grade, our staff observations of the parents and children working and playing together revealed that parents in the groups that focused more on parenting in the open-ended portion of the meetings were significantly warmer and more structured with their children than parents in the control condition. Their children showed fewer internalizing behaviors in their first-grade classrooms, as rated by teachers, and reported a greater sense of confidence and well-being in an individual puppet interview (Cowan, Cowan, & Heming, 2005). Parents in the groups that emphasized the couple and co-parenting relationship in the open-ended portion also showed significantly more effective parenting strategies than parents in the control condition—but in contrast with couples without a group intervention, they showed no increase in their level of couple conflict over the transition to school period. Reports from first-grade teachers revealed that children of the latter parents were less aggressive at school, and when tested individually by a member of the research team who had no knowledge of the condition to which the family had been assigned, showed significantly higher levels of academic achievement than children of parents in the control condition. Finally, in an unusually long-term follow-up assessment 10 years later, as the children made the transition to high school in ninth grade, positive intervention effects on mothers, fathers, and children were still apparent (C. P. Cowan et al., 2011).

Supporting Father Involvement

On the basis of the published positive results from the first two intervention trials, we were invited by the California State Office of Child Abuse Prevention to create and evaluate a group intervention with a large set of low-income families to see whether working on the same five aspects of family life would be effective for families with even fewer resources and greater relationship challenges than the couples in the first two intervention studies. The idea was also to increase the quantity and quality of fathers' involvement in their children's care and collaborative co-parenting as a preventive for potential abuse and neglect. During the first phase of the SFI study (P. A. Cowan, Cowan, Pruett, Pruett, & Wong, 2009), 279 Mexican American and European American couples were invited to take part in one of the following conditions on a randomly assigned basis, all with the same staff: (1) a one-time informational meeting for a group of couples (3 contact hours); (2) a 16-week group for fathers (32 contact hours); or (3) a 16-week group for couples (32 contact hours). The families had children ranging in age from 0 to 7 years, with the typical age of the youngest child 2–2.5 years, and some had older children as well. About two-thirds of the couples in each of these trials were married, most of the rest were cohabiting, and a few did not live together but were committed to collaboration in raising their child. These families were considered more at risk for child abuse and neglect, because two-thirds of them were at the lowest end of the income scale. In this first phase, none of the families was involved with the CWS when they entered the study. Couples were assessed with self-report questionnaires covering topics in the five-domain model at baseline, assessed 7 months later (2–3 months after the groups ended), and again 18 months later (more than a year after the intervention ended). Fathers and mothers who participated in the one-time informational meeting revealed no positive changes and some negative changes over 18 months—as individuals, couples, and parents—and they described increases in acting out, aggressive behaviors or shy, withdrawn, depressed behaviors in their children. Those who participated in the 16-week fathers-only groups showed increased father involvement and no increase in their children's problematic behaviors, but as in the control condition, these mothers and fathers showed declining satisfaction as a couple. By contrast, parents who participated in a couples group maintained their satisfaction as couples over those 18 months, showed reduced stress as parents, and their children's behaviors remained stable. So, as in our earlier interventions, a couples group for both parents resulted in keeping couple relationship satisfaction from declining and in boosting the individual well-being of the parents and their children.

We were encouraged by the funders to conduct a replication study, using the same procedures for recruitment, measurement, and follow-up, and adding another county with African American participants to our samples of Mexican American and European American couples (P. A. Cowan et al., 2014). In all, we served 236 couples from three ethnic backgrounds in five counties in the second trial. Of 11 measures used in the first phase, 10 revealed positive baseline-to-18-month changes in the second phase. Fathers' involvement in the care of their children increased significantly. The families showed positive changes similar to those in the earlier benchmark study results on six measures (decline in parenting stress; no decline in couple relationship satisfaction; no increase in children's hyperactivity, social withdrawal, or psychological symptoms; and increased income). On two measures, this second set of low-income families showed even greater positive change (reductions in parents' violent problem solving and children's aggression).

In a third clinical trial in the same five counties (being written up now), we conducted a new randomized clinical trial with 230 families that compared a community sample of low-income community parents as recruited before with families referred by CWS because they had been investigated for domestic violence, child abuse, or neglect. Approximately 60% of the 230 couples were randomly chosen and offered a chance to participate in a group immediately after recruitment, and 40% were offered a chance to participate in a group 7 months after recruitment, meanwhile receiving treatment as usual in the community, with the latter families constituting a delay control condition. Comparisons were made 7 months after all families entered the study, before those in the delay control condition had a chance to participate in a couples group. Preliminary as-yet unpublished results show that in comparison with the couples in the delay condition, couples who participated immediately showed a significant reduction in conflict and violence 2 months after the intervention, which was related to a significant reduction in harsh and anxious parenting 1 year later, which, in turn was related to fewer internalizing and externalizing problems in parents' descriptions of their children. While the CWS-referred parents at entrance to the study described themselves as showing higher risks for child abuse on a standardized questionnaire, there were no significant differences between CWS and non-CWS participants in the pattern of their intervention results.

We noted that the summary of results in Table 21.2 includes some findings that we did not have space to discuss in the text. One general conclusion from an examination of the table is that although the curriculum contains material from five domains of family risk, the intervention produced effects in three (individual parent and individual child, couple relationship, parent–child relationship). These changes occurred in spite of the fact that there were no statistically significant changes in life stressors or social supports; that is, both middle- and low-income families were developing skills to cope with external pressures, without being able to alter these pressures. Furthermore, the quantitative measure of the parents' relationships with their parents showed no change attributable to participation in the couples groups. Perhaps if we had been able to use the AAI both pre- and postintervention, we could have shown some increased understanding of both strengths and difficulties in the relationships across generations (i.e., it is possible that there could have been a move toward "earned security").

In our view, the results from these five clinical trials of our couples group intervention offered over many years to parents at increasing risk and distress provide strong evidence that (1) a couples group for parents of young children has positive outcomes for mothers and fathers, in that it decreases couple conflict, lowers parenting stress, and maintains relationship satisfaction over a substantial period of time; (2) a focus on the couple relationship provides a value-added component in comparison with a singular focus on parenting; (3) including both parents results in stronger effects than groups for fathers alone; and (4) parents' participation in a couples group with clinically trained leaders lowers the potential for problematic behaviors in the children.

Dissemination and Training

The SFI intervention is currently being disseminated in a number of new venues. For the past 3 years, staff members from Strategies, a training organization funded by the California Department of Social Services and trained by the Cowans and the

Pruetts, have been training local service providers to offer the SFI intervention in 13 new California counties.

In 2011, the Province of Alberta brought SFI to Canada and implemented the full program funded by the Norlien (now Palix) Foundation at four family resource centers, with a scaled-back evaluation component (M. K. Pruett, Gillette, Pruett, Cowan, & Cowan, in press). In 2013, the British government funded Parents as Partners (the renamed SFI program) for a 4-year trial, with a substantial evaluation component. Based at the Tavistock Centre for Couple Relationships in London, the project is now operating in more than a dozen London boroughs (Draper, 2015) and in other cities in Britain. A recent article (Casey et al., in press) based on the results from the first 100 couples showed results similar to, or stronger than, those in the California trials. In summary, the SFI interventions have been effective with families from a range of ethnic backgrounds and economic circumstances in all three countries. Additional expansions of the model include work with young (teen) parents (in Fresno, California, and New Haven, Connecticut) and replacing Case Managers with Home Visitors (in Massachusetts) to increase the latter's well-evaluated program outreach to be more inclusive of fathers.

The various iterations of our couples group intervention have used a training-of-trainers model in which the program creators (the Cowans and/or the Pruetts) trained new group leaders in sessions ranging from 2 to 4 days, and these leaders, after they have mastered the work of co-leading groups themselves, progress to training others. In every case, the initial training has been followed by ongoing supervision and consultation while the trainees conduct their first groups. Although the Cowans and the Pruetts have not established an infrastructure in which trainings take place on a regular basis, the group at the London Tavistock Centre for Couple Relationships (recently renamed Tavistock Relationships) has a nucleus of trainers now offering training workshops and supervision in many locales in the United Kingdom, with plans for further expansion. In this research building and dissemination process over 40 years, we have moved from "laboratory" university-based efficacy trials to community-based effectiveness trials for families in many locales, and from a range of socioeconomic and ethnic backgrounds in the "real world."[1]

Adult Attachment and Couple Attachment in the Family System

As we were conducting the intervention studies we have described here, we became increasingly interested in the role of attachment processes in family relationships, especially in the links between parents' working models of attachment and the quality of both their couple and parent–child relationships. In our recent studies, which included many hundreds of families, given the time and expense involved in coding the AAI, we were unable to administer AAI assessments both pre- and postintervention to determine whether the interventions alter men's or women's security of attachment over time. Instead, we began by examining links between parents' AAI measures of secure–insecure attachment and what we observed in couple

---

[1] Although a university-based intervention is often described as taking place in a "laboratory," and a community-based intervention, in the "real world," there are elements of both in each context.

and parent–child interactions in order to understand the connections among adult attachment, family relationship quality, and children's behavior. We describe those results here, and briefly touch on some relevant research from other investigators using either the AAI or attachment style questionnaires as a foundation for our speculations about how attachment principles help to explain the positive impact of our couples group interventions.

The application of attachment theory to couple relationships (Alexandrov, Cowan, & Cowan, 2005; Crowell & Owens, 1996; Dickstein, Seifer, St. Andre, & Schiller, 2001; Mikulincer & Shaver, 2007) takes as a basic assumption that an individual's mental model of intimate relationships formed in the family of origin will be expressed in behavior toward both romantic partners and children. In its most definitive version, this assumption describes the working model as a prototype in which early experiences form a template for all subsequent intimate relationships (Owens et al., 1995).

Pairing of Parents' Adult Attachment Classifications

We noted earlier that almost all studies of the connection between adult attachment and family relationships using the AAI have been conducted with mothers, with the result that the potential contribution of fathers' attachment models to their children's development has been ignored or minimized. In our first small-n study of adult attachment, we collected AAIs on 27 first-time mothers and fathers when their children were 3½ years old. What caught our attention was that the *pairing* of the two parents' attachment status seemed to make a difference in how they behaved in interaction with each other and with their children. As expected, and as others have found for mothers (van IJzendoorn, 1995), there were clear differences between pairs in which both parents were classified as secure and pairs in which both were classified as insecure, in both their couple interaction (Cohn, Silver, Cowan, Cowan, & Pearson, 1992) and their parent–child interactions (Cohn, Cowan, Cowan, & Pearson, 1992) as we observed them (see a schematic presentation of these results in Figure 21.1). However, if a wife classified as insecurely attached on the AAI had a husband classified as securely attached, the wife's parenting behavior and the quality of the couple and parent–child interaction were indistinguishable from those of the secure–secure pairs; that is, a husband with a secure working model of attachment appeared to buffer the potentially negative effects of his wife's insecure model on both their couple and parenting interactions. In this small sample there were too few examples of couples in which husbands had an insecure working model and wives had a secure working model to look at the reverse situation. However, in a larger sample of couples with a 5-year-old first child, Bradburn (1997) was able to assess all four combinations. She found that securely attached mothers did not buffer the negative impact of insecurely attached fathers on their couple and parent–child relationships; that is, the quality of wives' interactions with their 6-year-olds depended on whether their husbands were categorized as securely or insecurely attached on the AAI. One lesson from these results is that, contrary to the template theory in which individual working models of adult attachment shape later behavior, we may not be able to determine the impact of mothers' working model of attachment on their parenting without knowing about

Paired Attachment Category (AAI)	Cohn, Cowan, et al. (1992) Cohn, Silver, et al. (1992) Couple relationship quality and Mom's parenting quality	Bradburn (1997) Couple relationship quality and Mom's parenting quality
Mom securely attached Dad securely attached	+	+
Mom insecurely attached Dad insecurely attached	−	−
Mom insecurely attached Dad securely attached	+[a]	+[a]
		Couple relationship quality and Dad's parenting quality
Mom securely attached Dad insecurely attached	Not tested[b]	−[c]

[a]The question in the mixed pair "Mom insecurely attached, Dad securely attached" is whether the Dad's attachment security provides a buffer for the couple relationship and Mom's parenting (expected on the basis of her attachment classification to be negative).

[b]This combination was not tested in this study, because in 25 couples there was only one couple in this paired category.

[c]The question in the mixed pair "Dad insecurely attached, Mom securely attached" is whether the Mom's attachment security provides a buffer for the couple relationship and Dad's parenting (expected on the basis of his attachment classification to be negative).

FIGURE 21.1. Couple attachment pairing, couple relationship quality, and parenting quality: A schematic view of results.

the fathers' working model. Furthermore, the results suggest, but do not prove, that increasing men's security of attachment could possibly have a positive impact on the whole family system.

Predicting Child Outcomes: Adult Attachment and Couple Attachment Data from Both Parents

In another line of research that used data from our intervention studies, we investigated what van IJzendoorn (1995) has described as a "transmission gap"; that is, whereas a number of studies have found correlations among mothers' security of attachment, sensitivity of parenting, and children's development, this "transmission" model does not explain all of the variations in children's behavior and adaptation.

Adult Attachment and Child Behavior

In one study (P. A. Cowan, Bradburn, & Cowan, 2005), we used path analyses to trace the links among three AAI scale scores (Coherence, Parent Loving, Anger at Parent), observed and self-reported couple relationship quality, and observed parent–child interaction—all measured before children entered kindergarten—as predictors of children's internalizing and externalizing behaviors rated by their kindergarten teachers 1 year later. Separate models linking fathers' and mothers' AAI scores to externalizing behavior revealed that the data from parents explained large proportions of the variance in teacher-rated behavior in children's first year of school—as much as 53–63% of the links between both parents' attachment, marital, and parenting measures and daughter's externalizing behavior, and as much as 43% of the connections between fathers' scores and sons' externalizing behavior.

Couple Attachment and Child Behavior

Based directly on the questions in the AAI, the Cowans and two colleagues developed a Couple Attachment Interview (CAI; Silver, Cohn, Cowan, & Cowan, 1990). A coding system was created and validated (Alexandrov et al., 2005) to provide continuous scores based on the similarity of the overall transcribed CAI to three prototype descriptions: Secure, Dismissing, and Preoccupied. Using path models (P. Cowan, Cowan, & Mehta, 2009), we found that when parents are categorized as having secure working models of relationships with their parents and their partners, they tend to behave more positively with each other, and this, in turn, leads to more effective co-parenting of their child, and ultimately to more positive developmental outcomes in the child. The path models explained 20% of the variation in children's academic achievement, 33% of the variance in teacher-rated internalizing behavior, and 47% of the variance in children's externalizing behavior. Data from security of attachment in the couple relationship added significant predictive power to the data from the father–child and mother–child observations; that is, it is not only the mother's parenting behavior that links her working models of adult attachment to outcomes for the child: The father's parenting behavior, the quality of couple attachment, and observations of how parents treat each other are also involved in the intergenerational transmission of family patterns.

Attachment-Based Interventions for Couples

The data from correlational studies support the theoretical assumption that there are strong links among working models of couple relationships, observed behavior, and children's outcomes. They suggest that if an intervention enhances attachment security, positive changes in family relationships and children's adaptation ought to follow. The problem is that there are very few studies of couples interventions that actually measure changes in attachment security. We found one study that followed couples from pre- to posttherapy (Benson, Sevier, & Christensen, 2013) and another that used a randomized clinical trial design (Johnson et al., 2015). Neither found changes in adult attachment, but we wonder whether adult attachment was the most appropriate measure: We would expect *couple* attachment to change as a result of couples therapy, but not necessarily adult attachment based on relationships with one's parents.

Sue Johnson (2013) is a couples therapist who developed emotion-focused therapy (EFT)—an evidence-based intervention with a central emphasis on attachment theory. She theorizes that the anxiety, depression, and anger in couples coming for therapy have their source in perceived threats to the endurance of the relationship (fears of rejection or abandonment), or in attachment wounds that partners suffered when they were younger that are reevoked in the present couple relationship. The central goals of EFT are to help both partners to understand this process in order to deescalate negative cycles and to meet each other's attachment needs and build stronger couple bonds. Johnson's main technique is to focus on moments of emotional arousal when the attachment system is activated and to provide a therapeutic environment in which both partners can deescalate their anxiety or anger by coming to new understandings and expectations about what is leading to the arousal and what is possible in a less anxiety-ridden relationship. Moser and colleagues (2016) recently provided empirical support for Johnson's formulation in a study using EFT and a version of Brennan, Clark, and Shaver's (1998) Experiences in Close Relationships scale, modified so that all of the questions reflect attachment to the participant's current partner. Over the course of EFT, couples significantly decreased in relationship-specific attachment avoidance and anxiety, and these changes were associated with increases in relationship satisfaction. We cannot tell from this study whether the changes in attachment security caused the changes in relationship satisfaction, whether the changes in relationship satisfaction led to changes in attachment security, or whether it worked both ways. Nevertheless, the findings do provide support for the idea that attachment security may be an important ingredient of partners' satisfaction with their relationship. We are not aware of any couples intervention studies that have attempted to link *changes* in couple attachment security to benefits for the children.

Mechanisms Involved in Becoming Securely Attached

We know that attachment-based interventions are effective. The important question to be answered next is "How do they work?" We adopt several ideas about how people become securely attached to explain how our interventions may have produced the outcomes they did. We have argued that Bowlby never asserted that attachment security is stamped in during the early years of life and strongly resistant to change (P. Cowan & Cowan, 2007). Rather, he claimed that although the attachment system is a built-in evolutionary survival strategy, pathways leading to secure or insecure working models are a function of the child's cumulative experiences with one or more caregivers and whether he or she learns to expect that someone will be there to turn to for protection, comfort, and emotional support—to provide a *safe haven*. Less written about, but equally important to creating a secure working model of attachment relationships, is whether the child experiences encouragement and support for moving away from the caretaker to explore the world, with the expectation that the caregiver will be there when the child returns—that is, to provide a *secure base*.

An interesting line of research centers around safe haven and secure base concepts as helping to uncover the unique contribution of fathers in enhancing the development of their children. The literature on attachment is replete with claims of weak connections between fathers' behavior and whether their children are securely attached, as assessed in the separation and reunion procedures of the Strange Situation (see the meta-analysis by Lucassen et al., 2011). In a review of their own and others' studies (Grossmann et al., 2008), the Grossmanns have shown convincingly that the importance of fathers to their children's development may have been underestimated, because the Strange Situation emphasizes the function of the parent as a safe haven but does not assess the function of the parent, especially the father, in providing a secure base for exploration and play. The Grossmanns assessed both mothers and fathers in play with their 2-year-olds and found that fathers' sensitive and challenging behavior (providing a cooperative, accepting context that also encouraged mature play and autonomous behavior) predicted children's later attachment security, whereas mothers' behavior in a play context did not. A recent study (Kerns, Mathews, Koehn, Williams, & Siener-Ciesla, 2015) assessed both safe haven and secure base support through self-reports of 10- to 14-year-olds and found that both types of support from both parents were related to school outcomes, but that children reported greater safe haven support from mothers and greater secure base support from fathers.

The need for a figure or figures to provide a safe haven and secure base is lifelong (Mikulincer & Shaver, 2007). Adults, as well as children, need important people who listen when they are upset, tolerate their painful feelings, share experiences, and provide emotional support and comfort (a safe haven). They also need people who encourage exploration, trying new things, autonomous problem solving, self-soothing, and self-reflection (a secure base). For many contemporary adults, the expectation, at least at the beginning of a long-term committed romantic relationship, is that a primary safe haven and secure base figure will be one's romantic partner.

Interpretations of the attachment system as an emotion regulation system help to explain how attachment figures function as a safe haven and how a secure base promotes attachment security (Hill, Fonagy, Safier, & Sargent, 2003; Mikulincer, Shaver, & Pereg, 2003). The main function of the attachment system, which springs into action under the real or imagined threat of a loss of closeness or intimacy, is to regulate the emotional arousal (anxiety, depression, anger) triggered by the threat. In positive outcomes, the child seeks proximity to an attachment figure who is available and responsive when the child is upset, or relies on an attachment figure to be available after the child moves away to explore; this helps the child to self-soothe, down-regulate negative emotional arousal, and have the freedom to explore new things to enhance new learning. As children grow older, the emotion regulation function of the parents moves from sheer presence, touch, and reassurance, to listening, reflecting, encouraging talk about emotions, actively attempting to deal with the child's or adolescent's upsetting feelings, and allowing the child room to discover new coping strategies on his or her own (see also "meta-emotion coaching"; Gottman, Katz, & Hooven, 1997). In compelling examples of emotion regulation on the adult level, Coan, Kasle, Jackson, Schaefer, and Davidson (2013) demonstrated that when a husband holds the hand of his wife, who is told that she may be shocked in the process of being assessed in a functional magnetic resonance imaging (fMRI) machine, her physiological arousal is much reduced in comparison to a wife whose hand is held by a stranger. The partner's effect is even stronger when the couple is happily married. One study reported in the Coan et al. article indicates that for the emotion-regulating effect to occur, the woman's partner need only be present, not necessarily holding her hand.

A key component of the capacity to regulate emotion in oneself and others is what Fonagy and colleagues (Fonagy, Steele, Steele, Moran, & Higgitt, 1991) call *mentalisation*—the disposition and ability to be reflective about oneself and one's important relationships. Evidence summarized by Fonagy (2008) suggests that mothers with a secure working model of attachment are able to take a perspective on their child, be reflective, and use emotion language in responding to their child's distress; not surprisingly, their children are more likely to be securely attached and able to conceive that different people may have perspectives unlike their own (see Baradon et al., Chapter 8, this volume).

Our thoughts about the processes in the development of secure attachment in couples have also been shaped in part by the work of Shaver and Mikulincer (2008), who argue that the ability to confide in one's partner, to share vulnerabilities rather than attack or avoid, is a key aspect of establishing a secure model of relationships. More generally, following Fredrickson (2001), they proposed a "broaden and build" cycle of attachment security. Once the attachment system has been aroused in a child or adult, a positive response by an attachment figure augments the individual's resources for coping with stress. In turn, this alters the individual's working models of relationships concerning whether he or she can expect to receive support and nurturance. Of course, no single instance will have such long-lasting effects, but over time, both positive and negative events following attachment threats begin to have a cumulative, stabilizing influence on attachment security.

How Attachment Constructs Help to Explain Intervention Outcomes: Expanding the Constructs "Safe Haven" and "Secure Base"

Given our description of how attachment figures play a role in shaping the individual's developmental pathway toward or away from secure attachment, we can speculate about how this formulation works in the context of a couples group for parents. Although our couples group intervention is not therapy, some of the exercises explicitly raise attachment issues. Steele and Steele (2008), in discussing the clinical applications of the AAI, argue that the interview questions "activate the attachment system . . . by taking the adult back in his or her mind to childhood and earlier life circumstances, when the attachment system was previously activated" (p. 8). Our work in the couples groups and the exercises that examine family patterns, closeness, distance, and styles of caring (or not) evoke childhood memories for most parents in the groups. Encouraging them to describe these experiences—and their effect on them—helps some partners become more self-reflective; for them, this leads to the ability to think about those earlier experiences in the context of their current relationships as parents and partners. Over the months of the group, this encourages many participants to listen to other parents' experiences more openly, soften their reactions to their partners, and consider more consciously how they want to react as partners and parents.

Level 1: The Couple

Central to couples' reports and observations from videotapes of group meetings is the observation that a majority of the individual participants seem to develop more effective emotion regulation strategies, either an increased ability to self-soothe or an increased perception that when they are distressed, they can rely on their partner to tolerate their vulnerability and be supportive. In a qualitative study of the Canadian replication of SFI, the participants described themselves as having greater awareness of their own feelings, and greater empathy in their reactions to their partners and children (M. K. Pruett, Robins, Chen, Honig, & Lane, 2014). This increase in empathy may have been at least partly responsible for the quantitative results showing decreased conflict, more constructive problem-solving approaches, and healthier dynamics around division of labor and other parenting and co-parenting responsibilities. Participants also are more likely to expect that their partner will support their exploration of new things (work opportunities, new talents) outside the home; that is, they are more likely to find that their partners can function as a safe haven *and* a secure base. Following Shaver and Mikulincer (2008), we believe that there is a circular broaden-and-build process in which increases in the security of working models of couple relationships lead to greater relationship satisfaction and more positive interaction, while greater relationship satisfaction and positive interaction lead to greater security of couple attachment and the possibility that the couple relationship can buffer individual partners' insecure working models of attachment based on their family of origin relationships. Based on the path models we described earlier (P. A. Cowan, Bradburn, et al., 2005), we believe that this broadening and building of attachment security makes it more likely that both parents also act as a secure base and a safe haven for their children, and that this chain helps to explain how an intervention for couples results in important positive outcomes for their children. The research of P. A. Cowan, Bradburn, et al. on pairing of partners' attachment security suggests that the group experience may have a demonstrable effect on one partner's working model at first, and begin to affect the other partner's model later on.

Level 2: Other Couples as Attachment Figures

Because there are three to five other couples in the group, one or both partners typically find that others may also become a source of support, encouragement, and models for trying new and more adaptive behaviors. For example, even if one partner in a couple doesn't "get it" when the other expresses distress or anger, another group participant often becomes empathic, acts as an "interpreter," and provides a suggestion that may help deepen thinking about a problem. Over the course of 16 weeks, the couples in the group begin to be important to each other. This happens so often that the group leaders now caution against some couples getting together outside the group until the sessions are finished, to avoid the possibility of the exchange of important ideas and feelings that are not brought back to the group as a whole and may result in some members feeling left out.

Level 3: Group Leaders as Attachment Figures

Shaver and Mikulincer (2008) summarize a number of studies that provide evidence that clients perceive their therapist as a safe haven in times of distress, and that the therapist's role as an attachment figure has positive effects on the outcome of the therapy. In the SFI intervention, clinically trained male–female group leaders use their professional expertise to monitor the level of emotional arousal in the participants, help to up-regulate it in individuals or couples who tend to withdraw rather than engage, and down-regulate it in individuals or couples who find themselves becoming more upset, angry, or discouraged. While the leaders are not there to be "therapists," their clinical expertise informs their role of facilitating safe conversations about emotional issues, in which partners are encouraged to be self-reflective and to use mentalizing strategies (Fonagy & Target, 1997) to gain more perspective on knotty problems. The clearest examples of the leaders as potential attachment figures came in a number of groups in which one or more participants said to one of the leaders some version of "This week, I was at the end of my rope and about to explode at my wife when I felt you on my shoulder asking, 'What is hurting her to make her so uptight?'"

Level 4: The Group as a Safe Haven and Secure Base

Some years ago, John Byng-Hall (1999) advanced the idea that the family can operate as a safe haven and secure base for its members. Similarly, Shaver and Mikulincer (2008) have shown that people can use a group as a symbolic source of comfort, support, and safety in times of need, and as a secure base for exploration, skills learning, and task performance. Our observations over many years of working with couples groups are consistent with these ideas. Beyond the specific individuals and couples who are participants, the environment created by the group as a whole allows individual parents and partners to hold, respect, listen to, and express painful, fearful, worried emotions more than they typically do, to explore new ways of handling or avoiding distress as individuals and as couples, and to cope more thoughtfully and effectively with external stressors when they occur. Participants become more able to tolerate angry or attacking comments despite fearful or negative feelings, and to think about the source of their partners' vulnerabilities in an effort to understand what "pushes their buttons."

In this speculative section, we have argued that a number of constructs from attachment theory—safe haven, secure base, emotion regulation, empathy, mentalization, broaden and build—help to explain the positive outcomes of the SFI intervention, and our earlier interventions as well, as they play out between partners, between couples in the group, and between group members and the group leaders. These speculations require empirical testing, primarily by assessing attachment security both pre- and postintervention, and examining whether changes in attachment security are responsible for, or explain the variance in, the outcomes for couple relationships, parent–child relationships, and the children.

Conclusions

We have described a successful couples group approach to working with parents of young children. We have made a case for the added value of including fathers and focusing on the relationship between parents. We have outlined some of our own and others' evaluation research that reveals consistent links among adult and couple attachment, couple and parenting behavior, and children's development and adjustment. In the absence of empirical studies to explore *how* intervention-induced changes in working models of attachment affect family relationships and child outcomes causally, we have provided some speculations about how this could occur. Our speculations have been based on a synthesis of ideas from theories based on family systems, couples therapy, and attachment security. These ideas imply that multiple attachment figures beyond individual parents and the parents as couples have the potential to foster parents' and children's sense of security by providing both a secure base and a safe haven to break negative intergenerational relationship patterns and encourage healthy development in parents and their children. We await new studies to test whether our formulations can be supported empirically and to examine how concepts from attachment theory may contribute to an even more powerful intervention approach.

REFERENCES

Alexandrov, E. O., Cowan, P. A., & Cowan, C. P. (2005). Couple attachment and the quality of marital relationships: Method and concept in the validation of the new couple attachment interview and coding system. *Attachment and Human Development, 7*(2), 123–152.

Baumrind, D. (1966). Effects of authoritative parental control on child behavior. *Child Development, 37*(4), 887–907.

Benson, L. A., Sevier, M., & Christensen, A. (2013). The impact of behavioral couple therapy on attachment in distressed couples. *Journal of Marital and Family Therapy, 39*(4), 407–420.

Bradburn, I. (1997). *Attachment and coping strategies in married couples with preschool children.* Doctoral dissertation, University of California, Berkeley, Berkeley, CA.

Brennan, K. A., Clark, C. L., & Shaver, P. R. (1998). *Self-report measurement of adult attachment: An integrative overview.* New York: Guilford Press.

Brody, G. H., & Flor, D. L. (1997). Maternal psychological functioning, family processes, and child adjustment in rural, single-parent, African American families. *Developmental Psychology, 33*(6), 1000–1011.

Brody, G. H., & Forehand, R. (1985). The efficacy of parent training with maritally distressed and nondistressed mothers: A multimethod assessment. *Behaviour Research and Therapy, 23*(3), 291–296.

Byng-Hall, J. (1999). Family couple therapy: Toward greater security. In J. Cassidy & P. R. Shaver (Eds.), *Handbook of attachment: Theory, research, and clinical applications* (pp. 625–645). New York: Guilford Press.

Cabrera, N. J., & Tamis-LeMonda, C. S. (Eds.). (2013). *Handbook of father nvolvement: Multidisciplinary perspectives* (2nd ed.). New York: Routledge.

Carlson, M. J., McLanahan, S. S., & Brooks-Gunn, J. (2008). Coparenting and nonresident fathers' involvement with young children after a nonmarital birth. *Demography, 45*(2), 461–486.

Carlson, M. J., Pilkauskas, N. V., McLanahan, S. S., & Brooks-Gunn, J. (2011). Couples as partners and parents over children's early years. *Journal of Marriage and Family, 73*(2), 317–334.

Casey, P., Cowan, P. A., Cowan, C. P., Draper, L., Mwamba, N., & Hewison, D. (in press). Parents as partners: A U.K. trial of a U.S. couples-based parenting intervention for at-risk low-income families. *Family Process.*

Coan, J. A., Kasle, S., Jackson, A., Schaefer, H. S., & Davidson, R. J. (2013). Mutuality and the social regulation of neural threat responding. *Attachment and Human Development,* *15*(3), 303–315.

Cohn, D. A., Cowan, P. A., Cowan, C. P., & Pearson, J. (1992). Mothers' and fathers' working models of childhood attachment relationships, parenting styles, and child behavior. *Development and Psychopathology, 4*(3), 417–431.

Cohn, D. A., Silver, D. H., Cowan, C. P., Cowan, P. A., & Pearson, J. (1992). Working models of childhood attachment and couple relationships [Special issue]. *Journal of Family Issues, 13*(4), 432–449.

Conger, K. J., Rueter, M. A., & Conger, R. D. (2000). The role of economic pressure in the lives of parents and their adolescents: The family stress model. In L. J. Crockett & R. K. Silbereisen (Eds.), *Negotiating adolescence in times of social change* (pp. 201–223). New York: Cambridge University Press.

Conger, R. D., & Donnellan, M. B. (2007). An interactionist perspective on the socioeconomic context of human development. *Annual Review of Psychology, 58,* 175–199.

Cowan, C. P., & Cowan, P. A. (2000). *When partners become parents: The big life change for couples.* Mahwah, NJ: Erlbaum.

Cowan, C. P., Cowan, P. A., & Barry, J. (2011). Couples' groups for parents of preschoolers: Ten-year outcomes of a randomized trial. *Journal of Family Psychology, 25*(2), 240–250.

Cowan, C. P., Cowan, P. A., & Heming, G. (2005). *Two variations of a preventive intervention for couples: Effects on parents and children during the transition to school.* Mahwah, NJ: Erlbaum.

Cowan, P. A., Bradburn, I. S., & Cowan, C. P. (2005). Parents' working models of attachment: The intergenerational context of problem behavior in kindergarten. In P. A. Cowan, C. P. Cowan, J. Ablow, V. K. Johnson, & J. Measelle (Eds.), *The family context of parenting in children's adaptation to elementary school* (pp. 209–236). Mahwah, NJ: Erlbaum.

Cowan, P. A., Cohn, D. A., Cowan, C. P., & Pearson, J. L. (1996). Parents' attachment histories and children's externalizing and internalizing behaviors: Exploring family systems models of linkage. *Journal of Consulting and Clinical Psychology, 64*(1), 53–63.

Cowan, P. A., & Cowan, C. P. (2007). Attachment theory: Seven unresolved issues and questions for further research. *Research in Human Development, 4*(3–4), 181–201.

Cowan, P. A., & Cowan, C. P. (2012). Normative family transitions, couple relationship quality, and healthy child development. In F. Walsh (Ed.), *Normal family processes: Growing diversity and complexity* (4th ed., pp. 428–451). New York: Guilford Press.

Cowan, P. A., Cowan, C. P., Ablow, J. C., Johnson, V. K., & Measelle, J. R. (2005). *The family context of parenting in children's adaptation to elementary school.* Mahwah, NJ: Erlbaum.

Cowan, P. A., Cowan, C. P., & Mehta, N. (2009). Adult attachment, couple attachment, and children's adaptation to school: An integrated attachment template and family risk model. *Attachment and Human Development, 11*(1), 29–46.

Cowan, P. A., Cowan, C. P., Pruett, M. K., Pruett, K., & Gillette, P. (2014). Evaluating a couples group to enhance father involvement in low-income families using a benchmark comparison. *Family Relations, 63*(3), 356–370.

Cowan, P. A., Cowan, C. P., Pruett, M. K., Pruett, K., & Wong, J. J. (2009). Promoting fathers' engagement with children: Preventive interventions for low-income families. *Journal of Marriage and Family, 71*(3), 663–679.

Coyne, L. W., Low, C. M., Miller, A. L., Seifer, R., & Dickstein, S. (2007). Mothers' empathic understanding of their toddlers: Associations with maternal depression and sensitivity. *Journal of Child and Family Studies, 16*(4), 483–497.

Crowell, J. A., & Owens, G. (1996). *Current relationship interview and scoring system.* Stony Brook: State University of New York at Stony Brook.

Dadds, M. R., Sanders, M. R., Behrens, B. C., & James, J. E. (1987). Marital discord and child behavior problems: A description of family interactions during treatment. *Journal of Clinical Child Psychology, 16*(3), 192–203.

Dickstein, S., Seifer, R., St Andre, M., & Schiller, M. (2001). Marital Attachment Interview: Adult attachment assessment of marriage. *Journal of Social and Personal Relationships, 18*(5), 651–672.

Draper, L. (2015). "It seems so fair": Implementing "Parents as Partners" in the UK. *International Journal of Adolescent Medicine and Health, 2*(3), 36–39.

Elder, G. H., King, V., & Conger, R. D. (1996). Intergenerational continuity and change in rural lives: Historical and developmental insights. *International Journal of Behavioral Development, 19*(2), 433–455.

Feinberg, M. E., Jones, D. E., Kan, M. L., & Goslin, M. C. (2010). Effects of family foundations on parents and children: 3.5 years after baseline. *Journal of Family Psychology, 24*(5), 532–542.

Fivaz-Depeursinge, E. (2003). Coparental alliance and infant affective development in the primary triangle/L'alliance coparentale et le développement affectif de l'enfant dans le triangle primaire. *Therapie Familiale, 24*(3), 267–273.

Fonagy, P. (2008). The mentalization-focused approach to social development. In F. N. Busch (Ed.), *Mentalization: Theoretical considerations, research findings, and clinical implications* (pp. 3–56). New York: Analytic Press.

Fonagy, P., Steele, M., Steele, H., Moran, G. S., & Higgitt, A. C. (1991). The capacity for understanding mental states: The reflective self in parent and child and its significance for security of attachment. *Infant Mental Health Journal, 12*(3), 201–218.

Fonagy, P., & Target, M. (1997). Attachment and reflective function: Their role in self-organization. *Development and Psychopathology, 9*(4), 679–700.

Fraley, R. C., & Shaver, P. R. (2000). Adult romantic attachment: Theoretical developments, emerging controversies, and unanswered questions. *Review of General Psychology, 4*(2), 132–154.

Fredrickson, B. L. (2001). The role of positive emotions in positive psychology: The broaden-and-build theory of positive emotions. *The American Psychologist, 56*(3), 218.

George, C., Kaplan, N., & Main, M. (1985). *The Adult Attachment Interview.* Unpublished manuscript, University of California, Berkeley, Berkeley, CA.

Gottman, J. M., Katz, L. F., & Hooven, C. (1997). *Meta-emotion: How families communicate emotionally.* Hillsdale, NJ: Erlbaum.

Grossmann, K., Grossmann, K., E., Kindler, H., & Zimmerman, P. (2008). A wider view of attachment and exploration: The influence of mothers and fathers on the development of psychological security from infancy to young adulthood. In J. Cassidy & P. R. Shaver (Eds.), *Handbook of attachment: Theory, research, and clinical applications* (2nd ed., pp. 857–879). New York: Guilford Press.

Hill, J., Fonagy, P., Safier, E., & Sargent, J. (2003). The ecology of attachment in the family. *Family Process, 42*(2), 205–221.

Johnson, L. N., Tambling, R. B., Mennenga, K. D., Ketring, S. A., Oka, M., Anderson, S. R., . . . Miller, R. B. (2016). Examining attachment avoidance and attachment anxiety across eight sessions of couple therapy. *Journal of Marital and Family Therapy, 42*(2), 195–212.

Johnson, S. M. (2013). *Love sense: The revolutionary science of romantic relationships.* New York: Little, Brown.

Kerns, K. A., Mathews, B. L., Koehn, A. J., Williams, C. T., & Siener-Ciesla, S. (2015). Assessing both safe haven and secure base support in parent–child relationships. *Attachment and Human Development, 17*(4), 337–353.

Krishnakumar, A., & Buehler, C. (2000). Interparental conflict and parenting behaviors: A meta-analytic review. *Family Relations: An Interdisciplinary Journal of Applied Family Studies, 49*(1), 25–44.

Lamb, M. E., & Lewis, C. (2013). Father–child relationships. In N. Cabrera & C. S. Tamis-LeMonda (Eds.), *Handbook of father involvement: Multidisciplinary perspectives* (pp. 119–134). New York: Routledge/Taylor & Francis Group.

Larzelere, R. E., Morris, A. S., & Harrist, A. W. (2013). *Authoritative parenting synthesizing nurturance and discipline for optimal child development.* Washington, DC. American Psychological Association.

Levenson, R. W., & Gottman, J. M. (1983). Marital interaction: Physiological linkage and affective exchange. *Journal of Personality and Social Psychology, 45*(3), 587–597.

Lucassen, H., Tharner, A., van IJzendoorn, M. H., Bakermans-Kranenburg, M. J., Volling, B. L., & Verhulst, F. C. (2011). The association between paternal sensitivity and infant–father attachment security: A meta-analysis of three decades of research. *Journal of Family Psychology, 25,* 986–992.

Lundahl, B. W., Tollefson, D., Risser, H., & Lovejoy, M. C. (2008). A meta-analysis of father involvement in parent training. *Research on Social Work Practice, 18*(2), 97–106.

Masarik, A. S., Martin, M. J., Ferrer, E., Lorenz, F. O., Conger, K. J., & Conger, R. D. (2016). Couple resilience to economic pressure over time and across generations. *Journal of Marriage and Family, 78*(2), 326–345.

McHale, J. P., & Lindahl, K. M. (2011). *Coparenting a conceptual and clinical examination of family systems.* Washington, DC: American Psychological Association.

Mikulincer, M., & Shaver, P. R. (2007). *Attachment in adulthood: Structure, dynamics, and change.* New York: Guilford Press.

Mikulincer, M., Shaver, P. R., & Pereg, D. (2003). Attachment theory and affect regulation: The dynamics, development, and cognitive consequences of attachment-related strategies. *Motivation and Emotion, 27*(2), 77–102.

Miller, M., Drake, E., & Nafziger, M. (2013). *What works to reduce recidivism by domestic violence offenders?* (Document No. 13-01-1201). Olympia: Washington State Institute for Public Policy.

Moser, M. B., Johnson, S. M., Dalgleish, T. L., Lafontaine, M.-F., Wiebe, S. A., & Taska, G. A. (2016). Changes in relationship-specific attachment in emotionally focused couple therapy. *Journal of Marital Family Therapy, 42*(2), 231–245.

Owens, G., Crowell, J. A., Pan, H., Treboux, D., O'Connor, E., & Waters, E. (1995). The prototype hypothesis and the origins of attachment working models: Child–parent relationships and adult–adult romantic relationships. *Monographs of the Society for Research in Child Development, 60,* 216–233.

Panter-Brick, C., Burgess, A., Eggerman, M., McAllister, F., Pruett, K., & Leckman, J. (2015). Practitioner Review: Engaging fathers—recommendations for a game change in parenting interventions on a systematic review of the global evidence. *Journal of Child Psychology and Psychiatry, 22*(11), 1187–1212.

Parke, R. D. (2002). Fathers and families. In M. H. Bornstein (Ed.), *Handbook of parenting: Vol. 3. Being and becoming a parent* (2nd ed., pp. 27–73). Mahwah, NJ: Erlbaum.

Pruett, K. D. (2000). *Fatherneed: Why father care is as essential as mother care for your child.* New York: Free Press.

Pruett, K., & Pruett, M. K. (2009). *Partnership parenting: How men and women parent differently—Why it helps your kids and can strengthen your marriage.* Cambridge, MA: Da Capo Press.

Pruett, K. D., Pruett, M. K., Cowan, C. P., & Cowan, P. A. (2015). Supporting Father Involvement Project: A value-added co-parenting program. In J. Ponzetti (Ed.), *Evidence-based parenting education: A global perspective* (pp. 176–189). New York: Routledge/Taylor & Francis Group.

Pruett, M. K., Cowan, C. P., Cowan, P. A., & Pruett, K. (2009). Lessons learned from the Supporting Father Involvement study: A cross-cultural preventive intervention for low-income families with young children. *Journal of Social Service Research, 35*(2), 163–179.

Pruett, M. K., Insabella, G. M., & Gustafson, K. (2005). The Collaborative Divorce Project: A court-based intervention for separating parents with young children [Special issue]. *Family Court Review, 43*(1), 38–51.

Pruett, M. K., & Johnston, J. R. (2004). Therapeutic mediation with high-conflict parents: Effective models and strategies. In J. Folberg, A. L. Milne, & P. Salem (Eds.), *Divorce and family mediation: Models, techniques, and applications* (pp. 92–111). New York: Guilford Press.

Pruett, M. K., Gillette, P., Pruett, K., Cowan, C. P., & Cowan, P. A. (in press). Enhancing paternal engagement in a coparenting paradigm. *Child Development Perspectives.*

Schulz, M. S., Pape, C. P., & Cowan, P. A. (2006). Promoting healthy beginnings: A randomized controlled trial of a preventive intervention to preserve marital quality during the transition to parenthood. *Journal of Consulting and Clinical Psychology, 74*(1), 20–31.

Shaver, P. R., & Mikulincer, M. (2008). Augmenting the sense of security in romantic, leader–follower, therapeutic, and group relationships: A relational model of psychological change. In J. P. Forgas & J. Fitness (Eds.), *Social relationships: Cognitive, affective, and motivational processes* (pp. 55–74). New York: Psychology Press.

Silver, D. H., Cohn, D. A., Cowan, P. A., & Cowan, C. P. (1990). *Couple Attachment Interview.* Unpublished manuscript, University of California, Berkeley, Berkeley, CA.

Simons, R. L., Lorenz, F. O., Wu, C. I., & Conger, R. D. (1993). Social network and marital support as mediators and moderators of the impact of stress and depression on parental behavior. *Developmental Psychology, 29*(2), 368–381.

Steele, H., & Steele, M. (Eds.). (2008). *Clinical applications of the Adult Attachment Interview.* New York: Guilford Press.

Steele, H., Steele, M., & Fonagy, P. (1996). Associations among attachment classifications of mothers, fathers, and their infants. *Child Development, 67*(2), 541–555.

Steele, M., Steele, H., Woolgar, M., Yabsley, S., Fonagy, P., Johnson, D., & Croft, C. (2003). An attachment perspective on children's emotion narratives: Links across the generations. In R. Emde, D. Wolf, & D. Oppenheim (Eds.), *Revealing the inner worlds of young children: The MacArthur story-stem battery and parent–child narratives* (pp. 163–181). New York: Oxford University Press.

Stith, S. M., McCollum, E. E., Amanor-Boadu, Y., & Smith, D. (2012). Systemic perspectives on intimate partner violence treatment. *Journal of Marital and Family Therapy, 38*(1), 220–240.

Sturge-Apple, M. L., Davies, P. T., & Cummings, E. M. (2006). Impact of hostility and withdrawal in interparental conflict on parental emotional unavailability and children's adjustment difficulties. *Child Development, 77*(6), 1623–1641.

Twenge, J. M., Campbell, W. K., & Foster, C. A. (2003). Parenthood and marital satisfaction: A meta-analytic review. *Journal of Marriage and Family, 65*(3), 574–583.

van IJzendoorn, M. H. (1995). Adult attachment representations, parental responsiveness, and infant attachment: A meta-analysis on the predictive validity of the Adult Attachment Interview. *Psychological Bulletin, 117*(3), 387–403.

Watzlawick, P., Bavelas, J. B., & Jackson, D. D. (1967). *Pragmatics of human communication: A study of interactional patterns, pathologies, and paradoxes.* New York: Norton.

Webster-Stratton, C. (1985). The effects of father involvement in parent training for conduct problem children. *Journal of Child Psychology and Psychiatry, 26*(5), 801–810.

Author Index

Subject Index

Note. *f*, *n*, or *t* following a page number indicates a figure, a note, or a table.